CARS 2002

Computer Assisted Radiology and Surgery

Springer-Verlag Berlin Heidelberg GmbH

CARS 2002

Computer Assisted Radiology and Surgery

Proceedings of the 16th International Congress and Exhibition
Paris, June 26–29, 2002

Edited by
H. U. Lemke, M. W. Vannier, K. Inamura, A. G. Farman, K. Doi, and
J. H. C. Reiber

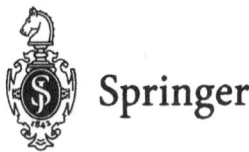 Springer

PROFESSOR HEINZ U. LEMKE, PhD
Technical University Berlin
Computer Graphics and
Computer Assisted Medicine
Secr. FR 3-3
Franklinstrasse 28–29
10587 Berlin, Germany

PROFESSOR KIYONARI INAMURA, PhD
Osaka University
Faculty of Medicine
School of Allied Health Sciences
Department of Radiological
Technology & Medical Engineering
1-7 Yamadaoka, Suita City
Osaka, 565-0871, Japan

PROFESSOR KUNIO DOI, PhD
University of Chicago Hospitals
Department of Radiology
Kurt Rossmann Laboratories
5841 S. Maryland Avenue, Mailcode 2026
Chicago, IL 60637, U.S.A.

PROFESSOR MICHAEL W. VANNIER, MD
The University of Iowa
College of Medicine
Department of Radiology
200 Hawkins Drive
Room 3966 JPP
Iowa City, IA 552242-1077, U.S.A.

PROFESSOR ALLAN G. FARMAN, PhD, DSc
University of Louisville
School of Dentistry
Department of Diagnosis and
General Dentistry
501 South Preston, Room 222E
Louisville, KY 40292, U.S.A.

PROFESSOR JOHAN H. C. REIBER, PhD
Leiden University Medical Center
Division of Image Processing
Department of Radiology
P. O. Box 9600
Albinusdreef 2
2300 RC Leiden, The Netherlands

This volume of the CARS proceedings is published simultaneously in print and on the web. The web edition contains colour images.

ISBN 978-3-642-62844-3   ISBN 978-3-642-56168-9 (eBook)
DOI 10.1007/978-3-642-56168-9

Library of Congress Cataloging-in-Publication Data

http://www.springer.de
http://www.cars-int.de

© Springer-Verlag Berlin Heidelberg 2002 and CARS
Originally published by Springer-Verlag Berlin Heidelberg New York in 2002
Softcover reprint of the hardcover 1st edition 2002

SPIN 10755372   31/3130 – 5 4 3 2 1 0 –

Honorary President

Kiyonari Inamura, PhD, Osaka University, Faculty of Medicine, Osaka (J)

Congress Organizing Committee

Ulrich Bick, MD
University of Chicago Hospitals (USA)

Kees de Wilde
Philips Medical Systems, Best (NL)

Kunio Doi, PhD
University of Chicago Hospitals (USA)

Allan G. Farman, PhD, DSc
University of Louisville (USA)

Guy Frija, MD
Société Francaise de Radiologie Médicale,
Paris (F)

Toyomi Fujino, MD, PhD, FACS
International Med. Information Center,
Tokyo (J)

Gary M. Glazer, MD
Stanford Univ. School of Med., Palo Alto,
CA (USA)

Kiyonari Inamura, PhD
Osaka University (J)

Takahiro Kozuka, MD
Kaizuka Municipal Hospital, Osaka (J)

J. Thomas Lambrecht, MD, DMD, PhD
University of Basle (CH)

Heinz U. Lemke, PhD
Technical University Berlin (D)

Roberto Passariello, MD
University "La Sapienza", Rome (I)

Pierre Rabischong, MD, PhD
Centre Propara, Montpellier (F)

Johan H.C. Reiber, PhD
Leiden University Medical Center (NL)

Hans G. Ringertz, MD, PhD
Karolinska Hospital, Stockholm (S)

Ramin Shahidi, PhD
Stanford University Medical Center (USA)

Nicola H. Strickland, MD
Hammersmith Hospital, London (UK)

Kintomo Takakura, MD, PhD
Tokyo Women's Medical University (J)

Michael W. Vannier, MD
The University of Iowa (USA)

Industrial Advisory Board

Chairman: Kees de Wilde, Philips Medical Systems, Best (NL)

Heinz-Christoph Blied
Siemens AG, MED, Erlangen (D)

Karel H.P. Cromzigt
IEARC, Den Hague (NL)

Gerhard Kacmaczyk
Image Devices GmbH, Taunusstein (D)

Annelies Kin
Agfa Europe NV, Mechelen (B)

Kenneth A. Marks, MBA
DOME Imag. Syst., Inc., Tiburon, (USA)

Willem Overlaet, PhD
Toshiba Medical Sys., Zoetermeer (NL)

Jürgen Reyinger
GE Medical Systems, Dornstadt (D)

Saeid Mitchell Seyedin
CBYON, Palo Alto, CA (USA)

Kurt R. Smith, DSc
Medtronics, Broomfield, CO (USA)

Chris Varian
Eastman Kodak Company, Hemel (UK)

Stefan Vilsmeier
BrainLAB GmbH, Heimstetten (D)

Program Committee

Andreas Adam, MB, RCP, FRCR
Guy's Hospital, London (UK)

Paul R. Algra, MD, PhD
Medisch Centrum Alkmaar (NL)

David J. Allison, MD
Hammersmith Hospital, London (UK)

Mostafa Analoui, PhD
Indiana University, Indianapolis, IN (USA)

Yutaka Ando, MD
Keio University, Tokyo (J)

Licinio Angelini, MD, FACS
Università "La Sapienza", Rome (I)

Takehide Asano, MD, PhD
Chiba University School of Medicine (J)

Hanna Bachtiar Iskandar, DDS
University of Indonesia, Jakarta (RI)

Frits H. Barneveld Binkhuysen, MD, PhD
Hospital Eemland, Amersfoort (NL)

Elizabeth Beckmann, BSc
Lanmark, Beaconsfield (UK)

Leonard Berliner, MD
Swissray Int., Staten Island, NY (USA)

Silvio Diego Bianchi, MD
Università degli Studi di Torino (I)

Josip S. Bill, MD, DDS
Julius-Maximillians-University, Würzburg (D)

Uldis Bite, MD
Mayo Clinic, Rochester, MN (USA)

Michel Bléry, MD
Hôpital de Bicêtre, Le Kremlin-Bicêtre (F)

Siegfried Bocionek, PhD
Siemens Health Services GmbH, Erlangen (D)

Hugo G. Bogren, MD, PhD
UC Davis Med. Center, Sacramento, CA (USA)

Nicolaas Bom, PhD
Erasmus Universiteit Rotterdam (NL)

Hans G. Bosch, MSc
Leiden University Medical Center (NL)

Carlos A. Bruguera, MD
Inst. de Ensenanza Audiovis., Buenos Aires (RA)

Jean Noel Bruneton, MD
Centre Antoine-Lacassagne, Nice (F)

Richard D. Bucholz, MD, FACS
Saint Louis University (USA)

Gerhard Buess, MD
Nova Med Klinik, München (D)

Jean-Marie Caillé, MD
Groupe Hospitalier Pellegrin, Bordeaux (F)

Davide Caramella, MD
University of Pisa (I)

Ernest V. Carcia, PhD
Emory Univ.., Atlanta, GA (USA)

Robert Cavézian, MD
Cabinet de Radiologie, Paris (F)

Curtis Ssu-Kuang Chen, DDS, MSD, PhD
National Taiwan University, Taipei (CHN)

S. James Chen, PhD
University of Colorado, Denver, CO (USA)

Kiyoyuki Chinzei, PhD
Mechanical Engineering Lab. AIST, Ibaraki (J)

John C. Chiu, MD
California Spine Inst., Thousand Oaks (USA)

Hiroaki Chiyokura, PhD
Keio University, Kanagawa (J)

Gary E. Christensen, PhD
University of Iowa (USA)

Philippe Cinquin, MD, PhD
CHU Grenoble, La Tronche (F)

Michel Claudon, MD
Hôpitaux de Brabois, Vandoeuvre (F)

Claus D. Claussen, MD
Eberhard-Karls-Univ. Tübingen (D)

Kevin Cleary, PhD
Georgetown Univ., Washington, DC (USA)

Alan C.F. Colchester, MD, PhD
University of Kent, Canterbury (UK)

Bernard L. Crowe, BA, MPH
Health Inf. Soc. of Australia, Canberra (AUS)

Jack T. Cusma, PhD
Mayo Clinic, Rochester, MN (USA)

Paolo Dario, PhD
Scuola Superiore S. Anna, Pisa (I)

Albert de Roos, MD
Leiden University Medical Center (NL)

Carlo del Favero, MD
Ospedale "Valduce", Como (I)

Anthony M. DiGioia III, MD
Shadyside Hospital, Pittsburgh, PA (USA)

Jouke Dijkstra, PhD
Leiden University Medical Center (NL)

Takeyoshi Dohi, PhD
The University of Tokyo (J)

Huilong Duan, PhD
Zhejiang University Hangzhou (RC)

André J. Duerinckx, MD, PhD
VA North Texas HC System, Dallas, TX (USA)

Masahiro Endo, PhD
National Inst. of Radiological Scie., Chiba (J)

Rolf Ewers, MD, DMD
Allg. Krankenhaus der Stadt Wien (A)

Aly A. Farag, PhD
University of Louisville (USA)

Taeko T. Farman, PhD, DMD, RT
University of Louisville (USA)

Allan G. Farman, PhD, DSc
University of Louisville (USA)

Eckhard Fleck, MD
Deutsches Herzzentrum Berlin (D)

Kevin T. Foley, MD
Image-Guided Surg. Res. Ctr.,Memphis, (USA)

Erik Fosse, MD, PhD
University of Oslo (N)

Bernard Fraysse, MD
Hôpital Purpan, Toulouse (F)

Hiroshi Fujita, PhD
Gifu University (J)

Günther Gell, PhD
Universität Graz - Landeskrankenhaus (A)

Bernard Gibaud
Université de Rennes I (F)

Maryellen L. Giger, PhD
The University of Chicago (USA)

Stephen Golding, FRCR
University of Oxford, Headington (UK)

Dietrich H.W. Grönemeyer, MD
Universität Witten-Herdecke (D)

Chiaki Hamanishi, MD
Kinki University School of Medicine, Osaka (J)

Daijo Hashimoto, MD, PhD
Tokyo Metropolitan Police Hospital (J)

Makoto Hashizume, MD, PhD, FACS
Kyushu University, Fukuoka (J)

Stefan Haßfeld, MD, MDS
Ruprecht-Karls-Universität, Heidelberg (D)

David Hatcher
Univ. of California, San Francisco, CA (USA)

David J. Hawkes, PhD
Guy's, Hospital, London (UK)

J.H.C. Hendriks, MD
University Hospital Nijmegen (NL)

Atsuko Heshiki, MD
Saitama Medical School (J)

Kenneth R. Hoffmann, PhD
University at Buffalo (USA)

Karl-Heinz Höhne, PhD
Universität Hamburg (D)

Steven C. Horii, MD
Univ. of Pennsylvania, Philadelphia, PA (USA)

Alexander Horsch, PhD
University of Munich (D)

Walter Hruby, MD
Sozialmedizinisches Zentrum Ost, Wien (A)

H.K. Huang, DSc, FRCR (Hon.)
Univ. of South. California, Los Angeles, CA (USA)

Junpei Ikezoe, MD
Ehime University (J)

Herwig Imhof, MD
Allgemeines Krankenhaus der Stadt Wien (A)

Hiroshi Iseki, MD, PhD
Tokyo Women's Medical College (J)

Takeo Ishigaki, MD, PhD
Nagoya University (J)

Akira Ito, PhD
Japanese Foundation for Cancer Res., Tokyo (J)

Ian T. Jackson, MD
Inst. f.Craniofacial a.R.Surg., Southfield (USA)

C. Carl Jaffe, MD
Yale Univ. School of Med., New Haven (USA)

Pierre Jannin, PhD
Université de Rennes I (F)

Werner Jaschke, MD
Univ-Klinik für Radiodiagnostik, Innsbruck (A)

Jack Jellins, PhD
Intern. Breast Ultrasound Sch., Sydney (AUS)

Peter Jensch, PhD
OFFIS e.V., Oldenburg (D)

Ferenc A. Jolesz, MD
Harvard Medical School, Boston, MA (USA)

Leo Joskowicz, PhD
The Hebrew University of Jerusalem (IL)

Willi A. Kalender, PhD
Friedrich-Alexander-Universität, Erlangen (D)

Shigenobu Kanda, DDS, PhD
Kyushu University, Fukuoka (J)

Kazuhiro Katada, MD
Fujita Health University, Aichi (J)

Amami Kato, MD, PhD
Osaka University Medical School (J)

Erwin Keeve, PhD
CAESAR, Bonn (D)

Ron Kikinis, MD
Harvard Medical School, Boston, MA (USA)

Reinhard Klette, PhD
University of Auckland (NZ)

Klaus Jochen Klose, MD
Universitäts-Klinikum, Marburg (D)

Goran Knezevic, DDS, PhD
University of Zagreb (HR)

Hidefumi Kobatake, PhD
Tokyo Univ. of Agriculture & Technology (J)

Masahiro Kobayashi, MD
Keio University, Tokyo (J)

Gerhard Koning, MSc
Leiden University Medical Center (NL)

Martti Kormano, MD, PhD
Turku University Central Hospital (FIN)

Uwe G. Kühnapfel, PhD
Forschungszentrum Karlsruhe GmbH (D)

Chikazumi Kuroda, MD
Osaka Medical Center for Cancer (J)

Axel Küttner, MD
Klinik. der Eberhard-Karls-Univ. Tübingen (D)

Frode Laerum, MD, PhD, MHA
University of Oslo (N)

J. Thomas Lambrecht, MD, DMD, PhD
University of Basle (CH)

Alexandra Lansky, MD
Cardiov.r Research Found., New York (USA)

Tore A. Larheim, PhD, DDS
University of Oslo (N)

Stéphane Lavallée, PhD
PRAXIM, La Tronche (F)

Swamy Laxminarayan, PhD
New Jersey Inst.of Techn., Newark, NJ (USA)

Lilian L.Y. Leong, MBBS
Queen Mary Hospital, Hong Kong (RC)

Yves Ligier, PhD
CareON S.A., Grand Saconnex (CH)

Jae Hoon Lim, MD
Sung Kyun Kwan University, Seoul (ROK)

Martin J. Lipton, MD
The University of Chicago Hospitals (USA)

Yu-Qing Liu, MD
FuWai Hosp. & Cardiovascular Inst., Beijing (RC)

Tim C. Lueth, PhD
Campus Virchow-Klinikum, Berlin (D)

Xiu-chen Ma, PhD
Peking Univ. Sch.of Stomatology, Beijing (RC)

Riley H. Lunn, DDS
Chattanoooga, TN (USA)

Heber MacMahon, MD
The University of Chicago (USA)

Sumio Makino, PhD
Yokohama-City (J)

Borut Marincek, MD
Universitätsspital Zürich (CH)

Steffen Märkle, PhD
Technical University Berlin (D)

Tom H. Marwick, MD
University of Queensland, Brisbane (AUS)

Herbert K. Matthies, PhD
Hannover Medical School (D)

Hans-Peter Meinzer, PhD
Deutsches Krebsforschungsz., Heidelberg (D)

Andreas Melzer, MD
Mühlheimer Radiologie Inst., Mülheim (D)

Reto A. Meuli, MD
CHUV, Lausanne (CH)

Kazuo Miyasaka, MD
Hokkaido University, Sapporo (J)

Kensaku Mori, PhD
Nagoya University (J)

Seong K. Mun, PhD
Georgetown University, Washington, DC (USA)

Eike Nagel, MD
Deutsches Herzzentrum Berlin (D)

K.S. Nagesh
R.V. Dental College, Bangalore (IND)

Hironobu Nakamura, MD, PhD
Osaka University Medical School (J)

Wolfgang Niederlang, PhD
Krankenhaus Dresden-Friedrichstadt (D)

Robert M. Nishikawa, PhD
The University of Chicago (USA)

Hiromu Nishitani, MD, PhD
The University of Tokushima (J)

Lutz-P. Nolte, PhD
Maurice E. Müller Institute , Bern (CH)

Fridtjof Nüsslin, PhD
Eberhard-Karls-Universität, Tübingen (D)

Takahiro Ochi
Osaka University (J)

Nagaaki Ohyama, PhD
Tokyo Institute of Technology, Yokohama (J)

Silas Olsson, MSc
Telia Research AB, Farsta (S)

Dietrich Onnasch, PhD
University of Kiel (D)

Stelios Orphanoudakis, PhD
Institute of Computer Science, Heraklion (GR)

Michel Osteaux, MD, PhD
Vrije Universiteit Brussels (B)

Helmut Oswald, PhD
T-Systems HCS AG, Bern (CH)

Hiroshi Oyama, MD
Kyoto University Hospital (J)

Paolo Pavone, MD
Università "La Sapienza", Rome (I)

Heinz-Otto Peitgen, PhD
University of Bremen (D)

Prem Pillay, MD
Asian Brain Spine Nerve Ctr., Singapore (SGP)

Gabriel E. Pislaru
Charlotte, NC (USA)

E. James Potchen, MD
Michigan State Univ., East Lansing, MI (USA)

Henri Primo
Siemens Medical Syst., Inc., Iselin, NJ (USA)

Osman M. Ratib, MD, PhD
Univ. of California, Los Angeles, CA (USA)

Hans F. Reinhardt, MD
Bethesda Spital, Basle (CH)

Maximilian Reiser, MD
Klinikum Großhadern, München (D)

Stephen J. Riederer, PhD
Mayo Clinic, Rochester, MN (USA)

Otto Rienhoff, MD
Georg-August-Universität, Göttingen (D)

Rainer K. Rienmüller, MD
Universitätskliniken Graz (A)

Richard A. Robb, PhD
Mayo Foundation, Rochester, MN (USA)

Ichiro Sakuma, PhD
The University of Tokyo (J)

Georges Salamon, MD
NW Univ. Med. School, Chicago, IL (USA)

Richard M. Satava, MD
Yale University, New Haven, CT (USA)

Ronald B. Schilling, PhD
PGI Corporation, Los Altos Hills, CA (USA)

Peter M. Schlag, MD, PhD
Robert-Rössle-Klinik, Berlin (D)

Wolfgang Schlegel, PhD
Deutsches Krebsforschungsz., Heidelberg (D)

Rainer M.M. Seibel, MD
Univ. Witten/Herdecke, Mülheim/Ruhr (D)

Wolfhard Semmler, MD
Deutsches Krebsforschungsz., Heidelberg (D)

Jean Sequeira, PhD
Laboratoire d'Informatique de Marseille (F)

Iekado Shibata, MD, PhD
Toho University, Tokyo (J)

Faina Shtern, MD
Harvard Medical School, Boston, MA (USA)

Robert Sigal, MD, PhD
Institut Gustave-Roussy, Villejuif (F)

Peter Sloot, PhD
University of Amsterdam (NL)

Milan Sonka, PhD
University of Iowa (USA)

Edward V. Staab, MD
National Cancer Inst., Rockville, MD (USA)

Gero Strauss, MD
University of Leipzig (D)

Nobuhiko Sugano, MD
Osaka University Med. School (J)

Predrag Sukovic, MS
University of Michigan, Ann Arbor, MI (USA)

Naoki Suzuki, MD, PhD
Jikei University School of Medicine, Tokyo (J)

Takashi Takahashi, PhD
Kyoto University Hospital (J)

Hiroshi Takeda, MD, PhD
Osaka University Medical School (J)

Past Honorary Presidents

CARS 2002 in cooperation with

AAOMR	American Academy of Oral and Maxillofacial Radiology
BAR	Bulgarian Association of Radiology
BIR	The British Institute of Radiology
CRS	Czech Radiological Society
CURAC	Deutsche Gesellschaft für Computer- und Roboterassistierte Chirurgie e.V.
DGBMT	Deutsche Gesellschaft für Biomedizinische Technik e.V.
DRG	Deutsche Röntgengesellschaft
ESCR	European Society of Cardiac Radiology
ESEM	European Society for Engineering and Medicine
EuroPACS	European Association for Promotion of Information Exchange on PACS Research
GI	Gesellschaft für Informatik
GMDS	Deutsche Gesellschaft für Medizinische Informatik, Biometrie und Epidemiologie e.V.
Hungarian Society for Computer Assisted Radiology	
IADMFR	The International Association of Dento-Maxillo-Facial Radiology
IEARC	International Exhibitors Association on Radiological Congresses
IEEE	The Institute of Electrical and Electronics Engineers
JCR	Japanese College of Radiology
JRS	Japan Radiological Society
JSOMR	Japanese Society for Oral and Maxillofacial Radiology
NVvR	Nederlandse Vereniging voor Radiologie
ÖRG	Österreichische Röntgengesellschaft
ÖWGTM	Österreichische Wissenschaftliche Gesellschaft für Telemedizin
Polish Section of the Polish-German Radiological Society	
PMSR	Polish Medical Society of Radiology
RCR	The Royal College of Radiologists
EFSUMB	European Federation for Ultrasound in Medicine and Biology
SFR	Société Française de Radiologie Médicale
SGR-SSR	Schweizerische Gesellschaft für Radiologie
SICTECA	Società Italiana di Chirurgia Tecnologica e Computer-Assistita
SIRM	Società Italiana di Radiologia Medica
Chinese Society for Computer Assisted Radiology	
SPIE	The International Society for Optical Engineering
SRS	Slovak Radiological Society
TU	Technische Universität Berlin
WABT	World Academy of Biomedical Technologies

ISCAS - International Society for Computer Aided Surgery

Administrative Council

President:
Kintomo Takakura, MD, PhD
Tokyo Women's Medical University,
Tokyo (J)

Past President:
Michael W. Vannier, MD
The University of Iowa (USA)

Vice Presidents:
J. Thomas Lambrecht, MD, DMD, PhD
University of Basle (CH)

Jeffrey L. Marsh, MD
St. Louis Children's Hospital (USA)

General Secretary:
Heinz U. Lemke, PhD
Technical University Berlin (D)

Adjoint Secretary:
Takeyoshi Dohi, PhD
The University of Tokyo (J)

Treasurer :
Toyomi Fujino, MD, PhD
International Med. Information Center,
Tokyo (J)

Adjoint Treasurer :
Rolf Ewers, MD, DMD
Allg. Krankenhaus der Stadt Wien (A)

Board Members

Richard D. Bucholz, MD, FACS
Saint Louis University (USA)

Alan C.F. Colchester, MD, PhD
University of Kent, Canterbury (UK)

Daijo Hashimoto, MD, PhD
Tokyo Metropolitan Police Hospital (J)

Richard A. Robb, PhD
Mayo Foundation, Rochester, MN (USA)

Russell H. Taylor, PhD
Johns Hopkins University, Baltimore,
MD (USA)

Jun-Ichiro Toriwaki, PhD
Nagoya University (J)

Honorary Board Member:
Pierre Rabischong, MD, PhD
Centre Propara, Montpellier (F)

Preface

Most, if not all, human knowledge is artificially divided into areas or fields by scientific culture and/or social convention. Professional disciplines are therefore man-made frameworks based on shared models, concepts and definitions. This is the ontological basis for communication and action for professionals in medical physics, radiology, surgery or computer science. In general, new knowledge is being squeezed into these existing boundaries or frames of fields of knowledge. Increasingly, however, this fitting process faces difficulties, particularly in rapidly evolving knowledge areas, such as information technology induced activities - to which CAR (Computer Assisted Radiology) and CAS (Computer Assisted Surgery) belong. Rather than allowing a simple fit into the traditional fields of mathematics, physics, engineering, informatics, medicine or management sciences, these new areas occupy knowledge subsets of two or more of these traditional disciplines. They may therefore be termed interdisciplinary. An example of such evolving interdisciplines is given in Figure 1.

Figure 1 shows the distribution of research and development activities in a number of new interdisciplinary fields or themes as demonstrated by the topics covered by the paper and poster abstract submissions to CARS 2002.

These CARS themes contribute towards the extension and/or fading of the boundaries of traditional disciplines, in particular Medical Physics, Informatics, and Medicine.

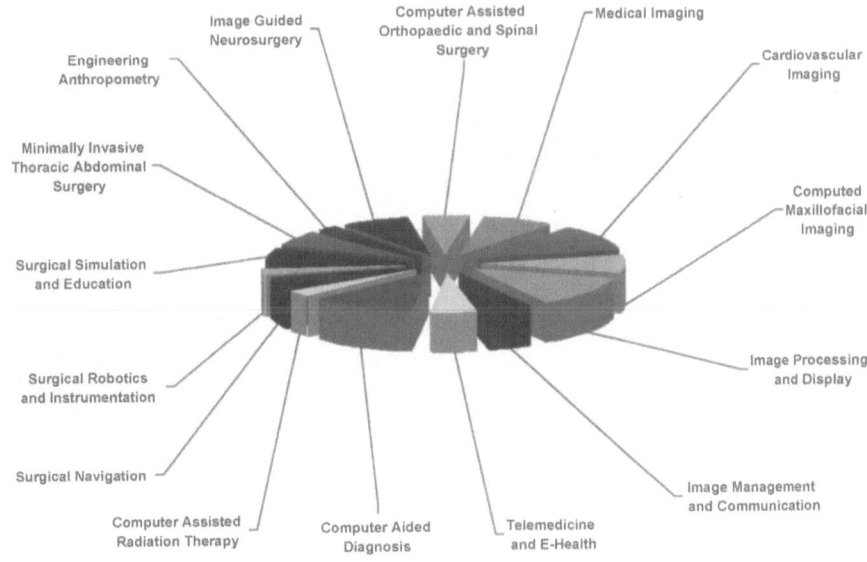

Fig. 1 Interdisciplinary themes of paper and poster abstract submissions for CARS 2002

The following brief definitions of the most important interdisciplines may serve as a guideline regarding the structure on which the CARS 2002 program has been compiled:

Medical Imaging (MI)
The science and engineering needed for the sourcing, acquisition, and processing of signals from the human body to generate multi-dimensional digital images.

Cardiovascular Imaging (CVI)
MI applied to the special requirements of the cardiovascular system and extended with IPD methods to allow quantitatively and qualitatively enhanced medical diagnosis.

Computed Maxillofacial Imaging (CMI)
MI applied to the special requirements of maxillofacial structures and extended with IPD methods to allow quantitatively and qualitatively enhanced medical diagnosis in this area.

Image Processing and Display (IPD)
Processing of elements/objects of images, e.g. pixels, voxels, regions and contours to enhance the quality, understanding, and representation of images. Image processing steps may include enhancement, restoration, registration, segmentation, analysis, interpretation, and multi-modality image fusion. Display steps may include various visualisation algorithms to represent data interrelationships or to enhance reality.

Image Management and Communication/PACS
Systems for storage, transmission, manipulation and display of digital images and the management of these images to enable an effective and hardcopyless (e.g. filmless) healthcare infrastructure.

Telemedicine and E-health (TMEH)
The use of information and communication technology to enable the transfer of medical data and programs to support healthcare activities between geographically separate locations.

Computer Aided Diagnosis (CAD)
MI and IPD methods applied to specific body parts to enable an image-guided diagnosis which enhances sensitivity and/or specificity of a diagnostic procedure carried out by humans.

Engineering Anthropometry (EA)
Acquisition, modelling, management and analysis of anatomic/physical landmarks and 3D surface data of different human populations. EA methods are based on data models, software tools and theoretical constructs and principles to support, for example, the searching and visualisation of 3D objects (human body scans). In healthcare, EA tools may also, for example, support anatomic atlas-based segmentation as well as the design of endoprosthetic devices and implants.

Surgical Navigation (SN)
IT-based systems to assist surgical procedures by guiding instruments within a surgical target volume to an operated volume with maximum accuracy and safety.

Surgical Robotics and Instrumentation (SRI)
IT and MEMS-based systems which use SN or SS to passively assist surgical activities semi-automatically or fully automatically.

Surgical Simulation (SS) and Education
IPD methods and simulation software applied to an surgical target volume to optimize surgical activities for the purpose of training and preoperative planning.

Image Guided Neurosurgery (IGNS)
The use of one or more methods derived from SN, SS or SRI, with a strong bias towards using images, to achieve minimally invasive interventions directed towards surgical target structures including the brain or spinal cord.

Computer Assisted Orthopaedic and Spinal Surgery (CAOS)
The use of one or more methods derived from SN, SS or SRI to achieve minimally invasive interventions directed towards surgical target volume including orthopaedic structures, such as the spinal vertebrae, hip, knee, ankle, or long bones. In a wider definition it may also include rapid prototyping and the design and manufacturing of endoprosthetic devices and implants.

Minimally Invasive Thoracic Abdominal Surgery (MITAS)
The use of one or more methods derived from SN, SS or SRI to achieve minimally invasive interventions directed towards surgical target volume within the thorax (excluding the cardiovascular structures) and the abdomen.

Computer Assisted Radiation Therapy (CART)
Modelling of radiation target structures with IPD methods and the application of radiation dose planning programs to optimize target volume (tumor) radiation treatment.

The subset of knowledge from the traditional fields of mathematics, physics, engineering, informatics, medicine, and management science required to advance the CARS interdisciplines given above is also subject of change. A proper understanding of this may illuminate which traditional profession comes closest to pursuing the respective activities within the CARS themes.

Results derived from CARS methods and applications provide valuable data, information, knowledge and even wisdom, and are changing medicine and associated professions. The impact this will have on current educational curricula as well as on changing the professional profiles of medical physicists, radiologists, surgeons, and computer scientists is substantial and requires further examination. As yet, few teaching institutions have responded to this challenge and are ready to offer appropriate educational courses and training. CARS 2002 and future CARS congresses are aimed at showing the direction into which a significant part of medicine will evolve in research, development and practice.

Heinz U. Lemke
Paris, June 2002

Acknowledgements

Once upon a time, back in the 1960s, when I first had to program a computer it was done in an assembler language. The good thing about this was that this language or interface to the computer, had a finite set of instructions and a finite set of combining these. The bad things were the lack of computational power of the workstation and the user interface to the assembler. On execution, however, the computer did more or less what one wanted it to do. Now, in 2002, times have changed. The good thing now is, that some twelve levels of hardware and software sophistication separate the assembler from the modern "easy to use" graphical user interfaces. Super computational power takes care of everything. The bad thing is, that the computer does not always do what one wants it to do.

Anyone who does not believe this, I should like to invite to do the electronic editing of the next CARS proceedings. The non-believers probably belong to the approx. 5% of authors who submitted their papers according to the author instruction for electronic submission for the CARS proceedings. These authors focused not only on providing excellent content but also on the structure and visual appearance of their papers. The other 95% obviously preferred to focus on content only and have worked, as I like to do, that is, leaving styling and layout of the paper to others.

The move into the electronic age was necessary in order to improve the quality and ensure the timely appearance of the CARS proceedings as a hardbound copy and also on the web. It has meant, however, a considerable amount of extra workload for Franziska Schweikert and her team, in particular Dagmar Harrison, in addition to the "usual" organizational and management work. During a two week period before and at the deadline of paper submission (i.e. 15th March, 2002) approx. 170 papers and 110 posters were received at the CARS Conference Office and electronically prepared and edited. The four weeks in March meant double-shift work for Franziska Schweikert and this is my written promise that next for year's CARS, we will engage additional assistance.

I also should like to acknowledge and thank for the continuing help received from the personnel of my department at the Technical University of Berlin, in particular from Helga Kallan, Steffen Märkle, Kai Köchy and René Tschirley. This is carried out in an environment marked by an increasing number of students in courses and for supervision, against a background of further cuts in teaching staff positions.

We are all delighted to have Prof. Kiyonari Inamura as the Honorary President of CARS 2002. I have known Kiyo Inamura for more than 10 years and had the pleasure to work closely together with him on a number of projects and many congress events. His contributions to research and development in many fields relating to CARS are documented in numerous publications. In particular, I treasure him for his engagement in advancing interdisciplinary and international cooperation. Through his remarkable selflessness, he is a great benefit not only for Japan but also for the rest of the world.

Heinz U. Lemke
Paris, June 2002

Prelude

CARS, Quo Vadis?

It is generally known that CARS involves a very wide spectrum of topics based on medicine, physics, computer science and even sociology. Since the first CAR Conference in 1985 up to the 16th CARS in 2002, there have been more than 60 topics. The terminology of these topics mainly came from the title of the sessions. However, I found that these topics could be grouped into 6 main categories, A to F, as shown below:

A. Modalities and their related topics
1 MRI, 2. CT, 3. Nuclear medicine, 4. Ultrasound, 5. Digital radiography involving a flat panel detector, 6. Angiography involving DSA, 7. Mathematical modeling for reconstruction etc., Multi-modality imaging and Medical imaging

B. Application of modalities
8. Radiation therapy and minimal invasive therapy, 9. Computer assisted radiology, Radiology diagnosis and Cardiology, Pediatric radiology, Neurology, IVR, Dosimetry in diagnosis and Computer assisted stereotaxy

C. Image processing, communication, display, interaction and related systems
10. PACS, RIS, HIS, Electronic med. record, Workflow, Standards such as DICOM, IHE (Integrating Healthcare Enterprise), 11. Telemedicine, 12. Image processing & display, Human-computer interaction and Virtual reality, 13. Workstation and Voice recognition applic., 14. Computer vision, 15. Computer graphics

D. Surgery, orthopaedics, maxillofacial and other related invasive topics
16. Surgery, Anthropometry, Surgical simulator, Surgical navigation, Neurosurgery, Spinal surgery, Thoracic and abdominal surgery, Standards in information-guided therapy, Surgical robotics, Optical diagnosis & in-situ tissue analysis, Ergonomics & motion analysis, Curved and steerable instr. and Endoluminal, 17. Orthopaedics, 18. Maxillofacial and Implantology, 19. Virtual endoscopy, 20. Cardio-vascular, Coronary and Medical innovation and technology

E. 21. Computer Aided Diagnosis

F. Surrounding and supporting infrastructure
22. Healthcare infrastructure, Interface between medicine and computer sciences, 23. Technology assessment and/or social implications, 24. Education, Knowledge based systems, Expert systems, Learning systems and Training systems, 25. Planning in the radiology department, 26. Strategic thinking, Decision making and Biointelligence

The chronological change in the number of presentations is shown in Table 1. The bracketed number indicates a double counted number. Example: (5) means that 5 presentations are double counted somewhere else in the same year. 16. Surgery in 2001 has 161 presentations and 72, the latter are broken down into I -VI. Also 16. Surgery in 2002 has 46 presentations and 56, the latter are composed of VII - XII. The features of CARS compared with those of other international conferences would be as follows:

1. Interdisciplinarity

   SPIE, SCAR, ICR and ECR cannot complete or bridge areas as CARS does in the categories shown in D and F in Table 1. Even RSNA is not as comprehensive as CARS.

2. Flexibility and elasticity

   CARS is sufficiently flexible to accept hot topics, new ideas, new concepts and different point of views. As shown in Table 1, sessions have been organized according to problem-oriented thinking. Session names have been revised rather frequently each year compared with other international conferences, because participants in CARS want different but the most appropriate solutions to chronologically changing problems. For example, the topics of "Computer vision" and "Computer graphics" which emerged in 1985 were revised to "Workstation" from 1991 and to "Image processing and display" from 1995, as shown in topics numbers 14, 15, 13 and 12 in Table 1.

3. Extension, penetration, but never fading out

   Depth and originality are respected, but they have often been driven by extension and penetration into other areas such as "medical innovation and technology".

I would like to point out the significance and importance of joint conferences. It was ten years ago, during his stay at Osaka Univ. as a visiting professor in 1992, that Prof. Heinz U. Lemke encouraged me to consider the extension of CAR topics, even outside conventional radiology. His idea was realized in 1995 when CAR collaborated with EuroPACS, ISPRAD, Telerad., The 2nd Congress of the Int. Society for Computer Aided Surgery-ISCAS 95, Computed Maxillofacial Imaging-CMI, and Image Guided Therapy.

In 1997, CAR, in collaboration with the 1st Annual Conference of the International Society for Computer Aided Surgery, was held in Berlin. However, the first CAR outside Europe was in Japan in 1998, and that was the beginning of a new era for CARS which had collaborated with more than 3 international formal annual conferences. Nowadays, for example in 2001, 6 international conferences joined with CARS and most enjoy exchanging common intellectual property. Efficacy, effectiveness and efficiency of knowledge communication as well as "aufheben" of new concepts and/or new ideas are the obvious advantages of joint international conferences. Especially young scientists, who accumulate a wealth of knowledge, will be stimulated intensively each June during 4 days in the last week.

I am sure that, in future, CARS will increasingly contribute to the education and training of young scientists, even though the development of new technologies and highly advanced medicine itself are the targets of CARS. In the field of radiology, the RSNA has its own education system with an educational fund, awards and credits etc, however, they have no consistent training. The disciplines and interdisciplines in CARS must be gradually focus and order to establish a training methodology to acquire and disseminate joint intellectual property among young scientists.

Kiyonari Inamura, PhD, Osaka University, Japan
Honorary President, CARS 2002

Table 1. Chronological change in the number of presentations for each topic in CAR and CARS

Cat	Topics	'85	''87	'89	'91	'93	'95	'96	'97	'98	'99	'00	'01	'02
A	1. MRI	12	14	12	14	6	10	16	13	10	9	16	21(5)	19
	2. CT	4	6	8	20	4	5	4	8	21	17	4	8	(19)
	3. Nuclear Medicine	9	6		2	4		5	1	8	2			
	4. UltraSound		5	4	8	2		6	4	4	4	2	34(13)	
	5. Digital Radiography	16	9	14	20	12	8	12	12	16	11	13	5	
	6. Angiography	5	6	5	6	11		5	8	1	12			
	7. Modeling	3	4		5									
B	8. Radiation Therapy	9	7	6	10	9	6	8	12	16	7	11	9	8
	9. Radiology & Diagnosis	10	12	19	17	17						1		
	10. PACS, RIS, HIS, EMR	10	16	30	38	44	33	33	54	41	51	36	45	17
C	11. Telemedicine	1			9	11	22	35	22	14	9	12	11	8
	12. Image Processing & Display	4	5	3	7	7	36	31	28	33	26	51	48	45
	13. Workstation				15	11	9	7	8	2	10	2	1	1
	14. Computer Vision	12	18	14	21	11								
	15. Computer Graphics	14	13	7		7			3			1		
	16. Surgery	3	1	3	8	8	30	60	82	65	76	78	161 72(I-VI)	46 56(VII-XII)
D	17. Orthopedics	4	10	8	6			19	7	15	31	16	16	10
	18. Maxillofacial						28	36		40	35	39	27	27
	19. Virtual Endoscopy							4		9	13	9	2	
	20. Cardiovascular	1		7	3									40
E	21. CAD						9	11	11	17	17	45	32	47
	22. Healthcare Infrastructure								9				5	
	23. Technology Assessment		6	7	7	9		3	4	4		(7)		
F	24. Education					2	10	7	15	7	7	12	15(4)	4
	25. Planning in Radiology Dept.						17			5	7			
	26. Strategic Thinking									1	1	2	9	
	Total	117	138	147	216	175	223	302	298	333	346	350	535	328

I Optical diagn.&in-situ tissue anal. 6 II Erg.&motion anal., curv. steer. instr. 10 III MedCapital 12 IV SMITIMAGE 13 V SMITEndol. 19 VI SMIT Poster 12 VII Anthropometry 9 VIII Surgical Simulator 11 IX Surgical Navigation 7 X Neurosurgery 13 XI Spine Surgery 6 XII Thoracic Abdominal Surgery 10

Contents

6th Annual Conference of the International Society for Computer Aided Surgery - ISCAS

Surgical Simulation

XXIV

Image Guided Neurosurgery

Robotics and Telesurgery

Surgical Robotics and Instrumentation

Minimally Invasive Spine Surgery

Computer Assisted Orthopaedic Surgery

**Special Session on Validation of Medical Image Processing in the Context
of Image-Guided Therapy**

Minimal Invasive Thoracic Abdominal Surgery

16th International Congress and Exhibition on Computer Assisted Radiology - CAR

Medical Imaging

Image Processing and Display

Image Management and Communication

Computer Assisted Radiation Therapy

Towards a World Engineering Anthropometry Resource

Telemedicine

Special Session on Electronic Health Record

4ᵗʰ International Workshop on Computer-Aided Diagnosis - CAD

Special Session on Breast CAD

XXXIV

Special Session on 3D CAD

2002 International Symposium on Cardiovascular Imaging - CVI

Invasive Coronary Imaging

Invasive Coronary and Vascular Imaging

Left and Right Ventricular Function

8th Computed Maxillofacial Imaging Congress - CMI

Image-Guidance in Implantology

Image-Guided Cranio-Maxillofacial Surgery

Poster Session

16th International Congress and Exhibition on
Computer Assisted Radiology - CAR

6th Annual Conference of the International Society for Computer Aided Surgery - ISCAS

4th International Workshop on Computer-Aided Diagnosis
Chairman: **Kunio Doi, PhD (USA)**

Special Session on Breast CAD

CARS 2002 – H.U. Lemke, M.W. Vannier; K. Inamura, A.G. Farman, K. Doi & J.H.C. Reiber (Editors)

Quantifying breast cancer risk from mammograms

Martin J. Yaffe[a], Norman F. Boyd[b]

[a] Imaging Research Program, Sunnybrook and Women's College Health Sciences
Centre and Department of Medical Biophysics, University of Toronto
2075 Bayview Avenue, Toronto Canada M4N 3M5

[b] Division of Epidemiology and Statistics, Ontario Cancer Institute and Division
of Preventive Oncology, Cancer Care Ontario, Toronto Canada

Abstract

Breast density, as assessed from the mammogram, is a strong risk factor for breast cancer. Both two and three-dimensional approaches to quantification of mammographic density are described. Potential applications of density measurement are discussed.

Keywords: Mammographic density, breast cancer risk

1. Introduction

Breast cancer is the second largest cancer killer of North American women. Its causes are largely not known and, therefore, currently, the most effective approach to reducing mortality is through early detection. Routine mammographic screening of women over 40 has been demonstrated to contribute to mortality reduction. The identification of risk factors for the disease is particularly important. Mammographic density has been shown to be a strong risk factor for breast cancer and, here, we describe methods for estimating breast cancer risk through quantitative analysis of mammographic density.

1.1 Mammographic density

The breast has a wide range of appearance on mammography, due to differences in composition. Radiographically, the breast consists mainly of two component tissues: fibroglandular tissue and fat. Regions of brightness on the mammogram, associated with the more x-ray attenuating fibroglandular tissue are referred to as <u>mammographic density</u>.

In the 1970's, Wolfe hypothesized that breast cancer risk is related to mammographic density [1]. He developed a qualitative scale, classifying the breast as being predominately composed of fat or belonging to one of three categories of increased mammographic density, due to the prominence of the ductal structures or diffuse areas of density. He correlated these categories to the subsequent development of breast cancer.

Several studies [2-4] have used multi-category quantitative classifications of dense tissue. Warner [5] performed a meta-analysis of these studies and compared quantitative versus strictly qualitative classifications of mammographic density. They found the former to give stronger predictions of risk. Breast density is an important risk factor for breast cancer, both because of the magnitude of the risk prediction, and because it is present in a

CARS 2002 – H.U. Lemke, M.W. Vannier; K. Inamura, A.G. Farman, K. Doi & J.H.C. Reiber (Editors)

large fraction of breast cancer cases. Another important and distinctive feature of mammographic density is that it appears to be modifiable. Density is known to regress with age, attributed to the hormonal changes associated with menopause and increase with hormone replacement therapy in peri- and post-menopausal women [6]. It is not yet known whether the reduction in density also reduces breast cancer risk. Nevertheless, the observation that a strong risk factor for breast cancer can be altered gives hope to the development of potential preventive strategies

2. Methods for characterizing mammographic density

Methods for characterizing mammographic density can be subjective, interactive or fully automatic. Subjective methods can provide strong risk predictions; however, several limitations have been identified, including considerable inter- and intra- observer variation in classification and limited ability to monitor small differences in mammographic density. This is particularly important in studies investigating changes in density with time, or with a potential intervention that may alter the breast tissue characteristics.

It is desirable to be able to measure mammographic density on a continuous, quantitative scale. To be useful in retrospective clinical studies, it is also important that all features to be used can be obtained from images without further information. Various approaches have been used to measure mammographic density quantitatively. For example, planimetry has been used to measure the area of dense tissue on the mammogram [4] and demonstrated risk factors on the order of 4. Generally, however, because the process is labour intensive, only a rather coarse outline of the areas of density is performed.

2.1 Interactive thresholding
A Windows-based interactive thresholding technique [7] has been developed for quantification of mammographically dense tissue. The user interface for this method is shown in Figure 1. An observer views the digitized mammogram and selects two grey levels: i_{EDGE}, which separates the of the breast from the background, and i_{DY}, the level above which all pixels are interpreted as representing mammographic density (solid bright area in Figure 1). From the grey-level histogram, h_i, the projected area of the breast, A, the projected area of dense tissue and their ratio, PD, are calculated as:

$$A = \sum_{i=i_{EDGE}}^{i_{MAX}} h_i \quad (1) \qquad PD = \frac{\sum_{i=i_{DY}}^{i_{MAX}} h_i}{A} \times 100\% \quad (2)$$

This method allows relatively simple decision criterion to be applied, which contributes to reproducible measures of A and PD, both within and between observers.

2.2 Automated analysis of mammographic densities
While interactive methods provide a continuous, quantitative scale for density assessment and have been shown to be quite reliable, they are still somewhat subjective and labour intensive. Several investigators have attempted to develop more objective techniques, using features, which can be calculated automatically and on a continuous scale [8-13]. Mammographic density can be distinguished on the basis of brightness or texture.

CARS 2002 – H.U. Lemke, M.W. Vannier; K. Inamura, A.G. Farman, K. Doi & J.H.C. Reiber (Editors)

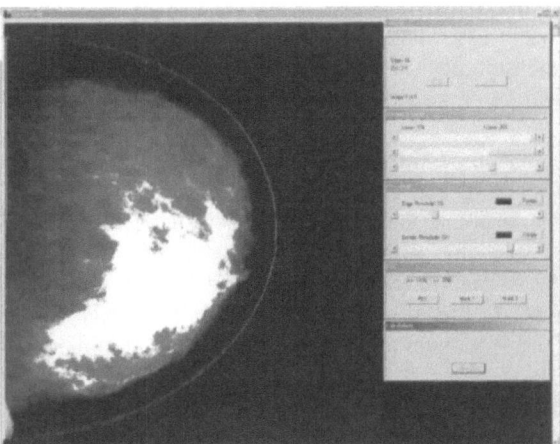

Fig. 1: User interface for interactive thresholding method.

Features for image segmentation can be based on the image itself, on transforms of the image, or on the grey level histogram.

In our work, we calculated a normalized skewness [8] in terms of the 3rd and 2nd moments of the histogram as $m_3/m_2^{3/2}$. This provided a unit-free measure. Normalization to the 3/2 power of m_2 removes the effect of the spread of the histogram, while preserving the skewness information. This facilitates comparisons of distributions with different variability. Local tissue composition is considered by calculating skewness for many individual, small regions of the breast and averaging the results.

Caldwell [10] found that a measurement based on fractal dimension correlated well with Wolfe's qualitative grades. The fractal dimension describes the texture of the image-dense breasts have a smoother texture and a lower fractal dimension, while fatty breasts exhibit greater local contrasts and a higher fractal dimension. We applied the technique of Lundahl [14] for calculating the fractal dimension on a set of 60 mammograms [8]. We found the mammograms to be highly fractal in nature with measured fractal dimension ranging between 2.23 and 2.54, similar to the range observed by Caldwell [10]. Taylor [12] also considered the fractal dimension and regional skewness measurements as features for characterizing breast composition and found that they successfully provide a two- category discrimination of dense from fatty mammograms.

3. Volumetric analysis of mammographic density

One of the major strengths of the PD method is that it can be employed in retrospective studies, where little information is available about how the mammographic exam is carried out. This eliminates most of the variables associated with the image acquisition procedure, however, has the significant disadvantage of treating the breast as a binary structure (dense or non-dense) and ignoring the variations in thickness of the dense tissue. Clearly, this is a three dimensional problem, which ideally should be treated as such.

CARS 2002 – H.U. Lemke, M.W. Vannier; K. Inamura, A.G. Farman, K. Doi & J.H.C. Reiber (Editors)

656

The mechanism linking density and risk is not yet known, however, it is logical that risk would be more closely associated with the actual amount of dense tissue than with its projected area. A measurement of volume of mammographic density may provide a more relevant characterization of density, and potentially a stronger risk prediction.

Volumetric density can be estimated by calibrating the mammography system [15,16]. This is done by including a test object, which allows the direct determination of the relationship between brightness (film optical density) and the thickness and composition of breast tissue. When this object is imaged adjacent to the breast, the empirical relationship obtained implicitly corrects for the effect of the x-ray exposure technique and processing variations. Composition at each point in the image can be determined by an inverse look-up of the brightness and thickness at that point in the breast.

A calibration object for this purpose is illustrated in Figure 2. It consists of steps of different thickness and compositions of breast-equivalent material. Using the digitized radiograph of this object, a relationship such as that illustrated in Figure 3 is obtained for each clinical image. For the exposure conditions used, a particular brightness could be obtained with many combinations of breast thickness and composition. However, if the total compressed breast thickness is known for a particular point in the image, then only a single combination of effective thicknesses of adipose and fibroglandular tissue adding to that total thickness is consistent with that image brightness.

4. Other imaging modalities: digital mammography ultrasound, MRI

In digital mammography, the image receptor has a linear response to the absorbed x-ray signal resulting from radiation transmitted by the breast. The response of the detectors is highly stable over time and the image is already in digital form. Therefore, it is much easier to make quantitative mammographic density measurements from digital mammograms than from film images [17,18].

Often, it is not practical to use the mammogram for assessment of breast density. Examples are young women (under age 40) who do not normally receive routine mammograms and high-risk women, where it may be advisable to monitor changes in the breast more frequently than is acceptable with mammography. In both cases, an imaging method such as ultrasound or MRI, that does not employ ionizing radiation, would be desirable. An additional advantage is that both produce three dimensional image data, thereby facilitating volumetric analysis.

With ultrasound, differences between the acoustic scattering properties within fibroglandular tissue and fat [19,20] give rise to differences in image texture. Work is currently underway to determine features that allow effective segmentation of dense tissue from fat and to reduce the high levels of speckle noise by averaging. It will also be necessary to adopt a mode in which machine settings are constant for the entire imaging procedure or else a method to correct for alterations in acquisition parameters.

CARS 2002 – H.U. Lemke, M.W. Vannier; K. Inamura, A.G. Farman, K. Doi & J.H.C. Reiber (Editors)

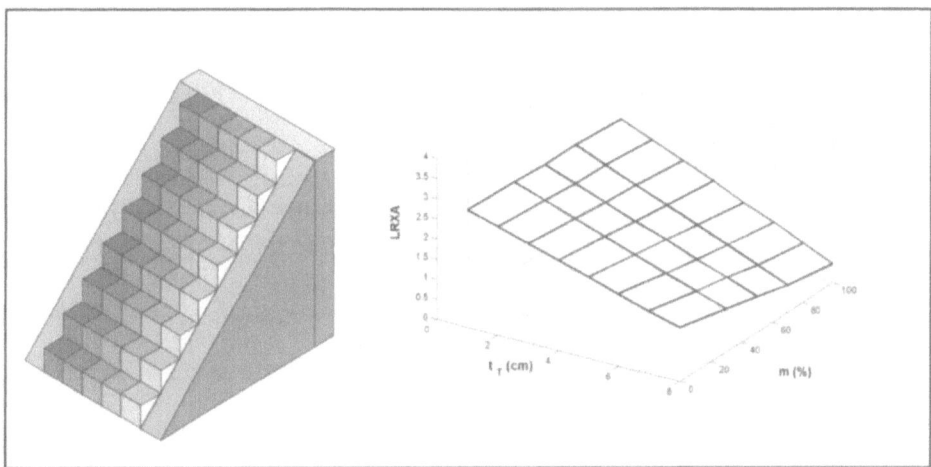

Fig. 2: Plastic device for calibration   Fig. 3: Calibration surface for volumetric density method.
of volumetric density technique.   (LRXA = log relative x-ray exposure, t_T= total breast
                                         thickness, m= % fibroglandular)

Some work has also been done to develop magnetic resonance imaging for characterizing the composition of the breast [21]. It has been shown that a pulse sequence that allows separate "fat" and "water" images to be produced provides data that correlate very well with x-ray mammographic density analysis [22].

5. Applications of mammographic density measurements

As a strong, potentially modifiable risk factor that is present in a large proportion of breast cancer cases, assessment of mammographic density could have important applications both to clinical practice and research. Women at increased risk due to high mammographic density may benefit from being screened more frequently. It may be possible to gain insight into the causes of breast cancer by finding the factors that are associated with density and determining whether they can be altered to reduce density and risk. Potential preventive strategies include manipulation of hormones, tamoxifen [23], or a dietary intervention [24].

Acknowledgements

This work was supported by a Program Project Grant from The Terry Fox Foundation.

References

1.   Wolfe JN, "Risk for breast cancer development determined by mammographic parenchymal pattern", *Cancer* ,37, 2486-92, 1976.
2.   Boyd NF, O'Sullivan B, Campbell JE, Fishell E, Simor I, Cooke G, Germanson T., "Mammographic signs as risk factors for breast cancer", *Br. J. Cancer*, 45, 185-93, 1982.
3.   Brisson J, Verreault R, Morrison A, Tennina S, Meyer F, "Diet, mammographic features of breast tissue, and breast cancer risk", *Am. J. Epidemiol.*,130, 14-24, 1989.

4. Byrne C, Schairer C, Wolfe J, Parekh N, Salane M, Brinton LA, Hoover R, Haile R, "Mammographic features and breast cancer risk: effects with time, age, and menopause status", *J. NCI* ,87, 1622-1629, 1995.

5. Warner E, Lockwood G, Math M, Tritchler D, Boyd NF, "The risk of breast cancer associated with mammographic parenchymal patterns: a meta-analysis of the published literature to examine the effect of method of classification", *Cancer Detection and Prevention*, 16, 67-72, 1992.

6. Laya MB, Gallagher JC, Schreiman JS, Larson EB, Watson P, Weinstein L, "Effect of postmenopausal hormonal replacement therapy on mammographic density and parenchymal pattern", *Radiology*,196, 433-437, 1995.

7. Byng JW, Boyd NF, Fishell E, Jong RA, Yaffe MJ, "The quantitative analysis of mammographic densities", *Phys. Med.Biol.*, 39, 1629-1638, 1994.

8. Byng JW, Boyd NF, Jong RA, Fishell E, Yaffe MJ, "Automated analysis of mammographic densities", *Phys. Med. Biol.*,41, 909-923, 1996.

9. Magnin IE, Cluzeau F, Odet CL, "Mammographic texture analysis: an evaluation of risk for developing breast cancer", *Optical Engineering*,25,780-4, 1985.

10. Caldwell CB, Stapelton SJ, Holdsworth DW, Jong RA, Weisser WJ, Cooke G, Yaffe MJ, "Characterization of mammographic parenchymal pattern by fractal dimension", *Phys. Med. Biol.*,35,235-47, 1990.

11. Miller P, Astley S, "Classification of breast tissue by texture analysis", *Image Vision and Computing*,10,277-82, 1992.

12. Taylor P, Hajnal S, Dilhuydy M-H, Barreau B, "Measuring image texture to separate 'difficult' from 'easy' mammograms" *Br. J. Radiol.*,67,456-63, 1994.

13. Kallergi M, Woods K, Clarke LP, Qian W, Clark RA, "Image segmentation in digital mammography: comparison of local thresholding and region growing algorithms", *Comput Med Imaging Graph.*,16,323-31, 1992.

14. Lundahl T, Ohley WJ, Kuklinski WS, Williams DO, Gewirtz H, Most AS, "Analysis and interpolation of angiographic images by use of fractals", *IEEE Computers in Cardiology*, 355-8, 1995.

15. Pawluczyk O, Yaffe MJ, "Field non-uniformity correction for quantitative analysis of digitized mammograms*" Med. Phys.*, 28; 438-444, 2001.

16. Pawluczyk O, Yaffe MJ, Boyd NF, Jong RA, "Estimation of volumetric breast density for risk prediction", In Dobbins JT III and Boone JM (Eds.) Medical Imaging 2000: Physics of Medical Imaging, Proc. SPIE 3977, 2000.

17. Yang J, Rico D, Mawdsley GE, Yaffe MJ, "Volumetric Breast Density Estimation Method for Full-Field Digital Mammography", *Radiology* 2001; 221P 192.

18. Kaufhold J, Thomas JA, Eberhard JW, Galbo CE, Gonzalez-Trotter DE, "Tissue composition determination in digital mammography", *Radiology* 2001; 221P 188.

19. Kaizer L, Fishell EK, Hunt JW, Foster FS and Boyd NF, "Ultrasonically defined parenchymal patterns of the breast: relationship to mammographic patterns and other risk factors for breast cancer", *British Journal of Radiology* 1988;61:118-124.

20. Blend R, Rideout DF, Kaizer L, Shannon P, Tudor-Roberts B, Boyd NF, "Parenchymal patterns of the breast defined by real time ultrasound", *Eur. J. Cancer Prev.*,4, 293-8, 1995.

21. Poon CS, Bronskill MJ, Henkelman RM, Boyd NF, "Quantitative magnetic resonance imaging parameters and their relationship to mammographic pattern", *J. NCI* , 84, 777-81, 1992.

22. Graham SJ, Bronskill MJ, Byng JW, Yaffe MJ, Boyd NF, "Quantitative correlation of breast tissue parameters using magnetic resonance and x-ray mammography", *British Journal of Cancer*,73, 162-168, 1996.

23. Nayfield SG, Karp JE, Ford LG, Dorr FA, Kramer BS, "Potential role of tamoxifen in prevention of breast cancer", *Journal of the National Cancer Institute*, 83, 1450-9,1991.

24. Boyd NF, Greenberg C, Lockwood G, Little L, Martin L, Byng J, Yaffe M, Tritchler D, "The effects at 2 years of a low-fat high-carbohydrate diet on radiological features of the breast: results from a randomized trial", *J. NCI*, 89, 488-96, 1997.

CARS 2002 – H.U. Lemke, M.W. Vannier; K. Inamura, A.G. Farman, K. Doi & J.H.C. Reiber (Editors)
©CARS/Springer. All rights reserved.

An automated detection method of mammographic masses based on adaptive threshold technique utilizing multi-resolution processing

Satoshi Kasai [a], Daisuke Kaji [a], Akiko Kano [a], Hiroshi Fujita [b], Takeshi Hara [b]
and Tokiko Endo [c]

[a] MI Solution Group, Medical & Graphic Company, Konica Corporation,
No.1 Sakura-machi, Hino-shi, Tokyo 191-8511 Japan
[b] Department of Information Science, Faculty of Engineering, Gifu University,
1-1 Yanagido, Gifu-shi, Gifu 501-1193 Japan
[c] Department of Radiology, National Hospital of Nagoya, 4-1-1Sannomaru,
Naka-ku, Nagoya-shi, Aichi 460-0001 Japan

Abstract

We have been developing an automated detection scheme for mass candidates on digital mammograms. However, this algorithm based on an adaptive thresholding technique showed somewhat lower detection performance for masses adjacent to skinlines. The technique also tended to produce less accurate segmentation between extremely low-contrast masses and surrounding mammary-gland tissues. The purpose of this study is to improve the detection rate for such masses so as to achieve a superior overall performance. We have developed a new detection alogorithm based on a multi-resolution processing, adaptive thresholding technique and discriminant analysis. By applying the new technique, our detection algorithm provided a sensitivity of 87.7% with 1.5 false-positive detections per image with a database of 626 digitized clinical mammograms. Eighteen masses were successfully detected among 23 masses that had not been detected by our previous method. The result demonstrates the effectiveness of the proposed method.

Keywords: Mammogram, CAD, mass detection

1. Introduction

The prevalence of breast cancer has recently been increasing. Mammography is considered to be a major significant way for detecting abnormalities in breast as early as possible. Breast cancer commonly presents masses. Currently there are a number of research groups who have been studying CAD systems to detect masses on digital mammograms. We also have been developing an automated detection scheme based on a thresholding technique for mass candidates[1,2]. In our previous method, digital mammograms were classified into four categories in accordance with glandular conditions.

For each category adapted thresholds were established. Candidate areas were then extracted and classified by feature analyses. However, this algorithm showed relatively low detection rate for masses adjacent to skinlines, because of steep density gradients on the background trends. Figure 1 illustrates (a) an example of a mass adjacent to the skinline and (b) the pixel value profile between A and B. The influence of background trend on the profile is obvious from this profile. Additionally, the technique had a difficulty in discriminating a mass from a surrounding normal tissue when there is only a slight difference of density between them.

The purpose of this study is to develop a new detection algorithm which can solve these two problems.

2. Materials and methods

Our new algorithm mainly consists of 4 steps:

2.1 Pre-processing by using a newly developed multi-resolution processing technique

A processing based on multi-resolution processing, which decomposes an image into plural frequency bands and enhances each frequency band independently, is applied. The algorithm is able to enhance masses, while suppressing low frequency component such as background trend and high frequency component such as mammary gland at the same time. We defined masses to detect as the size from 5 mm to 30 mm and designed a continuous frequency characteristic to selectively enhance

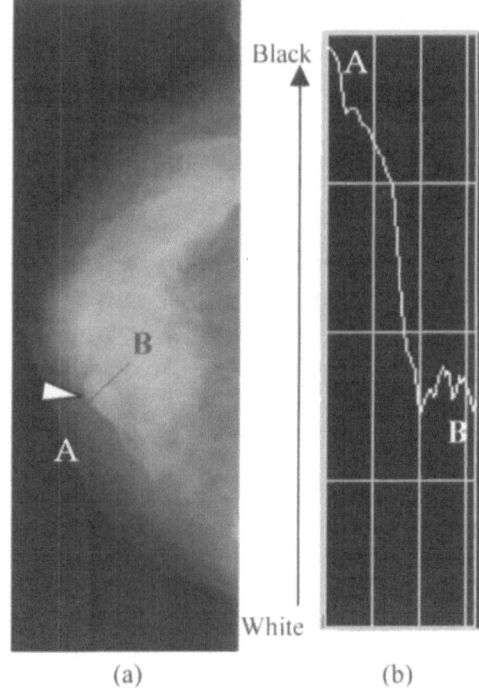

(a)   (b)

Fig.1 An example of mass adjacent to skinline (a) and profile of the pixel value between A and B (b) (an arrow indicates the mass)

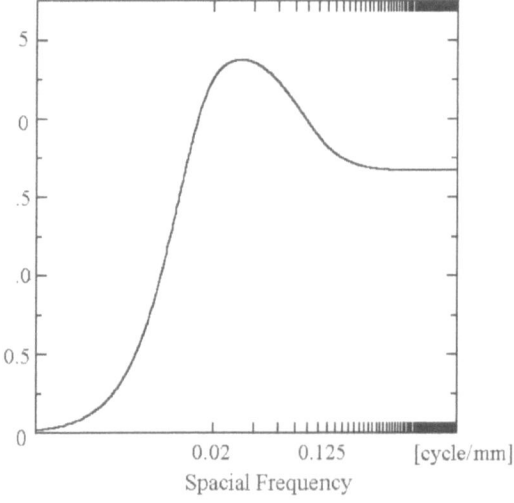

Fig.2 An example of frequency characteristic used in multi-resolution processing

CARS 2002 – H.U. Lemke, M.W. Vannier; K. Inamura, A.G. Farman, K. Doi & J.H.C. Reiber (Editors)

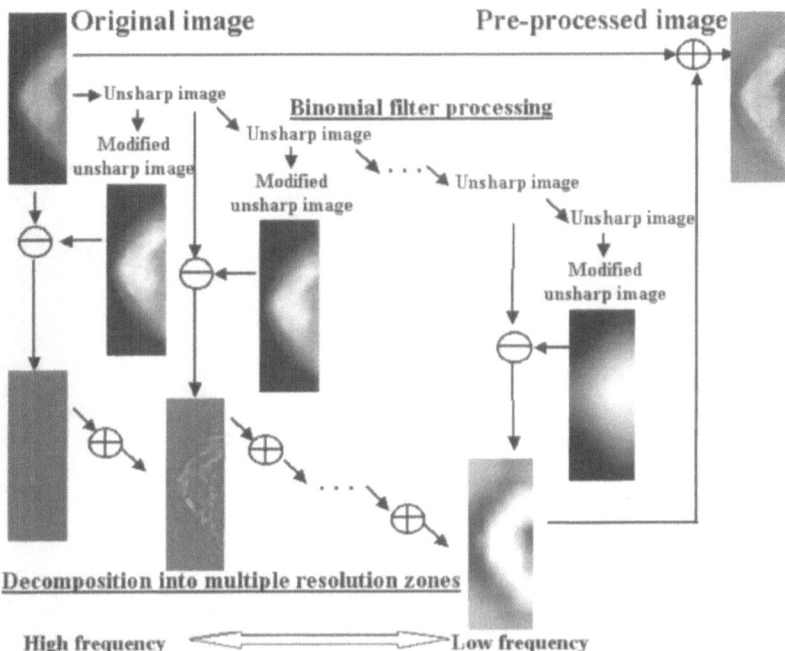

Fig.3 Pre-processing by using multi-resolution processing

them. The lowest frequency band which corresponds to background trend is designed to have nearly zero response. The frequency bands between 0.016 and 0.1 cycle/mm that involve potential mass candidates are enhanced so as to have a peak enhancement frequency with a response of 2.5. Frequency bands less than 0.016 cycle/mm and greater than 0.1 cycle/mm are relatively suppressed. Figure 2 shows a frequency characteristic which is used in this study.

A schematic diagram of the pre-processing process is shown in Fig.3.

On the decomposition stage, multiple unsharp images are created from the original image by using a binomial filter[3]. A binomial filtering is a fast filtering technique utilizing binomial distribution characteristics. Image data are subjected to repetitive 2x2 simple averagings to produce results equivalent to a Gaussian weighting filter.

Moreover, enhancement characteristic for each

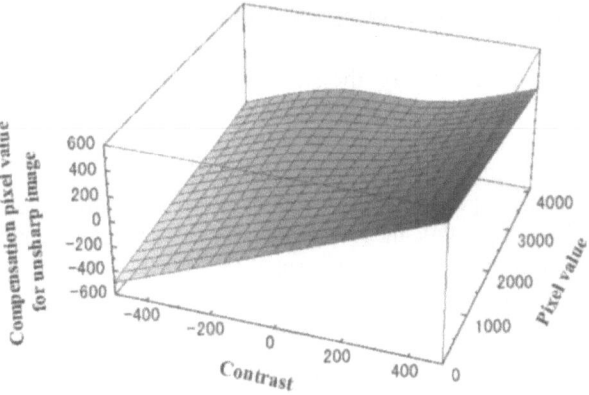

Fig.4 Compensation function for an unsharp image

CARS 2002 – H.U. Lemke, M.W. Vannier; K. Inamura, A.G. Farman, K. Doi & J.H.C. Reiber (Editors)

662

unsharp image is established based on a compensation function, which is determined by density and contrast of the unsharp image. An unsharp image is modified by adding compensation values to the corresponding pixel values. The compensation values are calculated based on a smooth function as shown in Fig.4. A subtraction image between the modified unsharp image and the unsharp image of adjoining frequency band is obtained. The resulting pre-processed image is reconstructed as the summation of all the subtraction images.

The enhancement characteristics employed in the proposed method enables a selective suppression of enhancement on tissues which have high contrast and low density. In consequence, artifacts due to overshoot and undershoot are prevented, as well as excessive granularity in low-density regions.

It was found that this process also improves the performance of the following false-positive elimination based on feature analyses. There are differences between features of masses

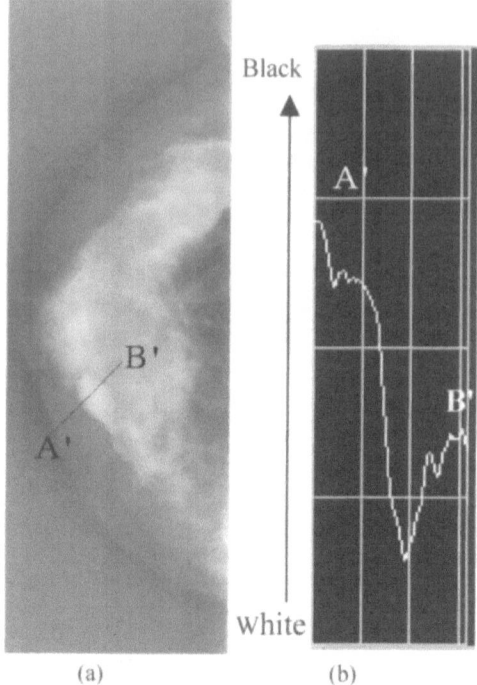

Fig.5 Pre-processed image(a) by a newly developed multi-resolution processing from the image in Fig.1, and a profile between A' and B' (b).

with microcalcifications and those of masses without microcalcifications. The proposed technique can reduce the amount of the differences which possibly produce misclassifications in multivariate analyses.

Figure 5(a) shows the pre-processed image obtained from the original image in Fig.1. The points A' and B' correspond to A and B in Fig.1, respectively. The profile shown in Fig.5(b) demonstrates the effective suppression of the background trend and enhancement of the mass.

2.2 Determination of candidate areas

Binary images are created by using different threshold values which correspond to pixel values of possible masses in the pre-processed image obtained in 1).

The threshold values vary from 10 % to 60 % of the pixel value distribution within the whole breast region, in order to minimize false-negative detections. The steps between the thresholds are set narrow enough to recognize mass contours precisely.

However, when there is little density difference between a mass and a surrounding normal tissue, it is often very difficult for a thresholding technique to distinguish them. In order to detect such masses, we employed a morphological opening processing with a structure factor of 1.2 mm (radius). This process consequently discriminates masses from linear mammary glands.

CARS 2002 – H.U. Lemke, M.W. Vannier; K. Inamura, A.G. Farman, K. Doi & J.H.C. Reiber (Editors)
'CARS/Springer. All rights reserved.

2.3 Multivariate analysis by nine features

Each candidate area in a multi-resolution processed image is labeled and feature analyses are applied. In the feature analyses, nine parameters are examined: size, contrast, two kinds of circularity, standard deviation, normalized average value, concentration, volume and representative pixel value of the candidate area. We employed two different definitions for circularity, one is based on comparison with a circle and the other is based on candidate's contour length. Volume is a feature value which represents the summation of difference between the threshold and every pixel value within a candidate area. Representative pixel value of the candidate area is defined as a normalized threshold between the minimum and the maximum pixel value within the breast region. First, an appropriate threshold is determined for each parameter with a rule-based method to distinguish masses from other tissues. For instance, when a candidate's circularity value is greater than the threshold, it will be classified as a mass candidate. For farther false-positive elimination, a discriminant analysis is applied to the nine features.

Seventy-nine masses and 3066 normal tissues which were selected from 63 images were used for making each variance-covariance matrix. The ratio of Mahalanobis distances was modified to provide a true-positive rate of 83.8% at an average number of 1.1 false positives per image with a training data set consisting of 63 mammograms.

2.4 Elimination of false-positive candidates

In order to eliminate false-positive candidates, co-occurrence matrix and gray level difference methods are employed. Co-occurrence matrix and gray level difference matrix from 0, 45, 90, 135 angles are made and angular second moment, inverse difference moment and entropy from co-occurrence matrix and contrast form gray level difference matrix are calculated. The averaged feature over the angles is used for discriminating mass candidates from other structures.

3. Results

The sensitivity of our improved detection algorithm was 87.7% (64/73) with 1.5 false-positive detections per image with our database of 626 digitized clinical mammograms, which includes extremely subtle masses in terms of density and masses adjacent to skinlines. It was possible to detect 18 out of 23 masses that had not been detected by our previous method.

Figure 6 shows the result of an FROC analysis by using the ratio of Mahalanobis distance as a parameter. It is apparent that the performance of the new algorithm is better than that of the previous one.

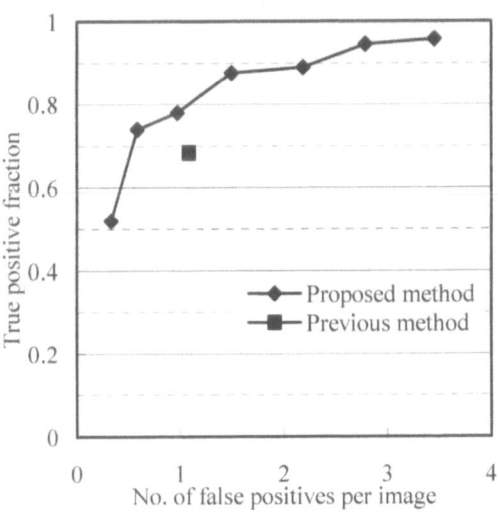

Fig.6 Result of FROC analysis

Most of the abnormalities which are missed even with this new algorithm are partial-loss masses locating near chest-wall regions or architectural distortions which do not form masses. We expect that the system performance will be improved by introducing a dedicated algorithm to the partial-loss masses locating near chest-wall regions, which our group has already developed and reported[4,5].

4. Conclusion

A new technique for detecting masses based on adaptive threshold technique utilizing multi-resolution processing was proposed and the algorithm has been developed. The new algorithm was able to detect 18 of 23 masses that were not detected with our previous method. A pre-processing technique by using a newly developed multi-resolution processing was found to be especially effective for thresholding technique. Furthermore, the technique is promising for other typical processes such as a template matching or a filtering, because background trends and high frequency components such as mammary glands also give undesirable influences on these processings. In addition, a morphological processing made it possible to detect mass candidates which have only a slight density difference from surrounding normal tissues. The result indicated that the new technique significantly improved the overall performance of our CAD system.

Acknowledgements

This work was supported in part by the Ministry of Health, Labour, and Welfare under a Grant-In-Aid for Cancer Research and in part by the Ministry of Education, Culture, Sports, Science and Technology under a Grant-In-Aid for Scientific Research.

References

1. T.Matsubara, H.Fujita, T.Endo, K.Horita, C.Kido, M.Ikeda, and T.Ishigaki, "Development of mass detection algorithm based on adaptive thresholding technique in digital mammograms", Proc. of 3rd International Workshop on Digital Mammography, 391-396, in Digital Mammography '96, Elsevier Science, Amsterdam, 1996.
2. Y. Hatanaka, T. Hara, H. Fujita, S. Kasai, T. Endo, and T. Iwase, "Development of an automated method for detecting mammographic masses with a partial loss of region", IEEE Trans. on Med. Imag., Vol. 20 No.12, 1209-1214, 2001.
3. B. Jahne, "Digital Image Processing Concepts, Algorithms, and Scientific Applications", 77-131, Springer-Verlag, Berlin, 1991.
4. S.Kasai, H.Fujita, T.Hara, T.Endo and H.Yoshimura, "Development of a detection algorithm for masses around thick mammary gland on mammograms", Proc. of the 12th International Symposium and Exhibition on Computer Assisted Radiology and Surgery CAR '98, 213-218, 1998.
5. Y. Hatanaka, T. Hara, H. Fujita, S. Kasai, T. Endo and T. Iwase, "An automated detection method of mammographic masses existing around thick-mammary-gland and near chest-wall regions", Proc. of the 15th International Congress and Exhibition CARS 2001, 527-532, Elsevier Science, Amsterdam, 2001.

CARS 2002 – H.U. Lemke, M.W. Vannier; K. Inamura, A.G. Farman, K. Doi & J.H.C. Reiber (Editors)

Image retrieval scheme for mammographic masses by using a local-pattern matching technique

Toshiaki Nakagawa[a], Takeshi Hara[a], Hiroshi Fujita[a]
Takuji Iwase[b], Tokiko Endo[c]

[a] Department of Information Science, Faculty of Engineering, Gifu University
Yanagido 1-1, Gifu 501-1193, Japan
[b] Department of Breast Surgery, Aichi Cancer Center Hospital
Kanokoden 1-1, Tikusa-ku, Nagoya 464-8681, Japan
[c] Department of Radiology, National Hospital of Nagoya
Sannomaru 4-1-1, Naka-ku, Nagoya 460-0001, Japan

Abstract

We proposed a concept of content-based image retrieval and demonstrated the potential usefulness in mammography. The approach incorporated a local-pattern matching method based on Nth-order autocorrelation features with KL expansion (principal components analysis) to retrieve similar mass shadows on digitized mammograms. The method can perform image retrieval without carrying out the image segmentation. We confirmed the tendency that similar mass images were retrieved as the initial studies by using the 30 simulated patterns and the 75 images of mammographic masses. The result showed that the image retrieval method might provide a new CAD system on mammograms.

Keywords: Image retrieval, mammogram, computer-aided diagnosis

1. Introduction

In recent years, large-scale databases of medical images were built for effective usage of information, and the technique was required to retrieve images from database as user's needs. Comparing the previous and similar images with current case is very effective procedure in interpreting by physicians. The purpose of this work is to develop an image retrieval system based on local-pattern matching technique, and to evaluate the performance by employing mammographic masses. The conceptual figure of the system is shown in Fig. 1.

This system searches out the image database for the image resembling to the entered one (query image) and outputs with diagnostic information. The information indicates whether the interpretation result is normal or abnormal, if the diagnosis is abnormal, the degree of malignancy is represented to determine the follow-up treatments. Recent researches on image retrieval technique are mainly categorized into two major approaches by using languages as a keyword of an image and by using a feature value of an image. Since the data in words or by numerical values are given in advance in the approach based on keywords, it is not so practical when the number of image in the database became larger.

CARS 2002 – H.U. Lemke, M.W. Vannier; K. Inamura, A.G. Farman, K. Doi & J.H.C. Reiber (Editors)

666

Moreover, if features of images are difficult to express by only language, this method is not effective.

Approaches of using image as key well employ the feature-extraction method in many researches [1-3]. Also in the field of a medical image, some researches are reported on retrieval of the similar image of a disease until now [4, 5]. In general studies, the image segmentation technique took an important role to distinguish the abnormal region from the background area. Various features based on the shape and the size were calculated from the result of the segmentation there. Therefore, since the retrieval results depend on the accuracy of the segmentation processing, it is not an effective approach to retrieve images that the object boundaries are difficult to determine strictly. In mammographic masses especially, the segmentation is not suitable because a part of boundary of the shade is not clear, or if the shade is malignant mass, determining the margin is often difficult.

In this research, the technique of extracting the feature from the whole image automatically and performing image retrieval without carrying out the image segmentation is proposed. To do this, we applied a local-pattern matching technique based on Nth-order autocorrelation features. The simulation experiment using the monochrome figures and the experiment using the mammographic mass images were conducted to examine the validity of this technique.

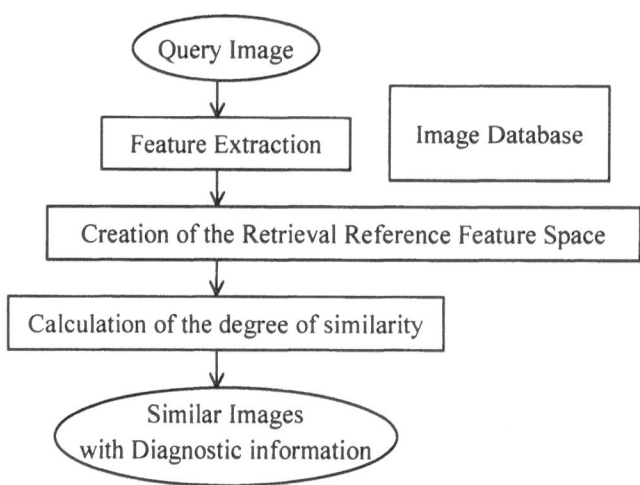

Fig. 1: Image retrieval system

2. Methods

2.1 Preprocessing
To raise the accuracy of retrieval results needs to perform the feature extraction using many local patterns from images with high resolution and high gray level. However, since those high qualities of image may be too fine in retrieval of similar images, even if shapes

CARS 2002 – H.U. Lemke, M.W. Vannier; K. Inamura, A.G. Farman, K. Doi & J.H.C. Reiber (Editors)

667

and density distributions of two images are slightly different, it is expected that the degree of similar may become low. Therefore, a preprocessing was performed to changes resolution and gray level into the optimal value judged from the amount of a database for the feature extraction.

2.2 Feature extraction

The features were extracted from the query image and the ones within whole database. The images including mass findings were simply cut from original digitized images in a square form. The autocorrelation features were extracted by counting patterns defined as local patterns consisted of some pixels with various gray level distributions. The example of the local pattern used for the feature extraction is shown in Fig. 2. The number of pixels classified the local patterns into several levels. The number was corresponding to the level indicated in the figure. For instance, the local pattern at level 2 consists of two pixels, the number is considered as the combination of a pixel value of each pixel and the joint direction. Although the kind of these patterns exists innumerably, a pixel value is prepared in the range of the gradation of the target image. If the feature extraction is carried out using N pieces of local patterns on each image, the feature vector with N elements is obtained. The number of those local patterns is considered as the feature values of the image in N-dimensional space. The feature values of all of the images in database were calculated, and the feature was expressed as a vector in N dimensions.

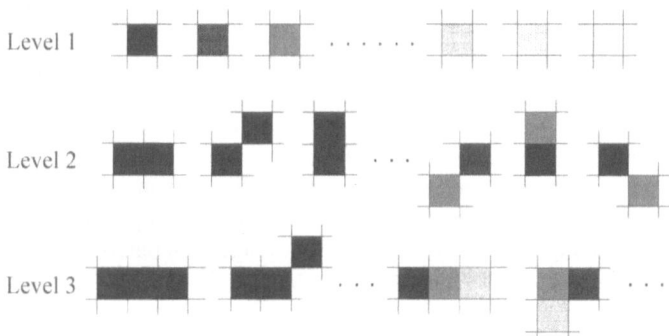

Fig. 2: Local pattern for feature extraction

2.3 Creation of the retrieval feature space using KL expansion

After storing the vector in each image, the KL expansion was used to decrease the number of dimension in feature space into from 4 to 10 axes to create the retrieval feature space that expressed effective feature values in retrieval using statistical character. The expanded feature vectors were newly stored to be retrieved. The accumulated rate of contribution of principal components becomes 90% or more was applied to reduction of the number of dimensions using KL expansion.

2.4 Calculation of the degree of similarity

To determine the similar image after the query one was given, the Euclid distance among the feature vectors measured on retrieval feature space evaluates the similarity between

CARS 2002 – H.U. Lemke, M.W. Vannier; K. Inamura, A.G. Farman, K. Doi & J.H.C. Reiber (Editors)

the query image and the others within the database. The nearest vector from the query image was employed as the retrieval result.

3. Simulation study

We evaluated the retrieval methods by using a database of 30 simulated patterns. Simulated-pattern group was based on handwriting and had 15-kind figure of two sheets each, and the same image did not exist within the data group. The feature vector based on local-pattern matching was determined after the preprocess, and the local patterns that consisted of up to 2 were employed for the definition of local patterns. That is, sixty-four kinds (8 at level 1, and 56 at level 2) of local patterns were defined to calculate the feature vectors.

KL expansion was performed to the extracted amount of the features, and the N-dimensional retrieval feature space was created from the 1st to Nth principal components of which the rate of accumulation contribution became 90%. One image in which the Euclid distance had the shortest feature in the retrieval feature space was determined the similar image about each image. As results of simulation study, it tended that the retrieved images were very similar to the query one in subjective opinions. The percentage of the correct answer was 77%.

4. Demonstration of similar image retrieval on mammographic masses

75 mass images digitized and clipped from mammogram taken by the screen/film system were used for similar image retrieval. Original digital data of the images had 4096 gray levels and 100-micrometer sampling pitch. To retrieval in a small-scale database, this quality of image might be too high. Therefore, the preprocess to changes gray level into 8 and resolution into 400 micrometers was performed for the mitigation of retrieval condition. The feature extraction based on local-pattern matching and KL expansion applied same procedure as the simulation study. One image was determined as a similar image to each image by the Euclid distance among the feature vectors measured on retrieval feature space.

5. Results

The retrieval results of the mammographic masses are shown in Fig. 3. The results indicated in the figure were chosen with degree of similar by subjective observation from 75 sets of retrieval results. The images of four sheets are a query image, a retrieved one, the sketch of the query image drawn by the physician, and the sketch of the retrieved image in an order from the left. Although there were many satisfied cases with the difference of density distribution between those images, there were a few results correspond to physician's opinion on the shape and the condition of margin of mass. The rate of coincidence was 29% on the shape, and was 34% on the margin.

CARS 2002 – H.U. Lemke, M.W. Vannier; K. Inamura, A.G. Farman, K. Doi & J.H.C. Reiber (Editors)

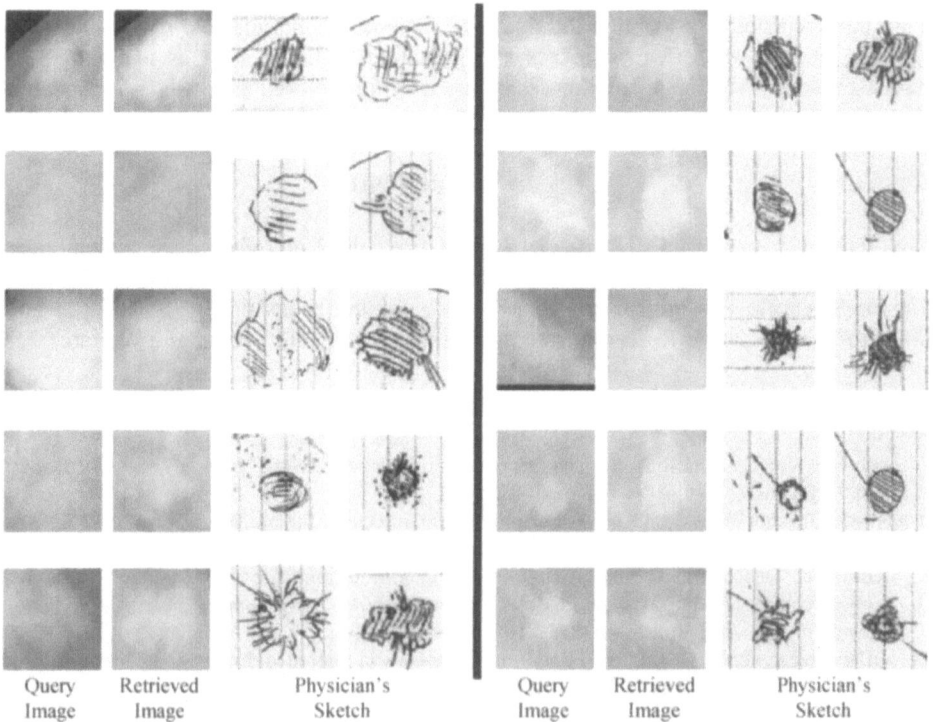

Fig. 3: 10 retrieval results of mammographic mass images. The images of four sheets are a query image, a retrieved one, the sketch of the query image drawn by the physician, and the sketch of the retrieved image in an order from the left.

6. Discussion

There was a difference in the classification of mass shade between retrieval results and physician's opinions. The reason of this was estimated that the signal-feature of an image is not in agreement with a physician's subjectivity measure. However, it can expect that the system to retrieve an image quantitatively by the degree of similar based on the feature analysis, and can reduce the variation in diagnosis of physicians, and it is estimated that it may be able to use as diagnostic support. Even when it was an inaccurate solution, the retrieved image has a similar impression in many cases. It is estimated that the feature vectors in the retrieval feature space were reflecting the shape of an object image well as this reason. The feature extracted by our method is shift-in-variant in the object position, but it depends on the density (pixel value) variance and the rotation of the images.

7. Conclusion

The retrieval technique based on local patterns existing in images was proposed. The degree of similarity was estimated by the difference among the Euclid distance of the feature vectors in the retrieval feature space created by KL expansion analysis. We confirmed the tendency that similar mass images were retrieved as the initial studies by

670

using the simulated patterns and the image of mammographic masses. It was concluded that our method was effective to retrieve gray-level patterns such as mammographic masses because image segmentation technique was not required and it did not depend on the accuracy of the determination of the margin.

Acknowledgements

This work was supported in parts by a grant from the Endo Saijirou commemorative foundation for the promotion of technology (KAI industries, Gifu, Japan), the Grant-In-Aid for Scientific Research from Japan Society for the Promotion of Science, and the Grant-In-Aid for Cancer Research from the Ministry of Health, Labour and Welfare.

References

1. Lee HK, Yoo SI, "Intelligent image retrieval using neural network", *IEICE Trans. Inf. & Syst.*, Vol. E84-D, No. 12, pp. 1810-1819, 2001.
2. Swets DL and Weng JJ, "Using discriminant eigenfeatures for image retrieval", *IEEE Trans. Pattern Analysis and Machine Intelligence*, Vol. 18, No. 8, pp. 831-836, 1996.
3. Kurita T, Otsu N and Sato T, "A face recognition method using highter order local autocorrelation and multivariate analysis", *Proc. of 11th International Conference of Pattern Recognition (ICPR)*, Vol. II, pp. 213-216, Hague, 1992.
4. Qi H and Snyder WE, "Content-based image retrieval in picture archiving and communications systems", *Journal of Digital Imaging*, Vol. 12, No. 2, Suppl 1, pp. 81-83, 1999.
5. Giger ML, Huo Z, Lan L and Vyborny CJ, "Intelligent search workstation for computer-aided diagnosis", *Proc. of the 14th International Symposium and Exhibition on Computer Assisted Radiology and Surgery (CARS2000)*, pp. 822-827, San Francisco, 2000.

CARS 2002 – H.U. Lemke, M.W. Vannier; K. Inamura, A.G. Farman, K. Doi & J.H.C. Reiber (Editors)

Segmentation of microcalcification in X-ray mammograms using entropy thresholding

Moti Melloul and Leo Joskowicz
School of Computer Science and Engineering
The Hebrew University of Jerusalem
Jerusalem 91904, ISRAEL
E-mail: moti@cs.huji.ac.il, josko@cs.huji.ac.il

Abstract

We describe a new algorithm for microcalcification segmentation in mammographic X-ray images. The algorithm detects microcalcifications in two steps. First, it removes background tissue with a multiscale morphological operation. Then, it applies entropy thresholding based on a 3-dimensional co-occurrence matrix. Unlike existing methods, ours is fully automatic, parameter-free, and independent of local statistics. To test its efficacy, we applied it to images from the Mammographic Image Analysis Society database and analyzed the results with the assistance of a clinician. We obtained detection rates of 93.75% of true positives, 6.25% of false positives, and 2% of false negatives.

Keywords: X-ray mammograms, microcalcification segmentation, entropy thresholding.

1. Introduction

Most early breast cancer can be diagnosed by detecting microcalcification clusters in mammographic X-ray images. The clusters appear as groups of small, bright particles with arbitrary shapes. Detecting microcalcifications is difficult because they are embedded in a non-homogeneous background. Many missed radiologist diagnoses can be attributed to human factors such as subjective or varying decision criteria, distraction by other image features, large number of images to be inspected, or simple oversight. Therefore, there is strong motivation to develop reliable and effective methods for automatic microcalcifications detection. While many methods for microcalcification segmentation have been developed in the past ten years, they either require manual thresholds adjustment or depend on local statistics to compute those thresholds. This paper presents a new fully automatic, parameter-free, and local statistics independent algorithm for microcalcification segmentation in mammographic X-ray images. For a detailed description of the method, see [1].

2. Previous work

Strickland and Hahn [2] describe a method that uses multiscale matched filters with wavelet transforms for enhancing and detecting calcifications. Nishikawa *et al* [3] use a difference technique to enhance microcalcifications. First, it extracts potential microcalcifications with global thresholding based on an erosion operator and local

CARS 2002 – H.U. Lemke, M.W. Vannier, K. Inamura, A.G. Farman, K. Doi & J.H.C. Reiber (Editors)

adaptive thresholding. False positives are then eliminated by texture analysis, and the remaining candidates are grouped with a non-linear clustering algorithm. Cheng *et al.* [3] propose a method based on fuzzy logic, which consists of image fuzzification, enhancement, irrelevant structure removal segmentation, and reconstruction. Chan *et al.* [4] investigate a convolution neural network based approach that is effective for reducing false positive detections. Nagel *et al.* [5] compare three feature analysis methods based on rules, artificial neural networks, and a combination of both. They report that the combined method performs best because each filter eliminates different types of false positives. McGarry and Deriche [6] use a hybrid model combining knowledge of mammographic imaging process and anatomical structure and Markov random fields. The drawbacks of these methods are that they either require manual adjustment of thresholds or depend on local statistics to compute the thresholds. This motivated our search for a parameter-free algorithm for threshold estimation.

3. Method

The algorithm detects microcalcifications in two steps. First, it removes background tissue with a multiscale morphological operation. Then, it applies entropy thresholding based on a third-order spatial gray-level dependence matrix.

Background tissue elimination is necessary to enhance the visibility and detectability of microcalcifications. We use a multiscale top hat morphological filtering to remove the slow rate of variation of the image intensity values and to enhance the image contrast. In morphology, filtering is performed using a kernel, and multi-scaling is performed by changing the size of the kernel. The top hat filter γ is a morphological opening operation. For a given image I, the multiscale top hat operator ρ removes objects whose size is larger than the given kernel size. The kernel is taken to vary from the smallest to the largest size of individual microcalcifications. The multiscale top hat equation is:

$$\rho_k(I) = I - \gamma_k(I)$$

where k is the kernel size.

The opening operation consists of erosion followed by dilation on a kernel that defines the size of the region over which pixel values are taken. Erosion replaces the pixel value at the center of the kernel by the minimum value of its neighborhood pixels, while dilation replaces it by the maximum value of its neighborhood pixels. The opened image is then subtracted from the original image. We use square kernels whose sizes vary between one and five pixels. For each scale, we obtain different filtered images with candidate microcalcifications.

To segment the resulting filtered images, we apply the following entropy-based thresholding method. First, we compute the spatial gray-level dependence matrix. This is a three-dimensional co-occurrence matrix T whose entries are the joint probabilities that pixel triplets' intensities (w_i, w_j, w_k) are in a rectangular region of width s and height h. The entries of the third-order entropy matrix of the image are then obtained by summing the pixel triplet probability times its logarithm over all regions of size sxh. We choose to use

CARS 2002 – H.U. Lemke, M.W. Vannier; K. Inamura, A.G. Farman, K. Doi & J.H.C. Reiber (Editors)
°CARS/Springer. All rights reserved.

the third-order space mean over the more commonly used second order matrix because our experiments indicated that higher order correlations improved the discrimination capabilities. The (i,j,k)th entry of the 3D co-occurrence matrix, denoted by T_{ijk}, is defined by:

$$T_{ijk} = \sum_{m=1}^{M} \sum_{n=1}^{N} \delta(m,n)$$

where

$$\delta(m,n) = \begin{cases} 1 \text{ if } I(m,n) = i \text{ and } I(m,n+1) = j \text{ and } I(m+1,n) = k \\ 0 \text{ otherwise} \end{cases}$$

Next, we partition the resulting matrix into two regions: the background information B, which appears in the upper left corner of the matrix, and the microcalcification information O, which appears in the rest of the matrix. Each region defines a distribution of the of gray-levels transitions. Then, we build for each region the probability P based on the distribution of the pixels transitions in the given region of the 3D co-occurrence matrix. By normalizing the total number of transitions in the given region of the co-occurrence matrix, we obtain the desired transition probability P.

$$P_{ijk} = \frac{T_{ijk}}{\sum_{i=0}^{L-1} \sum_{j=0}^{L-1} \sum_{k=0}^{L-1} T_{ijk}}$$

The size of the regions B and O is adjusted dynamically by changing the position of the boundary between the two regions. We compute the entropy of each region according to the boundary position. The boundary separating background and microcalcifications is the one that gives the maximum sum of the entropies. The optimal threshold is the one that maximizes the sum the entropies of the background and microcalcification regions defined by this boundary

Formally, let t be the threshold of the two groups the foreground and the background in the image. The background entropy $H_B(t)$ and the objects entropy $H_O(t)$ are computed on the volumes B and O. The entropies quantify the background-to-background transitions and objects-to-objects transitions. The image entropy is obtained by

$$H(t) = H_B(t) + H_O(t)$$

The optimal threshold is the value t that yields the maximum of the image entropies

$$T_{optimal} = \arg\max_t (H(t))$$

Then, we segment the filtered image according the optimal threshold. The fusion of the different scale segmented images produces the final mammogram segmentation.

CARS 2002 – H.U. Lemke, M.W. Vannier; K. Inamura, A.G. Farman, K. Doi & J.H.C. Reiber (Editors)
°CARS/Springer. All rights reserved.

674

4. Results

We applied the algorithm to a database consisting of a few dozen images from the Mammographic Image Analysis Society (MIAS) database and our own clinical images. We then performed a quantitative analysis of the results with the assistance of a radiologist. Images are of size *1024x1024* pixels with *8*-bit gray-values. We use a morphological multiscale top hat with 1x1 pixels to 5x5 pixels kernels for background filtering and applied entropy thresholding as described above to detect individual microcalcifications. The algorithm was able to detect subtle microcalcifications and its results were deemed highly accurate. The microcalcifications were then are grouped into clusters based on their proximity using the Cluster Affinity Search Technique. The intermediate steps of the algorithm are illustrated in Fig. 1 on a sample mammogram.

We obtained mean detection rates of *93.75%* of true positives, *6.25%* of false positives, and *2.0%* of false negatives (ranging from *0%* to *3.75%*). The results were evaluated and confirmed by a radiologist. These are considered very low false positive and false negative rates. We noted some variance depending on the size of the region of interest and the texture of the mammogram in the region. Running times on a Pentium III *700* MHz PC with *256*MB of main memory and no code optimization average *20* minutes per image. This was deemed acceptable based on the quality of the results.

To further evaluate our algorithm, we compared it to three state of the art algorithms. Yu and Guan [7] compute statistical features and report *90%* mean true positives at the cost of *0.5%* false positives per image. On our data set, our implementation of the algorithm produced *92%* mean true positives and *8%* false positives, which is significantly worse than our results. Its drawbacks are that it has many statistical features and parameters to adjust, and is very computation-intensive. Vilarras et al. [8] use morphological operations to remove noise background and report a true positives rate of only *85%* on the MIAS data set. Karssemeijer and Barke [9] apply a statistical method and report a mean of *93%* true positives for a cost of two false positives per image.

5. Conclusion

We have presented a new algorithm for microcalcification segmentation in mammographic X-ray images. The algorithm uses a multiscale morphological operation and entropy thresholding based on a three dimensional co-occurrence matrix. Unlike existing methods, ours is fully automatic, parameter-free, and independent of local statistics. We are currently applying our algorithm to a larger data set and investigating the causes for the small percentage of false positives and false negatives. To improve these results, we plan to perform an analysis of the extracted microcalcifications in the morphological and texture feature spaces.

675

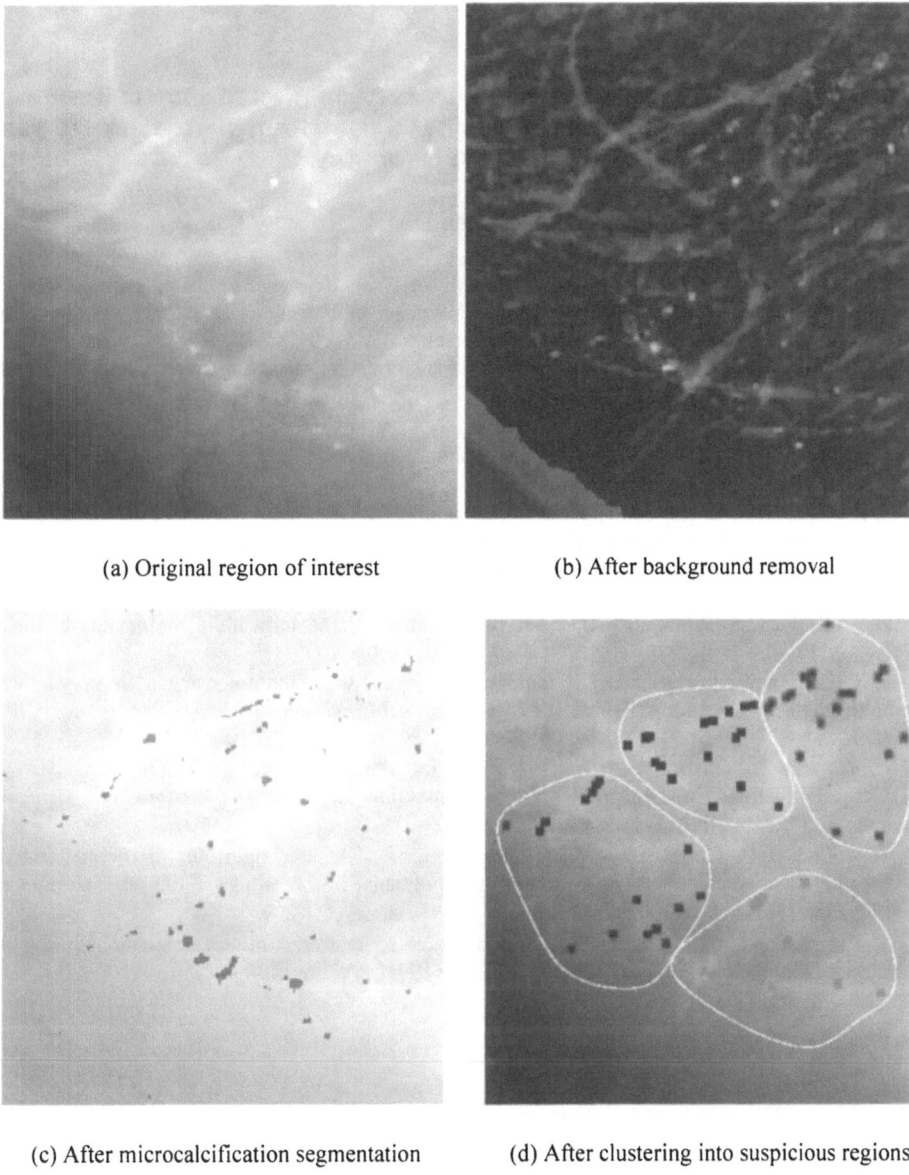

(a) Original region of interest (b) After background removal

(c) After microcalcification segmentation (d) After clustering into suspicious regions

Fig. 1: Illustration of the algorithm steps on a sample mammogram

Acknowledgments

This research was supported in part by a grant from the Israel Ministry of Trade and Industry under the IZMEL consortium on Image-Guided Therapy. We thank Dr. Miri Sclair for qualifying and quantifying the results of our analysis.

References

1. M. Melloul, *Segmentation of Microcalcifications in X-ray Mammograms using Entropy Based Thresholding*, Masters Thesis, The Hebrew University of Jerusalem, Dec. 2001. Available in http://www.cs.huji.ac.il/~josko/cas-publications.html

2. R.N. Strickland and H. I. Hahn, ``Wavelet transforms for detecting microcalcifications in mammograms'', *IEEE Transactions on Medical Imaging*, Vol. 15(2), pp. 218-229, April 1993.

3. H-D. Cheng, Y. M. Lui, and R. I. Freimanis, ``A novel approach to microcalcification detection using fuzzy logic technique'', IEEE Transactions on Medical Imaging, Vol. 17(3), pp. 442-450, June 1998.

4. H.-P. Chan, S.-C. B. Lo, B. Sahiner, K.L. Lam, and M.A. Helvie. ``Computer-aided detection of mammographic microcalcifications: Pattern recognition with an artificial neural network'', *Medical Physics*, Vol. 22(10), pp. 1555-1567, October 1995

5. R. H. Nagel, R. M. Nishikawa, J. Papaioannou, and K. Doi, "Analysis of methods for reducing false positives in automated detection of clustered microcalcifications in mammograms'', *Medical Physics*, Vol. 25(8), pp. 1502-1506, August 1998.

6. G.McGarry and M. Deriche, ``Mammographic image segmentation using a tissue-mixture model and Markov random fields'', *IEEE International Conference on Image Processing*, ICIP, 2000.

7. S. Yu and L. Guan , ``A CAD System for the Automatic Detection of Clustered Microcalcifications in Digitized Mammogram Films'', *IEEE Transactions on Medical Imaging*, 19(2) 115-126, February 2000.

8. A. Vilarrasa, V. Gimenez, D. Manrique, J. Rios , ``A new algorithm for computerized detection of microcalcifications in digital mammograms'', Proceedings of the Int. Conference on Computer-Aided Radiology and Surgery, CARS'98, pp. 224-229.

9. N. Karssemeijer and G.M. Barke, ``Recognition of clustered microcalcifications using a random field model'', *Proceedings of SPIE*, Vol. 1905, 1993, pp. 776-786.

CARS 2002 – H.U. Lemke, M.W. Vannier; K. Inamura, A.G. Farman, K. Doi & J.H.C. Reiber (Editors)

On the problem of breast compression modelling

Fredrik Georgsson[a], Niklas Björnestål[a]
[a] {fredrikg,nb}@cs.umu.se
Department of Computing Science, Umeå University
SE-901 87 Umeå, Sweden

Abstract

Simple models for breast compression are investigated and it is concluded that tissue movements in homogenous bodies is not uniform making it highly unlikely that tissue movements in breasts is uniform. By calculating the anatomical axis of rotation, it is concluded that the tissue tends to move in a direction between the true axis of rotation and perpendicular to the pectoralis muscle. This is verified by using the model to reconstruct three-dimensional points in the breast based on two-view mammography.

Keywords: Breast compression, mammography, Hough transform

1. Introduction

A mammogram is an x-ray image of a female breast. Like all x-ray images, the intensity in a point corresponds to the accumulated attenuation of the x-rays along a line through the image point and the x-ray foci, see Figure 1. In order to minimise the dosage for the woman and optimise the image quality the breast is compressed when the image is acquired. The effects of the compression makes it very hard to determine what points in the uncompressed breast that are projected onto a specific image point. If the tissue movement inside the breast while under compression could be modelled, it would be possible to calculate, for instance, three-dimensional coordinates based on the images taken from different angles. When combined with models for anatomical symmetry it would also allow for a sound approach to bilateral comparison of mammograms, one of the key issues in incorporating domain specific knowledge into computer aided judging of mammograms. In other words, it could be argued that breast compression modelling is one of the most important fields within modern mammographic image processing.

2. Methods

The heterogeneity of the female breast makes it hard to make accurate models for breast compression. In fact, little is known about how the tissue moves inside the breast as it is compressed. Novak [1] studied how hook wires and biopsy needles as well as how skin markers moved while compressing the breast. More recently Azar et. al [2] have modelled the breast using finite elements methods by studying the movements of cysts with MRI.

CARS 2002 – H.U. Lemke, M.W. Vannier; K. Inamura, A.G. Farman, K. Doi & J.H.C. Reiber (Editors)

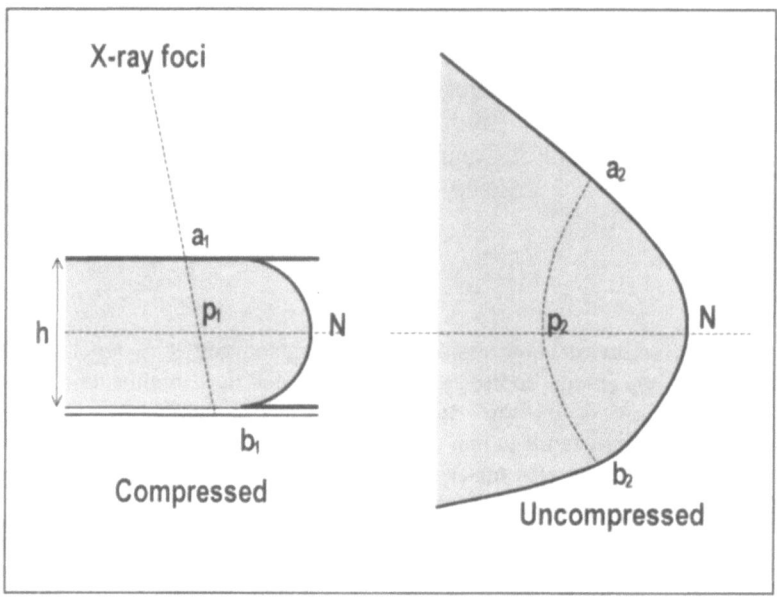

Figure 1. Geometrical modelling

2.1 Geometrical modelling

The first approach to breast compression modelling is to make simple geometrical assumptions, such as: the volume of the breast is constant, the skin does not move in relation to the compression paddles, the skin is elastic, the tissue can not move backwards past the pectoralis, and that all breast tissue have the same compression properties. Similar assumptions are found in [3]. Of the assumptions taken, the one of the homogeneity of the tissue is the least realistic since it is quite clear that the different tissue types in the breast have very different properties. Furthermore, the tissue types are connected anatomically to each other in a way that effects the movement. For instance, the glandular tissue is attached to the mamilla that in turn is attached to the skin. Since the skin is forced to bulge outwards during the compression the glandular tissue will follow. The effect of this is that the central part of the breast moves more outwards than one would first expect. Another anatomical issue to remember is that malignant tumours are connected with the surrounding tissue and this may cause it to move significantly and unpredictably. One conclusion regarding the geometrical approach is that we do not have the knowledge to model such a complex organ as the female breast but it still holds as a first approximation.

To verify the geometrical assumptions for homogeneous bodies a simple clay model were constructed. This clay model was a cylinder built of identical circular disks of clay. The disks were of different colours. The cylinder was then compressed radially between two plates to a specific thickness. Several identical cylinders were built and compressed to different thickness. Each compressed cylinder was then cut in half perpendicular to the compression plates, in other words the cylinder was cut sagitally. Since the cylinder was composed of different coloured layers of clay, it was possible to gain an understanding of how the movement depend on the distance to the compression plate see Figure 2 left.

CARS 2002 – H.U. Lemke, M.W. Vannier; K. Inamura, A.G. Farman, K. Doi & J.H.C. Reiber (Editors)
ᶜCARS/Springer. All rights reserved.

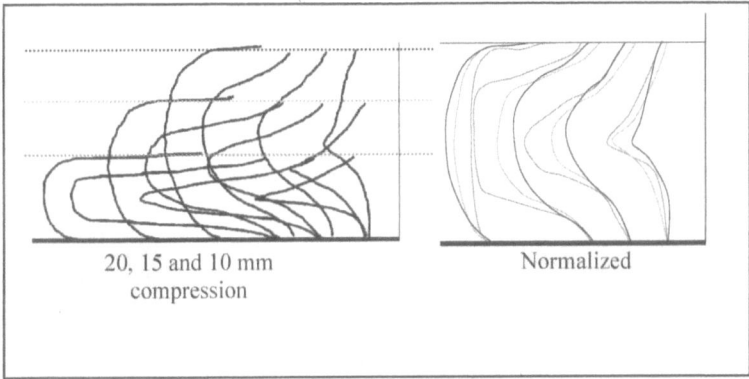

Figure 2. Sagital movements

Another clay model was constructed to investigate whether or not the 'tissue' radiate outwards at compression. This model was constructed by using small clay bricks of different colour to build a cube that was compressed to a specific thickness and then cut in half. This time the clay model was cut in a transversal manner. As in the previous case, several identical cubes were built and compressed to different thickness to gain an understanding of the 'tissue' movement as a function of compression.

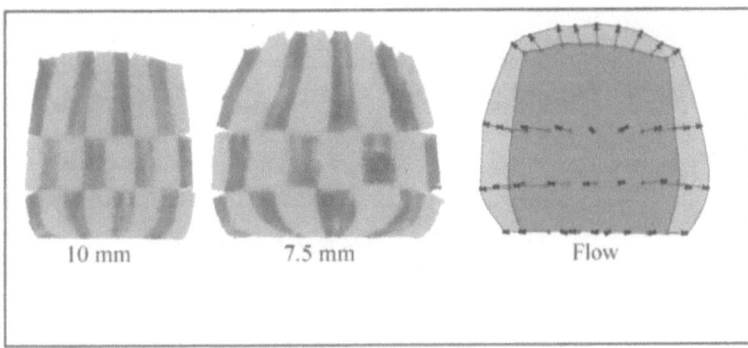

Figure 3. Transversal movements

3. Anatomical markers

Some insight to how breast tissue actually moves is to study two projections of the same breast. If some kind of markers could be introduced in the breast, it would be possible to observe how these markers are projected and use this knowledge to build a compression model. It turns out that calcifications are excellent markers since they occur naturally in the breast, they are easy to locate, they are well defined, and unlike hook wires and biopsy needles they do not have an influence in how the surrounding tissue moves.

CARS 2002 – H.U. Lemke, M.W. Vannier; K. Inamura, A.G. Farman, K. Doi & J.H.C. Reiber (Editors)

680

3.1 The direction of distance preservation

Given a pair of images of the same breast but taken from different projections and asked to mark the same calcification in both views an expert radiologist measured the distance from the nipple perpendicular to the pectoralis muscle and used this as a view invariant measurement. If the direction of distance preservation could be established it would give some information on the tissue movement in the breast. Since the images are acquired from different angles, it would be expected that only distances in the direction that is

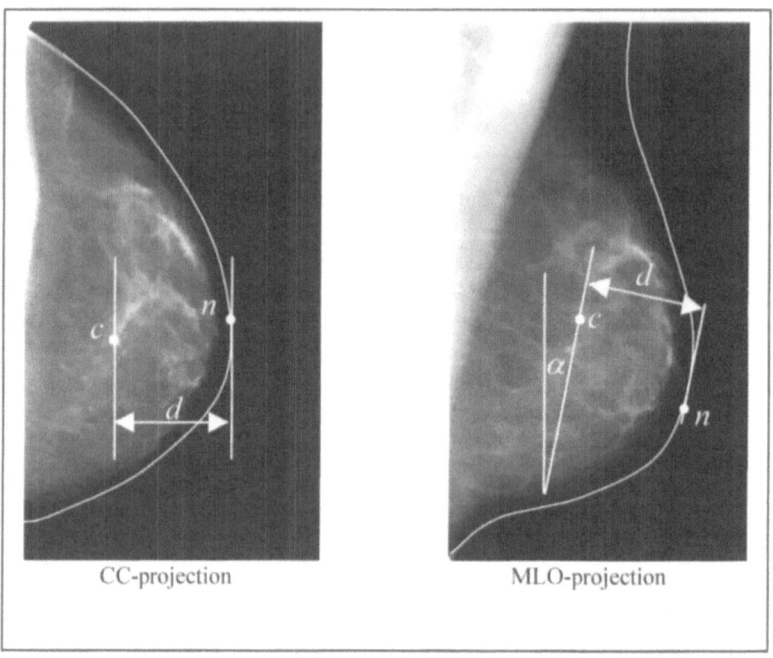

CC-projection   MLO-projection

Figure 4. Direction of preserved distances

perpendicular to the rotation axis would be preserved. Of course, the axis of rotation is well known in the case of mammography, since it is fixed with the x-ray machine.

However, if this were the true anatomical axis of rotation the distance measured along the coordinate fixed to the image frame would be preserved. This is because the image frame is fixed in relation to the x-ray machine. The observation of how the radiologist measured the distance indicates that the anatomical axis of rotation, that is the combination of the geometrical axis of rotation and the effect of the compression of the breast, is not aligned with the image frame.

To find this anatomical axis of rotation we used images from the Digital Database for Screening Mammography, University of South Florida. Only images showing calcifications in two views (CC and MLO) were used. The CC-image was used as a reference and the distance from the calcification c to the nipple n along the coordinate system of the image, i.e. perpendicular to the chest wall, was measured, see Figure 4. We

CARS 2002 – H.U. Lemke, M.W. Vannier; K. Inamura, A.G. Farman, K. Doi & J.H.C. Reiber (Editors)

call this distance *d*. Then it was calculated in which direction in the MLO image this distance was preserved. This was done by plotting the two points, the calcification and the nipple, as points and then calculating the Hough transform of these points. The Hough transform of a point is a sine curve and consequently two sine curves were obtained for each pair of points. To find the angle α that gives a distance *d* between the points we only have to find the angles were the distance between the sine waves are *d*. There will be two of these distances symmetrically distributed around the point were the sine waves intersect. The angle of intersection of the sine waves corresponds to the angle of a straight line from the two points.

3.2 Verification of model

A problem with a breast compression model is how to evaluate it. As stated earlier very little is known about the tissue movements, so there is no easy accessible way to verify the model. However, it is possible to evaluate models by using it to reconstruct the three-dimensional curve of points that are projected onto a specific image point [4]. If a point is visible in two projections taken at the same time the distance at some point between two curves should be small, even zero, if the compression is modelled correctly. Of course, the point where the curves intersect corresponds to the three-dimensional coordinate of the projected point.

4. Results

4.1 Clay-model

The results of the clay models were the following. To investigate whether of not the sagital movement could be modelled as being the same in the entire 'breast' the line separating each layer of clay was approximated by a spline and all splines associated with a specific compression thickness was normalised by using only using scaling and translation. If the movement were uniform in the entire breast, all splines associated with a specific height in the breast would align after normalisation. This was not the case as seen in Figure 2, right. Near the compression plates, the movement can be assumed uniform but closer to the centre of the 'breast' the movement is larger, relatively speaking, for larger compression. The result was consistent for all heights except for the skin-air interface where larger compression implies smaller relative movements. Why this is, we do not know.

In the case of the transversal model, it was clearly seen that homogenous tissue radiates perpendicular to the surface. The amount of movement seems to be linearly dependent on the distance to the central line of the model.

4.2 Direction of anatomical rotational axis

The direction of distance preservation was measured in 45 cases of calcifications from 38 different breasts with the following result. It was shown that the angle of the anatomical rotational axis was 7.4 degrees below the x-axis in the MLO-image. The standard deviation was 16.7 degrees.

CARS 2002 – H.U. Lemke, M.W. Vannier; K. Inamura, A.G. Farman, K. Doi & J.H.C. Reiber (Editors)
ᶜCARS/Springer. All rights reserved.

5. Conclusions

5.1 Clay-model
The clay models are, of course, very simplified models of the real breast. Mostly they differ in the fact that the clay is homogenous and the breast is not. Furthermore, the present clay models do not have the connective properties as real tissue has. Still, many of the characteristics of the clay model are expected to be present in the movement of the real breast tissue.

5.2 Direction of anatomical rotational axis
It seems that the direction of the anatomical rotational axis is somewhere between that of the geometrical axis of rotation and the direction of the normal of the pectoralis muscle, as seen in the MLO projection. This indicates that the direction of tissue movement tend to be in the direction of the normal to the pectoralis plane.

5.3 Model verification
The experiences from the clay models and the direction of the anatomical rotational axis were combined and verified by calculating the distances between the three-dimensional curves as described above. In this implementation, we used the simplified assumption from the experience with the clay model that the movement is uniform in the entire breast. We also investigated two different sagital movements: perpendicular to the pectoralis and radiating outwards from a central line. The results was that to use the direction perpendicular to the pectoralis yielded an average error of 0.75 cm while assuming radiating sagital movement yielded an error of 1.05 cm. The results are based on 6 calcifications from 4 breasts.

These preliminary results are consistent with the direction of the anatomical rotational axis.

Acknowledgements

The authors are grateful to radiologist Stina Carlson at the Mammographic Unit at the University Hospital of Northern Sweden.

References

1. R. Novak, *Transformation of the female breast during compression at mammography with special reference to the importance for localization of a lesion*, Ph.D.-thesis, Stockholm, 1988
2. F.S. Azar, D.N. Metaxa and M.D. Schnall, "Methods for Modelling and Predicting Mechanical Deformations of the Breast under External Perturbations", *Medical Image Analysis*, 6, 1-27, 2002
3. M. Yam, M. Brady, R. Highnam, C. Behrenbruch, R. English, and Y. Kita, "Three-Dimensional Reconstruction of Microcalcification Clusters from Two Mammographic Views", *IEEE Transactions on Medical Imaging*, 20, 479-489, 2001
4. F. Georgsson, "Multi View Three Dimensional Reconstructions of Points in Mammograms", Proceedings of SSAB, pp. 41-44, 2001

Special Session on Thoracic CAD

CARS 2002 – H.U. Lemke, M.W. Vannier, K. Inamura, A.G. Farman, K. Doi & J.H.C. Reiber (Editors)

Automatic segmentation and texture analysis of PA chest radiographs to detect abnormalities related to interstitial disease and tuberculosis

Bram van Ginneken[a], Bart M. ter Haar Romeny[b], Max A. Viergever[a]

[a] Image Sciences Institute, University Medical Center Utrecht,
Utrecht, The Netherlands

[b] Faculty of Biomedical Engineering, Medical and Biomedical Imaging,
Eindhoven University of Technology, Eindhoven, The Netherlands

Abstract

We present an automatic system for detecting diffuse abnormalities in chest radiographs. The system starts with segmentation, subdivides the lung fields in smaller, overlapping regions and extract texture features from each ROI. Using these features, the probability that each ROI contains abnormalities is estimated with a k-nearest-neighbour classifier. The classification of all regions is pooled into an overall abnormality indicator. Evaluation on databases containing cases of interstitial disease and tuberculosis shows promising results. Directions for further research are briefly discussed.

Keywords: Computer-aided diagnosis, chest radiography, texture analysis

1. Introduction

Around thirty percent of all radiological examinations are conventional chest radiographs. Given this huge number of studies, and the fact that they may contain extremely subtle abnormalities, it is not surprising that computer-aided diagnosis (CAD) in chest radiography is an active research area with serious potential for clinical applications [1]. We are developing a system for CAD in chest radiographs. It currently focuses on the detection of interstitial abnormalities, and could be used in tuberculosis screening.

Broadly speaking, abnormal signs in chest images can be subdivided in two categories: signs independent of location, and those signs whose appearance depends on their location in the lung field. Lung nodules are an example of the former, and most existing algorithms for lung nodule detection perform an analysis independent of the location of a candidate lesion. Diffuse abnormalities that characterize interstitial disease are examples of the latter. Consequently, algorithms to detect such signs can benefit from a specific analysis for each lung region.

CARS 2002 – H.U. Lemke, M.W. Vannier; K. Inamura, A.G. Farman, K. Doi & J.H.C. Reiber (Editors)

2. Methodology

2.1 Algorithm outline

In order to perform a regional analysis of chest images, we propose the following multi-stage approach. The first step is an automatic segmentation of both lung fields. Subsequently, the lung fields are divided into smaller regions of interest (ROIs). Each region is searched for abnormal signs. Because we focus on diffuse abnormalities, we perform texture analysis and extract a set of features from each ROI. In an off-line stage, the results for each region on images with known locations of abnormalities are used to construct a training set of reference cases. In the on-line analysis, a statistical classifier estimates the likelihood that a specific ROI is abnormal. The system could stop here and present the possibly abnormal regions to a radiologist. Optionally, the results of all regions can be pooled in a final stage into a single score for the complete image.

2.2 Segmentation

Currently we employ a modified version [2] of Active Shape Models [3] to extract the lung fields from a chest radiograph. This method is very robust and trainable, making it easy to adjust it to other databases with different image characteristics. The segmentation result is generally sufficiently accurate for our purposes.

2.3 Subdividing the lung fields

Each lung fields is divided into an upper, middle and lower part (6 regions). Each region is subdivided into a medial and lateral part (12 region), each of which is finally divided into an upper and lower part again (24 regions). Thus the total number of - overlapping - regions is 42. The exact subdivision used is not critical. The notion of overlapping regions is important though, it may allow detection of both small and large abnormal regions. Alternatively, a subdivision into costal and intercostal space could be beneficial, but would require an accurate algorithm for delineating the rib cage.

2.4 Texture feature extraction

A filter-bank texture analysis method that extracts multi-scale texture features from local histograms is used (see e.g. [4]). The set of filters is given by the Gaussian and its derivatives up to second order, at multiple scales. The histogram per region of the filtered image is computed, from which the first four moments are extracted. Density features are added and the difference between corresponding regions in the left and right lung field is used to construct additional 'difference' features, in order to mimic right-left comparisons as they are made routinely by radiologists.

2.5 Region classification

The features are each scaled to zero mean and unit variance. A simple k-nearest neighbour classifier is used to estimate the probability that a region is abnormal. Different sets of features (different scales, different moments, whether or not to include the difference features, etc.) have been tested on several databases. A selection of features for each region separately could be employed, but the size of our databases is currently rather small (for some regions the number of features is much larger that the number of abnormal cases), therefore we currently do not perform feature selection.

2.6 Region pooling

For each region, the performance of the system can be measured in terms of A_z, the area under the ROC curve. Using A_z, we perform a weighted average of all regions to arrive at a final abnormality score of the complete image. The exact way in which the weighting is implemented is ad hoc, but turns out to have little effect on the overall performance of the system. The weighting procedure ensures that regions for which no reliable estimate can be made have only a small influence on the total abnormality estimate.

3. Results

We show results of the system on two databases. The first database, referred to as the TB database, contains 279 abnormal and 290 normal posterior-anterior (PA) chest radiographs collected from a tuberculosis screening program for people seeking political asylum in The Netherlands [5]. The second database, the ID database, contains 100 normal and 100 abnormal PA chest radiographs with interstitial disease obtained at the University of Chicago Hospitals [6].

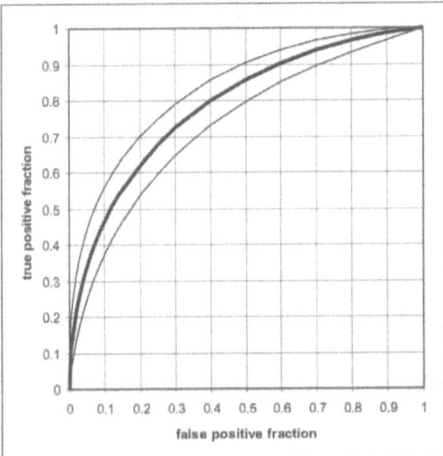 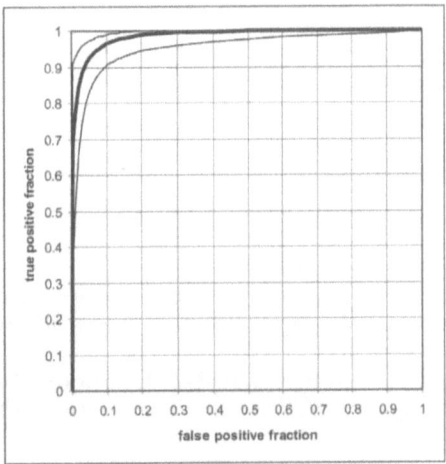

Fig. 1: ROC curves for both databases. The thin lines below and above the curve denote the asymmetric 95% confidence intervals. (Left) The TB database. The area under the curve is 0.820. (Right) The ID database. The area under the curve is 0.986.

Figure 1 shows ROC curves. For the ID database, the results are near perfect. The TB database contained many subtle abnormalities, which are not easily detected by the system. Furthermore, the abnormal areas were often small (in the order of a few percent of the area of a single lung field) and since the system averages the results over all regions, it is not very sensitive to small abnormalities.

CARS 2002 – H.U. Lemke, M.W. Vannier; K. Inamura, A.G. Farman, K. Doi & J.H.C. Reiber (Editors)

4. Discussion

The use of the system has not yet been evaluated in clinical practice. There are several ways in which such a system could be used in practice: (a) As a stand-alone filtering stage in which each image in a mass chest screening is processed and only sent to a radiologist if it is possibly abnormal; (b) As a computer-aided diagnosis module that the radiologist can use as a second opinion; (c) To highlight possibly abnormal areas during reading; (d) To retrieve images with similar textural appearance in abnormal regions as reference cases. This enumeration is by no means exhaustive.

To make the system more powerful, it should be trained with substantially larger database. This may allow it to catch more subtle abnormal sign that occur over small areas only. A range of improvements and extensions could be integrated into the system. Current research areas are (a) Integration of previous chest radiographs using temporal subtraction techniques; (b) Integrating clinical information (patient history) into the classification stage; (c) Include a dedicated algorithm for the detection of lung nodules and dense infiltrates, for which texture analysis is not the most suitable approach; (d) Detection of the rib cage, the heart and the clavicles prior to analysis; (e) Including shape analysis of segmented objects in the images – abnormalities such as blunting of the costophrenic angle can be handled in this way .

References

1. B. van Ginneken, B.M. ter Haar Romeny, M.A. Viergever, "Computer-aided diagnosis in chest radiography: a survey", *IEEE Trans. on Medical Imaging*, 20(12):1228-1241, 2001.
2. B. van Ginneken, A.F. Frangi, J.J. Staal, B.M. ter Haar Romeny, M.A. Viergever, "A non-linear gray-level appearance model improves active shape model segmentation", in *IEEE Workshop on Mathematical Models in Biomedical Image Analysis (MMBIA 2001)*, pp. 205-212.
3. T.F. Cootes, C.J. Taylor, D. Cooper, J. Graham, "Active shape models - their training and application", Computer Vision and Image Understanding, 61(1):38-59, 1995.
4. M. Unser. and M. Eden, "Multi-resolution feature extraction and selection for texture segmentation", *IEEE Trans. on Pattern Analysis and Machine Intelligence*, 11(7):717-728, 1989.
5. B. van Ginneken, S. Katsuragawa, B.M. ter Haar Romeny, K. Doi, M.A. Viergever, "Automatic detection of abnormalaties in chest radiographs using local texture analysis", *IEEE Trans. on Medical Imaging*, 21(2), to appear, 2002.
6. T. Ishida, S. Katsuragawa, K. Ashizawa, H. MacMahon, K.Doi, "Application of artificial neural networks for quantitative analysis of image data in chest radiographs for detection of interstitial lung disease", *Journal of Digital Imaging*, 11(4):182-192, 1998.

CARS 2002 – H.U. Lemke, M.W. Vannier; K. Inamura, A.G. Farman, K. Doi & J.H.C. Reiber (Editors)

Clinical usefulness of temporal subtraction technique for detection of interval changes on digital chest radiographs

S. Katsuragawa[a], T. Uozumi[b], S. Kakeda[b], H. Watanabe[b], H. Nakata[b], K. Doi[c]

[a] General Research Centre, Nippon Bunri University,
1727 Ichigi, Oita, 870-0397, Japan

[b] Department of Radiology, University of Occupational and Environmental Health,
1-1 Iseigaoka, Yahatanishi-ku, Kitakyusyu, 807-8555, Japan

[c] Department of Radiology, The University of Chicago
5841 South Maryland Avenue, Chicago, Illinois 60637, USA

Abstract

The temporal subtraction image which is obtained by subtracting a previous chest radiograph from a current one, can enhance interval changes considerably. In this article, we provide an overview of the scheme and the clinical usefulness of the temporal subtraction technique for the detection of interval changes on digital chest radiographs. Observer performance studies with ROC analyses clearly indicated that the radiologists' detection accuracy of pulmonary nodules was significantly improved when the temporal subtraction images were used. In addition, the temporal subtraction technique was applied to screening chest radiography with a mobile computed radiography system for a mass survey of lung cancer. Our result indicates that the lung cancer, which was not detected with current and previous images alone, was correctly detected by using the temporal subtraction image in the lung cancer screening program. Therefore, we strongly believe that the temporal subtraction technique is clinically useful for radiologists to detect interval changes in digital chest radiographs.

Keywords: Temporal subtraction, chest radiography, computer-aided diagnosis

1. Introduction

The evaluation of interval changes between temporally sequential chest radiographs is necessary for the detection of new abnormalities or for follow-up of changes in known abnormalities, such as pulmonary nodules and interstitial diseases. However, it is difficult for radiologists to detect subtle interval changes when the lesions are low contrast and/or overlap with ribs and large pulmonary vessels. Therefore, we have been developing a fully automated temporal subtraction technique based on a nonlinear image warping to assist radiologists in detection of interval changes in digital chest radiographs [1, 3, 4]. The temporal subtraction image which is obtained by subtraction of a previous image from a current image of the same patient can enhance interval changes [2]. In this article, we provide an overview of the scheme and the clinical usefulness of the temporal subtraction technique for the detection of interval changes in digital chest radiographs. In addition, an application of the temporal subtraction scheme to screening chest radiography with a mobile computed-radiography (CR) system for a mass survey of lung cancer was described.

2. Temporal subtraction technique

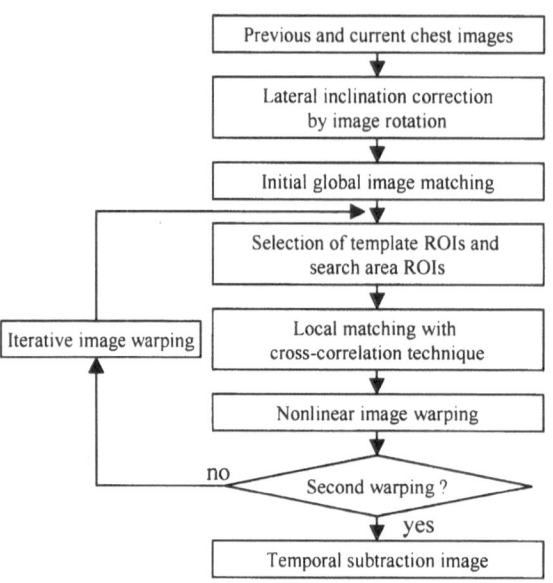

Figure 1. Overall scheme of temporal subtraction technique.

The overall scheme of the temporal subtraction technique is shown in Fig. 1. First, the matrix size of the previous and the current chest radiographs is reduced to 586 x 586 by subsampling. Then each image is segmented into lung fields, mediastinum and diaphragm by detection of ribcage edges, cardiac boundaries and diaphragm boundaries. This image segmentation is based on analysis of image profile. The lateral inclination caused by variation in patient positioning between the previous and the current images is corrected by an image rotation technique based on the midline determined from the ribcage edges. For initial global matching, the previous image is shifted in two orthogonal directions to match the current image by use of a cross-correlation between the two blurred low-resolution images [3].

For detailed local matching, approximately 300 template regions of interest (ROIs) with a 32 x 32 matrix size and the corresponding search area ROIs with a 64 x 64 matrix size are selected automatically in the lung fields and the mediastinum on the current and the previous images, respectively. The local shift vectors, which indicate the shifts in locations for all pairs of selected ROIs, are determined by use of the cross-correlation technique for finding the best-matched areas in the search area ROIs [1]. The local shift vectors for each pixel in the previous image are obtained from a two-dimensional surface fitting with a polynomial function. The previous image is nonlinearly warped according to the local shift vectors. For further reduction of misregistration artifacts in the subtraction image, the local image matching and the image warping are performed again for the first warped previous image and the current image [4]. Finally, the subtraction image is obtained by subtraction of the second warped previous image from the current image as shown in Fig. 2. This method is called an iterative image-warping technique.

CARS 2002 – H.U. Lemke, M.W. Vannier; K. Inamura, A.G. Farman, K. Doi & J.H.C. Reiber (Editors)

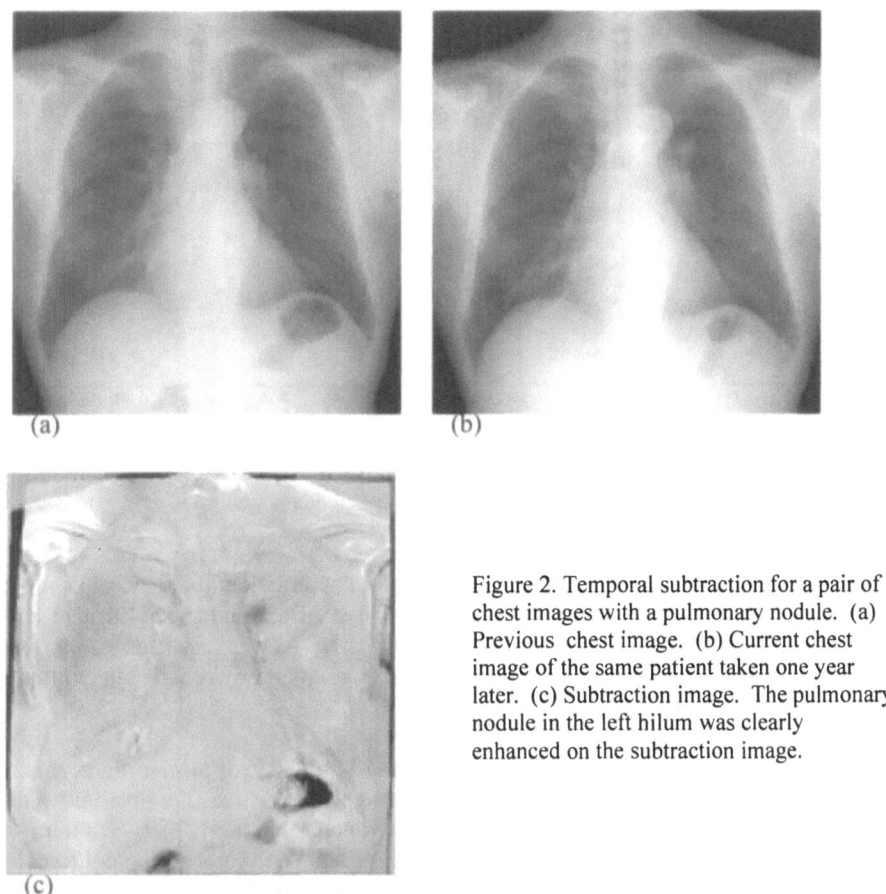

Figure 2. Temporal subtraction for a pair of chest images with a pulmonary nodule. (a) Previous chest image. (b) Current chest image of the same patient taken one year later. (c) Subtraction image. The pulmonary nodule in the left hilum was clearly enhanced on the subtraction image.

3. Observer performance studies

In order to evaluate the usefulness of the temporal subtraction images in radiologists' diagnoses of lung nodules, we performed two observer performance studies; one for the detection of nodules of primary lung cancer and various benign diseases [5], and another for the detection of metastatic lung nodules [6]. All chest radiographs used in the observer performance studies were obtained with a computed radiography (CR) system. In the first observer performance study, 20 cases with solitary lung nodules less than 30 mm in diameter, including 10 lung cancers and 10 benign nodules were used as nodule cases. For non-nodular cases, 20 cases without interval changes were selected. Eight radiologists including four attendings and four residents participated as observers in this study. In the second observer performance study, 21 cases with metastatic lung nodules and 21 cases without nodules were employed, and eleven radiologists including three attendings and eight residents participated as observers. In both observer performance studies, radiologists' confidence level regarding presence or absence of a lung nodule was marked on a continuous rating scale with a line-checking method. The current and previous radiographs were first shown for conventional interpretation, and the radiologist

692

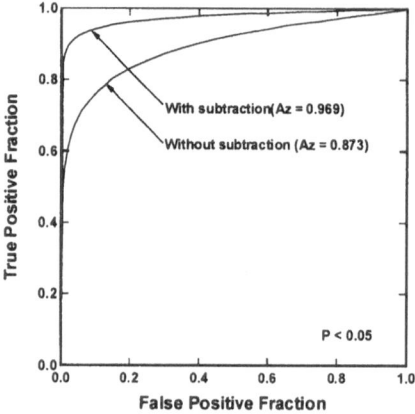

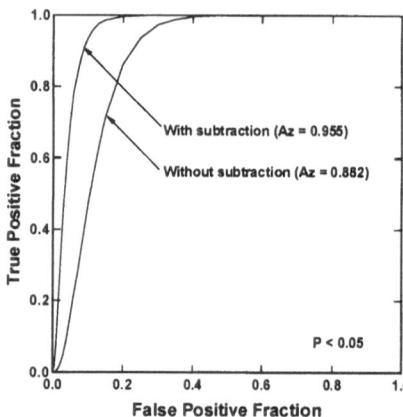

Figure 3. ROC curves for detection of nodules of primary lung cancer and various benign diseases.

Figure 4. ROC curves for detection of metastatic lung nodules.

marked his or her confidence level. Then, the temporal subtraction image was displayed on a CRT monitor additionally, and the radiologist marked his or her confidence level again, if different from the first confidence level. ROC analyses were used for comparison of the observer performance for the detection of lung nodules without and with the temporal subtraction images.

From the observer performance study for the detection of nodules of primary lung cancer and various benign diseases, it was found that the average Az value (the area under the ROC curve) for eight radiologists was significantly increased from 0.873 without, to 0.969 with the temporal subtraction images ($P < 0.05$) as shown in Fig. 3. In addition, the average Az value for the eleven radiologists for detection of metastatic lung nodules was also significantly increased from 0.882 to 0.955 ($P < 0.05$) as shown in Fig. 4. Therefore, these results of observer performance studies indicated that the detection accuracy of lung nodules was significantly improved, when the temporal subtraction images were employed.

4. Application of temporal subtraction to screening chest radiography

Since 1997, we have been performing a screening chest radiography for a mass survey of lung cancers in eight communities in Iwate Prefecture, Japan by using a trailer with a CR system and a digital archive system [7]. Approximately 10,000 digital chest radiographs per year were taken with a 1760 x 1760 matrix size and a 10-bits gray scale during the past five years. The previous, current and subtraction images were displayed on two CRT monitors for radiologists' interpretation.

For 4173 examinations performed from May 1999 to July 1999, we investigated the effect of temporal subtraction images on radiologists' diagnostic decision. In this period, radiologists read current and previous images alone first; then the subtraction images were

CARS 2002 – H.U. Lemke, M.W. Vannier; K. Inamura, A.G. Farman, K. Doi & J.H.C. Reiber (Editors)
ⓒCARS/Springer. All rights reserved.

Table 1. Effect of temporal subtraction images on radiologists' diagnostic decision in the lung cancer screening program.

		current, previous and subtraction images	
		normals and others*	suspicious lung cancer
current and previous images alone	normals and others*	4058	80
	suspicious lung cancer	9	26

*include benign abnormality and lung disease except for lung cancer.

interpreted, together with all other images. Only those cases for which the radiologists' diagnostic decision was altered in the second reading were recorded.

Table 1 shows the effect of temporal subtraction images on radiologists' diagnostic decision in the lung cancer screening program. Note that the diagnostic decision of 80 cases was altered from normals and others to suspicious lung cancer by using the temporal subtraction images. The lung cancer was confirmed for one case out of the 80 cases by an advanced CT examination and an operation. Therefore, our result indicates that the temporal subtraction images may be useful in the lung cancer screening program.

5. Conclusion

We have developed the temporal subtraction technique based on nonlinear image warping for detection of interval changes in digital chest radiographs. The radiologists' detection accuracy of lung nodules was significantly improved when the temporal subtraction images were used. In addition, the lung cancer, which was not detected with current and previous images alone, was correctly detected by using the temporal subtraction image in the lung cancer screening program. Therefore, we strongly believe that the temporal subtraction technique is clinically useful for radiologists to detect interval changes in chest radiographs.

Acknowledgements

This work was supported by USPHS grants CA62625 and CA64370. S. Katsuragawa and K. Doi are shareholders of R2 Technology, Inc., Los Altos, CA, and K. Doi is a shareholder of Deus Technologies, Inc., Rockville, MD. It is the policy of the University of Chicago that investigators disclose publicly actual or potential significant financial interests that may appear to be affected by research activities.

References

1. Kano A, Doi K, MacMahon H, Hassell DD, and Giger ML: Digital image subtraction of temporally sequential chest images for detection of interval change. Med Phys, 21:453-461, 1994.

CARS 2002 – H.U. Lemke, M.W. Vannier; K. Inamura, A.G. Farman, K. Doi & J.H.C. Reiber (Editors)

2. Difazio MC, MacMahon H, Xu XW, Tsai P, Shiraishi J, Armato III SG, and Doi K: Digital chest radiography: effect of temporal subtraction images on detection accuracy. Radiology **202**:447-452, 1997.

3. Ishida T, Ashizawa K, Engelmann R, Katsuragawa S, MacMahon H, and Doi K: Application of temporal subtraction for detection of interval changes on chest radiographs: Improvement of subtraction images using automated initial image matching. J Digtal Imag, **12**: 77-86, 1999.

4. Ishida T, Katsuragawa S, Nakamura K, MacMahon H, and Doi K: Iterative image warping technique for temporal subtraction of sequential chest radiographs to detect interval change. Med Phys **26**: 1320-1329, 1999.

5. Kakeda S, Nakamura K, Kamada K, Watanabe H, Nakata H, Katsuragawa S, and Doi K: Improved detection of lung nodules with temporal subtraction technique. Radiology (in press).

6. Uozumi T, Nakamura K, Watanabe H, Nakata H, Katsuragawa S, and Doi K : ROC Analysis of detection of metastatic pulmonary nodules on digital chest radiographs with temporal subtraction. Acad Radiol **8**: 871 - 878, 2001.

7. Katsuragawa S, Sasaki Y, MacMahon H, Ishida T, and Doi K: Application of temporal subtraction to screening chest radiographs with a mobile computed radiography system. Computer-Aided Diagnosis in Medical Imaging, Elsevier, Amsterdam, 51-56, 1999.

CARS 2002 – H.U. Lemke, M.W. Vannier; K. Inamura, A.G. Farman, K. Doi & J.H.C. Reiber (Editors)

Update on the development of an automated lung nodule detection method for CT scans

S. G. Armato III

Department of Radiology, The University of Chicago, MC 2026,
5841 S. Maryland Ave, Chicago, Illinois 60637, USA

Abstract

The expanded use of thoracic computed tomography (CT) for diagnostic purposes and as a screening tool, combined with the increased number of sectional images generated by each CT scan, has resulted in a rapid increase in the amount of image data that must be interpreted by radiologists. Automated, computerized analyses of these images could serve as a valuable aid to radiologists and complement their medical decision-making process. One such computerized analysis technique we have been developing is automated lung nodule detection, which has demonstrated promising performance in its ability to detect nodules in both diagnostic and low-dose screening CT scans. The process begins with the creation of a segmented lung volume. Multiple gray-level thresholds are applied so that three-dimensionally contiguous structures "dissolve" into multiple smaller structures at increasing gray-level thresholds. A volume criterion is used to qualify structures as nodule candidates. Features computed for each candidate are used as input to classifiers that categorize candidates as "nodule" or "non-nodule." Detection results may then be displayed through a computer interface for radiologist assessment. The method has been applied to several databases of diagnostic and low-dose CT scans.

Keywords: Computer-aided diagnosis (CAD), image processing, computed tomography

1. Introduction

Computed tomography (CT) of the thorax has earned an expanded role as a diagnostic imaging modality and as a viable screening tool. Perhaps impelled by the greater use of CT scans worldwide, CT technology has advanced significantly over the past decade, with scanners generating a greatly increased number of images for each examination. The net result of these two factors—an expanded role for CT and the acquisition of more sectional images per scan—has been a rapid increase in the amount of image data that must be interpreted by radiologists. Automated analyses of these CT scans could become a valuable aid to radiologists as a computerized "second opinion." One such automated analysis application that has been explored at The University of Chicago is automated lung nodule detection. The automated lung nodule detection method we have developed has demonstrated promising performance in its ability to detect nodules in both diagnostic CT scans and low-dose CT scans acquired as part of a lung cancer screening program.

A number of investigators have reported progress in the development of automated methods for lung nodule detection in CT based on a wide range of image processing and computer vision techniques [1-13]. In particular, the methods that have been and continue to be developed at The University of Chicago have undergone an evolution of approach and application [1,14-17,10,18]. These methods have developed from the analysis of individual CT sections (and immediately adjacent sections) combined with a rule-based approach for nodule detection [1] to the analysis of three-dimensionally contiguous structures within the lung volume combined with linear discriminant analysis for nodule detection [10]. Moreover, these methods have been applied to several databases of CT scans, including (1) diagnostic scans with contiguous reconstruction of image data acquired with 10-mm collimation [10] and image data acquired with 7-mm collimation with a 5-mm reconstruction interval and (2) low-dose scans with contiguous reconstruction of image data acquired with 5-mm collimation [17] and with 10-mm collimation [18]. The methods have demonstrated a robustness with regard to these different CT databases, and overall performance measures continue to show improvement.

2. Methodology

The automated lung nodule detection method is depicted in Figure 1 [10]. Lung segmentation is performed for each section of a CT scan based on a threshold identified for that section from gray-level histogram analysis. The lung segmentation regions that result from this straightforward approach (see Figure 2) are modified to (1) separate left and right lungs that thresholding may have merged at the anterior junction, (2) eliminate the trachea and main stem bronchi that thresholding may have included within the lung segmentation regions, and (3) include dense juxta-pleural or perihilar structures that thresholding may have excluded from the lung segmentation regions. The collection of lung segmentation regions for all sections in the scan constitutes the segmented lung volume.

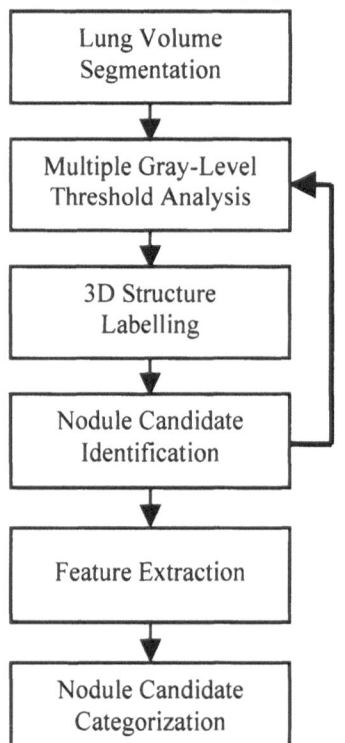

Figure 1. Automated nodule detection method.

A series of gray-level thresholds is applied to the pixels within the segmented lung volume. The bold arrow in Figure 1 represents an iterative process that begins with a low gray-level threshold and is repeated for each of 36 increasingly larger threshold values. At each iteration, pixels with gray levels less than the threshold are turned off in the segmented lung volume to produce a thresholded lung volume. A region-labelling technique is used to inventory all three-dimensionally contiguous groups of remaining pixels ("structures") within the thresholded lung volume, and those structures that satisfy a maximum-volume criterion are designated nodule candidates. This process is repeated for each successively larger gray-level threshold, with correspondingly fewer pixels remaining in the thresholded lung volume. At each iteration, structures that satisfy the maximum-volume criterion become lung

CARS 2002 – H.U. Lemke, M.W. Vannier; K. Inamura, A.G. Farman, K. Doi & J.H.C. Reiber (Editors)

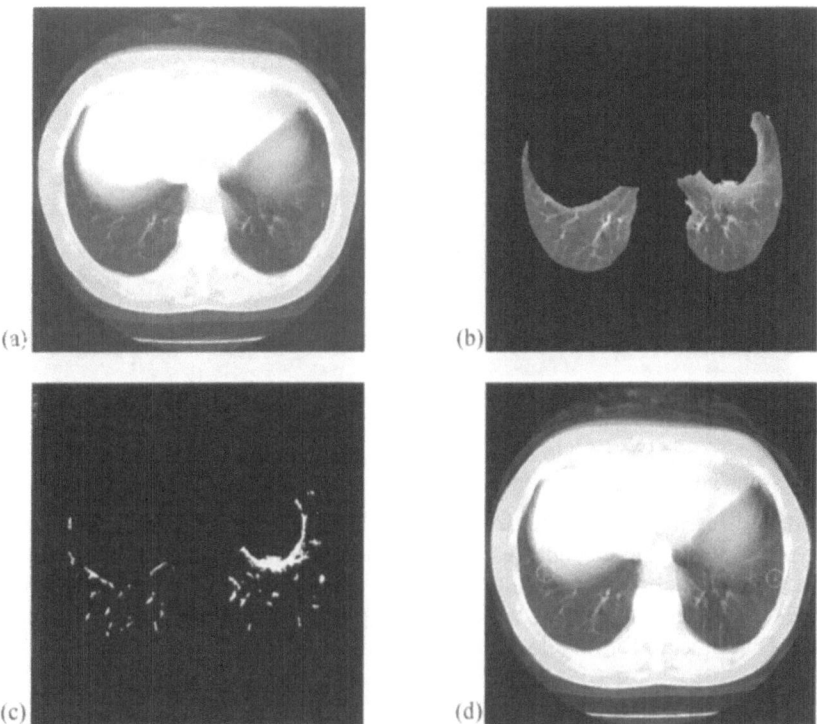

Figure 2. Images depicting different stages of the automated lung nodule detection method. (a) An original CT section image. (b) The segmented lung regions for this section. (c) A binary image representing the structures that were identified as nodule candidates. (d) The final nodule detection results presented as circles superimposed on the original CT section indicating one true positive in the left hemithorax and one false positive in the right hemithorax.

nodule candidates. The effect of this iterative process is illustrated in Figure 3. The single structure present in Figure 3(a) is comprised of one set of three-dimensionally contiguous pixels that remained in the thresholded lung volume generated at a low gray-level threshold. The large volume of this structure prevents its inclusion as a nodule candidate. At a higher gray-level threshold, the pixels that had belonged to a single structure at the lower threshold have disassociated into multiple smaller structures (Figure 3(b)), many of which will satisfy the volume criterion to become nodule candidates.

The multiple gray-level thresholding process generates an initial set of nodule candidates, which is captured in Figure 2(c) for one section. For each candidate in the initial set, a nine-dimensional feature vector is computed which includes the three-dimensional features (1) mean gray level of the candidate, (2) gray-level standard deviation, (3) gray-level threshold at which the candidate was identified, (4) volume, (5) sphericity, and (6) radius of the sphere of equivalent volume and the two-dimensional features (1) eccentricity, (2) circularity, and (3) compactness. An empirically determined rule-based scheme obtained with two of these features is used to substantially reduce the number of

CARS 2002 – H.U. Lemke, M.W. Vannier; K. Inamura, A.G. Farman, K. Doi & J.H.C. Reiber (Editors)
ⓒCARS/Springer. All rights reserved.

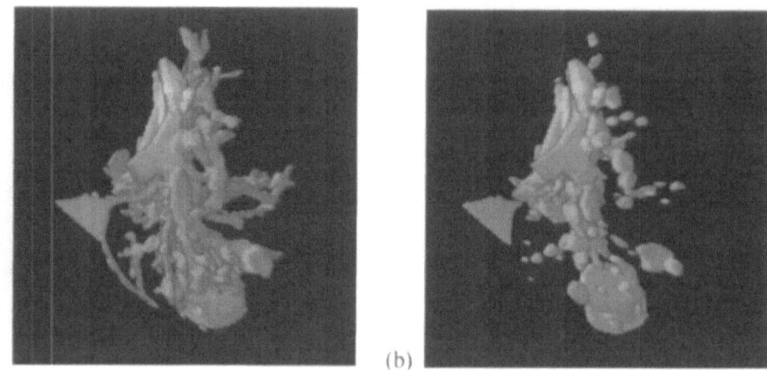

(a)   (b)

Figure 3. A single structure identified at a low gray-level threshold (a) decomposes into multiple smaller structures at a higher gray-level threshold (b). Reprinted with permission from reference [14].

nodule candidates that correspond to "non-nodule" structures (i.e., false positives). The features of the remaining candidates are merged through linear discriminant analysis [19] to further reduce the number of false positives. The output of the method at this stage constitutes the "detection results," which may be presented as circles superimposed on the original section images for radiologist review (Figure 2(d)).

3. Results

The automated lung nodule detection method has been applied to several databases of CT scans, including diagnostic scans and low-dose scans obtained from lung cancer screening programs, since computerized nodule detection methods are expected to contribute to both of these clinical scenarios. In the realm of diagnostic CT scans, a database of 43 scans was collected. These scans had been acquired with 10-mm collimation and a 10-mm reconstruction interval at a helical pitch of 1 on a GE HiSpeed Advantage scanner (GE Medical Systems, Milwaukee, WI). The scans contained a total of 171 lung nodules with a median effective diameter of 6.5 mm. The method achieved an overall nodule detection sensitivity of 70% with an average of 1.5 false-positive detections per section. Within the subset of 20 cases with at most two nodules, a corresponding sensitivity of 89% was achieved with an average of 1.3 false-positive detections per section [10].

Nodule size has an effect on the nodule detection method. For example, if the "detection task" is specified only for nodules with an effective diameter greater than 5 mm, the method detected 81% of such nodules at the same rate of 1.5 false positives per section, or, alternatively, the method generated only 0.6 false positives per section at the same detection sensitivity of 70% when nodules greater than 5 mm were the detection target. We are currently investigating the performance of the method on a database of diagnostic CT scans acquired with 7-mm collimation and 5-mm reconstruction interval.

The method has been applied to databases of low-dose CT scans. The first such database we used contained 13 scans that had been performed on a Philips Tomoscan SR 7000

CARS 2002 – H.U. Lemke, M.W. Vannier; K. Inamura, A.G. Farman, K. Doi & J.H.C. Reiber (Editors)
ᶜCARS/Springer. All rights reserved.

scanner (Philips, Eindhoven, The Netherlands) with 1.5:1 helical pitch, 5-mm collimation, and a 5-mm reconstruction interval. These scans contained 255 lung nodules with a median effective diameter of 5.0 mm. An automated nodule detection performance of 71% sensitivity was achieved with an average of 1.2 false positives per section [17].

A second database of low-dose CT scans has been investigated more recently. This database consisted of 38 CT scans obtained from a lung cancer screening program with 10-mm collimation, 10-mm reconstruction interval, and a helical pitch of 2. These scans contained a total of 50 lung nodules, including 38 nodules that represented cancers that had been "missed" by radiologists during initial clinical interpretation [18]. The automated method attained a nodule detection sensitivity of 80% with an average of 1.3 false-positive detections per section. We are currently investigating the performance of the method on a larger database of low-dose screening CT scans.

4. Summary

We have developed a fully automated method for the detection of lung nodules in diagnostic and screening CT scans. The method has been applied to a number of different databases of CT scans acquired with various imaging protocols and has demonstrated promising results. Such computerized nodule detection methods are expected to become essential elements of the CT interpretation process in the future.

Acknowledgments

This work was supported in part by USPHS grant CA83908, funding from The University of Chicago Cancer Research Center, funding from the Grant Healthcare Foundation through The University of Chicago Medical Imaging Research and Education Foundation, and a grant from the American Lung Association of Metropolitan Chicago. S. G. Armato is a shareholder in R2 Technology, Inc. (Los Altos, CA).

References

1. M. L. Giger, K. T. Bae and H. MacMahon, "Computerized detection of pulmonary nodules in computed tomography images", *Investigative Radiology*, 29, 459–465, 1994.
2. K. Kanazawa, M. Kubo, N. Niki, H. Satoh, H. Ohmatsu, K. Eguchi and N. Moriyama, "Computer assisted lung cancer diagnosis based on helical images", *Image Analysis Applications and Computer Graphics: Proceedings of the Third International Computer Science Conference*, R. T. Chin, H. H. S. Ip, A. C. Naiman and T.-C. Pong (eds.), 323–330, Springer-Verlag, Berlin, 1995.
3. W. J. Ryan, J. E. Reed, S. J. Swensen and P. F. Sheedy, Jr, "Automatic detection of pulmonary nodules in CT", *Proceedings Computer Assisted Radiology*, H. U. Lemke, M. W. Vannier, K. Inamura and A. G. Farman (eds.), 385–389, Elsevier Science, Amsterdam, 1996.
4. T. Okumura, T. Miwa, J. Kako, S. Yamamoto, M. Matsumoto, Y. Tateno, T. Iinuma and T. Matsumoto, "Image processing for computer-aided diagnosis of lung cancer screening system by CT (LSCT)", *SPIE Proceedings*, 3338, 1314–1322, 1998.
5. M. Fiebich, C. Wietholt, B. C. Renger, S. G. Armato, III, K. R. Hoffmann, D. Wormanns and S. Diederich, "Automatic detection of pulmonary nodules in low-dose screening thoracic CT examinations", *SPIE Proceedings*, 3661, 1434–1439, 1999.

6. S.-L. Lou, C.-L. Chang, K.-P. Lin and T.-S. Chen, "Object-based deformation technique for 3-D CT lung nodule detection", *SPIE Proceedings*, 3661, 1544–1552, 1999.

7. H. Satoh, Y. Ukai, N. Niki, K. Eguchi, K. Mori, H. Ohmatsu, R. Kakinuma, M. Kaneko and N. Moriyama, "Computer aided diagnosis system for lung cancer based on retrospective helical CT image", *SPIE Proceedings*, 3661, 1324–1335, 1999.

8. H. Taguchi, Y. Kawata, N. Niki, H. Satoh, H. Ohmatsu, R. Kakinuma, K. Eguchi, M. Kaneko and N. Moriyama, "Lung cancer detection based on helical CT images using curved surface morphology analysis", *SPIE Proceedings*, 3661, 1307–1314, 1999.

9. D. Wormanns, M. Fiebich, C. Wietholt, S. Diederich and W. Heindel, "Automatic detection of pulmonary nodules at spiral CT—first clinical experience with a computer-aided diagnosis system", *SPIE Proceedings*, 3979, 129–135, 2000.

10. S. G. Armato, III, M. L. Giger and H. MacMahon, "Automated detection of lung nodules in CT scans: Preliminary results", *Medical Physics*, 28, 1552–1561, 2001.

11. M. S. Brown, M. F. McNitt-Gray, J. G. Goldin, R. D. Suh, J. W. Sayre and D. R. Aberle, "Patient-specific models for lung nodule detection and surveillance in CT images", *IEEE Transactions on Medical Imaging*, 20, 1242–1250, 2001.

12. J. P. Ko and M. Betke, "Chest CT: Automated nodule detection and assessment of change over time—preliminary experience", *Radiology*, 218, 267–273, 2001.

13. Y. Lee, T. Hara, H. Fujita, S. Itoh and T. Ishigaki, "Automated detection of pulmonary nodules in helical CT images based on an improved template-matching technique", *IEEE Transactions on Medical Imaging*, 20, 595–604, 2001.

14. S. G. Armato, III, M. L. Giger, J. T. Blackburn, K. Doi and H. MacMahon, "Three-dimensional approach to lung nodule detection in helical CT", *SPIE Proceedings*, 3661, 553–559, 1999.

15. S. G. Armato, III, M. L. Giger, C. J. Moran, J. T. Blackburn, K. Doi and H. MacMahon, "Computerized detection of pulmonary nodules on CT scans", *RadioGraphics*, 19, 1303–1311, 1999.

16. S. G. Armato, III, M. L. Giger and H. MacMahon, "Analysis of a three-dimensional lung nodule detection method for thoracic CT scans", *SPIE Proceedings*, 3979, 103–109, 2000.

17. S. G. Armato, III, M. L. Giger, K. Doi and H. MacMahon, "Computerized lung nodule detection: Comparison of performance for low-dose and standard-dose helical CT scans", *SPIE Proceedings*, 4322, 1449–1454, 2001.

18. S. G. Armato, III, F. Li, M. L. Giger, H. MacMahon, S. Sone and K. Doi, "Performance of automated CT nodule detection on missed cancers from a lung cancer screening program", *Radiology*, (accepted), 2002.

19. R. A. Johnson and D. W. Wichern, *Applied Multivariate Statistical Analysis*, Prentice Hall, Englewood Cliffs, NJ, 1992.

CARS 2002 – H.U. Lemke, M.W. Vannier; K. Inamura, A.G. Farman, K. Doi & J.H.C. Reiber (Editors)

A CAD system for lung cancer based on 3D CT images

Noboru Niki[a], Yoshiki Kawata[a], Mitsuru Kubo[a], Hironobu Ohmatsu[b],
Ryutaro Kakinuma[b], Masahiro Kaneko[c], Masahiko Kusumoto[c],
Noriyuki Moriyama[c]

[a] Dept. of Optical Science and Technology, Univ. of Tokushima, Japan
[b] National Cancer Center Hospital East, Chiba, Japan,
[c] National Cancer Center Hospital, Tokyo, Japan

Abstract

This paper presents a prospective evaluation of lung cancer screening based on low-dose single helical 3D CT images. This CT screening uses a computer-aided diagnosis (CAD) system to efficiently detect lung nodules from 3D images. The performance of this screening is evaluated by over 5,000 cases for 5 years. The effectiveness of the screening using the CAD system is certified from a large data test.

Keywords: CAD system, lung cancer screening, prospective evaluation

1. Introduction

Lung cancer is the leading cause of cancer deaths in the world. Early detection and treatment of lung cancers are crucially important to achieve high survival rate. A trial of early detection of lung cancer using a promising low-dose CT has been starting since 1993 1, 2. The screening requests a digital diagnosis environment to efficiently read a number of 3D images. Therefore we are studying a detection system for lung cancer screening based on thoracic 3D CT images. We developed a CAD system in 1996 3, 4, and the prospective study was started in July 1997. In this paper, we show the prospective evaluation and we evaluate the detection ability of the CAD system and its availability from the result of the evaluation.

2. Lung cancer screening using CT

In the conventional screening, first two physicians check CT images cooperatively. This double reading are effectively decreased the number of false negatives and false positives of the abnormal shadows. Next, the comparative reading is executed using each personal time-series CT images. Suspicious malignant shadows are selected using the temporal change from abnormal shadows checked by the first reading. The flow of these reading is shown in Figure 1 (a). However, these film-based reading is a burden on physicians and the performance of reading is not clinical. We present an efficient screening using CAD system as shown in Figure 1 (b). A physician executes a twice reading. A first reading is to check 3D CT images. A second reading is to recheck with CAD results. This reading by a physician and CAD is expected to be equal and superior to the cooperative reading by two physicians. Using the CAD system, a physician only is efficiently read with high diagnostic accuracy.

CARS 2002 – H.U. Lemke, M.W. Vannier; K. Inamura, A.G. Farman, K. Doi & J.H.C. Reiber (Editors)

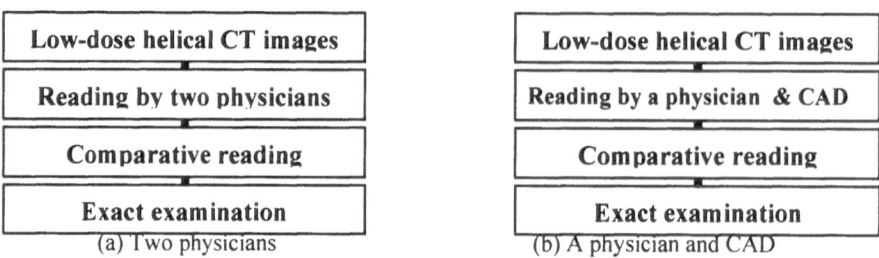

Figure 1: Flow of reading

Table 1. Criterion of judgment

Judgment E	Suspicious malignant lesion
Judgment D	Abnormal lesion with exact examination
Judgment C	Abnormal lesion without exact examination
Judgment B	Normal case

The diagnostic criterion is shown in Table.1. In case of judgment E or D, these shadows are exactly examined using high-resolution CT images.

3. Prospective evaluation

From July 1997, we have been starting a clinical trial of a reading using the CAD system. We have applied our system to 4,602 cases from July 1997 to December 2000. The results are shown in Table.2. The first reading suspects 925 cases and the second reading suspects 1053 cases. 128 cases were added by rechecking abnormal cases detected by the CAD system. Comparative reading is executed to historically check on time-series images of each abnormal shadow. The final results indicated 514 cases. These 514 cases were evaluated based on judgment results of second reading. 290 cases were judgment results of E or D and 224 cases were judgment results of C or B. The 224 cases were added by the comparative reading. By exact examination using high-resolution CT images, 154 cases were judgment results of suspicious malignant cases. Finally 16 cases were cancer cases and its detection rate was 0.35%.

Figure 2 shows the contribution of the CAD to reading. The correction ratio of the CAD is 5.4 %, 4.5 %, and 6.3 % on each reading stage. This figure shows that the CAD system assisted by almost equivalent rates on each inspection and these rates were about 10 % of the detection ratio of a physician. 28 of 128 cases, which were assisted by the CAD on the second reading, were carried out the exact examination. Its rate was 21.88%. 262 of 925 cases, which are detected by a physician at first reading, were carried out the exact

CARS 2002 – H.U. Lemke, M.W. Vannier; K. Inamura, A.G. Farman, K. Doi & J.H.C. Reiber (Editors)
°CARS/Springer. All rights reserved.

examination. The rate was 28.32%. These results showed that the reading using a physician and CAD has the same detection capability of the double reading by two physicians.

Table 2. Results of each diagnosis stage from July 1997 to December 2000

Total	4602 cases	Rate
First reading	925 cases	20.10 %
Second reading	1053 cases	22.88%
Comparative reading (Exact examination is requested)	514 cases (290 + 224 cases)	11.17%
Exact examination (Suspicious malignancy is indicated)	154 cases	3.35 %
Lung cancer	16 cases	0.35 %

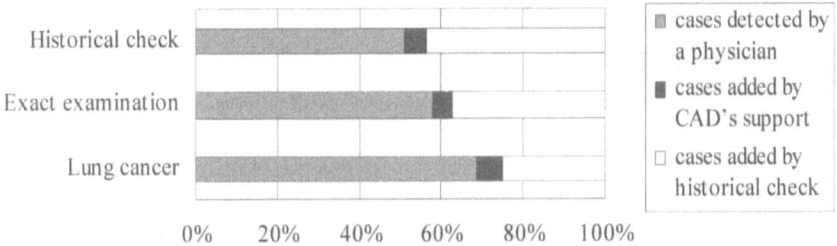

Figure 2: The shadow corrected by CAD

17 cancers of 16 cases are evaluated in detail. The results of the reading using the CAD system are shown in Table.3. At first reading the physician did not detect six cancers. One cancer was judgment B and five cancers were judgment C. At second reading one cancer was changed from judgment B to judgment E. This change was assisted by the CAD system. Other five cancers were judgment C as well as the first reading. The five cancers were added by the comparative reading and these four cancers were also detected by the CAD system. The CAD system is expected for developing an image retrieval function to efficiently execute the comparative reading. The CAD system did not detect 4 cancers of 17. The detection rate was 76.5% and the number of false positives was 0.30 per slice. Size and average CT value of 17 cancers are shown in Figure 3. These cancer areas were detected by manual operation. The size is a diameter of the circle equivalent to the area of the detected field. All cases were small cancers of 20 mm or less. This fact shows that the

704

CAD system can detect lung cancer at an early stage successfully. Within 17 cancers, two small cancers are shown in Figure 4. A cancer of Fig. 4 (a) was judgment E but the CAD system did not detect it. The cancer of Fig. 4 (b) was judgment B and the cancer was assisted by the CAD system. This fact is expected that the CAD system is effective on clinic.

Table 3 The detection results of lung cancer

	First reading			Second reading			Comparative reading			CA
Total	E or D	C	B	E or D	C	B	E or D	C	B	TP
17	11	5	1	12	5	0	17	0	0	13

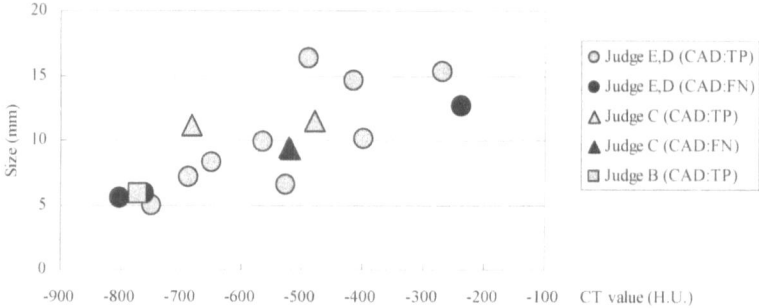

Fig. 3 Size and average CT value of 17 cancers

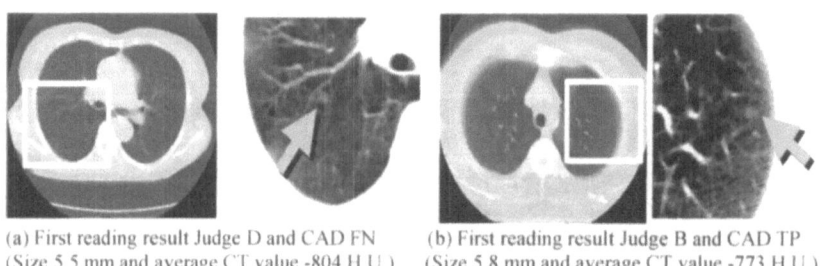

(a) First reading result Judge D and CAD FN   (b) First reading result Judge B and CAD TP
(Size 5.5 mm and average CT value -804 H.U.)   (Size 5.8 mm and average CT value -773 H.U.)

Fig. 4 Judgment of two small cancers

CARS 2002 – H.U. Lemke, M.W. Vannier; K. Inamura, A.G. Farman, K. Doi & J.H.C. Reiber (Editors)
ᶜCARS/Springer. All rights reserved.

4. Conclusion

We described a lung cancer screening using the CAD system based on 3D CT images. The screening using the CAD system detected lung cancers at an early stage efficiently and the performance was validated by the prospective evaluation. From these results, the CAD system could show a reduction of physician labor and a uniformity of diagnostic results sufficiently. The presented system promoted an expectation of CT screening for lung cancer. But, the CAD system did not detect all cancers. It is necessary to improve its detection ability. A function of comparative reading is also requested. Furthermore, a high-performance screening for lung cancer will be developed by an effective combination of multi-slice CT with digital diagnosis environment.

Acknowledgements

This works ware supported in part by Dr. Kenji Eguchi of the Tokai University, Dr. Kiyoshi Mori of the Tochigi Cancer Center, Dr. Hiroyuki Nishiyama of the Social Health Insurance Medical Center, Kenichiro Katsumata of the Toshiba Cop. and Dr candidate students of Niki laboratory of the Univ. of Tokushima.

References

1. N.Moriyama, R.Iwata, F.Wako, M.Ohtani, and H.Ohmatsu, "Helical computed tomography scanning of the thorax and abdomen," Jpn.J.Clin.Oncol.,vol.23, pp.156-161,1993.
2. M.Kaneko, K.Eguchi, at al., "Peripheral Lung Cancer: Screening and Detection with Low-Dose Spiral CT versus Radiography," Radiology, vol.201, pp.798-802, 1996.
3. K.Kanazawa, N.Niki, at al.,"Computer Assisted Diagnosis of Lung Cancer Using Helical X-Ray CT," IEEE Workshop on Biomedical Image Analysis, pp.261-267,1994.
4. K.Kanazawa, N.Niki, at al., "Computer-aided diagnosis for pulmonary nodules based on helical CT images," Comput. Med. Imag. Graph., 22, pp.157-167, 1998.

CARS 2002 – H.U. Lemke, M.W. Vannier; K. Inamura, A.G. Farman, K. Doi & J.H.C. Reiber (Editors)

706

Optimal image feature set for detecting lung nodules on chest X-ray images

Jun Wei, Yoshihiro Hagihara, Akinobu Shimizu, Hidefumi Kobatake
Graduate School of Bio-Applications and Systems Engineering
Tokyo University of Agriculture and Technology
2-24-16, Naka-cho, Koganei, 184-8588, Tokyo, Japan

Abstract

The performance of a computer-aided diagnosis system depends on the feature set used in it. This paper shows the results of image feature selection experiments. We evaluated 210 features to look for the optimum feature set. For the purpose, a forward stepwise selection approach was employed. The area under the receiver operating characteristic (ROC) curve was adopted to evaluate the performance of each feature set. Analysis of the optimally selected feature set is given and the experiments using 247 chest x-ray images are also shown.

Keywords: Computer aided diagnosis, lung cancer, feature selection

1. Introduction

Lung cancer is one of the most serious cancers in the world. Survival from lung cancer is directly related to its growth at its detection. The earlier the detection is, the higher the chances of successful treatment are. Chest X-ray image has been used for detecting lung cancer for a long time. The early detection and diagnosis of pulmonary nodules in chest X-ray image are among the most challenging clinical tasks performed by radiologists. Computer-aided diagnosis (CAD) has been proven to be a very effective approach as assistant to radiologists for improving diagnostic accuracy. Numerous systems were reported for detecting lung nodules on chest X-ray images [1-3]. However, the strong concern of almost all of them is that the false positives per image are too large. How to reduce the number of false positives while maintaining a high true positive detection rate is the most important work in realizing a chest CAD system[4].

Most of the proposed computer-aided diagnosis systems (CAD systems) adopt a two-step pattern recognition approach, which is a combination of a feature extraction process and a classification process using neural network classifier or statistical classifier. The performance of the classifier depends directly on the ability of characterization of candidate regions by the adopted features. Many kinds of features have been proposed for discriminating between normal tissues and abnormal ones. However, there have been a few researches on comparing the effectiveness of those features[5-9]. The numbers of features used in those researches are not sufficiently large. The purpose of our research is to find the optimal feature set from a large number of features which enable a CAD

CARS 2002 – H.U. Lemke, M.W. Vannier; K. Inamura, A.G. Farman, K. Doi & J.H.C. Reiber (Editors)
'CARS/Springer. All rights reserved.

system for lung cancer screening to take large step toward a practical application. And this paper shows the results of the preliminary experiments of this project.

2. CAD system and the optimal feature set

Our CAD system consists of four processing steps: 1) location of tumor candidates by using adaptive ring filter, 2) extraction of the boundaries of tumor candidates, 3) extraction of feature parameters, and 4) discrimination between the normal and the abnormal regions. Fig. 1 shows the configuration of the CAD system. Adaptive ring filter, which is a kind of convergence index filter (CI filter) [10], is employed to extract tumor candidates. It evaluates the degree of convergence of gradient vectors to the pixel of interest. Its output does not depend on the contrast of the region of interest to its background. Actually, we have found highly ranked local peaks of the outputs of the adaptive ring filter correspond to the summit of tumors. In this work, the top 25 peaks on each X-ray image are detected as the tumor candidate location.

At each tumor candidate location, the boundary of the candidate is estimated by using a two-step process. In the first step, Iris filter, which is another kind of CI filter, is used to estimate the fuzzy boundary [11]. Then, SNAKES algorithm is applied to the output image of the Iris filter to obtain the boundary of the tumor candidate. It is called a suspicious region (SR) in the following. Feature parameters are calculated for each SR.

The discrimination between the normal and the abnormal regions is performed using a statistical method based on the Maharanobis distance measure. Fig. 2 shows the whole story of the project of our research. Features are extracted from each of multi-resolution images. Various kinds of filtering or transformation such as Fourier transform, Wavelet transform, spatial difference, Iris filtering, adaptive ring filtering, et al. can be applied to each image. Those transformed images give another various kinds of features. The total number of features extracted from the multi-scale images and their transformed ones can be well over one thousand. Among them we can expect to derive the optimal feature set by which the performance of the CAD system can be vastly improved. This project is the work-in-progress and this paper shows the results of the preliminary study using the original images reduced by 1/4. Spatial resolution of the original image is 0.175mm per pixel and that of the reduced image is 0.7mm per pixel.

3. Feature selection

3.1 Method

Feature selection is a very important step in organizing a classifier. Theoretical approach cannot be applied to determine the optimal combination of features, and the only way to select the optimal feature subset is to evaluate all possible combinations of the features. Moreover, sufficient numbers of test materials are necessary to evaluate the performance of

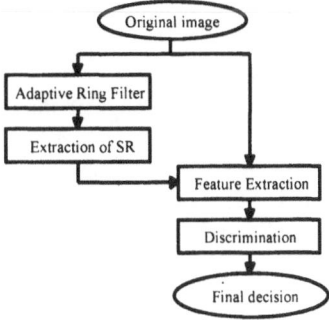

Fig. 1 Processing flow of the CAD system

708

each feature combination. It means that the number of combinations and the total amount of computation time become impractically huge. Therefore, it is acceptable to adopt heuristic algorithms such as a genetic algorithm, a forward stepwise and a backward stepwise selections which need much smaller computational loads. These algorithms give not a really optimal feature set but a sub-optimal one because only a part of possible combinations of features are evaluated. The sub-optimal feature set is referred to as the optimal feature set for simplicity in the following. In this work, we adopted the forward stepwise selection method to obtain the optimal feature set. The area under ROC curve was adopted as the criterion to evaluate the performance of feature sets.

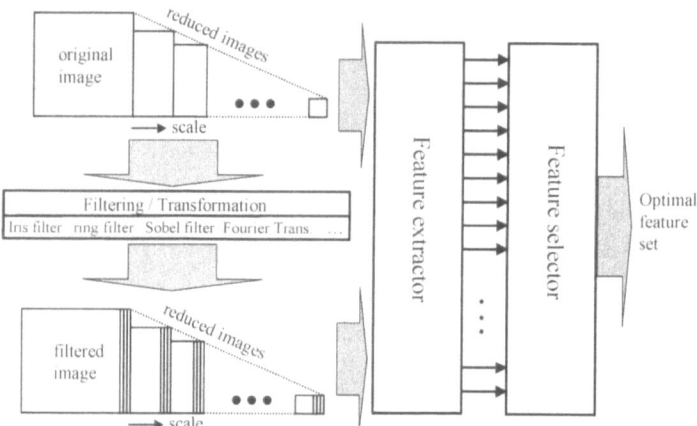

Fig. 2 The scheme to obtain the optimal feature set

3.2 Features

Four kinds of filtered images, that is, the original image reduced by 1/4, the output images of the iris filter and the adaptive ring filter, and the difference image obtained by applying the Sobel filter were used to extract features, and the number of features examined in the following experiments is 210. These features can be categorized into four types as follows.

(1) Geometric Features

Six geometric features are calculated from the binary SR region. They are Spreadness, Circularity, Area, Equivalent radius, Distance from the candidate point to the pulmonary hilum, and Flatness.

(2) Contrast Features

Generally, tumor region is brighter than its background on x-ray image. So, the contrast information can be used as features. In this work, nine kinds of features [12] are calculated from SR regions on each of 4 kinds of filtered images. The total number of features related to the contrast is 36.

(3) First-Order Statistics

First-order statistics are calculated from two histograms of the grey-scale values. They are obtained from two regions. One is called the inner region which covers the core region of SR. The other one is called the outer region which corresponds to the boundary area of SR. The histograms are obtained from 4 kinds of filtered images. Features calculated from

CARS 2002 – H.U. Lemke, M.W. Vannier; K. Inamura, A.G. Farman, K. Doi & J.H.C. Reiber (Editors)
©CARS/Springer. All rights reserved.

each histogram include mean, standard deviation, contrast, skewness, kurtosis, energy and entropy. The total number of first-order statistical features is 56.

(4) Second-Order Statistics

Co-occurrence matrix method has been adopted to extract features of second-order statistics. They are obtained by using Haralick transformation. Co-occurrence matrix is the two-dimensional histograms of the frequency of the joint occurrences of two pixels with a displacement and an orientation. In this work, they were set to 2 pixels and 90°, respectively. Co-occurrence matrices are obtained from the inner and the outer regions of each SR. The fourteen scalar statistical properties were calculated from a co-occurrence matrix. Four kinds of filtered images were used to calculate it. Therefore, the total number of features related to the second-order statistics is 112.

4. Experiments

4.1 Experimental materials

Two hundred and forty-seven chest x-ray images included in JSRT Database were used as test materials. They include 154 malignant tumors whose difficulty of detection distributes almost equally from rank 1 (hard to detect) to rank 5 (easy to detect). The spatial resolution of the original x-ray image is 0.175 mm and the size of each image is 2048 x 2048 pixels with 12-bits accuracy. Using our CAD system, 6175 candidate regions (SR) were detected. Several malignant tumors split into two or three candidate regions and 187 SR's correspond to malignant tumors. The other 5988 SR's correspond to normal tissues. The forward stepwise selection method was adopted to find the optimal combination of features among 210 features. The leave-one-out method was employed to evaluate the performance of each combination of features. In reference [13], CAD system based on the optimal feature set obtained from 55 features is described. These features are included in 210 features. For comparing the performance changes by increasing the number of features, experiments using 55 features have been also performed.

4.2 Experimental results

Fig. 3 shows the relationship between the area under the ROC curve (Az) and the number of features (the dimension of the feature vector) selected by the forward stepwise selection method. Among 210 features there were 8 features which are highly correlated with other ones and they were excluded from the experiments. Therefore the total number of features is 202. The area Az increases gradually as the increase of the number of features and it keeps almost the maximum (Az = about 0.85) where the number of features is over 30. The maximum of Az was attained by the combination of 98 features. Table 1 shows the contribution of 4 kinds of filtered images to the optimal feature set with 98 features. We can say that the 4 kinds of filtered images almost equally contain information effective in discriminating between malignant and normal tissues. The relationship between Az and the number of features for the case of 55 features is also shown in Fig. 3. Experimental results showed that the performance attained by the optimal subset of 202 features is much better than that of 55 features.

The relationship between the number of false positives per image and the number of features was also analyzed, where the true positive detection rate is 80%. We can say that by using optimally selected feature set the number of false positives per image can be as

710

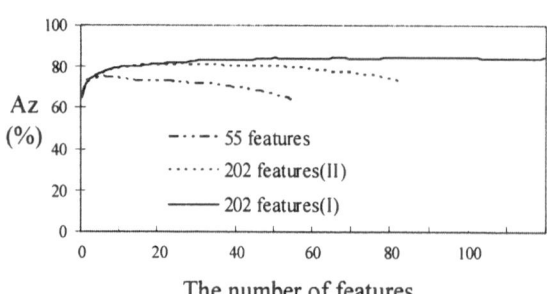

The number of features

Fig. 3 The relationship between the number of features
and the area Az.

low as 5.4 per image. Another optimal feature selection procedure has been applied to features belonging to the types (2), (3) and (4). First, the optimal feature set for each of 4 kinds of filtered images was determined using the forward stepwise selection method. The numbers of the features consisting of the optimal feature sets are 25, 24, 13 and 16 for the original image, the output image of the iris filter, the output image of the adaptive ring filter and the difference image, respectively. Totally 78 features were selected. By adding six geometrical features of the type (1), the total number of features becomes 84. Then, the forward stepwise selection method was applied to obtain the optimal feature set among 84 features. Experimental results as shown in Fig. 3 showed that the area Az attained by the feature set obtained by this procedure is slightly smaller than that of the optimal feature set among 202 features.

5. Conclusion

The optimal feature set among 210 features has been identified using the forward stepwise selection method. The average number of false positives per image attained by the optimal feature set is as low as 5.4 per image where the true positive detection rate is 80%. The spatial resolution of the X-ray images used in this paper is 0.7mm per pixel. It is low enough to remove fine structures of candidate regions. However the experimental results shown in this paper is promising. Experiments using images with higher spatial resolution and much more features are now in progress.

Table 1 The contribution of 4 kinds of filtered images to the optimal feature set.
Arabic numerals show the number of selected features.

Filtered image	Geometric Features	Contrast Features	First-Order Statistics	Second-Order Statistics	Total
-	3	-	-	-	3
Reduced original image	-	6	4	8	18
Output image of the Iris filter	-	7	5	15	27
Difference image	-	8	6	8	22
Output image of the ring filter	-	6	6	16	28
Total	3	27	21	47	98

CARS 2002 – H.U. Lemke, M.W. Vannier; K. Inamura, A.G. Farman, K. Doi & J.H.C. Reiber (Editors)

Acknowledgements

This work was supported in part by the Grant-in-Aid for Scientific Research from the Ministry of Education, Culture, Sports, Science and Technology, Japan and the Grant-in-Aid for Cancer Research from the Ministry of Health, Labour and Welfare, Japan.

References

1. H. Suzuki, N. Inaoka, H. Takabatake, M. Mori, H. Natori and A. Suzuki, "An experiment system for detecting lung nodules by chest x-ray image processing," SPIE. Biomedical Image Processing II, Vol.. 1450, pp. 99-107, 1991.
2. J. Lin, S. B. Lo, A. Hasegawa, M. T. Freedman and S. K. Mun, "Reduction of false positives in lung nodule detection using a two-level neural classification," IEEE Trans. On Med. Imag., Vol.. 15, pp. 206-217, 1996.
3. Xin-Wei. Xu, K. Doi, T. Kobayashi, H. MacMahon and M. L. Giger, "Development of an improved CAD scheme for automated detection of lung nodules in digital chest images," Med. Phys., Vol..24, No. 9, pp. 1395-1403, 1997.
4. H. Yoshida and K. Doi, "Computerized detection of pulmonary nodules in chest radiographs: reduction of false positives based on symmetry between left and right lungs," Proc. SPIE in Medical Imaging 2000, pp. 97-102, 2000.
5. Y.Wu, M.L.Giger, K.Doi, C.J.Vyboorny, R.A.Schmidt, C.E.Metz, "Artificial Neural Networks in Mammography: Application to Decision Making in the Diagnosis of Breast Cancer," Radiology, Vol..187, pp.81-87, 1993.
6. M.Kupinski, M.L.Giger, P.Lu, and Z.Huo, "Computerized detection of mammographic lesions: Performance of artificial neural network with enhanced feature extraction, " Proc. of SPIE, Vol..2434, pp.598-605, 1995.
7. B.Sahiner, H P Chan, D.Wei, N.Petrick, M.A.Helvie, D.D.Adler, and M.M.Goodsitt, "Image feature selection by a genetic algorithm: Application to classification of mass and normal breast tissue, " Med. Phys. Vol..23, No.10, pp.1671-1683, 1996.
8. M.A.Kupinski, M.L.Giger, "Feature selection and Classifiers for the Computerized Detection of Mass Lesions in Digital Mammography," IEEE International Congress on Neural Networks, Houston, Texas, June, pp. 2460-2463, 1997.
9. G.D.Tourassi, E.D.Frederick, M.K. Markey, C.E.Floyd, Jr., "Application of the mutual information criterion for feature selection in computer-aided diagnosis," Med. Phys., Vol..28, No.12, pp.2394-2402, 2001.
10. Jun Wei, Yoshihiro Hagihara and Hidefumi Kobatake: Detection of Cancerous Tumors on Chest X-ray Images - Candidate Detection Filter and Its Application -, Proc. of ICIP, Paper No. 27AP4.2, 1999.
11. H. Kobatake and S. Hashimoto, "Convergence Index Filter for Vector Fields," IEEE Trans. on Image Processing, Vol. 8, No. 8, pp.1029-1038, 1999.
12. Guido M te Brake, Nico Karssemeijer, et al, "An automatic method to discriminate malignant masses from normal tissue in digital mammograms," Phys. Med. Biol., 45, pp. 2843-2857, 2000.
13. J. Wei, Y. Hagihara, H. Kobatake, "Detection of lung nodules on digital chest radiographs," Med. Imag. Tech., Vol. 19, No. 6, pp. 468-476, 2001. (in Japanese)

CARS 2002 – H.U. Lemke, M.W. Vannier; K. Inamura, A.G. Farman, K. Doi & J.H.C. Reiber (Editors)

712

Effect of the computer output on radiologists' decision-making for classification of solitary pulmonary nodules in chest radiographs

Junji Shiraishi[a], Hiroyuki Abe[a], Roger Englemann[a], Masahito Aoyama[b], Heber MacMahon[a], and Kunio Doi[a]

[a] Kurt Rossmann Laboratories for Radiologic Image Research
Department of Radiology, The University of Chicago
[b] Department of Intelligent Systems, Faculty of Information Sciences, Hiroshima City University

Abstract

We examined the usefulness of an automated computerized scheme for distinction between benign and malignant solitary pulmonary nodules in chest radiographs, based on ROC analysis of radiologists' performance. The average performance (Az = 0.817) of all radiologists with the computer output was significantly improved compared to that (Az = 0.743) without the computer output (p < 0.01). However, the performance (Az = 0.889) of the computer result was much better than these results. The effect of the computer output on radiologists' decision-making was clearly demonstrated by the high correlation coefficient (R = 0.845) between the average change (%) in radiologists' confidence level from without to with the computer output and the likelihood measures of malignancy (%). In other words, radiologists tended to change their confidence level to be consistent with the likelihood measure of malignancy presented. This effect tended to be greater in a group of attending radiologists (R = 0.872) compared with a group of residents (R = 0.714). These results indicated that this automated computerized scheme for distinction between benign and malignant solitary pulmonary nodules has a high potential to improve the diagnostic accuracy of radiologists' decision-making when the radiologist uses the computer output as a "second opinion. "

Keywords: CAD, receiver operating characteristic (ROC) analysis, lung nodule

1. Introduction

It has been well demonstrated that radiologists' performance with use of computer-aided diagnosis (CAD) can be improved significantly in the detection of abnormalities and also in the distinction between benign and malignant lesions [1-5]. However, it is still unclear how radiologists use the output from the CAD scheme in their decision-making. In this study, we examined the usefulness of an automated computerized scheme for distinction between benign and malignant solitary pulmonary nodules in chest radiographs, based on ROC analysis of radiologists' performance. In addition, we examined the relationship between the radiologists' rating score in an observer study and the computer output, and then we analyzed how observers were influenced by the CAD.

CARS 2002 – H.U. Lemke, M.W. Vannier; K. Inamura, A.G. Farman, K. Doi & J.H.C. Reiber (Editors)
^{c}CARS/Springer. All rights reserved.

2. Materials and methods

2.1 Automated computerized scheme

Our automated computerized scheme [6,7] was based on linear discriminant analysis (LDA) applied to seven features including the age, the root-mean-square value of the power spectrum, an overlap measure on histograms, full width at half maximum (FWHM) for the outside region of the segmented nodule on the background corrected image, degree of irregularity, FWHM for the inside region of the segmented nodule on the original image, and the contrast of the segmented nodule on the background-corrected image. These seven features were selected from two clinical parameters (age and sex) and seventy-five image features as an optimal combination of parameters for the LDA [7]. Seventy-five features were demonstrated from the outline and image analysis of regions inside and outside of automatically segmented nodules. The computer output indicates the likelihood measure of malignancy (%).

2.2 Observer performance study

Sixteen radiologists participated in this observer study, including 9 attendings and 7 residents. They were asked to give the confidence level on their judgment of benign/malignant nature of lesions included in fifty-three chest radiographs (31 primary lung cancers and 22 benign nodules) [6,7]. For the observer study, we used a continuous rating scale with a PC-based observer interface by using a CRT monitor [2]. Radiologists' ratings without and with the computer output were obtained sequentially for each case [1,8]. Both the original chest image and the enlarged image of the area of the nodule on the monitor were first presented to a radiologist for his/her decision-making. After the radiologist marked the initial level of confidence, the computer output of the likelihood measure of malignancy was shown on the monitor. The radiologist was asked

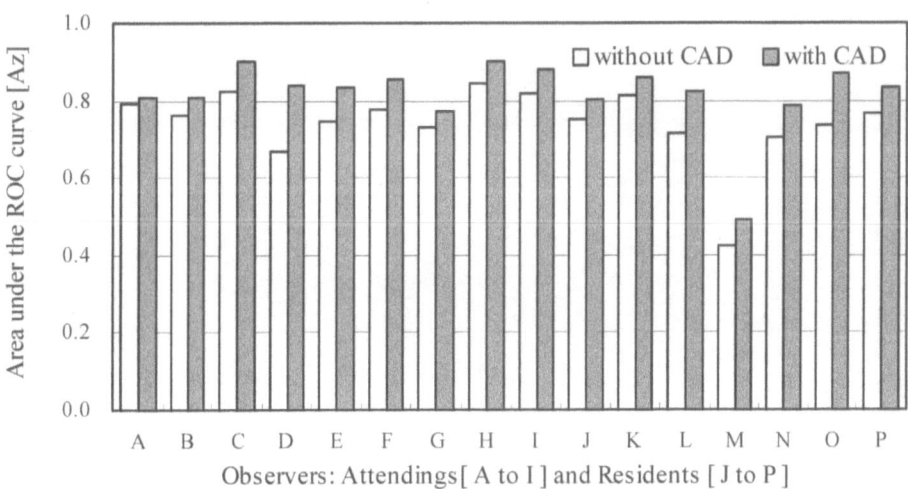

Fig. 1 Area under the ROC curves obtained without and with CAD by each radiologist

again to mark his/her confidence level, if the level was changed from the initial result. ROCKIT [9] and LABMRMC [10] programs (CE. Metz, The University of Chicago) were

CARS 2002 – H.U. Lemke, M.W. Vannier; K. Inamura, A.G. Farman, K. Doi & J.H.C. Reiber (Editors)
ᶜCARS/Springer. All rights reserved.

714

used for ROC curve fitting and the testing of statistical significance on the difference in Az values obtained without and with the computer output.

3. Results

Figure 1 shows the area under the ROC curve (Az) values obtained with and without the computer output for each radiologist. The average performance (Az = 0.817) of all radiologists with the computer output was improved significantly compared to that (Az = 0.743) without the computer output (p=0.002). Furthermore, all radiologists improved their diagnostic accuracy by use of the computer output. However, the performance (Az = 0.889) of the computer result was much better than these results. The average performance (Az = 0.845) of attendings with the computer output was better than that (Az = 0.781) of residents with the computer output, but there was no statistical significance in the difference between them.

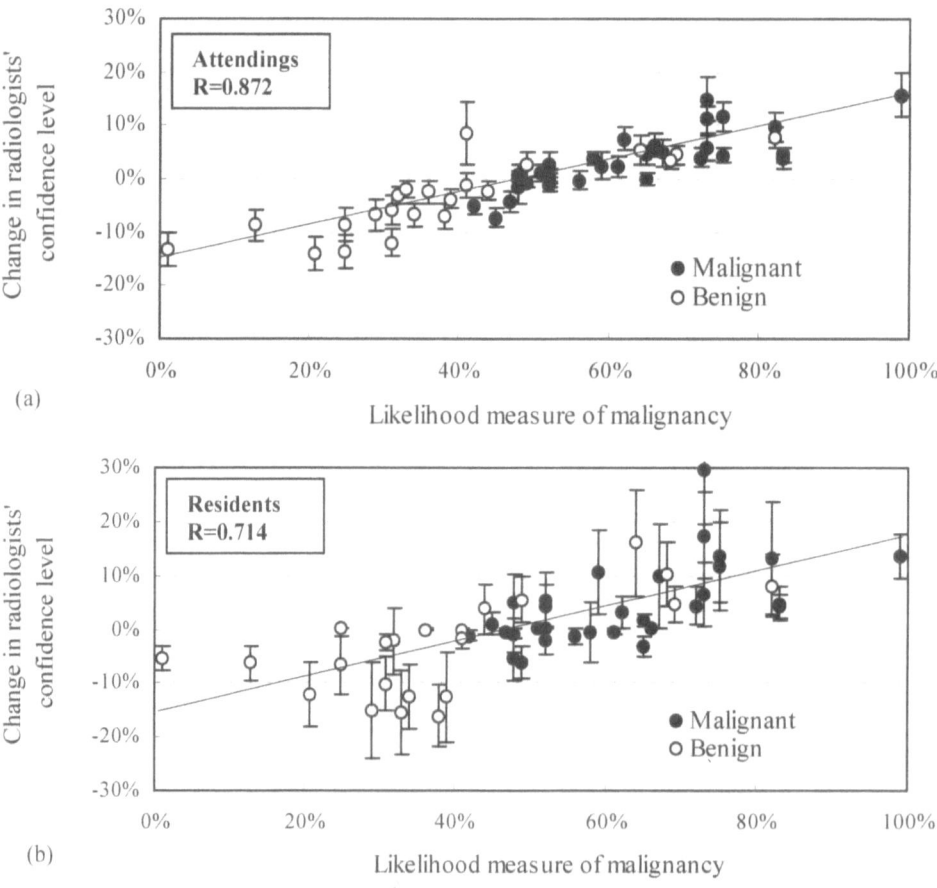

Fig.2   Relationship between the likelihood measure of malignancy and the average change (%) in radiologists' confidence level from without to with the computer output for attendings (a) and residents (b).

The average change (%) in radiologists' confidence level from without to with the computer output was highly correlated (R = 0.845) with the likelihood measures of malignancy. It should be noted that radiologists tend to be more confident toward malignant decisions when the likelihood measure of malignancy is greater than 50%, and benign decisions when the likelihood measure of malignancy is smaller than 50%. This effect tended to be greater in the group of attendings (R = 0.872) compared with the group of residents (R = 0.714), as shown in Fig.2 (a) and (b).

Figure 3 shows the number of benign cases identified correctly as benign by each radiologist. The number of benign cases was determined with the assumption that the minimum rating score for malignant cases used by each radiologist was considered as the threshold value, such that cases with rating scores below and above this threshold would be classified as benign and malignant, respectively, by each radiologist. Thus, all malignant cases would be identified correctly as malignant by each radiologist. The average number of correctly identified benign cases increased significantly from 4.9 to 9.0 when the computer output was used as a "second opinion" for radiologists' decision-making. There was a statistically significant difference (p = 0.005) between the numbers of correctly identified benign cases without and with CAD for all radiologists. Furthermore, sixteen benign cases of twenty-two actually benign cases were identified correctly as benign by the computer, whereas all of the malignant cases were identified correctly as malignant.

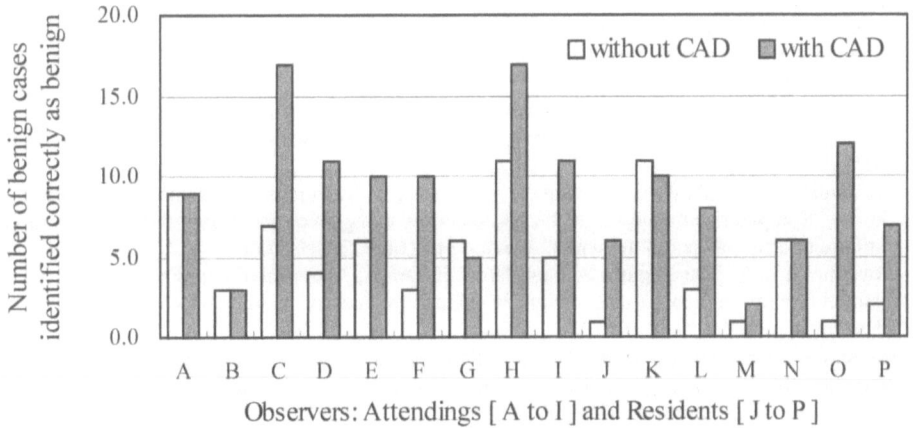

Fig. 3 Number of benign cases identified correctly as benign by each radiologist

4. Conclusion

This automated computerized scheme has great potential to improve the diagnostic accuracy of radiologists' decision-making when the radiologists use the computer output as a "second opinion."

716

Acknowledgments

The authors are grateful to Carl J. Vyborny, MD, PhD, Ulrich Bick, MD, Bonnie Fines, MD, J. Herman Kan, MD, Richard Kim, MD, Feng Li, MD, PhD, Peter MacEneaney, MD, Laurence Monnier-Cholley, MD, Katsunori Oikado, MD, Brian O'Rourke, MD, Yasuo Sasaki, MD, Christopher Straus, MD, George Vatakencherry, MD, Vishal Verma, MD, and Doris Yip, MD, for participating as observers; to Charles E. Metz, PhD, for his useful suggestions and discussions; and to Elisabeth Lanzl for improving the manuscript. This work is supported by USPHS Grant CA62625. K. Doi and H. MacMahon are shareholders in R2 Technology, Inc., Los Altos, CA.

References

1. Kobayashi T, Xu XW, MacMahon H, Metz CE, Doi K, "Effect of a computer-aided diagnosis scheme on radiologists' performance in detection of lung nodules on radiographs", *Radiology*, 199, 843-848, 1990.
2. MacMahon H, Engelmann R, Behlen FM, Hoffmann KR, Roe C, Metz CE, Doi K, "Computer-aided diagnosis of pulmonary nodules: Results of a large-scale observer test", *Radiology*, 213, 723-726, 1999.
3. Ashizawa K, MacMahon H, Ishida T, Nakamura K, Vyborny CJ, Katsuragawa S, Doi K, "Effect of an artificial neural network on radiologists' performance in the differential diagnosis of interstitial lung disease using chest radiographs", *AJR*, 172, 1311-1315,1999.
4. Difazio M, MacMahon H, Xu XW, Tsai P, Shiraishi J, Armato SG, Doi K, "Digital chest radiography: Effect of temporal subtraction images on detection accuracy", *Radiology*, 202, 447-452, 1997.
5. Monnier-Cholley L, MacMahon H, Katsuragawa S, Morishita J, Ishida T, Doi K, "Computer-aided diagnosis for detection of interstitial opacities on chest radiographs", *AJR*, 171, 1651-1656, 1998.
6. Nakamura K, Yoshida H, Engelmann R, MacMahon H, Katsuragawa S, Ishida T, Ashizawa K, Doi K, "Computerized analysis of the likelihood of malignancy in solitary pulmonary nodules with use of artificial neural networks", *Radiology*, 214, 823-830, 2000.
7. Aoyama M, Li Q, Katsuragawa S, MacMahon H, Doi K, "Automated computerized scheme for distinction between benign and malignant solitary pulmonary nodules on chest images", *Med Physics* (in press).
8. Uozumi T, Nakamura K, Watanabe H, Nakata H, Katsuragawa S, Doi K, "ROC analysis of detection of metastatic pulmonary nodules on digital chest radiographs with temporal subtraction", *Acad Radiol*, 8, 871-878, 2001.
9. Metz CE, Herman BA, Shen J-H, "Maximum-likelihood estimation of receiver operating characteristic (ROC) curves from continuously distributed data", *Statistics in Medicine*, 17, 1033-1053, 1998.
10. Dolfman DD, Berbaum KS, Metz CE, "ROC rating analysis: generalization to the population of readers and cases with the jackknife method", *Invest Radiol*, 27, 723-731, 1992.

CARS 2002 – H.U. Lemke, M.W. Vannier; K. Inamura, A.G. Farman, K. Doi & J.H.C. Reiber (Editors)

An efficient recognition method of lung nodules from X-ray CT images using 3-D object models

Kanae Shigemoto, Hotaka Takizawa, Shinji Yamamoto (*1), Tohru Nakagawa (*2), Tohru Matsumoto, Yukio Tateno, Takeshi Iinuma (*3), Mitsuomi Matsumoto (*4)
*1) Toyohashi University of Technology
*2) Hitachi Health Care Center
*3) National Institute of Radiological Sciences
*4) Tokyo Metropolitan University of Health Sciences

Abstract

In this paper, we propose an efficient algorithm to detect candidates of nodule shadows from X-ray CT images using 3D geometric object models of cancers and blood vessels. By using such 3D geometric object models, the anatomical knowledge about the 3D structures of nodules and blood vessels can be reflected in recognition process. Additionally, we improve the performance of the recognition method using template matching techniques. The template images are generated from the object models before the recognition process, and all of the template images can be memorized in the computers. As a result of the improvement of the performance, the calculation time of the recognition method is decreased drastically. By applying our new method to actual CT images (38 patient images), a good result has been acquired.

1. Introduction

In Japan, recently, the death rate by lung cancer is increasing rapidly. To cope with this problem, mass screening for lung cancer is widely performed by simple chest X-ray films with sputum cytology. At present, however, the detection ability of the observation by the simple X-ray film is not sufficient yet. It is known that the false negative ratio of the observation is considerably high.

From such a viewpoint, we proposed a lung cancer screening system by CT (LSCT) for the mass screening.[1]. By using the new screening system, the false negative ratio can be decreased. In this system, however, one problem is the increase of the number of the images to be diagnosed by a doctor to about 30 slices per patient from 1 X-ray film. To

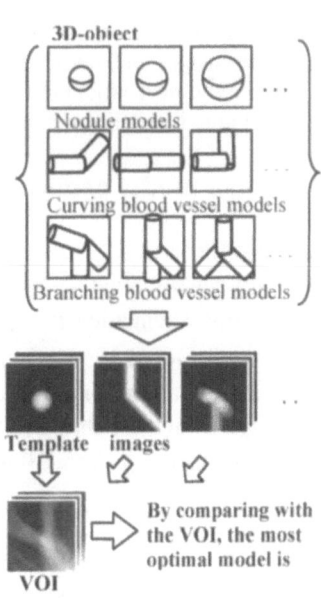

Figure 1: Recognition process.

718

overcome such problems, we have to develop an automatic recognition algorithm of pathological shadow candidates, which can reduce the number of the images to be diagnosed by a doctor.

First, we developed an image filter called quoit filter [2], which is a kind of mathematical morphology filter. This filter can detect pathological shadow candidates with the sensitivity over 95[%], but a lot of false positives are also detected yet. Thus, for the next step, we developed a recognition method [3] of shadow candidates using 3D Markov random field (MRF) models with geometric object models such as nodules (which are candidates of cancers) and blood vessels. This model-based recognition method can reduce the number of the false positives only about to 5 [shadow/patient] without any additional false negatives, but it needs a lot of calculation times, about 120[min/shadow]. In order to make this accurate method more practical, we increase the performance of the method. In this paper, we propose an efficient recognition method of lung nodules using template matching techniques. The detail of this new method is described below.

Figure 1 shows the recognition process described in this paper. First, we use our quoit filter to detect pathological shadow candidates, and extract volume-of-interest (VOI) areas, which include the detected shadow candidates. We represent nodules as sphere models and blood vessels as connected cylinder models respectively. By changing the parameters of these object models such as radii of the sphere models and angles of the blood vessel models, a certain number of nodule and blood vessel models are generated. From these object models, artificial CT images are generated by using computer graphics techniques. These artificial CT images are used as template images in the next recognition process. For each template image, we calculate a sum value of the squared differences (SSD) of the corresponding voxel values between the VOI area and the template image, and search for the optimal object model minimizing the SSD value. If the optimal object model obtained by this template matching process is a nodule model, the VOI area is determined to be abnormal. Otherwise it is determined to be normal.

2. Object model generation

2.1 Nodules
We represent a nodule as a sphere model whose radius is
r and X-ray attenuation is A_x as shown in Figure 2. The
center point is fixed at the center of the VOI, which
include the shadow candidate detected by quoit filter. By
changing the radius r from 2[mm] to 9[mm] by 1[mm] and
X-ray attenuation A_x from 30 to 100 by 10 independently,
we generate 40 nodule models and memorize them into
the calculation computer.

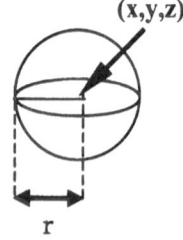

Figure 2: Nodule model

2.2 Curving blood vessels
We represent straight and curving parts of blood vessels using two joining circular cylinder models as shown in Figure 3. This curving blood vessel model is represented

CARS 2002 – H.U. Lemke, M.W. Vannier; K. Inamura, A.G. Farman, K. Doi & J.H.C. Reiber (Editors)
©CARS/Springer. All rights reserved.

using two radii of the cylinders r_1 and r_2, the directions θ_1, ϕ_1, θ_2 and ϕ_2. By changing the radii r_1 and r_2 from 1[mm] to 2[mm] by 1[mm], the directions θ from 0[deg] to 360[deg] by 22.5[deg] and the directions ϕ from 0[deg] to 180[deg] by 45[deg] independently, we generate 4704 curving blood vessel models and memorize them into the computer.

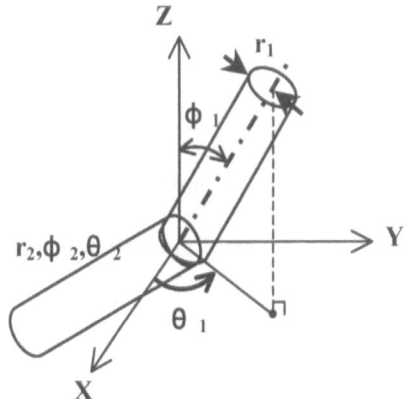

Figure 3: Curving blood vessel model

2.3 Branching blood vessels

We represent branching parts of blood vessels using three joining circular cylinder models. We generate 71664 branching blood vessel models and memorized them into the computer in the same way as Sec.2.2.

3. Generation of template images from object models

From the object models memorized in Sec.2, we generate artificial CT images (whose sizes are same as those of the VOI's) using a ray tracing method [4], which is a kind of computer graphics techniques. We utilize the generated artificial CT images as template images. Figure 4 shows an example of template images generated from a nodule model whose radius is 5 [mm]. Figure 5 shows another example of template images generated form a curving blood Bessel model.

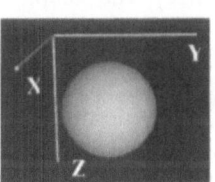

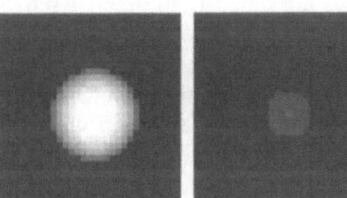

(a) A nodule model
whose radius is 5[mm]   (b) The template mages generated from Fig.4 (a)

Figure 4: A nodule model and the generated template images

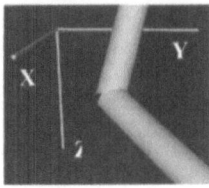
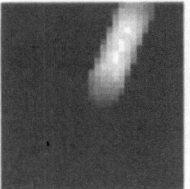
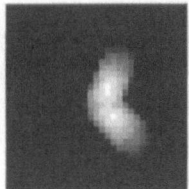
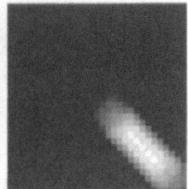

(a) A curving blood vessel   (b) The template images generated from Fig.5 (a)

Figure 5: A curving blood vessel model and the generated template images

CARS 2002 – H.U. Lemke, M.W. Vannier; K. Inamura, A.G. Farman, K. Doi & J.H.C. Reiber (Editors)

720

4. Recognition by template matching

Let VOI (x, y, z) be a voxel value at (x, y, z) in the VOI area, $TMPL_i^{ND}$ (x, y, z) a value at (x, y, z) in the template image generated from the i-th nodule model, and $TMPL_j^{BV}$ (x, y, z) a value at (x, y, z) in the template image generated from the j-th blood vessel model, respectively. We evaluate the similarity using a sum of squared differences (SSD) of the corresponding voxel values between the VOI and the template images :

$$SSD_i^{ND} = \sum_{x,y,z} \{VOI(x,y,z) - TMPL_i^{ND}(x,y,z)\}^2 \quad (1)$$

$$SSD_j^{BV} = \sum_{x,y,z} \{VOI(x,y,z) - TMPL_j^{BV}(x,y,z)\}^2 \quad (2)$$

We search for the optimal object models by minimizing the SSD values. If the ratio

$$\gamma^* = \frac{\min_j SSD_j^{BV}}{\min_i SSD_i^{ND}} \quad (3)$$

is larger than a certain threshold T, the VOI area is determined to be abnormal. Otherwise it is determined to be normal.

5. Experimental results

We use 38 actual CT images, which are low-dose CT images. A CT image is composed of about 30 slices. One slice cross section has 512×512 pixels. The resolutions of the CT images are 0.625 [mm/pixel] $\times 0.625$ [mm/pixel] $\times 10$ [mm/slice]. The sample CT images include 30 typical lung cancer shadows.

First we apply our quoit filter [2] to these sample CT images, and 547 pathological shadow candidates are extracted with the sensitivity over 95[%]. The ratio of the false positives is 13.6 [shadow/patient]. Next, we apply the method [3] and the method described in this paper to these shadow candidates. Table 1 shows the ratios of the false positives obtained by these methods, and their calculation times (the both methods have no additional false negatives). The calculation time is decreased drastically with keeping the accuracy.

Figure 6 shows an example of a VOI area of a candidate shadow detected by our quoit filter. Figure 7(a) and (b) show the optimal nodule model and the optimal blood vessel model, respectively. Figure 8 shows the template images of these object models. Since the ratio of the SSD values $\gamma^* = 1.27 \times 10^7$, the candidate shadow is correctly determined to be abnormal. Figure 9 shows another example of a VOI area of a candidate shadow detected by our quoit filter. Figure 10(a) and (b) show the optimal nodule model and the optimal blood vessel model, respectively. Figure 11 shows

CARS 2002 – H.U. Lemke, M.W. Vannier; K. Inamura, A.G. Farman, K. Doi & J.H.C. Reiber (Editors)
©CARS/Springer. All rights reserved.

template images of these object models. Since the ratio of the SSD values $\gamma^* = 0.82 \times 10^7$, the candidate shadow is correctly determined to be normal.

Table 1. Ratios of the false positives and the calculation times

	FP[shadow/patient] Smaller than 10[mm]	FP[shadow/patient] Larger than 10[mm]	Calculation time per patient
The method [3]	2.82	1.94	30 [min]
The proposed method	3.65	1.78	0.3 [sec]

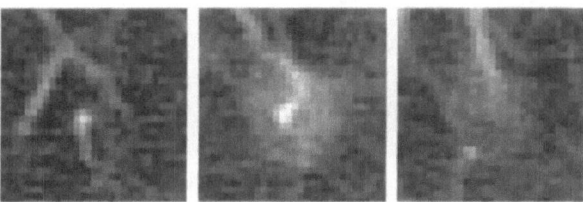

Figure 6: A sequence of a VOI area. The middle figure shows a shadow candidate.

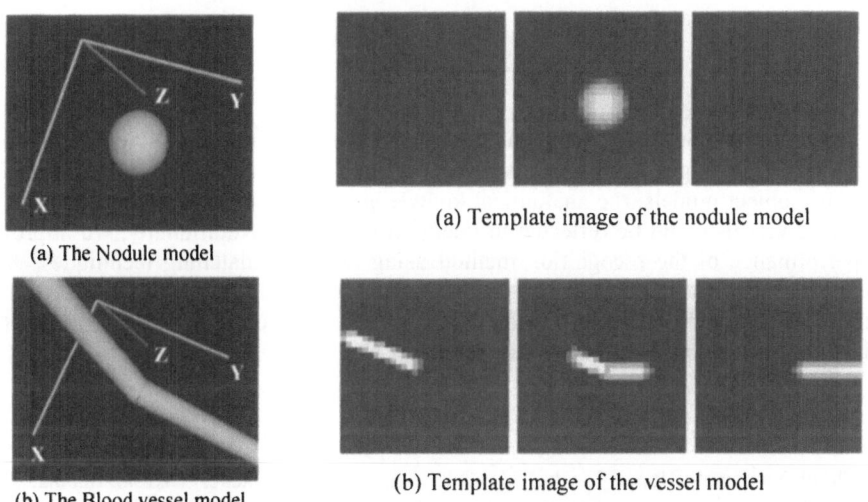

(a) The Nodule model

(a) Template image of the nodule model

(b) The Blood vessel model

(b) Template image of the vessel model

Figure 10: The optimal object model

Figure 11: The template image

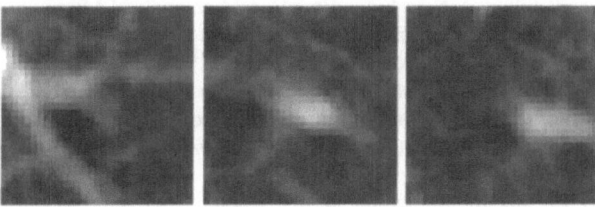

Figure 9: A sequence of a VOI area. The middle figure shows a shadow candidate.

CARS 2002 – H.U. Lemke, M.W. Vannier; K. Inamura, A.G. Farman, K. Doi & J.H.C. Reiber (Editors)

722

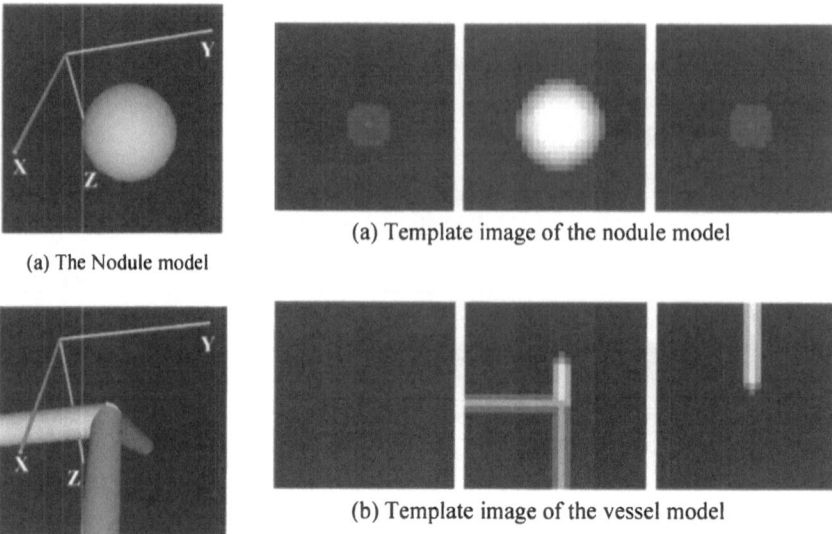

(a) The Nodule model

(a) Template image of the nodule model

(b) The Blood vessel model

(b) Template image of the vessel model

Figure 7: The optimal object model

Figure 8: The Template image

6. Conclusion

In this paper, we proposed an efficient algorithm to detect candidates of nodule shadows from X-ray CT images using models of cancers and blood vessels. By using such 3D geometric object models, the anatomical knowledge about the 3D structures of nodules and blood vessels could be reflected in recognition process. Additionally, we improved the performance of the recognition method using template matching techniques. As a result of the improvement of the performance, the calculation time of the recognition method is decreased drastically. By applying our new method to actual CT images (38 patient images), a good result has been acquired.

References

1. Shinji Yamamoto, Ippei Tanaka, Masahiro Senda, Yukio Tateno, Takeshi Iinuma, Toru Matsumoto, and Mitsuomi Matsumoto. "Image Processing for Computer-Aided Diagnosis of Lung Cancer by CT(LSCT)". *Systems and Computers in Japan*, Vol.25, No.2, pp.67-80, 1994.
2. Shinji Yamamoto, Mitsuomi Matsumoto, Yukio Tateno, Takeshi Iinuma, and Toru Matsumoto. "Quoit Filter: A New Filter Based on Mathematical Morphology to Extract the Isolated Shadow, and Its Application to Automatic Detection of Lung Cancer in X-Ray CT". In Proc. *13 th Int. Conf. Pattern Recognition II*, pp.3-7, 1996.
3. Hotaka Takizawa, Shinji Yamamoto, Tohru Matsumoto, Yukio Tateno, Takeshi Iinuma, and Mitsuomi Matsumoto. "Recognition of Lung Nodules from X-ray CT Images Using 3D MRF Models". In Proc. *15 th Int. Congress and Exhibition Computer Assisted Radiology and Surgery*,pp.570-575,2001
4. S.D.Roth, "Ray Casting for Modeling Solids", Computer Graphics and Image Processing, Vol.18, pp.109-144, 1982.

CARS 2002 – H.U. Lemke, M.W. Vannier; K. Inamura, A.G. Farman, K. Doi & J.H.C. Reiber (Editors)

Network based CAD system
for lung cancer screening by X-ray CT

Hiroshi Emoto[a], Shinji Yamamoto[b], Mitsuomi Matsumoto[c], Toru Matsumoto[d],
Yukio Tateno[d], Takeshi Iinuma[e]

[a] Communications Research Laboratory,
2-2-2 Hikaridai, Seika-cho, Kyoto 619-0286, Japan
[b] Toyohashi University of Technology, Aichi, Japan
[c] Tokyo Metropolitan College of Allied Medical Sciences, Tokyo, Japan
[d] National Institute of Radiological Science, Chiba, Japan
[e] Saitama Institute of Technology, Saitama, Japan

Abstract

This paper presents a network based CAD system for lung cancer screening by LSCT based on our proposed system. The system is server client style, and running on PC (Personal Computer). The system consists of two parts, automatic processing part and image based diagnosis part. The two parts are connected with network. The data of CT images are processed by automatic processing part in server, and have data transferring with client. The client of image based diagnosis part is constructed for radiologists. Radiologists operate the client to make screening works, and give final clinical records.

Keywords: Image processing, network based CAD, lung cancer screening

1. Introduction

The development of Computer-Aided Diagnosis (CAD) for pulmonary diseases can be loosely grouped into two categories based on the past researches, by using digital chest radiography [1-3] and CT [4-9]. Recently, automatic detection of pulmonary nodules by CT and CAD system constructions have been reported [4-9].

We are developing a CAD system for lung cancer screening by using X-ray CT (LSCT). The LSCT is a mobile-type CT scanner for mass screening of lung cancer, and the images from LSCT are round 30 slices per person. We have constructed a CAD system for radiologists to support the mass screening works [10-13].

On the other hand, as the progress of network technology including broadband communication and computer performance including the personal computer, telemedicine become an important task to provide high quality of medical services. There are reports to present the methods of data transferring and archiving, platform and application construction, and so on [14]. However, the construction of network based CAD system needs new concepts and methods based on conventional technologies.

This paper presents a network based CAD system for lung cancer screening by LSCT based on our proposed system. The system consists of two parts, automatic processing part and image based diagnosis part. The two parts are connected with network. The

724

system is server client style, and running on PC (Personal Computer). The data of CT images are processed by automatic processing part in server, and have data transferring with client. The client of image based diagnosis part is constructed for radiologists. Radiologists operate the client to make screening works, and give final clinical records.

2. Overview

2.1 Concepts of network based CAD system

Generally, network based CAD system should consider the following conditions. Processing time and high performance computer are needed to provide screening support data obtained from CT data in large quantities, database is required for data store and reference, multiple users can use the system from the places which are connected with network. The server client style is better to satisfy the above conditions. The server can respond the requests from clients with physical distance, and provide collaboration services for multi-user. The client is set at hand of doctor, can use personal computer, and has the functions of screening support and data transferring. The concepts of network based CAD system are shown in Figure.1.

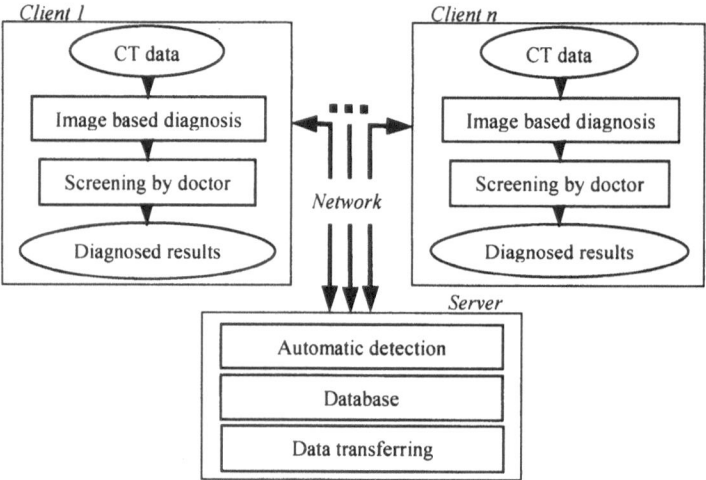

Figure.1 Concepts of network based CAD system

2.2 Configuration of the CAD system

The system we proposed is designed based on two concepts, network based and PC based system construction. Server client style is applied to the system construction, and both of server and client is connected with network. The server has the functions to store the data transferred from client, detect the candidate regions of lung cancer, generate the support information and transfer back the data to client. The client has the functions of data transferring, communication with server, screening support, and other options. Based on above considerations, the CAD system is separated into two parts, automatic processing part running on server and image based diagnosis part running on client. The server generates the screening support data, and the client is used for screening. The results obtained by automatic processing part are provided to image based diagnosis part through

CARS 2002 – H.U. Lemke, M.W. Vannier; K. Inamura, A.G. Farman, K. Doi & J.H.C. Reiber (Editors)

network as support information for increasing the performance of screening. The configuration of the CAD system is shown in Figure.2.

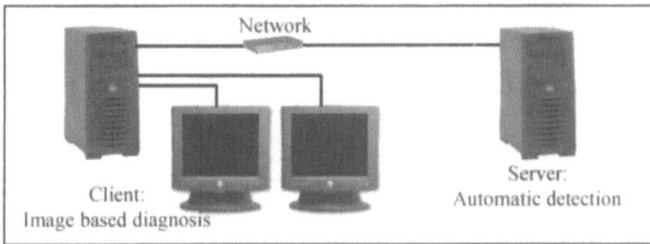

Figure.2 Configuration of the CAD system

3. Server: Automatic detection part

The automatic processing part running on server is including three functions, storing the data transferred from a client, automatic processing to obtain the candidate regions of lung cancer, and transfer back the results to client. The CT data are stored into the server after the server received a signal of data transferring from a client. Image processing procedure is prepared for candidate region detection of lung cancer such as lung region extraction, noise remove, and isolated shadow detection. The results of processing are including size, shape, position, and screening support images. The progress of processing is transferred to client for confirmation. After the processing finished, a signal is sent to client, and all of results are transferred to client when the server received the command of result transfer.

4. Client: Image based diagnosis part

The image based diagnosis part running on client is a visual interface, and uses two monitors to support screening. One monitor is the main monitor to display a main window, and the other is the support monitor to display sub-windows. The main window has two functions, one is to display system menu including data file operation, automatic processing selection, screening support selection, and other options. The other is that the main window is displaying original images slice by slice along with body-axis as an animation. The speed of the animation displaying can be selected by request, of course including the display slice by slice through one mouse click. Several functions are directly displayed with the original image including measurement, selection of ROI (Region Of Interest), and changing of window level and width.

Several sub-windows are displayed on the support monitor, they are MIP window, front view window, result window, comparison window, and clinical record window, we called. Namely, they are displaying MIP (Maximum Intensity Projection) image, front view of lung region and the result images detected automatically, respectively. The MIP window shows MIP image from different angle as an animation. The front view window shows a 2D image of displaying the form of the lung region like X-ray film. The result window shows images of the detected results as an animation along with body-axis like main window. Comparison window can show the past image to compare two or three images, and search the changing of candidate regions. All comments for diagnosis can be written into clinical record form, and the comments are set with all results of images.

726

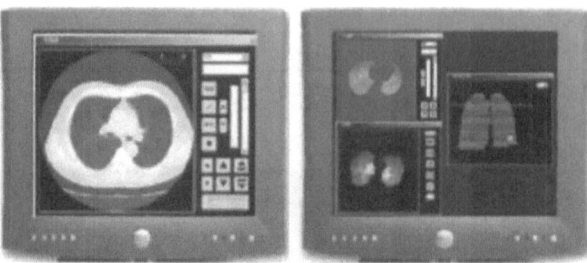

Figure.3 Layout of screening support mode

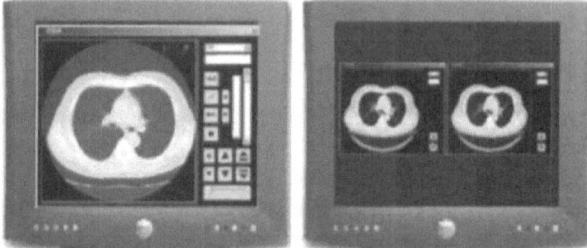

Figure.4 Layout of comparison mode

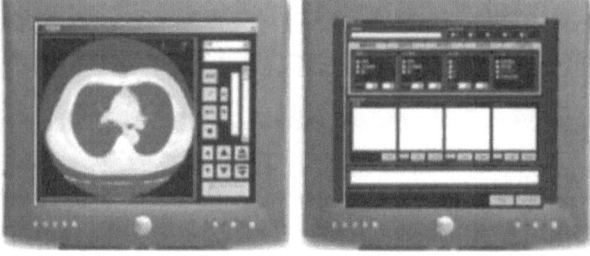

Figure.5 Layout of clinical record writing mode

Based on the request of screening work, we provide three modes to supporting, screening support mode, comparison mode, and clinical record writing mode. The layout of screening support mode is shown in Figure.3, result window, MIP window, and front view window are displayed on support monitor to help the screening work. The layout of comparison mode is shown in Figure.4, the past images are displayed on support monitor to search the changing of candidate regions. Of course, the animation of past images on the support monitor is linked with the main window on the main monitor. The layout of clinical record writing mode is shown in Figure.5, the form of clinical record is displayed on support monitor. The diagnosed results can be recorded by character and figure, which are inputted by key broad and mouse drawing, and the form is stored with images as a data set.

5. Screening support

The results obtained by automatic processing part are provided to image based diagnosis part as support information for radiologists to make screening. The position and number of candidate slices are displayed on the main window and the result window, and colour rings indicating candidate slices are superimposed on the grey image of result window. By clicking the indicator, which indicates the position of candidate slices, the window shows directly the next candidate slice. The animation of result window is linked with main window for displaying the same slice.

In the front view window, the candidate slices obtained by automatic processing part are indicated by colour lines, and superimposed on the image of front view of lung region. The MIP window shows an animation of MIP images from different angle, and the animation is repeated during diagnosis of this sample. It can roughly provide the 3D position, shape and size of the cancer region if there is a cancer in this sample.

All of the resources described above are provided to radiologist as support information for screening, and final result of diagnosis is given by integrating all of the resources.

6. Experiments

We are applying samples including cancer samples to this CAD system for evaluating each function with radiologists. The radiologists found it easy to use, the animation displaying is valuable for mass screening, and the results of automatic detection are helpful as support information.

The data transfer is evaluated using two kinds of network, private network and intranet, and 100BASE-TX is used for the experiments. Data transfer time is measured for small data, 1 patient, and large data, 100 patients. Transfer time of sending back the results from server to client is also measured. Compressed and uncompressed conditions are considered. Transfer time is measured 5 times, and we show the mean.

Table 1 Transfer time from client to server using private network

	1 patient		100 patient	
	Compressed (6.59MB)	Uncompressed (12.5MB)	Compressed (659MB)	Uncompressed (1250MB)
Mean (sec.)	0.68	1.35	67.99	142.04

Table 2 Transfer time from server to client using private network

	1 patient		100 patient	
	Compressed (4.01MB)	Uncompressed (24.6MB)	Compressed (401MB)	Uncompressed (2460MB)
Mean (sec.)	0.43	2.64	44.20	264.44

Table 3 Transfer time from client to server using intranet

	1 patient		100 patient	
	Compressed (6.59MB)	Uncompressed (12.5MB)	Compressed (659MB)	Uncompressed (1250MB)
Mean (sec.)	0.88	1.75	89.69	182.55

Table 4 Transfer time from server to client using intranet

	1 patient		100 patient	
	Compressed (4.01MB)	Uncompressed (24.6MB)	Compressed (401MB)	Uncompressed (2460MB)
Mean (sec.)	0.51	3.17	51.41	311.45

Table 1and 2 show the time transferring image data from client to server, and the results data from server to client. The both experiments are using a private network.

Table 3 and 4 show the time transferring image data from client to server, and the results data from server to client. The both experiments are using an intranet.

According to the results above, data transfer is not a heavy charge to the CAD system although the transfer time is increasing as the data in quantities are increasing. On the other hand, the transfer time using private network is different from intranet, but we can accept the difference between both. We can also recognize that the transfer time is dependent on the traffic of network. The time of automatic detection of cancer candidate region is longer than the data transfer [13], but we can carry out the processing of automatic detection off line, namely, after received the original image data from client, the server can detect the candidate in background, send message to client if the detection is finished.

We can say that the stress is not felt if the server has few accesses. On the other hand, the time of automatic processing is increasing as the accesses are increasing, so that it is better to construct a server of clustering of PC. As the performance of computer is increasing and broadband of network are used wildly, the above points are improved.

7. Conclusion

We have described the network based CAD system for lung cancer screening by using X-ray CT (LSCT) and the radiologists found it easy to use. The system consists of two parts, automatic processing part and image based diagnosis part. The two parts are connected with network. The system is server client style, and running on PC. The data of CT images are processed by automatic processing part in server, and have data transferring with client. The client of image based diagnosis part is constructed for radiologists.
. Radiologists operate the client to make screening works, and give final clinical records.

The experimental results show that the data transfer is not a heavy charge to the system, so that the system can be applied to the application from multiple points connected with network. We are evaluating the system with radiologists continually, and improve this system based on comments. We also construct a database for reference, and consider the feasibility study.

References

1. F.M.Carrascal, M.Cabrera, J.M.Carreira, et al, Proc. CAR'96, pp.368-373 (1996)
2. S.Katsuragawa, H.MacMahon, T.Ishida, et al, Proc. CAR'96, pp.380-384 (1996)
3. K.R.Hoffmann, R.Engelmann, H.MacMahon, et al, Proc. CAR'97, pp.337-341 (1997)
4. W.J.Ryan, J.E.Reed, S.J.Swensen, et al, Proc. CAR'96, pp.385-389 (1996)
5. K.R.Heitmann, H.-U.Kauczor, T.Uthmann, et al, Proc. CAR'97, pp.331-336 (1997)
6. M.S.Brown, M.F.McNitt-Gray, J.G.Goldin, et al, Proc. ICIP'97, Vol.III, pp.516-519 (1997)
7. Y.Kawata, N.Niki, H.Ohmatsu, et, Proc. ICIP'97, Vol.III, pp.528-530 (1997)
8. N.Niki, Y,Kawata, and M,Kubo, Proc. CARS 2001, pp.593-598 (2001)
9. C.L.Novak, L.Fan, J.Z.Qian, and et al, Proc. CARS 2001, pp.599-604 (2001)
10. S.Yamamoto, M.Matsumoto, Y.Tateno, et al, Proc. ICPR'96, Vol.II-B, pp.3-7 (1996)
11. S.Yamamoto, H.Jiang, M.Matsumoto, et al, Proc. IEEE 3rd WACV, pp.236-241 (1996)
12. H.Jiang, N.Masuto, S.Yamamoto, et al, Proc.WCAD, pp.125-130 (1998)
13. S.Yamamoto, H.Takizawa, H.Jiang, et al, Proc. CARS 2001, pp.605-610 (2001)
14. T.M.Buzug, H.Handels, and D.Holz, Kluwer Academic/Plenum Publishers, New York, (2001)

CARS 2002 – H.U. Lemke, M.W. Vannier, K. Inamura, A.G. Farman, K. Doi & J.H.C. Reiber (Editors)

Computer classification of lung tumors from chest CT images according to the types of tissue using 3D extended Voronoi diagram

Yasushi Hirano[a], Jun-ichi Hasegawa[b], Junichiro Toriwaki[a], Hironobu Ohmatsu[c] and Kenji Eguchi[d]

[a] Faculty of Engineering, Nagoya University,
Furo-cho, Chikusa-ku, Nagoya, Aichi 464-8603, Japan

[b] School of Computer and Cognitive Sciences, Chukyo University,
101 Tokodachi, Kaizu-cho, Toyota, Aichi 470-0393, Japan

[c] National Cancer Center Hospital East,
6-5-1 Kashiwanoha, Kashiwa, Chiba 277-0882, Japan

[d] School of Medicine, Tokai University,
143 Shimokasuya, Isehara, Kanagawa, 259-1193, Japan

Abstract

A method to quantify the shrinkage of lung lobe using chest X-ray CT images is proposed in this paper. The shrinkage of lung lobe is caused by the convergence concerning the interstitium. It is known that the existence of the convergence gives us useful information about the malignancy of tumor. If the convergence occurs, vessels are distributed densely in the neighborhood of tumor. In this paper, the volume of the Voronoi diagrams using the vessel regions are calculated. We propose two features using the difference of the volumes of the Voronoi regions near the tumor region and apart from the tumor region. Features are calculated using seventy-eight cases. First, as the result of the significance test using twenty-nine cases for which the degree of the convergence was evaluated by medical doctors, it is shown that both the two features tend to have high values when the convergence exists. Next, using other twenty-five cases, the proposed feature cans classify the cases into types of the tissue which tend to cause the convergence or not. Finally, The result of benign/malignant discrimination using seventy-eight cases was performed. False positive rate was $0.26(7/27)$ and false negative rate was $0.14(7/51)$.

Keywords: 3D extended Voronoi diagram, classification of tumor, chest CT image

1. Introduction

In this paper, we propose a new method to quantify the shrinkage of the lung lobe caused by the convergence of tissues using three-dimensional (3D) chest X-ray CT images. The convergence is the phenomenon that tissues (blood vessels, bronchus, interstitium, etc.) around the tumor are pulled toward the tumor. The convergence is often observed when the tumor is malignant, especially adenocarcinoma. It is known that the existence of the convergence gives us useful information to discriminate benign tumors from malignant ones. Although, in the computer classification, the existence of the convergence also

730

provides useful information, the convergence has not been quantified except for the convergence concerning blood vessels and bronchus[1,2]. Here we propose a method to quantify the convergence concerning the interstitium using the 3D extended Voronoi division. It is thought that the convergence concerning the interstitium causes the shrinkage of the lung lobe in which tumor exists. Lung lobes consist of small regions which are called the pulmonary segments and each pulmonary artery dominates a pulmonary segment. The dominative relationship will not change even if the shrinkage of the lung lobe may occur. In the meanwhile, the pulmonary veins exist on the boundary of the pulmonary segments. It is thought that the blood vessels (pulmonary arteries and veins) are distributing densely, if the shrinkage of the lung lobe occurs. Therefore, if we calculate the Voronoi diagrams using the vessel regions as seeds after grouping them by the radius of vessels, the volumes of the Voronoi regions near the tumor will be smaller than the volumes of the Voronoi regions apart from the tumor in the lung with tissue convergence. We propose two features measuring such property. The features are calculated for seventy-eight cases of the chest X-ray CT images. It is shown that the proposed features significantly related to the convergence, the types of the tissue which construct the lung tumors, and malignancy of tumor.

2. Method

Lung regions, vessel regions, and tumor regions are extracted from chest X-ray CT images using the threshold operation against CT values and the distance transformation[1,3]. The vessel regions are linearized by the 3D thinning method using the Euclidean distance transformation[4]. Each voxel on the line figures which are transformed from the vessel region is given the radius of the vessel. The voxels are classified into groups according to radius values. The 3D extended Voronoi division[5] is performed using the group or the groups as seeds. The average volumes of the Voronoi regions near the tumor (M_{Tr}) and in the lung regions (M_{Lr}) are calculated. The vessel regions and the tumor regions are not included to the volumes of the Voronoi regions. Finally, two features, $M_r = M_{Lr}/M_{Tr}$ and $M'_r = M_r/L$ are calculated, where r and L is the radius of the vessel and the volume of the lung region, respectively. If the convergence occurs, the vessels are distributing densely near the tumors. This leads to the result which

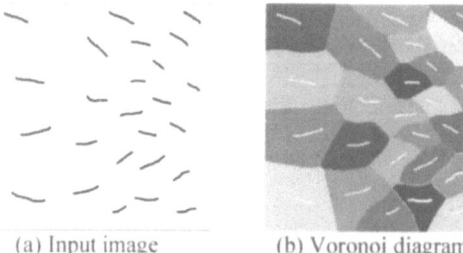

(a) Input image   (b) Voronoi diagram

Fig.1 Example of the Voronoi diagram
The line segments distributes densely in the right half of
the input image and the Voronoi regions are small in that part.

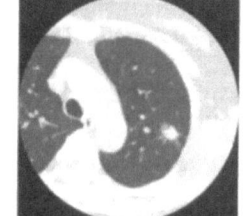

Fig.2 Example of CT images

the volumes of Voronoi regions near the tumor become smaller in comparison with those apart from the tumor. As the result, the features M_r and M'_r become larger, if the

CARS 2002 – H.U. Lemke, M.W. Vannier; K. Inamura, A.G. Farman, K. Doi & J.H.C. Reiber (Editors)

convergence occurs. Fig.1 shows an example using an artificial figure in two-dimensional space. The feature M_r will be close to 1.0, when the distribution of vessels is uniform over the whole lung region, in other words, when the convergence does not occur.

Table 1 Specification of CT images used in the experiments

Size of a slice [*pixels*]	512 x 512
Number of slices per image	43 ~ 65
Size of pixel in slice [*mm*]	0.29 x 0.29 ~ 0.43 x 0.43
Reconstruction pitch [*mm*]	1.0
Thickness [*mm*]	2.0

Table 2 Details of CT images

	Degree of convergence					Total
	Nil	Slight	Moderate	Intense	Unknown	
Benign	6	1	0	0	20	27
Malignant	5	6	7	4	29	51
Total	11	7	7	4	49	78

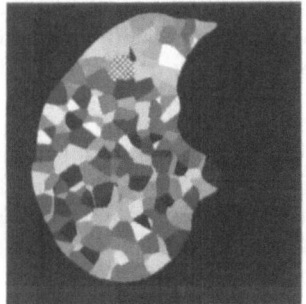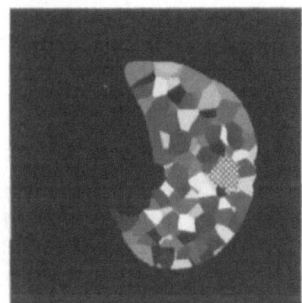
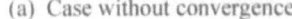

(a) Case without convergence   (b) Case with intense convergence

Fig.3 Voronoi diagrams obtained from CT images

3. Results

Fig.2 shows an example of CT images used in this experiment. The specification and details of CT images are shown in Table 1 and 2, respectively. Two features M_r and M'_r were calculated for seventy-eight cases of thin slice chest X-ray CT images, where $r = 0.4$ ~ $0.6mm$. The twenty-nine cases were given the degree of the convergence by medical doctors. Fig.3 shows the Voronoi diagrams obtained from actual CT images. The Voronoi diagram was calculated in 3D space in this experiment. Cross sections of Voronoi diagrams at the center of tumor are shown in Fig.3. As we mentioned above, vessel regions and tumor regions are not used for the calculation of volumes of Voronoi regions, but the vessel regions are not removed in Fig.3 for the easiness of understanding. The hatched regions mean tumor regions. It is confirmed that in the case without the

CARS 2002 – H.U. Lemke, M.W. Vannier; K. Inamura, A.G. Farman, K. Doi & J.H.C. Reiber (Editors)

732

convergence, volumes of Voronoi regions are almost uniform over the whole lung region(Fig.3(a)), while in the case with the intense convergence the Voronoi regions near the tumor are smaller than those apart from the tumor(Fig.3(b)).

Scatter diagrams of features were calculated using the twenty-nine cases with the degree of the convergence(Fig.4). It was confirmed that the cases with the convergence tend to have larger values of M_r and M'_r. The Mann-Whitney test was applied to the distributions of M_r and M'_r. The null hypothesis H_0 : "There is no difference between the distributions of the cases with the convergence and the cases without the convergence." was assumed. Concerning both two features the hypothesis was rejected with the level of significance 0.05. This means that the features tend to be significantly smaller in the cases without the convergence than in the cases with the convergence.

The feature M_r was calculated for the twenty-five cases which consist of two groups : the type of tissue which tends to cause the convergence(Type A), and the type of tissue which does not tend to cause the convergence(Type B). The former contains the well differentiated (w/d) adenocarcinoma(malignant), and the latter contains the squamous cell carcinoma(malignant) and the hamartoma(benign). In this experiment, we used fourteen cases of the w/d adenocarcinoma, five cases of the squamous cell carcinoma, and six cases of the hamartoma. The Nearest-Neighbor decision rule was used for the classification and the leave-one-out method was employed for performance evaluation. The two features, variance of CT values in the peripheral region of tumor and M_r, were used in this classification. The false negative rate(FN) was defined as the ratio of the number of the misclassified Type A(That is, classified as Type B) to the number of all Type A cases, and the false positive rate(FP) was defined as the ratio of the number of the misclassified Type B to the number of all Type B cases. FN was 0.07(1/14), and FP was 0.09(1/11). The scatter diagram is shown in Fig.5.

Finally, the benign/malignant discrimination was performed by the Nearest-Neighbor decision rule using seventy-eight cases. As the result, FN was 0.14(7/51) and FP was 0.26(7/27). The used features were M_r, the entropy of CT values in a tumor, and the variance of CT values in peripheral region of a tumor. Here FN was defined as the ratio of the number of misclassified malignant tumors to the number of all malignant tumors, and

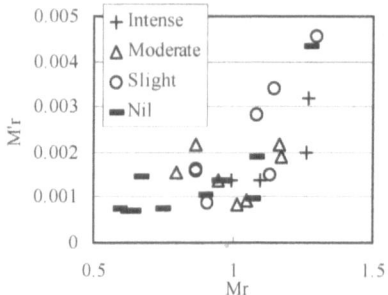
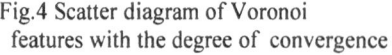
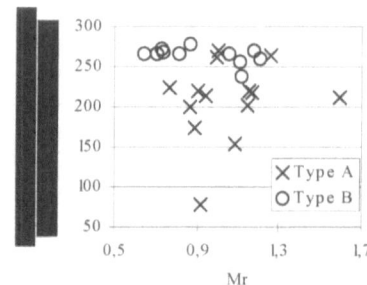

Fig.4 Scatter diagram of Voronoi features with the degree of convergence

Fig.5 Scatter diagram of Voronoi features with tissue type

FP was defined as the ratio of the number of misclassified benign tumors to the number of all benign tumors.

4. Conclusion

In this paper, two features using the 3D extended Voronoi diagram were proposed. It was shown that the proposed features significantly related to the degree of the convergence and types of tissue. This means that proposed features are useful to quantify the convergence and classify the tissue type, and could be used for the benign/malignant discrimination. Because the accuracy of benign/malignant discrimination was not so high, the optimization of the features will be needed.

Future work includes the improvement of the ability of the proposed features, development of better features for the benign/malignant discrimination, and development of the CAD system for the discrimination of lung tumor from chest X-ray CT images.

Acknowledgements

Authors thank colleagues of Prof. Toriwaki's Laboratory of Nagoya University for useful discussions. The data conversion program developed in Prof. Niki's laboratory of Tokushima University was used to transfer CT images. Parts of this research were supported by the Grant-in-Aid for Scientific Research from the Ministry of Education, Culture, Sports, Science and Technology, the Grant-in-Aid for Private University High-Tech Research Center from Ministry of Education, Culture, Sports, Science and Technology and the Grant-in-Aid for Cancer Research from the Ministry of Health, Labor and Welfare, Japanese Government.

References

1. Y.Hirano, Y.Mekada, J.Hasegawa, J.Toriwaki, H.Ohmatsu and K.Eguchi : "Three Dimensional Concentration Index -A Local Feature for Analyzing Three Dimensional Digital line Patterns and Its Application to Chest X-ray CT Images-", *Proc. of International Conference on Pattern Recognition (ICPR) '98*, A.K.Jain, S.Venkatesh and B.C.Lovell, pp.1040-1043, IEEE Computer Society, Los Alamitos, 1998
2. H.Shikata, H.Kitaoka, B.Keserci, Y.Sato and S.Tamura : "Quantitative evaluation of the spatial distribution of vessels surrounding pulmonary nodules", *Proc. of Computer Assisted Radiology and Surgery (CARS) 2000*, H.U.Lemke, M.W.Vannier; K.Inamura, A.G.Farman and K.Doi, pp.761-766, ELSEVIER, Amsterdam, 2000
3. Y.Hirano, J.Hasegawa, J.Toriwaki, H.Ohmatsu and K.Eguchi : "Extraction of tumor regions keeping boundary shape information from chest X-ray CT images and benign/malignant discrimination", *Proc. of Computer Assisted Radiology and Surgery (CARS) 2001*, H.U.Lemke, M.W.Vannier; K.Inamura, A.G.Farman and K.Doi, pp.617-622, ELSEVIER, Amsterdam, 2001
4. T.Saito and J.Toriwaki : " Sequential thinning algorithm for three dimensional digital pictures using the Euclidean distance transformation", *Proc. of 9th Scandinavian Conference on Image Analysis*, Borgefors G , pp.507-516, Swedish Society for Automated Image Analysis, Göteborg, 1995
5. T.Saito and J.Toriwaki : "Algorithms of three dimensional Euclidean distance transformation and extended digital Voronoi diagram, and analysis of human liver section images", *Journal of the Institute of Image Electronics Engineering of Japan*, Vol.21, No.5, pp.468-474, 1992 (In Japanese)

Special Session on 3D CAD

CARS 2002 – H.U. Lemke, M.W. Vannier; K. Inamura, A.G. Farman, K. Doi & J.H.C. Reiber (Editors)

Visualization and segmentation techniques in 3-D ultrasound images

Aaron Fenster and Dónal B. Downey
The John P. Robarts Research Institute
100 Perth Drive, London, ON, N6G 4N9 Canada, and
Department of Diagnostic Radiology & Nuclear Medicine
The University of Western Ontario, London, ON, Canada

Abstract

2-D viewing of 3-D anatomy, using conventional ultrasound (US), limits our ability to quantify and visualize complex pathology. Efforts have focused on overcoming this deficiency by developing 3-D US imaging techniques that are capable of rapidly producing 3-D images on inexpensive computers. The availability of 3-D US images has allowed the development of techniques to segment and quantify organs and structures such as the prostate and carotid plaque volume and surface morphology. In this paper, we describe 3-D US visualization techniques in common use as well as techniques to segment the carotid arteries and the prostate. For the segmentation approaches we used both a 2-D and 3-D Discrete Dynamic Contour, in which internal contour and image based forces drive the boundary to edges. Results and applications of the segmentation in monitoring carotid disease progression/regression and in prostate brachytherapy will be described.

Keywords: 3-D ultrasound, segmentation, rendering

1. Introduction

Developments in CT and MRI over the past 2 decades have greatly accelerated the use of 3-D visualization and quantification. Medical ultrasound (US) has also benefited from major advances in technology and has become an indispensable imaging modality. In the last decade, US has further advanced with the development of 3-D US, in which existing ultrasound technology is combined with advances in 3-D image visualization [1-5]. In addition, advanced computational techniques have led to development of segmentation algorithms allowing quantitative analysis of volume and shape. This paper discusses 3-D US visualization techniques and recent advances in 3-D US segmentation.

2. Advantages of 3-D ultrasound

Because 2-D US images represent thin planes, and their location/orientation is controlled manually by the user, it is difficult to reproduce a particular view at a later time and it is difficult to form a mental impression of complex 3-D anatomy. 3-D US provides a volume image that can be registered to an image obtained at a later time and allows the use of viewing techniques to demonstrate complex anatomy. In addition, the availability

CARS 2002 – H.U. Lemke, M.W. Vannier; K. Inamura, A.G. Farman, K. Doi & J.H.C. Reiber (Editors)

738

of a complete 3-D image of an organ or the pathology allows the development of segmentation approaches for use in rapid automated or semi-automated measurements.

3. 3-D ultrasound visualization

Many algorithms are available to visualize 3-D CT, MRI and US images. Due to the variety in the methods used to acquire 3-D US images, the quality and geometric accuracy of the 3-D US image can vary. Never the less, the 3-D display technique often plays a dominant role in the ability to obtain the desired information from the 3-D US image. Over the past decade, many 3-D US display techniques have been employed, the two used most often used are: multi-planar reformatting (MPR) and volume rendering (VR) [6].

3.1 Multi-Planar Reformatting (MPR)

The MPR technique reformats the 3-D US image to a display of 2-D planes by extracting any desired plane from the 3-D data set and displaying it with 3-D cues. Three approaches have been used. In the **crossed-planes** approach, the extracted planes are presented in their correct relative 3-D position and orientation as shown in Fig. 1a. The user can move each plane to reveal desired views of the anatomy. A second technique uses the **cube-view** approach (Fig. 1b), in which the extracted 2-D US images are texture-mapped onto the faces of a polyhedron. The user can select any face and move it, while the appropriate 2-D US image is texture-mapped in real-time on the new face [5]. In a third approach, the **extracted planes** (typically 3 orthogonal) are shown beside each other with lines drawn on each extracted plane to designate their intersection with the other planes [7,8].

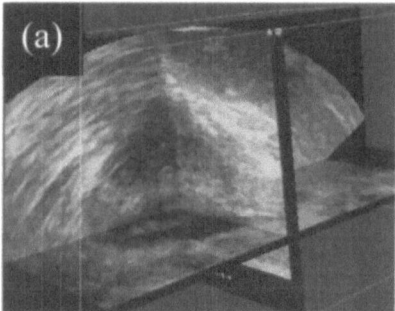 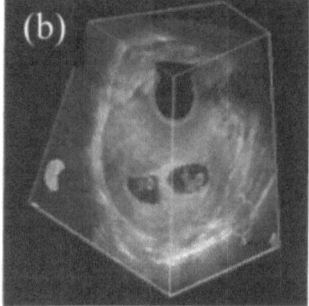

Figure 1. Two MPR techniques are shown: a) Crossed planes view of a prostate, in which the extracted planes are orthogonal and intersecting with each other. b) Cube-view approach of first trimester twins, in which the extracted planes are texture mapped onto the faces of a polyhedron.

3.2 Volume Rendering Techniques (VR)

Although the MPR technique is the most common visualization method used to view 3-D US images, it is limited because it only provides 2-D images with 3-D cues and not the complete 3-D information. Volume-rendering approaches are frequently used to view 3-D CT and MRI images by projecting the entire 3-D image onto a 2-D plane. Typically, this is accomplished using ray-casting techniques, in which a 2-D array of rays is projected through the 3-D image [6-8]. The volume elements (voxels) intersecting each ray are weighted and then summed in various ways to produce the desired effect. 3-D US imaging has made effective use of three VR techniques: maximum intensity projection,

CARS 2002 – H.U. Lemke, M.W. Vannier; K. Inamura, A.G. Farman, K. Doi & J.H.C. Reiber (Editors)
^cCARS/Springer. All rights reserved.

translucency rendering and surface enhancement as shown in Fig. 2. Interpretation of complex images is difficult in VR images because all the 3-D information is projected onto a 2-D plane. Thus, viewing subtle contrast differences between different soft tissues is difficult. It has been used most successfully to view surfaces, which are clearly distinguishable, such as fetal structures surrounded by amniotic fluid [9,10] tissue/blood interfaces, and power or color Doppler 3-D images [11].

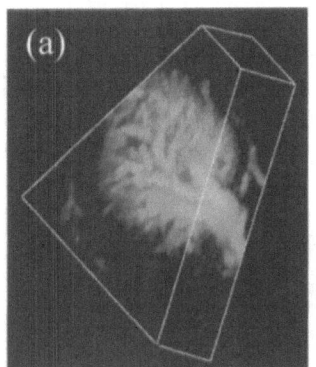 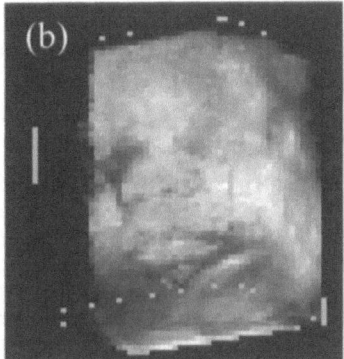

Figure 2. Two VR techniques of 3-D US images. a) Maximum intensity projection of a human kidney power Doppler image. b) Volume rendering with enhancement of surfaces of the fetal face.

4. Segmentation using 3-D ultrasound images

Because 3-D US images provide the user with a complete view of the organ or pathology, accurate measurement of its volume is possible. Because the use of manual planimetry technique for measuring volume is time-consuming and tedious, investigators are developing automated or semi-automated segmentation techniques.

4.1 The need for 3-D US-guided prostate brachytherapy

The most common form of prostate brachytherapy involves the implantation of about 80 radioactive seeds (*e.g.*, ^{125}I) into the prostate. Accurate positioning of the seeds within the prostate first involves pre-implantation dose planning (pre-plan), in which CT or US is used to determine the prostate geometry and the location of radiation sensitive structures. The pre-plan is then used at a later outpatient visit to implant the seeds, while the patient is positioned in the approximate same position as in the pre-plan. Since it is difficult to position the patient for pre-implantation and implantation procedures in the same way, errors in seed placement can occur. Performing the procedure with 3-D US imaging with rapid scanning and immediate viewing of the prostate anatomy permits pre-implant dose planning and seed implantation at the same session thereby avoiding problems of repositioning, prostate motion, and prostate size changes. Thus, an efficient procedure requires integration of 3-D US imaging with efficient prostate segmentation.

We reported on our development of a prostate 3-D US imaging technique [12,13] and used it for prostate cryosurgery [14]. We have been extending this approach to 3-D US guided prostate brachytherapy with the development of prostate, needle and seed segmentation. In the following section we describe our prostate segmentation approach.

740

4.2 3-D Segmentation of the prostate

Our approach is to segment the prostate boundary in sequential 2-D image slices and join these to provide the complete 3-D shape of the prostate. We used the Discrete Dynamic Contour (DDC), which is a sequence of points connected by straight-line segments that deforms automatically to fit the desired boundary [15-17]. Our used two phases: in the first, the DDC is initialized by an approximate outline of the object; and in the second, the initial outline is deformed automatically to fit the desired prostate boundary [15].

Initialization: In the initialization phase, the operator selects 4 points on the boundary of the prostate in a 2-D image slice of the 3-D image. We use two points in the midline defining an axis of symmetry and two points at both sides of the base defining the width (Fig. 3a). Using these points, which define the size of the prostate, we calculate an initial boundary based on a model equation of the prostate as in Fig. 3a [15].

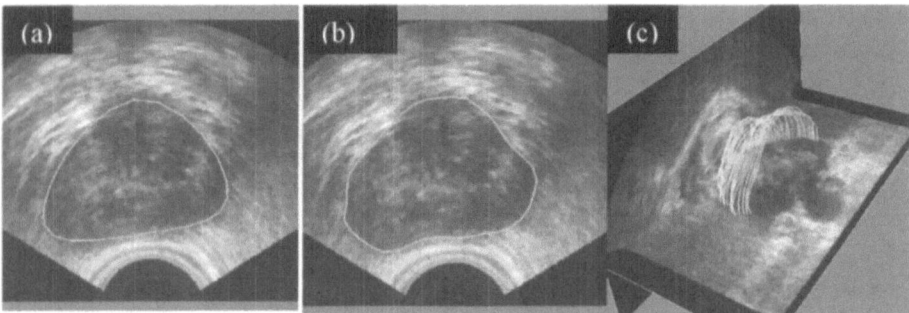

Figure 3. Prostate segmentation procedure steps. a) 4 points identified by the user on the prostate boundary initialize the DDC. b) The initial boundary is refined using the DDC approach. c) The 3-D segmentation is completed by repeatedly using one boundary to initialize an adjacent section.

Refinement: The boundary refinement phase uses the initial contour in the operation of the DDC, which is based on simple dynamics, as described by Eq. 1. A weighted combination of internal ($\vec{f}_i^{int}$), image ($\vec{f}_i^{img}$) and damping ($\vec{f}_i^{d}$) forces are applied to each vertex i of the DDC, resulting in a total force, $\vec{f}_i^{tot}$. This boundary evolves by the movement of the vertices until the total force acting on each vertex is zero.

$$\vec{f}_i^{tot} = w_i^{int} \vec{f}_i^{int} + w_i^{img} \vec{f}_i^{img} + \vec{f}_i^{d}, \qquad (1)$$

where w_i^{img} and w_i^{int} are weights for the image and internal forces, respectively [15,17].

The external force is proportional to the local image gradient, causing the vertex to seek the prostate boundary. The internal force mimics an elastic force and is proportional to edge length, causing the boundary to be smooth. We have found that a choice of $w_i^{img} = 1.0$ and $w_i^{int} = 0.3$ results in optimal segmentation. Fig. 3b shows the result of the boundary refinement with the prostate image, demonstrating good results. To segment the complete prostate, we used this contour to initialize images from adjacent slices repeatedly, 1 mm apart, until the complete prostate was segmented as shown in Fig. 3c.

CARS 2002 – H.U. Lemke, M.W. Vannier; K. Inamura, A.G. Farman, K. Doi & J.H.C. Reiber (Editors)
©CARS/Springer. All rights reserved.

5. Need for segmentation of carotid plaques

Improved strategies to treat atherosclerosis non-surgically require sensitive non-invasive imaging techniques to monitor carotid disease progression and regression. Use of 2-D US demonstrated mixed results in quantifying changes in plaque morphology. 3-D US of the carotid plaque may allow quantitative monitoring of plaque changes in volume and morphology, providing important information about the plaque's response to therapy.

5.1 Segmentation of carotid plaques from 3-D US images

We developed a semi-automated segmentation algorithm based on 3-D deformable models requiring minimal user interaction and processing time to obtain surface of plaques [18,19]. We used a 3-D deformable model, in which the boundary was defined as a series of vertices. This allows internal and external forces to be calculated at each vertex, using image information, and moved iteratively until the forces acting on the vertices are zero. We used 3 steps: placement of the initial mesh inside the vessel; model inflation towards the plaque surface; and refinement to localize the mesh at the plaque surface.

Dynamics of the 3-D mesh model are given by the equation of motion for vertex "i":

$$m_i x''_i(t) + v_i x'_i(t) + g(x_i(t)) = f(x_i(t)) \qquad (2)$$

where $x_i(t)$ is the position of vertex "i", $x'_i(t)$ and $x''_i(t)$ are its velocity and acceleration, m_i is its mass, v_i is the damping coefficient, $g(x_i(t))$ is the resultant surface tension at the vertex, and $f(x_i(t))$ is a "driving" force. Equilibrium is reached when both $x'_i(t)$ and $x''_i(t)$ become zero. To simplify and speed the calculations, we assume that the mesh has no inertia ($m_i = 0$) and the damping coefficient is one ($v_i = 1$).

The equilibrium position is computed iteratively by updating the time in Eq. 2. After the driving force is used to obtain an approximate plaque surface, the inflation is stopped and the driving force is replaced by an image-based force, which uses a potential function (P) based on the image gradient, causing the mesh to fit the plaque surface details.

$$P(x_i(t)) = 1/[\|\nabla G_\sigma * I\| + \varepsilon] \qquad (3)$$

where G_σ is a 3-D Gaussian of width σ, and ε is a small constant to prevent division by zero. The potential function produces a force field, which deforms the model thus: $f(x_i(t)) = -k\nabla P(x_i(t))$. The adjustable term k controls the strength of the force and is optimized.

Acknowledgements

The authors gratefully acknowledge the financial support of the Canadian Institutes of Health Research and the Ontario R & D Challenge Fund. The first acknowledges the support of the Canada Research Chair program.

References

1. Nelson TR, Downey DB, Pretorius DH, Fenster A. *Three-Dimensional Ultrasound.* Lippincott, Williams, and Wilkins, Philadelphia, 1999.
2. Fenster A, Downey DB. 3-D ultrasound imaging: A review. IEEE Eng in Med and Biol 1996; 15:41-51.
3. Fenster A, Downey D, Cardinal N. Review: 3-dimensional Ultrasound Imaging. Physics in Medicine and Biology 2001; 46:R67-R99.
4. Fenster A, Downey D. Three-Dimensional Ultrasound Imaging. *Handbook of Medical Imaging, Volume I, Physics and Psychophysics.* Beutel J, Kundel H, Van Metter R (eds.). SPIE Press, Bellingham, Washington, p. 433-509, 2000.
5. Downey DB, Fenster A, Williams JC. Clinical utility of 3-D US. Radiographics 2000; 20:559-571.
6. Robb RA, *Three-dimensional biomedical imaging: Principles and practice.* VCH Publishers, N.Y., 1995.
7. Nelson TR, Pretorius DH, Sklansky M, Hagen-Ansert S. Three-dimensional echocardiographic evaluation of fetal heart anatomy and function: Acquisition, Analysis, and Display. J Ultrasound Med 1996; 15:1-9.
8. Pretorius DH, Nelson TR. Fetal face visualization using three-dimensional ultrasonography. J Ultrasound Med 1995; 14:349-356.
9. Nelson TR, Pretorius DH, Sklansky M, Hagen-Ansert S. Three-dimensional echocardiographic evaluation of fetal heart anatomy and function: Acquisition, Analysis, and Display. J Ultrasound Med 1996; 15:1-9.
10. Pretorius DH, Nelson TR. Fetal face visualization using three-dimensional ultrasonography. J Ultrasound Med 1995; 14:349-356.
11. Downey DB, Fenster A. Vascular imaging with a 3-D power Doppler system. AJR 1995; 165:665-668.
12. Tong S, Downey DB, Cardinal HN, Fenster A. A three-dimensional ultrasound prostate imaging system. Ultrasound Med Biol 1996; 22:735-746.
13. Tong S, Cardinal HN, Downey DB, Fenster A. Analysis of Linear, Area, and Volume Distortion in 3D Ultrasound Imaging. Ultrasound in Med and Biol 1998;24:355-373.
14. Chin JL, Downey DB, Mulligan M, Fenster A. Three-dimensional transrectal ultrasound guided cryoablation for localized prostate cancer in nonsurgical candidates: A feasability study and report of early results. J of Urology 1998; 159:910-914.
15. Ladak H, Mao F, Wang Y, Downey D, Steinman D, Fenster A, "Prostate Boundary Segmentation from 2D Ultrasound Images. Medical Physics 2000; 27:1777-1788.
16. Lobregt S, Viergever MA. A discrete dynamic contour model. IEEE Trans in Med Imaging, 1995; 14:12-24.
17. T. McInerney, D. A. Terzopoulos. A dynamic finite element surface model for segmentation and tracking in multidimensional medical images with applications to cardiac 4D image analysis. Comput. Med. Imaging Graph 1995; 19, 69-83.
18. Mao F, Gill J, Downey D, Fenster A. Segmentation of carotid artery in ultrasound images: method development and evaluation techniques. Med Phys 2000;27:1961-1970.
19. Gill J, Ladak H, Steinman D, Fenster A. Accuracy and variability assessment of semi-automatic technique for segmentation of the carotid arteries from 3D ultrasound images. Medical Physics 2000; 27: 1333-1342.

CARS 2002 – H.U. Lemke, M.W. Vannier; K. Inamura, A.G. Farman, K. Doi & J.H.C. Reiber (Editors)

Current concepts and future directions in computer-aided diagnosis for CT colonography

Ronald M. Summers

Department of Radiology, National Institutes of Health

Building 10 Room 1C660, Bethesda, MD 20892-1182, USA

Abstract

This review summarizes recent progress in computer-aided detection for CT colonography.

Keywords: Colonic polyps, colon cancer, shape detection

1. Introduction

Beginning in approximately 1997, we began an investigation of automated diagnosis for CT bronchography ("virtual bronchoscopy") [1-3]. In our study published in 1998, we found that 100% of airway lesions 5mm in size or larger could be detected using a shape-based detection algorithm [4]. The specificity was 80%. This technology transferred readily to CT colonography, and in association with colleagues at Stanford University, we published a feasibility study showing that colonic polyps could be detected in a phantom model [5]. More recently, we published the first study of computer-aided polyp detection for CT colonography to appear in a peer-reviewed journal, in association with colleagues at Mayo Clinic [6]. These early results showed the feasibility of CT colonography computer-aided diagnosis. In addition, they suggested that computer-aided diagnosis might become an important part of the radiologist's assessment of CT colonography studies. In this review article, I present a brief overview of the current status of CT colonography computer-aided diagnosis.

2. Rationale for computer-aided diagnosis

The rationale for computer-aided diagnosis or detection (CAD) is to reduce both perceptual error and interpretation times. It has been shown that perceptual error reduces the sensitivity of CT colonography by 14% for polyps 1 cm in size or larger [7]. Given the multitude of images in a CTC study, the causes of perceptual error are not mysterious. Depending upon the reconstruction interval, there can be 1,200 images or more to interpret. For example, images in the prone and supine position must be interpreted. Some investigators examine the colon antegrade and retrograde and in lung and soft tissue windows. When needed for problem solving, three dimensional virtual endoscopic views may also be used. Interpretation times ranging from 10 – 60 minutes per study have been reported in the literature. Many reported studies used consensus readings of two radiologists, further lengthening interpretation time. Consensus readings are usually impractical in most busy clinical radiology departments.

CARS 2002 – H.U. Lemke, M.W. Vannier; K. Inamura, A.G. Farman, K. Doi & J.H.C. Reiber (Editors)

3. Principles of CAD

The purpose of CAD is to locate possible polyps automatically and either annotate the images or present a list of image locations. The radiologist reviews the output of the CAD and makes the final diagnosis. he main functions of the CAD software are to identify features that characterize polyps and classify sites of detection as polyps or false positive diagnoses [8]. A suitable CAD system has high sensitivity for detection of clinically significant polyps (those over a size threshold, e.g. 0.5 or 1.0 cm) and a low number of false positive detections. All current CTC CAD systems produce on average at least one false positive detection per CTC examination.

Two useful features for CAD are surface shape and CT attenuation. Surface shape is an intuitive feature to identify polyps, and is an essential feature in the definition of a polyp. Colonic polyps protrude inward from the wall of the colon toward the air-filled lumen of the colon and are characteristically rounded in contour. In contrast, haustral folds tend to be circumferential and ridge-shaped.

CT attenuation has also been shown to be useful for CAD, particularly for distinguishing polyps from false positive diagnoses. False positive diagnoses tend to have low CT attenuation and polyps tend to have soft tissue attenuation. Residual stool may mimic a polyp but stool can sometimes be distinguished by the presence of tiny gas bubbles within it.

There are many ways to mathematically describe surface shape. A mathematical algorithm for computing shape is necessary since the computer must be instructed how to recognize such shapes. While there are a number of different methods for quantifying shape, we have found curvature to be an excellent shape descriptor [4]. The principle behind curvature assessment is that each point on the surface of the colon can be described as having one of six elemental shapes: elliptical pit, elliptical peak, hyperbolic, cylindrical valley, cylindrical ridge and plane. Elliptical peak shapes are like the top of an ice cream cone. Elliptical pit shapes are like the inside of a hollow ball. Hyperbolic shapes are like a saddle. Cylindrical valley and ridge shapes are like the inside and outside of a pipe, respectively. Plane shapes are flat.

Polyps tend to have elliptical peak shape [5]. Haustral folds tend to have cylindrical curvature. Normal colon between haustral folds tends to have plane, cylindrical, or elliptical pit curvature. We have found that approximately 91% of the colonic surface can be safely excluded from further analysis using this shape classification system [5]. The remaining 9% of the colonic surface contains polyps and other structures, some of which the radiologist needs to review. Further processing can reduce the area of interest to only 0.4% of the colonic surface. In a study of ten simulated 1 cm polyps inserted into a CT colonography study of an adult patient we found that all 10 polyps could be detected using the shape based algorithm. When further processing was applied to reduce false positives, 8 of the polyps could be located without any false positive diagnoses.

Once potential polyps are detected by CAD, they must be shown to the radiologist who makes the final diagnosis. There are a number of ways to do this. We have found it useful to label sites directly on CT colonography images to show the radiologist where the tentative polyp detections may be found [9]. These labels can be turned on or off so that

CARS 2002 – H.U. Lemke, M.W. Vannier; K. Inamura, A.G. Farman, K. Doi & J.H.C. Reiber (Editors)
^cCARS/Springer. All rights reserved.

they do not obscure the original images. To save time, the radiologist can jump directly to the labeled images. To evaluate the potential time efficiency of CAD, we applied CAD to a CT colonography study consisting of 161 images. The CAD software placed 7 CAD detections on 22 of the 161 images. Some of the CAD detections spanned more than one image. The total interpretation time was only two minutes to locate a colonoscopically proven 1.5 cm polyp in the rectosigmoid colon. This result suggests that CAD may be able to sharply reduce interpretation times.

4. Current status of CTC CAD

CT colonography computer-aided detection is in a preliminary stage of development. It is in early clinical trials at several academic centers. In this section, I summarize the published results of these trials. Particular attention is paid to whether statistical analyses are performed (such as cross-validation) that correct the overestimate of CAD performance on data from which it has been developed and optimized.

Our first clinical trial, performed in collaboration with colleagues at Mayo Clinic, was a study of 20 high risk subjects with known polyps [6]. There were 28 polyps 1 cm or larger, 26 of which could be found in retrospect. The sensitivity of the CAD algorithm was 64%, using a classification scheme that minimized the false positive detections to on average 6 false positive detections per colon. Note that these results were obtained using supine CTC only. The sensitivity would be higher if prone CTC was added although the number of false positive detections would also be higher. The sensitivity could be improved at the expense of an increase in false positive detections. When only polyps in well distended colonic segments were considered, the sensitivity increased to 71%. In this study, CT attenuation was used to reduce the number of false positive detections by 39% (to 3.5 false positive detections per colon). Processing took about 2 minutes on a common desktop computer.

The University of Chicago group assessed curvature in a thin layer that included the colonic wall [10-12]. They analyzed "directional gradient concentration" and applied linear and quadratic discriminant analyses. They used a "leave-one-out" analysis to validate their results. In a study of 14 patients having 15 polyps less than or equal to 1 cm and 6 polyps greater than 1 cm, they found 100% sensitivity per patient. Their average false positive rate was 2.0 per patient. At a false positive rate of 2.0 per patient, their sensitivity for polyps was 90% (19 of 21).

Stanford University researchers have used a shape analysis of the colonic wall based upon the Canny edge detector and Hough transform operator [13, 14]. In a study of 14 polyps greater than 8.5 mm in 9 patients, they found a sensitivity of 92.9% and 7.9 false positives per colon. In a refinement of their algorithm, they developed a random orthogonal shape selection (ROSS) technique based on statistical pattern recognition [15]. In this method, randomly selected volumes in coronal, sagittal, and axial orientations are taken through potential polyps and then analyzed using statistical pattern recognition. The ROSS method included additional shape signatures which identified elliptical and linear shapes. The researchers utilized ten-fold cross validation and found that the ROSS method

CARS 2002 – H.U. Lemke, M.W. Vannier; K. Inamura, A.G. Farman, K. Doi & J.H.C. Reiber (Editors)

746

reduced false positives by 62%. However, this technique was time consuming, requiring hours of processing per subject. This group has also published preliminary results of an optical flow technique to reduce false positive detections [16].

Wake Forest University researchers published a shape and wall thickness analysis for CTC CAD in a conference proceeding article [17]. They found 11 of 15 polyps measuring 0.5 to 4.0 cm in 10 patients (sensitivity 73%) with an average of 49 false positives per patient. Researchers from Leuven in a conference proceedings article used a shape analysis based on convexity and sphericality [18]. They found all 10 polyps 1 cm or larger in 18 patients. There were 8 false positives per CT colonography scan.

5. Challenges ahead

CT colonography computer-aided detection research is in an early stage but already is producing exciting results. There are many challenges ahead and one anticipates new and useful results in the near future [19]. The two most exciting research challenges are determination of useful features and improvement in classification strategies. The key to this research is to identify features that describe polyps so they cluster together and away from false positives in feature-space.

Another challenge is how to properly match polyps on conventional colonoscopy and on CT colonography. Typically, conventional colonoscopy identifies polyps to within a colonic segment and even then considerable errors in location can occur. Such errors can impair CAD research.

Additional challenges are the trade-off between sensitivity and specificity and the limited amount of available data to train and test CAD. While initial results often report high sensitivity and few false positives, when presented with new data CAD will typically have lower sensitivity with more false positives. This fact highlights the need for suitable training databases that researchers can use to validate the robustness of their CAD algorithms.

Polyp camouflage is another important problem. Polyp camouflage includes residual fluid, stool, and bulbous haustral folds, and can mimic or hide true polyps. CAD needs to see through camouflage that hides polyps and distinguish camouflage that mimics polyps. Stool subtraction techniques may play a role here.

Another challenge is to use the supine and prone CTC images together to find polyps and reduce false positives. For example, if a polyp is found in the same location on both supine and prone CTC, the confidence is high that this represents a true polyp. CAD may need to recognize such concordances.

Cancer detection, while feasible with CAD, may be a less important use for CAD. It has been shown in a number of studies that CTC without CAD already has 100% sensitivity for detecting colon cancers [20].

CARS 2002 – H.U. Lemke, M.W. Vannier; K. Inamura, A.G. Farman, K. Doi & J.H.C. Reiber (Editors)
© CARS/Springer. All rights reserved.

Other challenges include how to deal with artifacts, poor colonic distention, image noise, and low image resolution. A most important challenge will be how to show the impact of CAD in an actual clinical interpretive setting. Studies will need to be done showing that CAD improves clinical sensitivity without an undue burden in terms of reduced specificity or an increase in interpretation time.

6. Conclusion

Preliminary results in CT colonography CAD are encouraging. There is evidence that high sensitivity and a low number of false positive detections per examination are possible in the foreseeable future. However, these early results need to be confirmed on larger image databases. The application of CAD to clinical practice is also sure to provide interesting results that will propel further research.

Acknowledgements

Andrew Dwyer, M.D., is thanked for critical review of the manuscript.

References

1. Summers RM, Selbie WS, Malley JD, et al. Computer-assisted detection of endobronchial lesions using virtual bronchoscopy: application of concepts from differential geometry. In: Conference on mathematical models in medical and health sciences. Nashville, TN: Vanderbilt University, 1997.
2. Summers RM, Pusanik LM, Malley JD. Automatic detection of endobronchial lesions with virtual bronchoscopy: comparison of two methods. In: Medical Imaging 1998: Image Processing. San Diego, California: SPIE, 1998; 3338:327-335.
3. Summers RM. Chapter 45. Morphometric Methods for Virtual Endoscopy Reconstructions. In: I. N. Bankman, ed. Handbook of Medical Imaging: Processing and Analysis. San Diego, Calif.: Academic Press, 2000; 747-755.
4. Summers RM, Selbie WS, Malley JD, et al. Polypoid lesions of airways: early experience with computer-assisted detection by using virtual bronchoscopy and surface curvature. Radiology 1998; 208:331-337.
5. Summers RM, Beaulieu CF, Pusanik LM, et al. Automated polyp detector for CT colonography: feasibility study. Radiology 2000; 216:284-90.
6. Summers RM, Johnson CD, Pusanik LM, Malley JD, Youssef AM, Reed JE. Automated polyp detection at CT colonography: feasibility assessment in a human population. Radiology 2001; 219:51-59.
7. Fletcher JG, Johnson CD, Welch TJ, et al. Optimization of CT colonography technique: prospective trial in 180 patients. Radiology 2000; 216:704-11.
8. Summers RM, Jerebko AK, Franaszek M, Malley JD. An integrated system for computer-aided diagnosis in CT colonography: Work-in-progress. In: Computer Assisted Radiology and Surgery (CARS). Berlin, Germany: Elsevier Science, 2001; 629-634.
9. Summers RM, Pusanik LM, Malley JD, Reed JE, Johnson CD. Method of labeling colonic polyps at CT colonography using computer-assisted detection. In: Computer Assisted Radiology and Surgery (CARS). San Francisco, CA: Elsevier Science, 2000; 785-789.
10. Yoshida H, Nappi J. Three-dimensional computer-aided diagnosis scheme for detection of colonic polyps. IEEE Transactions on Medical Imaging 2001; 20:1261-1274.

748

11. Yoshida H, Masutani Y, MacEneaney P, Rubin DT, Dachman AH. Computerized detection of colonic polyps at CT colonography on the basis of volumetric features: pilot study. Radiology 2002; 222:327-36.

12. Yoshida H, Nappi J, MacEneaney P, Rubin DT, Dachman AH. Computer-aided diagnosis scheme for the detection of polyps in CT colonography. Radiographics 2002; in press.

13. Paik DS, Beaulieu CF, Jeffrey RB, Yee J, Steinauer-Gebauer AM, Napel S. Computer aided detection of polyps in CT colonography: Method and free-response ROC evaluation of performance. Radiology 2000; 217:704.

14. Paik DS, Beaulieu CF, Mani A, Prokesch RW, Yee J, Napel S. Evaluation of computer-aided detection in CT colonography: Potential applicability to a screening population. Radiology 2001; 221:332-332.

15. Gokturk SB, Tomasi C, Acar B, et al. A statistical 3-D pattern processing method for computer-aided detection of polyps in CT colonography. IEEE Transactions on Medical Imaging 2001; 20:1251-1260.

16. Acar B, Napel S, Paik DS, Gokturk B, Tomasi C, Beaulieu CF. Using optical flow fields for polyp detection in virtual colonoscopy. In: MICCAI. Utrecht: Springer-Verlag, 2001; LNCS 2208:637-644.

17. Vining DJ, Ge YR, Ahn DK, Stelts DR. Virtual colonoscopy with computer-assisted polyp detection. In: K. Doi, H. MacMahon, M. L. Giger and K. R. Hoffmann, ed. Computer-aided diagnosis in medical imaging: proceedings of the first international workshop on computer-aided diagnosis. Chicago: Elsevier, 1999; 445-452.

18. Kiss G, Van Cleynenbreugel J, Thomeer M, Suetens P, Marchal G. Computer aided diagnosis for virtual colonography. In: MICCAI. Utrecht: Springer-Verlag, 2001; LNCS 2208:621-628.

19. Summers RM. Challenges for computer-aided diagnosis for CT colonography. Abdominal Radiology 2002; in press.

20. Summers RM, Hara AK, Luboldt W, Johnson CD. Computed tomographic and magnetic resonance colonography: summary of progress from 1995 to 2000. Current Problems in Diagnostic Radiology 2001; 30:141-168.

CARS 2002 – H.U. Lemke, M.W. Vannier; K. Inamura, A.G. Farman, K. Doi & J.H.C. Reiber (Editors)

Computer-aided detection of polyps in CT colonography: effect of feature-guided polyp segmentation

J. Näppi and H. Yoshida

The University of Chicago, Department of Radiology

5841 S. Maryland Avenue, MC 2026, Chicago, IL 60637, USA

Abstract

We evaluated the effect of our novel feature-guided polyp segmentation technique on the reduction of false-positive (FP) colorectal polyp findings generated by our computer-aided diagnosis (CAD) scheme for the detection of colonic polyps in CT colonography (CTC). A total of 72 patients, including 14 patients with 21 colorectal polyp findings, were used in the evaluation. At a 100% (95%) by-patient (by-polyp) sensitivity level, the FP rate was 1.9 FPs (1.9 FPs) per patient for the round-robin analysis. The results indicate that our CAD scheme has the potential of making CTC a viable option for screening of colonic polyps in large patient populations.

Keywords: Computer-aided detection, colorectal cancer, CT colonography

1. Introduction

Colorectal cancer is the second leading cause of cancer-related deaths in the United States [1,2]. Most colorectal cancers develop in polyps, and therefore early detection and removal of colorectal polyps can reduce the risk of developing colorectal cancer [3].

Radiologists have been reported to detect large colorectal polyps and masses in CT colonography (CTC) at 90-100% sensitivity with a low false-positive (FP) rate [4]. However, the detection of polyps that are smaller than 10 mm in diameter is time-consuming and prone to interpretation errors. To assist radiologists in the detection task, we are developing a fully automated CAD scheme for the detection of colonic polyps that indicates the locations of suspicious polyps to radiologists. The CAD scheme could help radiologists to detect colorectal polyps faster and with higher accuracy than previously.

The initial steps of the CAD detection process generate several FP findings that need to be differentiated from true-positive (TP) polyp findings. In our previous study, we differentiated the FP findings by using feature values that were computed directly from the regions identified as polyp candidates by use of hysteresis thresholding and fuzzy clustering [5]. However, these regions are not necessarily representative of the findings in terms of individual features, because the region that is most representative of one feature may occupy a spatially different region than that for another feature (Fig. 1). Therefore, if we compute the feature values from the single region identified as a polyp candidate, the discrimination performance of the features may be degraded. This degradation may occur if some of the voxels included in the computation of a feature are redundant for the

CARS 2002 – H.U. Lemke, M.W. Vannier; K. Inamura, A.G. Farman, K. Doi & J.H.C. Reiber (Editors)

feature. Moreover, because the segmentation of the polyp region is often based on features that are not necessarily used for the differentiation step, voxels that carry important information for other features could be excluded in the segmented region.

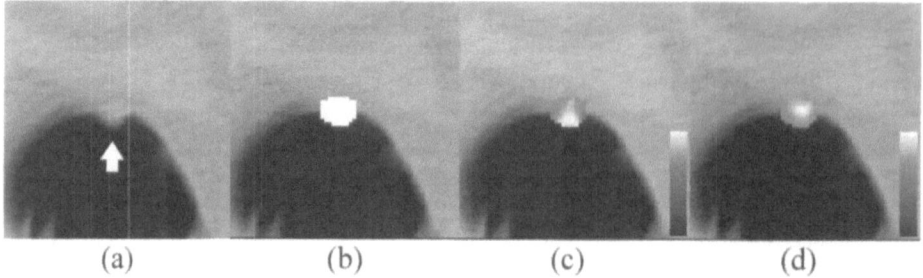

(a)   (b)   (c)   (d)

Fig. 1: (a) Axial view of a region of interest including a polyp indicated by white arrow. (b) Region of a polyp candidate segmented by CAD is colored white. (c) Highest shape index feature values (white color; see color bar in the bottom right corner) concentrate on the cap-like part of the segmented region. (d) Highest gradient concentration feature values (white color) concentrate on the center of the segmented region.

In this study, we developed a novel technique of feature-guided polyp segmentation that extracts the most representative region of a polyp candidate for each feature. The feature values are then characterized by statistics such as the mean and variance. The resulting feature vectors are subjected to quadratic discriminant analysis to reduce FPs and to determine the final output of the CAD scheme.

2. Material

We used CTC data obtained in clinical CTC examinations at the University of Chicago. The CT scanning was performed in the supine and prone positions with a helical CT scanner by use of a collimation of 2.5-5.0 mm, pitch of 1.5-1.7, and reconstruction intervals of 1.5-2.5 mm. Optical colonoscopy had been performed on the same day as the CTC. The patients underwent standard pre-colonoscopy cleansing, and the colon was insufflated with room air. For the present study, we used 72 patients (144 data sets). A total of 21 colonoscopy-confirmed polyps were present in 14 patients (27 data sets). Seventeen of the polyps were 5-10 mm, three polyps were 11-12 mm, and one polyp was 25 mm in diameter.

3. Methods

3.1 Detection of polyp candidates

The CAD scheme first generates an isotropic volume by interpolating linearly between the original CT slices, after which the visible colonic wall is extracted by application of a *knowledge-guided colon segmentation* (KGS) technique [6]. First, the KGS removes the region outside the body, the osseous structures, and lung bases, and then extracts the colonic wall with a thickness of approximately 4 mm. Because the extracted region could contain extracolonic components such as the small bowel and stomach, the second step of

CARS 2002 – H.U. Lemke, M.W. Vannier; K. Inamura, A.G. Farman, K. Doi & J.H.C. Reiber (Editors)

KGS implements a self-adjusting volume-growing process to segment the colonic lumen by using the region extracted in the first step. The third step removes the extracolonic components by retaining only the region of the extracted colonic wall that is associated with the colonic lumen. On average, more than 98% of the visible colonic surface is covered by the region segmented by the KGS technique [6].

The polyps are detected from the extracted colonic wall by use of *hysteresis thresholding* [7] based on two volumetric features called the *shape index* (SI) and *curvedness* (CV) [8]. The SI classifies the topological shape located at a voxel into five classes: cup, rut, saddle, ridge, or cap. The CV characterizes the flatness, or scale, of the shape indicated by the shape index (Fig. 2).

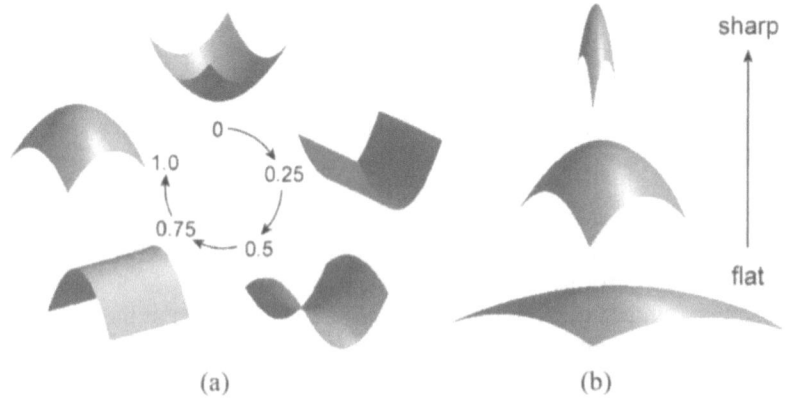

(a)   (b)

Fig. 2: (a) The shape index characterizes the local volumetric shape located at a voxel. (b) Curvedness characterizes the scale of the shape.

3.2 Reduction of false positives

In this study, we used three features to differentiate between TP and FP polyp candidates: the mean value of the SI, the mean value of the *modified gradient concentration* (MGC), and the *variance of the CT value*. The SI feature was described above. The MGC feature is a novel feature that is based on the gradient concentration (GC) and directional gradient concentration (DGC) features developed in our previous study [9]. These two features characterize the variation of the 3-dimensional gradients around an operating point, so that the highest values of the GC and DGC occur in spherical and hemispherical objects, respectively. The MGC feature combines these properties of the GC and DGC by mapping the values of GC through a sigmoid function. As a result, the MGC feature produces a high response to both spherical and hemispherical objects, which are similar to pedunculated and sessile polyps.

3.3 Segmentation of polyp candidate region

Hysteresis thresholding (section 3.1) extracts regions that have polyp-like values of SI and CV. However, these regions do not necessarily cover the visually perceived region of a detected lesion completely, and they could exclude voxels that contain representative

CARS 2002 – H.U. Lemke, M.W. Vannier; K. Inamura, A.G. Farman, K. Doi & J.H.C. Reiber (Editors)
©CARS/Springer. All rights reserved.

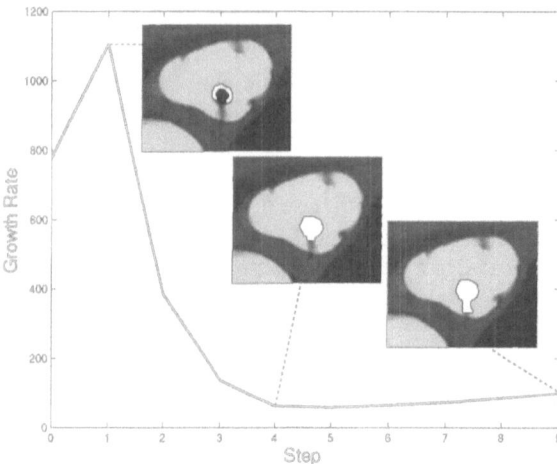

Fig. 3: Plot of the growth rate of a conditionally dilated region. The three sample images show an axial view of the dilated region (white) of steps 1, 4, and 9 of the dilation process. Here, step 4 determines the final region of the polyp candidate.

information for other features. Therefore, we segment the entire region of a polyp candidate as described below.

The region extracted by hysteresis thresholding is considered as a seed region R_0. A step-wise *conditional morphological dilation* [10] $R_i = (R_{i-1} \oplus B) \backslash L$ is then performed. Here, R_{i-1} is the previous region, $\oplus$ indicates morphological dilation, B is a morphological structuring element, \ indicates the set difference, and L is the region of the colonic lumen determined by the KGS colon segmentation technique. In each step, the dilation extends the boundary surface of R_{i-1} by Δs mm within the colonic wall. The maximum number of dilations, D, is bounded by $D\Delta s \leq 7.5$ mm, i.e., the boundary surface may extend at most 7.5 mm from its starting position in R_0. Therefore, the technique can extract the complete region of polyps up to 15 mm in diameter.

One of the dilated regions, R_C, is chosen to represent the region of the polyp candidate. To determine this region, we record the amount of voxels, N_i, which were added to R_{i-1} to yield R_i in each step of the conditional dilation. The region of polyp candidate R_C is the one for which dN_i/ds, i.e., the growth rate of the conditional dilation, is smallest. As shown in Fig. 3, the growth rate first increases, and then decreases as the dilated region becomes bounded by the visually perceived shape of the polyp. Afterwards, the growth rate increases again as the dilated region starts to expand into the colonic wall. Therefore, the region corresponding to the minimum of the growth rate provides the complete region of the polyp candidate.

3.4 Analysis of histogram of features
By studying the histograms of feature values within TP polyp candidates, we can find signature patterns that are different from those appearing in the histograms of FP polyp candidates (Fig. 4). Based on a study of these histograms, we thresholded the region of polyp candidate by using the following threshold values: $SI \in [0.7, 1.0]$, $GC \in [0.7, 1.0]$, and $CT \in [-300, \infty($. Here, the CT values are given in Hounsfield units. The mean values of SI and MGC, and the variance of CT values, were then computed from their corresponding thresholded regions.

CARS 2002 – H.U. Lemke, M.W. Vannier; K. Inamura, A.G. Farman, K. Doi & J.H.C. Reiber (Editors)
^cCARS/Springer. All rights reserved.

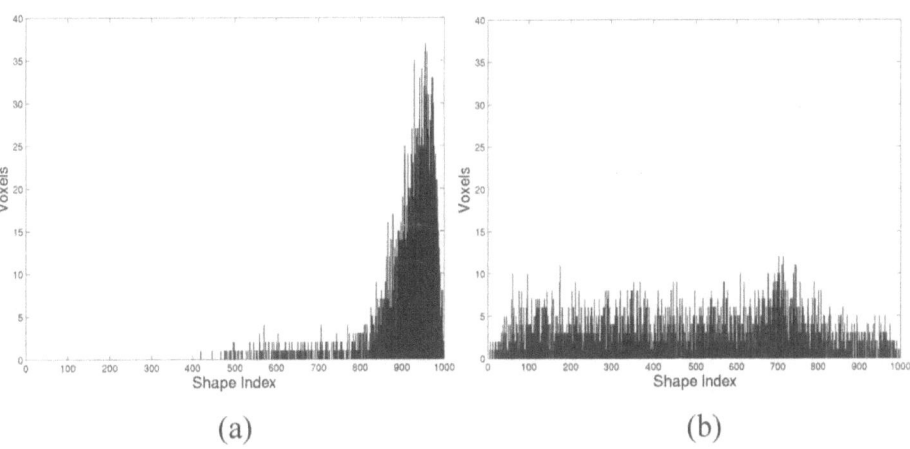

(a)   (b)

Fig. 4: Histograms of shape index values (scaled to [0,1000]) within a polyp candidate region. (a) Typical histogram of a TP polyp candidate. (b) Histogram of a FP polyp candidate.

3.5 Quadratic discriminant analysis

The combination of the mean value of SI, the mean value of MGC, and the variance of the CT value, was used as input to a quadratic classifier that differentiated the polyp candidates into TP and FP candidates. The TP candidates define the final output of the CAD scheme. The sensitivity and specificity of the polyp detection were computed for each combination by use of all available data ("consistency") and by use of round-robin analysis. The detection results were compared to the results obtained by use of our previously developed polyp segmentation technique, in which all features are computed from the same fixed region of a polyp candidate as determined by hysteresis thresholding and fuzzy clustering based on SI, CV, and spatial coordinates [5].

4. Results

We evaluated the performance of the polyp detection using *by-patient* and *by-polyp* analysis. In by-patient analysis, a patient with one or more polyps is considered detected correctly if at least one polyp is detected from the prone or supine data set of the patient. In by-polyp analysis, a polyp is considered detected correctly if it is detected from either the prone or the supine data set of a patient.

For the consistency results, the application of the feature-guided polyp segmentation technique yielded a 100% sensitivity at a FP rate of 1.72 FPs per patient in a by-patient analysis. In a by-polyp analysis, the same FP rate was obtained at a sensitivity of 95%. For the round-robin results, the sensitivity was 100% at a FP rate of 1.88 FPs per patient in a by-patient analysis. The same FP rate was obtained at a sensitivity of 95% in a by-polyp analysis.

These results are a substantial improvement over those obtained by the application of our previously developed technique for polyp segmentation. When the number of discriminative features is limited to three at most, the use of the previous technique, with the same 72 patients that were used in this study, yielded a FP rate of 4 detections per patient at a 100% sensitivity in a by-patient analysis. Although the FP rates could be improved to 2.0-2.5 FPs per patient, this would have required the use of more than three features [11]. Therefore, the application of our new technique of feature-guided polyp segmentation appears more promising.

5. Conclusion

Our novel feature-guided polyp segmentation technique is effective in improving the specificity of our CAD scheme for detecting colorectal polyps. Because of its high sensitivity and low false-positive rate, our CAD scheme has the potential of making CTC a viable option for screening of large patient populations for colorectal cancer.

Acknowledgments

This work was supported in part by the University of Chicago Cancer Research Center, the Cancer Research Foundation of America, and the Paul C. Hodges Alumni Society.

References

1. M. O'Brien, S. Winawer, A. Zauber, et al., "The national polyp study: patient and polyp characteristics associated with high-grade dysplasia in colorectal adenomas", *Gastroenterology* 98, 371-379, 1990.
2. J. Potter, M. Slattery, R. Bostick, and S. Gapstur, "Colon cancer: a review of the epidemiology", *Epidemiol Rev* 15, 499-545, 1993.
3. S.Winawer, A. Zauber, M. Ho, et al., "Prevention of colorectal cancer by colonoscopic polypectomy. The National Polyp Study Workgroup", *N Engl J Med* 329, 1977-1981, 1993.
4. J. Yee, G. A. Akerkar, R. K. Hung, et al., "Colorectal neoplasia: performance characteristics of CT colonography for detection in 300 patients", *Radiology* 219, 685-692, 2001.
5. H. Yoshida, Y. Masutani, P. MacEneaney, D. T. Rubin, and A.H. Dachman, "Computerized detection of colonic polyps at CT colonography on the basis of volumetric features: pilot study", *Radiology* 222, 327-336, 2002.
6. J. Näppi, A. Dachman, P. MacEneaney, and H. Yoshida, "Effect of knowledge-guided colon segmentation in automated detection of polyps in CT colonography", *Proc SPIE*: 4683, 2002 (in press).
7. G. Lohmann, *Volumetric Image Analysis*, John Wiley & Son Ltd., New York, 1998.
8. H. Yoshida and J. Näppi, "Computer-aided diagnostic scheme for the detection of colonic polyps", *IEEE Trans Med Imaging* 20, 1261-1274, 2001.
9. J. Näppi and H. Yoshida, "Automated detection of polyps in CT colonography: evaluation of volumetric features for reduction of false positives", *Acad Radiol* 9, 386-397, 2002.
10. R. Gonzalez and R. Woods, *Digital Image Processing*, Addison-Wesley, 1992.
11. H. Yoshida, J. Näppi, P. MacEneaney, D. Rubin, and A.H. Dachman, "Computer-aided diagnosis scheme for the detection of polyps in CT colonography", *RadioGraphics*, 2002 (in press).

CARS 2002 – H.U. Lemke, M.W. Vannier; K. Inamura, A.G. Farman, K. Doi & J.H.C. Reiber (Editors)

Feature-based approach toward computer aided detection and diagnosis

Zhengrong Liang, Zigang Wang, Lihong Li, and Donald P. Harrington

Dept. of Radiology, State University of New York, Stony Brook, NY 11794, USA

Abstract

We present a framework for computer aided detection and diagnosis based on segmented tissue mixtures in each voxel of the image. Detection is based on both the geometry and texture. Diagnosis is based on both the texture and feature extracted from the mixture segmentation.

Keywords: Mixture segmentation, feature extraction, feature-based visualization

1. Introduction

With advance of medical imaging technologies (including instrumentation, computer and algorithm), the acquired data information is getting so rich toward beyond the human's capability of visual recognition and efficient use for clinical assessment. The concept of computer or ideal interpreter has been around for many years. Computer technologies can make somewhat simple abnormality detection and disease diagnosis from the images, but could not replace the human ability to analyze complex information. On the other hand, computer technologies can "see" some details inside the images, while human might not be able to see. A computer interpreter can efficiently and consistently "read" many images, while human might make inconsistent assessments in an inefficient manner. Therefore, computer aided detection (CAD) and computer aided diagnosis (CADx) become more desirable and are now under development by many research groups in the world. The former one aims to detect any abnormality from the images, while the later one intends to differentiate the detected abnormality as either benign or malignance or to identify the detected abnormality as a most possible disease.

We view image-based CAD and/or CADx more generally as a computer-aided procedure to assist physicians for medical diagnosis, treatment/surgical planning, and follow-up evaluation of disease management. This process is thought as an information processing.

Images acquired from a patent carry all the subjective and objective information. This information itself may or may not be enough to make a decision. For this reason, physicians' input as additional information would be useful to the decision-making. However, in more cases, presentation of the patient image information to the physician for clinical assessment is limited by currently available technologies and, therefore, results in many undetermined cases. With advent of advanced computer technologies and sophisticated image processing algorithms, those detailed information beyond human visual ability to acquire from the images can be extracted and displayed in real time for physician's assessment. With both physician's input of additional information and computerized extraction of more details from the images, it is expected to decrease dramatically the number of undetermined cases. In this paper, we present a unique CAD/CADx system, which addresses both the information processing and information visualization issues for medical diagnosis, treatment/surgical planning, and follow up evaluation. The information processing is detailed by the following two sections of (i) mixture-based image segmentation and (ii) featture analysis of the mixture segmentation with the options of physician's editing. The editing integrates physician's experience into the clinical assessment. The information visualization is detailed in the third section of feature-based volumetric/surface rendering.

2. Mixture-based image segmentation

Given an acquired image or a series of images with finite voxel size (voxel is an image element in three dimensions and is called as pixel in two dimensions), conventional segmentation algorithms label each voxel as a single class or tissue type or object [2, 5, 10]. This kind image classification limits quantitative accuracy on the contents inside the voxels and on the spatial location of tissue boundaries. Our segmentation method not only labels each voxel as the conventional algorithms do, but also quantifies the contents as percentages of tissues inside that voxel [3, 4, 6]. (The percentage vector of tissues inside a voxel is called as mixel). This later kind image segmentation has unlimited spatial resolution on the tissue boundaries and achieves the most accurate measurement on the voxel contents. Furthermore, the neighborhood system of mixture segmentation can provide tissue growth tendency, in addition to the anatomical structure of the tissues. Presentation of both the anatomical structure and growth tendency of a tissue type with accurate quantification of the tissue contents shall improve the clinical assessment for diagnosis, treatment/surgical planning, and follow-up evaluation. Our CAD/CADx system is based on the mixture segmentation.

3. Mixture-based feature analysis

3.1 Feature extraction from mixture segmentation

User Edited Texture Extraction: Given the mixture segmentation or mixel volume data, we extract a tissue structure based on the similarity of mixels. First, a seed point or voxel is selected by the user for a specific tissue type or object. The percentage of this specific tissue must be greater than other tissue types inside that voxel. The percentage proportion of all tissue types in the mixel provides a characteristic vector reflecting the specific tissue type. All mixels with similar percentage proportions will be grouped together by utilizing region-growing strategies with modification by adding neighbor mixels into consideration. Those mixels with noticeable variation by vector similarity threshold measure will be labeled as layer mixels. Any unexpected small variation in the fully automated segmentation will be corrected at this stage by the physician.

Volumetric Analysis: For volumetric quantification on different tissues, the layer mixels provide a blurred boundary to separate two tissues. The volumetric measures of these two tissues will include the blurred boundary and count their percentages respectively. Volumetric analysis has a wide application in neural disorder diagnosis. One example is the diagnosis of multiple sclerosis (MS) and evaluation of a treatment means by measuring the brain atrophy [1, 3]. If we do not provide any treatment during a time course, the volumetric variation or atrophy measure itself will be an effective means for

CARS 2002 – H.U. Lemke, M.W. Vannier; K. Inamura, A.G. Farman, K. Doi & J.H.C. Reiber (Editors)

757

the MS diagnosis. Differentiation of benign or malignance of a detected pulmonary module by the volumetric measures in a time period is another example for diagnosis of a specific disease by volumetric analysis. The unique aspect of our CAD/CADx system is its accuracy due to the mixture segmentation.

Treatment/Surgical Planning: For surgical planning, the layer mixels will be colored as differently from the two or more tissues invading the layer. The portion of the layer with lesion percentage will be operated [7]. The mixer layer provides the most accurate reference to the surgeon to operate on the target.

Surface Geometric Analysis: Based on the mixture segmentation, a tissue/object boundary can be extracted from the mixel layer with high accuracy. By utilizing the neighboring mixels, the tendency of the surface movement can be quantified. The accurate surface geometry provides a means for CAD on abnormality; and the tendency of the surface movement, combining the texture of the mixel layer, provides a means for CADx on the detected abnormality.

For visualization purpose, we shall identify some area with high suspicious for physicians' inspection. Presenting accurately the features on these suspected areas is another key point of our CAD/CADx system. As we pointed out before, we will provide not only the tissue structure, but also the tissue growth tendency by analyzing the features of the mixture segmentation. In the followings, we present our CAD/CADx system for visualization-based clinical applications.

3.2 Principal direction feature of mixture segmentation

One feature in the segmented mixture data volume is the principal direction. Principal direction is an important attribute to describe the tissue/object surface. In our method, we modify the definition of the principal direction to fit the segmented mixel volume. For object/tissue l in a given mixel $M_{i,j,k}$ (or voxel with mixture tissues inside), there exists a percentage $P^l_{i,j,k}$ of object l inside the mixel, provided by the segmentation. Thus, there exists an iso-surface in the mixture volume across all mixels $M^l_{k,s,t}$ with percentage $P^l_{k,s,t} = P^l_{i,j,k}$. The principal direction of tissue l at $M_{i,j,k}$ is defined as the principal direction of this iso-surface. To calculate the principal direction of each mixel, we have developed a neighbor matrix method to extract the principal direction from the mixture volume rapidly. Firstly, we use the discrete difference method to obtain the normal vector of object/tissue l in mixel $M_{i,j,k}$

$$N^l_{i,j,k} = (\, P^l_{i-1,j,k} - P^l_{i-1,j,k} \,,\, P^l_{i,j+1,k} - P^l_{i,j-1,k} \,,\, P^l_{i,j,k+1} - P^l_{i,j,k-1} \,). \qquad (1)$$

Secondly, for each object l in mixel $M_{i,j,k}$, we create a 3D neighbor array A. Thus A can be represented as

$$\{\, A_{k,s,t} \,|\, A_{r,s,t} = (\, P^l_{r,s,t}, N^l_{r,s,t}) \,\} \quad r \in [i\text{-}1, i\text{+}1], s \in [j\text{-}1, j\text{+}1], t \in [k\text{-}1, k\text{+}1]. \qquad (2)$$

According to the similarity between the percentages of the neighboring mixels, we assign a value to each element/voxel in the neighbor array A. Collecting all value in the array, an index is constructed. Using this index, we can search, in a check-list, for several candidate directions, along one of which the maximum curvature will occur. Using the position and the normal information of Eqns.(1) and (2), we can figure out the principal direction among these candidate directions. This method only uses the neighboring mixel information to calculate the principle direction. It needs a little calculation effort. Furthermore, the neighbor arrays A of two adjacent mixels are similar, so we can use this

CARS 2002 – H.U. Lemke, M.W. Vannier; K. Inamura, A.G. Farman, K. Doi & J.H.C. Reiber (Editors)
°CARS/Springer. All rights reserved.

fact to speed up the algorithm. Collecting all the principal direction information, a feature based vector volume is then constructed.

4. Feature-based volume rendering

Our presented rendering algorithm is composed of three sections: (1) converting feature vector volume to stroke based scale volume; (2) constructing the mixture scale color volume; and (3) rendering the final mixture scale color volume. The flow chart is shown by Figure 1 below.

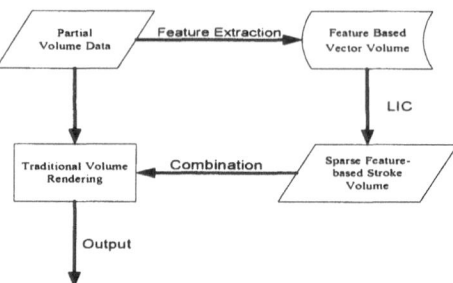

Figure 1. The flowchart of our feature-based rendering algorithm.

4.1 Converting feature vector volume to stroke scale volume

For the feature vector volume, we need to convert the feature vector volume to stroke volume. In the latter volume, all vector are classified and quantatized. The continuous vector volume is rendered as a 3D texture volume -- stroke based scale volume. To accomplish this objective, we utilize two methods: (i) modified line integral convolution (LIC) method and (ii) streamline method.

Modified Line Integral Convolution (LIC) Method: The LIC method is a popular method to display the vector volume by the texture analysis. This method utilizes the vector field V and the input texture data Tex to create another texture data $Output$, whose pattern can describe the vector field clearly. The crucial conversion function is

$$output_{i,j,k} = \int_{s_{i,j,k} - L}^{s_{i,j,k} + L} k(s - s_{i,j,k})Tex(\sigma(s))ds . \qquad (3)$$

In the original method, the input texture data volume Tex is a continuous white noise texture volume. We utilize a sparse cluster texture as the input texture Tex. The texture volume is composed of a given number of clusters. Using this texture, the output texture volume will be a sparse stroke volume. The strokes can describe the vector field very well. The distribution of the clusters is controllable. This means that by adjusting the corresponding variable, we can control the distribution and the position of the strokes.

Streamline Method: Streamline method is another method to describe the vector field. At first, we select several seed points in the vector volume. These seed points can move along a curve whose gradient at a given position is equal to the vector value at that location. By recording the moving track of the seed point, a sparse stroke volume, which is composed of the track voxels, is created. Same as the modified LIC method, the distribution of the seed points can be controlled by the feature and mixel information. Thus the surface information is converted into the volume information. By controlling the distribution of the seed points and the other attributes of the LIC algorithm, different

CARS 2002 – H.U. Lemke, M.W. Vannier; K. Inamura, A.G. Farman, K. Doi & J.H.C. Reiber (Editors)
©CARS/Springer. All rights reserved.

stroke volumes can be generated in which different interesting feature sections are focused at different "directions".

These two methods have their own advantages. The modified/advanced LIC method can describe the details of the vector volume, and its implementation is simple. The streamline method can save a great calculation cost, so it is more suitable for the non-dense vector volume. If the distribution of the strokes is dense and the vector field is continuous, we prefer to utilize the LIC algorithm. If the distribution of the strokes is sparse, we may use the streamline method.

4.2 Constructing mixture scale volume

The sparse stroke based volume is a scale color volume has the same dimension as the original mixture volume. We integrate the stroke based volume S with the original mixture volume O into a final mixture volume M

$$M^l_{i,j,k} = S^l_{i,j,k} \oplus O^l_{i,j,k} \qquad i, j, k \in [1, n], \quad l \in [1, t] \qquad (4)$$

where n is the dimension of the data volume, t is the number of tissues in a mixel, and $\oplus$ is the interpolation operator.

The information of two volumes includes color, opaque and so on. The interpolation operator can be overlay, addition, minus, line interpolation, and so on. Using the interpolation operator, the strokes, which describe the feature in the volume, can be embedded into the original volume. Thus all information can be synthesized into a scale volume. Using different operator, we can get different effect.

4.3 Rendering the integrated volume by volume rendering

For the final integrated volume, we use volume-rendering algorithm to render the final projected image. Volume rendering is a popular and efficient method to render the scale volume. Before volume rendering, we construct a non-mixture scale color volume C

$$C_{i,j,k} = \sum_{l=1}^{t} f(M^l_{i,j,k}) \cdot p^l_{i,j,k} \qquad (5)$$

where $p^l_{i,j,k}$ is the percentage of tissue/object l in mixel (i,j,k), and f is the illumination function.

After computed the color volume and assigned each voxel the corresponding opaque, a conventional volume rendering can calculate the color of each voxel on the projected image. Because a conventional volume rendering needs much calculation time, instead we used the latest 3D texture-based and hardware assisted volume rendering [8]. The rendering time was noticeably shortened. We also developed a new image based volume rendering algorithm -- sphere light field algorithm to further improve the speed of volume rendering [9]. By constructing a sphere light field, this algorithm can achieve the real time rendering of the volume data.

An example of demonstrating our feature-based visualization is illustrated using a 3D elliptical sphere volume image, as shown by Figure 2 below. There are two objects or tissues in the volume dataset: the inner one is object 1 (red); and the outer one is object 2 of white color. All the partial/mixture volume image and stroke volume are rendered by a traditional volume rendering method. As shown in Figure 2(a), the rendered original image without the stroke volume shows only an outline of the two objects with some

CARS 2002 – H.U. Lemke, M.W. Vannier; K. Inamura, A.G. Farman, K. Doi & J.H.C. Reiber (Editors)

760

degree of blurring. The rendering of the combination of the partial/mixture volume image and the stroke volume shows clearly the features of tissue/object growth tendency as seen in Figure 2(b), i.e., after invoking the strokes into the rendering of the partial/mixture volume image.

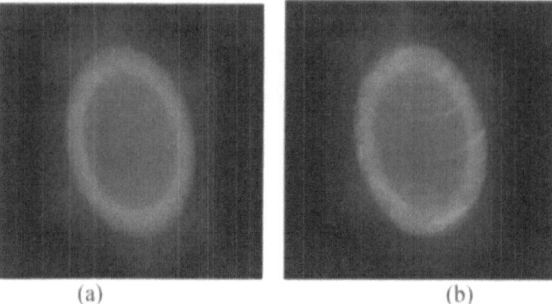

(a)   (b)

Figure 2. (a) The original 3D partial volume image. (b) The rendering result with feature extracted from the partial volume image data.

References

1. Christodoulou, C., Krupp, L., Huang, W., Chen, D., Melville, P., Scherl, W., Perone, P., Morgan, T., Liang, Z., Roche, P., Peyster, R., and Roque, C. (2001), "Cognitive correlates of quantitative MRI and MRS in MS," *Neurology*, **56**: A191-192.
2. Clark L., Velthuizen R., *et al.* (1995), "MRI segmentation: methods and applications," *J of MRI*, **13**: 343-368.
3. Li, L., Li, X., Huang, W., Christodoulou, C., Chen, D., *et al.* (2002), "A novel mixture-based segmentation algorithm for quantitative analysis of MS using multi-spectral MR images," *10th Intl Soc MR in Medicine*, to appear.
4. Liang, Z., Jaszczak, R., & Coleman, R. (1992), "Parameter estimation of finite mixtures using the EM algorithm and information criteria with application to medical image processing," *IEEE Trans Nucl Science*, **39**: 1126-1133.
5. Liang, Z. (1993), "Tissue classification and segmentation of MR images: research on statistical approaches offers avenue toward automation," *IEEE Engin. in Medicine and Biology*, pp. 81-85.
6. Liang, Z., MacFall, J., & Harrington, D. (1994), "Parameter estimation and tissue segmentation from multispectral MR images," *IEEE Trans on Medical Imaging*, **13**: 441-449.
7. Smouha, E., Chen, D., Li, B., and Liang, Z. (2001), "Computer-aided virtual surgery for congenital aural atresia," *Otology and Neurotology*, **22**: 178-182.
8. Wang, Z. and Liang, Z. (2002), "Feature based rendering for 2D/3D partial volume segmentation datasets," *SPIE Medical Imaging*, to appear.
9. Wang, Z. and Liang, Z. (2002), "Sphere Light Field Rendering," *SPIE Medical Imaging*, to appear.
10. Young & Fu (1986), *Handbook of Pattern Recognition and Image Processing*, New York: Academic Press.

CARS 2002 – H.U. Lemke, M.W. Vannier; K. Inamura, A.G. Farman, K. Doi & J.H.C. Reiber (Editors)

Clinical potential of CT colonography in the diagnosis of pelvic lymph node metastasis for patients with rectal cancer

Gen Iinuma [a], Takayuki Akasu[b], Noriyuki Moriyama[a]
[a] Department of Diagnostic Radiology
[b] Department of Colorectal Surgery
National Cancer Center Hospital
1-1 Tsukiji 5-chome, Chuo-ku, Tokyo, Japan

Abstract

We conducted an evaluation of the accuracy of multi-planar reconstruction (MPR) views of 3-dimensional volumetric data generated by helical computed tomography (CT) in the diagnosis of pelvic lymph node metastases in rectal cancer patients. From December 1998 to November 1999, 57 patients with rectal cancer underwent helical CT scanning for evaluation of preoperative staging of lymph node metastases. Three radiologists evaluated the staging based on consensus by use of MPR views of the 3-dimensional volumetric data reconstructed from CT slices. Then the staging was rated by use of the pathologic findings of the surgically resected specimens as gold standard. In this study, lymph nodes larger than or equal to 6 mm in size were defined as metastases. The detection sensitivity, specificity, and accuracy were 96.4%, 51.7%, and 73.7%, respectively, which were substantially higher than those reported previously. Thus, the MPR view is an excellent method for recognizing each organ consecutively and for discriminating lymph nodes from vascular structures. CT colonography with MPR has the potential of being a modality for computer-assisted diagnosis (CAD) of not only colorectal polyps but also lymph node metastases. Use of CAD is expected to improve radiologists' performance in the diagnosis of colorectal cancers, including lymph node metastases.

Keywords: Colorectal cancer, lymph node metastasis, multi-planar reconstruction.

1. Introduction

Computed tomography (CT) is an effective procedure for staging rectal carcinomas involving lymph node metastases. For establishing the surgical treatment of patients with rectal cancer, it is important to evaluate not only the extension of the primary lesion, but also that of node metastases. Currently, pelvic lymph node resection has been performed widely for reduction of the local recurrence rate and for improvement of the survival rate. Determination of accurate preoperative staging is essential for appropriate therapy and for avoidance of insufficient or excessive surgery, leading to maximal survival and functional results such as urinary and sexual function.

Normal pelvic lymph nodes are either invisible or recognized to be less than 1 cm in diameter on CT images. They are of intermediate attenuation, and are best seen after the intravenous administration of contrast medium, which results in increased attenuation of

CARS 2002 – H.U. Lemke, M.W. Vannier; K. Inamura, A.G. Farman, K. Doi & J.H.C. Reiber (Editors)

blood vessels and thus allows accurate differentiation between blood vessels and lymph nodes. When enlargement occurs due to metastasis, they can be identified by their relationship to normal vascular structures. CT has been advocated as a screening tool for the evaluation of lymph node metastases for rectal cancer patients; however, its accuracy in the diagnosis of metastases is still uncertain.

Recent advances in computer technology allow us to use multi-planar reconstruction (MPR) views of 3-dimensional volumetric data generated by helical CT for diagnosis of abdominal lymph nodes [1,2]. Currently, however, the diagnosis of lymph nodes on helical CT images is still performed by hardcopy images reconstructed with a thickness of 1 cm or less. Because of the partial volume effect, it is difficult to identify small lymph nodes of less than 1 cm. Given this limitation, we regard MPR views on the video monitor as an effective method for evaluation of lymph nodes accurately.

Therefore, we conducted a study to evaluate the accuracy of MPR views of 3-dimensional volumetric data generated by helical CT in the diagnosis of preoperative staging for pelvic lymph node metastases in rectal cancer patients. From December 1998 to November 1999, 57 patients with rectal cancer underwent helical CT scanning for evaluation of preoperative staging of lymph node metastases with the following parameter settings: 120 kV, 250 mA, 3 mm beam width, a table speed of 5 mm/sec, and bolus injection of contrast medium. Three radiologists evaluated the staging based on consensus by use of MPR views of the data reconstructed from CT slices. Then the staging was rated by use of the pathologic findings of the surgically removed specimens as gold standard.

Lymph nodes larger than or equal to 6 mm in size were defined as metastases in this study. The detection sensitivity, specificity, and accuracy for the metastases were 96.4%, 51.7%, and 73.7%, respectively, which were substantially higher than those reported previously. These results shows that, by use of the MPR view, we can observe subtle changes in image density in coronal and sagittal slices as well as in axial slices. Thus, the MPR view is an excellent method for recognizing each organ consecutively and for discriminating lymph nodes from vascular structures.

Recently, 3-D images generated by CT colonography have been recognized as an effective option for evaluating colorectal polyps [3-6]. Both 3-D images and MPR views can be generated from the same CT colonographic data acquired by helical CT scanning. It is expected that, by combining these two techniques, we can diagnose colorectal cancers more accurately and more easily. Some studies have assessed an application of computer-assisted diagnosis (CAD) in the detection of colorectal polyps for reduction of the interpretation time and for improvement of the diagnostic accuracy of radiologists [7,8]. MPR views can potentially be added to the CAD program in order to improve radiologists' performance in the diagnosis of colorectal cancers, including lymph node metastases.

CARS 2002 – H.U. Lemke, M.W. Vannier; K. Inamura, A.G. Farman, K. Doi & J.H.C. Reiber (Editors)
°CARS/Springer. All rights reserved.

Acknowledgements

The work was supported in part by a Grant for Scientific Research Expenses for Health and Welfare Programs and the Foundation for the Promotion of Cancer Research in Japan, and by 2nd-term Comprehensive 10-year Strategy for Cancer Control in Japan.

References

1. Seltzer SE, Judy PF, Adams DF, et al., Helical CT of the Chest: Comparison of Cine and Film-Based Viewing. Radiology 197:73-78, 1995

2. Bonaldi VM, Bret PM, Atri M, et al., Helical CT of the pancreas: A Comparison of Cine Display and Film-Based Viewing. AJR 170:373-376, 1998

3. Hara AK, Johnson CD, Reed JE, et al., Detection of colorectal polyps with CT colography: Initial assessment of sensitivity and specificity. Radiology 205: 59-65, 1997.

4. Farrell RJ, Morrin MM, McGee JB. Virtual colonoscopy: A gastroenterologist's perspective. Dig Dis 17: 185-193, 1999.

5. Miao YM, Amin Z, Healy J, et al., A prospective single center study comparing computed tomography pneumocolon against colonoscopy in the detection of colorectal neoplasms. Gut 47: 832-837, 2000.

6. Fenlon HM, Nunes DP, Schroy PC, et al., A comparison of virtual and conventional colonoscopy for the detection of colorectal polyps. N Engl J Med 341: 1496-1503, 1999.

7. Yoshida H, Masutani Y, MacEneaney P, et al., Computerrized detection of colonic poyps at CT colonography on the basis of volumetric features: Pilot study. Radiology 222:327-336, 2002

8. Summers RM, Johnson CD, Pusanik LM, et al., Automated polyp detection at CT colonography: feasibility assessment in a human population. Radiology 2001; 219:51-59.

Three-dimensional computer-aided diagnosis schemes for classification of benign and malignant pulmonary nodules

Y. Kawata, N. Niki, H. Ohmatsu[a], M. Kusumoto[b], R. Kakinuma[a],
K. Mori[c], H. Nishiyama[d], K. Eguchi[e], M. Kaneko[b], N. Moriyama[b]

Dept. of Optical Science, Univ. of Tokushima, [a]National Cancer Center Hospital
East, [b]National Cancer Center Hospital,[c]Tochigi Cancer Center, [d]The Social
Health Insurance Medical Center, [e] Univ. of Tokai

Abstract

We present an example-based assisting approach for classifying pulmonary nodules in 3-D thoracic CT images. The technique represents the internal and surrounding structures of the nodule by means of the distribution pattern of CT density and 3-D curvature indexes. When given an unknown nodule image, the images of lesions with known diagnoses (e.g. malignant vs. benign) are retrieved from a 3-D nodule image database. The malignant likelihood of the unknown case is estimated by the difference between the representation patterns of the unknown case and the retrieved lesions. In the present study, we adopt the Mahalanobis distance as the difference measure and then, explore the feasibility of the classification based on patterns of similar lesion images.

Keywords: CAD, pulmonary nodule, classification.

1. Introduction

(CAD) has the potential to increase the diagnostic accuracy by reducing the false-negative rate while increasing the positive predictive values of abnormalities in three-dimensional (3-D) thoracic images. The interpretation of the pulmonary nodule images often involves the matching features extracted from a database of the nodules with associated clinical information. When the matching procedure is performed well, the database can provide physicians more information concerning the diagnosis and prognosis of the queried nodule. Moreover, the corresponding structures retrieved from the database may help to design the CAD scheme for the distinction between benign and malignant nodules.

In this paper, we formulate the nodule-classification problem as one of learning to recognize nodule patterns from examples. Each nodule pattern is represent by the extracted internal and surrounding features based on CT density and 3-D curvature indexes. We use an initial database of 248 nodule images (malignant case: 179 and benign case : 69) to search similar malignant and benign lesion patterns and construct a distribution-based local lesion model in a high-dimensional image vector space of the nodule representation. We then estimate the likelihood of the malignancy by computing the difference between representation patterns of the unknown case and the retrieved lesions. In this study, we used the Mahalanobis distance as the difference measure and then, explore the feasibility of the classification based on patterns of similar lesion images. We first describe the representation method used as a pre-process of the data and

CARS 2002 – H.U. Lemke, M.W. Vannier; K. Inamura, A.G. Farman, K. Doi & J.H.C. Reiber (Editors)

then give the definition of the similarity criteria. We are then showing results of similar nodule images and estimation the malignant likelihood.

2. Methods

2.1 3-D nodule images

The 3D chest image used in this paper was a stack of thin-section CT images obtained by the helical CT scanner (Toshiba TCT900S Superhelix and Xvigor). The thin-section CT images were measured under the following conditions; beam width: 2mm, table speed: 2mm/sec, tube voltage: 120kV, tube current : 250mA or 200mA. For the scan duration, patients held their breath at full inspiration. Per patient, about 60 slices at 1mm intervals were obtained to observe whole nodule region and its surroundings. The range of pixel size in each square slice of 512 pixels was between 0.3×0.3 mm^2 and 0.4×0.4 mm^2, and the slice contains an extended region of the lung area. The 3D chest image was reconstructed from the thin-section CT images by a linear interpolation technique to make each voxel isotropic. The data set in this study included 248 3-D chest images from 248 patients provided by National Cancer Center Hospital East and Tochigi Cancer Center. Of the 248 cases, 179 contained malignant nodules, and 69 contained benign nodules. Whole malignant cases and part of benign cases were proved by cytologically or histologically diagnosis. In benign cases lesions showed no change or decreased in size over a 2-year period were considered benign nodules.

2.2 Nodule representation

We build a 3-D nodule image database from the data set. The database consists of two types elements, such as text-based elements and image-based elements. The text-based elements of the database are as follows, ID number, measurement conditions, sex, age, diagnosis result, nodule diameter and volume that compute from the segmented nodule image. The image-based elements are as follows, the 3-D ROI image with a nodule of interest, the segmented nodule image, the representation of local density pattern inside the nodule and nodule surroundings. Because of perception subjectivity, there exist multiple representations that characterize the feature from different perspectives for any give features [3]. Since the internal and surrounding structures of the nodule are important cues to distinct malignancy from benign cases, we concentrate on the feature representation inside the nodule and the nodule surroundings. We present the representation procedure as well as the pre-processing of the representation such nodule segmentation, feature extraction.

2.2.1 Pre-processing of the nodule representation

The segmentation of the 3D pulmonary nodule image consists of three steps [2] ;1) extraction of lung area, 2) selection of the region of interest (ROI) including the nodule region, and 3) nodule segmentation based on a deformable surface approach. The lung area extraction step plays an essential role when the part of a nodule in the peripheral lung area touches the chest wall. The ROI including the nodule was selected interactively. A pulmonary nodule was segmented from the selected ROI image by the deformable surface approach. The nodule surrounding region was computed by the distance from the nodule surface. The distance was obtained by applying the Euclidean distance transformation approach proposed by Saito et al. [7] to the nodule surrounding region.

CARS 2002 – H.U. Lemke, M.W. Vannier; K. Inamura, A.G. Farman, K. Doi & J.H.C. Reiber (Editors)

766

Each voxel in the region of interest (ROI) including the pulmonary nodule is locally represented by CT density and curvature index. By assuming that each voxel in the ROI lies on the surface which has the normal corresponding to the 3-D gradient at the voxel, we computed directly the curvatures on each voxel from the first and the second derivatives of the gray level image of the ROI. At each voxel two principal curvatures and directions of principal curvatures are computed by using the approach proposed by Thirion [4]. As the curvature index at each voxel in the ROI image, we use the shape index that is computed from two principal curvatures [5],[6]. The continuous surface type is mapped on the interval [0, 1] of the shape index value.

To quantify the relationship between the nodule and its surrounding structure such as vessel and pleura, we focus on two indicators of malignancy, which are denoted as vascular convergence and pleural retraction. In the 3-D thoracic CT images, these findings are observed so that the vessel and pleura images are drawn in the nodule. We assumed that the shape of the vessel and the pleura images are similar to cylindrical or conic structures. Therefore, we measure an amount of the vascular convergence and pleural retraction by computing the absolute value of the inner product of the directions of cylindrical or conic structures and the normal directions of the nodule surface. For the representation of the directions, we compute two vector fields that consist of the directions of the maximum principal curvature and normal vector of the nodule surface. The vector field is denoted as the maximum principal curvature vector (MPV) field. The normal directions of the nodule surface at the vicinity of the nodule are estimated by a diffusion procedure proposed by Xu [8]. The approach is to keep the desirable property of the gradients near the nodule edges, but to expand the gradient away from the edges into homogeneous regions of the nodule surrounding using the computational diffusion process. The vector field obtained by the normal vector of the nodule surface is denoted as gradient vector (GV) field.

2.2.2 Joint-histogram based representation
In order to characterize the distribution pattern of the CT density and the shape index inside nodule, we compute two types of joint histogram using the distance value from the nodule center. Since the distance value depends on the nodule size, the first type is directly derived from the distance value and used to search similar lesions. Once obtained similar lesions, the variation of internal structure provides more important information to classify nodule patterns rather than the nodule size. Therefore, the second type is derived from the normalized distance value which ranges between zero and one value and used to evaluate the likelihood of the malignancy. To compute the distance value at each voxel, we apply the Euclidean distance transformation technique [7] to the segmented nodule image and obtain the maximum distance value inside the nodule.

For the representation of the nodule surrounding region, we compute the absolute value (F) of the inner product between MPV and GV fields at each voxel in surrounding region of the nodule. Then, we represent the nodule surrounding by using the joint histogram of the distance value from the nodule surface and the absolute value of the inner product. To select the part of cylindrical or conic structures in the surrounding region, we specified two threshold values T_{SH} for the shape index value (SH) and then

CARS 2002 – H.U. Lemke, M.W. Vannier; K. Inamura, A.G. Farman, K. Doi & J.H.C. Reiber (Editors)
ᶜCARS/Springer. All rights reserved.

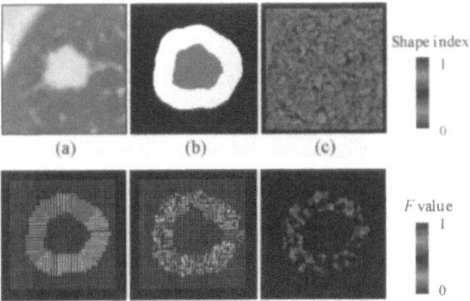

Fig. 1: Feature extraction result of a malignant nodule. (a) Slice image of ROI. (b) Segmentation results of the nodule and its surrounding regions. (c) Shape index distribution. (d) GV field. (e) MPV field. (f) F value distribution.

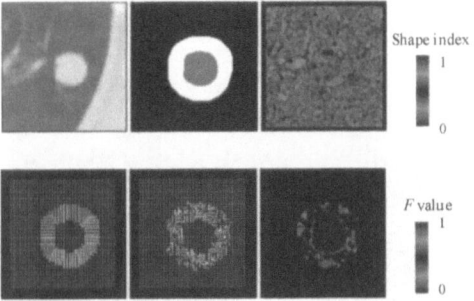

Fig. 2 : Feature extraction result of a benign nodule. (a) Slice image of ROI. (b) Segmentation results of the nodule and its surrounding regions. (c) Shape index distribution. (d) GV field. (e) MPV field. (f) F value distribution.

obtained the region consisting of voxels which satisfied with a condition of $SH < T_{SH}$. The value of T_{SH} was set to 0.5. This process means that the surface types of cylindrical or conic structures are extracted by the shape index value. Two types of joint histogram are computed for the selected region in the similar equation of the computation the joint histogram of the CT density value and the distance value.

2.3 Searching similar nodule images
It is a possible way to directly apply a similarity measure to the 3-D nodule image. However, this approach requires solving the registration between two images. In this study, we apply a simple similarity measure, which is the correlation coefficient (CC) to the nodule representation based on the joint histogram. At the first glance of a given nodule image, it is thought of that the nodule size and nodule density are important indexes for the visual assessment. Then, the features with respect to the local intensity structure are examined in detail to search similar patterns. In this study, we generate the list of similar nodule image by the searching process based on the similarity. We apply the and then sort the CC value from more to less of similar patterns.

CARS 2002 – H.U. Lemke, M.W. Vannier; K. Inamura, A.G. Farman, K. Doi & J.H.C. Reiber (Editors)
ᶜCARS/Springer. All rights reserved.

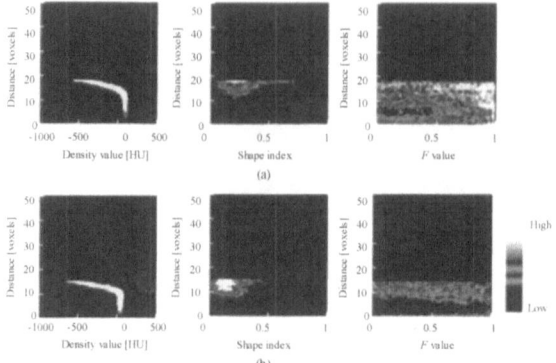

Fig. 3 : Joint histogram-based representations of the malignant and benign cases shown in Figs. 1 and 2, respectively. (a) Malignant case. (b) Benign case. From left to right, representation with respect to the CT density value, shape index value, and F value, respectively.

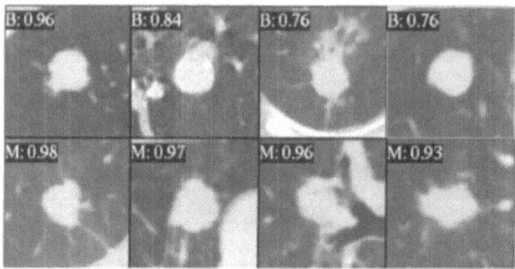

Fig. 4 : Similar image of the unknown case. First row: similar image obtained from the benign group (B). Second row: similar images obtained from the malignant group (M). From left to right: sorting result from more to less similar pattern. The fraction number denotes the CC value.

2.4 Difference measure for classifying nodule patterns

We select respectively the M examples from each list of the malignant and benign similar pattern to construct local two malignant and benign clusters that are similar to the unknown case concerning the CT density distribution pattern and the nodule size. The second type of the joint-histogram is used to model the distributions of the retrieved malignant and benign examples. Each malignant and benign example is represented by two 20x20 pixel images of the joint histograms regarding the shape index and F values and treated as 800-dimensional feature vector space. The Mahalanobis distance is used as a distance measure between the unknown pattern and each local model. In this preliminary study, we classify the unknown case into the cluster with small Mahalanobis distance.

3. Results and Conclusion

Fig. 1 presents an application result of the feature extraction procedure to a malignant case. Fig.1 (f) shows the F value distribution computed from the GV and MPV fields as

CARS 2002 – H.U. Lemke, M.W. Vannier; K. Inamura, A.G. Farman, K. Doi & J.H.C. Reiber (Editors)

shown in (d) and (e), respectively. Compared Fig.1 (a) with (f), it is observed that Fig 3 presents the first joint histogram-based representations of the malignant and benign cases shown in Figs. 1 and 2, respectively. Compared malignant with benign cases, it is observed that there is a few difference pattern between the joint histogram based representations with respect to CT density and distance except for the different expansion along the distance axis. While, it can be observed that there are difference patterns of the first joint histogram-based representations concerning the shape index and the F value. Compared the malignant case with the benign case, the benign case has extremely high frequency of the shape index value around zero. This means that peak surface type occupies the inner structure of the benign case. Owning to the component of vessels and speculations, it seems that malignant case has larger amount of the component radiating from the nodule than the benign case.

We considered the malignant nodule shown in Fig. 1 as an unknown case and applied our approach to this case. Fig. 4 presents the searching similar images of the unknown case. Fig. 4 shows sorting results of similar images obtained from benign and malignant groups in our database. Fig. 5 presents the first joint histogram-based representations of the most similar benign and malignant nodules to the unknown case. The Maharanobis distance of the unknown case was more close to the malignant cluster.

More research requires building a classifier between malignant and benign cases based on the similar patterns feature spaces. Still, we believe that the searching similar image approach would provide a better understanding for any given nodule in assisting physician's diagnostic decisions.

References

1. M. Kaneko, K. Eguchi, H. Ohmatsu, R. Kakinuma, T. Naruke, K. Suemasu, N. Moriyama "Peripheral lung cancer: Screening and detection with low-dose spiral CT versus radiography", *Radiology*, vol.201, pp.798-802, 1996.
2. Y. Rui, T.S. Huang, S.-F. Chang, "Image retrieval: current techniques, promising directions and open issues", *Journal of Communication and Image Representation*, vol. 10, pp.39-62, 1999.
3. Y. Kawata, N. Niki, H. Ohmatsu, R. Kakinuma, K. Eguchi, M. Kaneko, N. Moriyama, "Quantitative surface characterization of pulmonary nodules based on thin-section CT images", *IEEE Trans. Nuclear Science*, vol. 45, pp.2132-2138, 1998.
4. J.-P, Thirion and A. Gourdon, "Computing the differential characteristics of isointensity surfaces", *Computer Vision and Image Understanding*, vol.6, pp.190-202, 1995.
5. J. J. Koenderink and A. J. V. Doorn, "Surface shape and curvature scales", *Image and Vision Computing*, vol.10, pp.557-565, 1992.
6. Y. Kawata, N. Niki, H. Ohmatsu, "Curvature based internal structure analysis of pulmonary nodules using thoracic 3-D CT images", *IEICE Trans., vol.J-83-D-II*, pp.209-218, 2000.
7. T. Saito and J. Toriwaki, "Euclidean distance transformation for three-dimensional digital images", *Trans. IEICE, vol.J76-D-II*, pp.445-453, 1993.
8. C. Xu and J.L. Prince, "Snake, shape, and gradient vector flow", *IEEE Trans. Image Processing*, vol. 7, pp.359-369, 1998.

CARS 2002 – H.U. Lemke, M.W. Vannier; K. Inamura, A.G. Farman, K. Doi & J.H.C. Reiber (Editors)

Pulmonary nodule detection using cartwheel projection analysis

Li Fan[a], Jianzhong Qian[a], Guo-Qing Wei[a], David P. Naidich[b]

[a]Siemens Corporate Research, 755 College Road East, Princeton, NJ 08540
[b]New York University, Medical Center, New York, NY 10016

Abstract

In this paper, we propose a novel method, called cartwheel projection analysis (CWPA), to automatically detect lung nodules in high-resolution multi-slice CT images. First, a nodule candidate generation algorithm is applied to examine the whole lung volume and record only structures that are potentially nodules. This step quickly excludes small and large sized vessels from further analysis, so that computation can be saved dramatically. Then, cartwheel projection analysis is applied to examine the shape characteristics of the structures corresponding to the nodule candidates. CWPA is based on 1-dimensional curves obtained from a series of 2D cutting planes centered at the structure of interest in the volume. Finally, a set of criteria is applied for identifying the existence of nodules based on shape analysis of the 1-D shape curves.

Keywords: Lung nodule detection, computed tomography (CT), lung cancer

1. Purpose

Lung cancer has been reported as the second most commonly diagnosed cancer for both men and women, as well as the leading cause of cancer death in America [1]. Meanwhile, resection of certain lung cancer at early stage has been shown to significantly improve the five-year survival rate [2]. Therefore, as a sensitive sign of lung cancer, nodules are very much desirable to be detected via non-invasive methods at their early stages. Multi-slice CT puts precision imaging into practice and provides such a way in which nodules from 2 to 30 mm in diameter can be imaged. However, the large amount of HRCT data presents formidable challenges to physicians. A typical multi-slice CT scan with slice thickness of 1 to 1.5 mm may have 300 or more image slices. If CT for lung cancer screening becomes widespread, there will be a tremendous demand for such examinations. Clearly, it would be time consuming and impractical for physicians to study every single slice image. Automatic detection therefore has attracted tremendous interests recently. However, with certain degree of success, most of the existing automatic detection has the drawback of high false positive rate, and low sensitivity in detecting nodules attached to vessels.

In this paper, we propose a novel approach to automatically detect pulmonary nodules with low false positive rate and high sensitivity. First, the lung volume is extracted and a nodule candidate generation algorithm is applied to record the structures that are potentially nodules. This step quickly excludes small and large sized vessels from further analysis, and computation can therefore be saved dramatically. Next, cartwheel projection analysis (CWPA) is applied to each of the structure of interest corresponding to the nodule candidates. This is done by analyzing the shape characteristics of the structure of interest

CARS 2002 – H.U. Lemke, M.W. Vannier; K. Inamura, A.G. Farman, K. Doi & J.H.C. Reiber (Editors)

on a series of 2D spinning planes. One-dimensional curves representing the shape of the structure is computed and analyzed based a set of criteria to identify the existence of a nodule.

2. Methods

Currently, one of the widely applied approach for radiologists to detect nodules from CT images is to read hard copies of axial 2D slices. Images are reconstructed at low axial resolution (5 to 10mm thick slices) for practical reasons, so that there will usually be about 30 slices per patient study for manual examination. Physicians examine every slice to find bright, round-shaped objects that suddenly appear and disappear in consecutive slices. However, radiologists probably find it easier to detect nodules in peripheral areas of the lungs. CT values of blood vessels are very similar to those of pulmonary nodules. Moreover, blood vessels may have similar shapes as nodules on 2D slices when they lie perpendicular to the imaging plane. In addition, radiologists cannot obtain enough information about the 3D connectivity information of the structure of interest. These facts make it hard for physicians to detect nodules in central areas where many vessels exist, and to detect nodules that are attached to vessels.

To overcome the existing problems and to free physicians from the heavy burden of reading through hundreds of image slices every day, algorithms that can automatically detect pulmonary nodules with reasonable confidence are highly desirable. Such an algorithm should have the following features:

- Sensitive to nodules. This feature actually corresponds to the two problems that radiologist are encountering now. To be a real assistance to physicians, the detection algorithm should be able to find nodules, even when they are attached to vessels.

- Low false-positive rate. The detection algorithm should have an acceptable false positive rate while keeping a high sensitivity. If there are too many false positive, physicians will lose faith in the system and find it tedious to use.

- Computationally efficient. The detection should be finished in a reasonable amount of time, so that physicians may validate the results without adding a significant time burden.

In this section, we describe a novel approach that meets these requirements. The proposed automatic detection scheme incorporates *a priori* knowledge of pulmonary structures, and makes full use of intensity and shape information. It consists of four main steps:

2.1 Lung area extraction
The major purpose of this step is to locate and separate lung region from chest wall. Morphological operations combined with simple thresholding can extract the lung region from chest wall, while keeping the nodules and vessels attached to the chest wall.

2.2 Nodule candidate generation
In this step, structures with high likelihood to be nodules are identified and recorded for much detailed examination. To do so, we apply the Euclidean distance map (EDM) in a way that most vessel structure can be quickly excluded. This step also dramatically saves the computational cost [3]. A previously proposed automatic method for solitary nodule

772

detection can also be applied [4]. The herein proposed CWPA approach can reduce false positives by distinguishing small nodules from weak vessels.

2.3 Cartwheel projection analysis (CWPA)

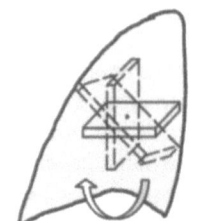

Figure 1. An illustration of the cartwheel projection (CWP).

Cartwheel projection (CWP) is a cine loop with each frame of the cine representing a small cutting slice of the data, taken at slightly different angles, centered at the point of interest. It was reported in our pervious work as 'Fly Around' [5]. An illustration can be seen in Figure 1. On the CWP slices of each nodule candidate generated, the shape characteristics and 3D connectivity information can be revealed and examined. 1-dimensional curves representing the shape of the structure are computed along the principle axis direction first on binary CWP slices and then weighted by the corresponding intensity values.

2.4 Decision making

Representing the shape characteristics of the anatomical structures, the weighted 1-D shape curves exhibit distinct difference in their shape features between the curves of nodules and those of vessels. Usually, the weighted 1-D shape curve of a nodule is Gaussian shaped with its variation proportional to the nodule size, no matter the nodule is isolated or attached to vessels, while that of a vessel does not possess such a property. The difference can be observed in Figures 2 and 3. Therefore, multiple criteria are set to check the shape of the curves and decision is made on whether or not the nodule candidate represents a nodule.

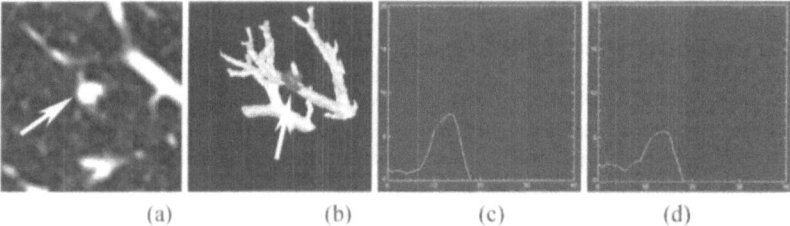

(a)   (b)   (c)   (d)

Figure 2. A nodule attached to vessels. (a) Axial view of the nodule on 2D slice; (b) 3D shaded surface rendering of the nodule; (c) and (d) two examples the 1-D shape curves of the cartwheel projection analysis which are of Gaussian shape with the variations proportional to the nodule size.

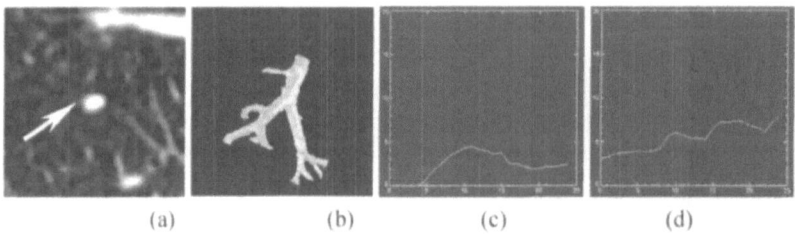

(a)   (b)   (c)   (d)

Figure 3. A vessel. (a) Axial view of the vessel on 2D slice; (b) 3D shaded surface rendering of the vessel; (c) and (d) two examples the 1-D shape curves of the CWP analysis. It can be observed that although at certain angles of the CWP spinning plane, the 1-D shape curve appears to be a Gaussian, on some other angles, it does not.

CARS 2002 – H.U. Lemke, M.W. Vannier; K. Inamura, A.G. Farman, K. Doi & J.H.C. Reiber (Editors)
ᶜCARS/Springer. All rights reserved.

3. Results

We applied the proposed method to 10 CT screening studies of smokers. The data sets were all low dose multi-slice high resolution CT images, with dosages from 20 to 40 mAs, in-plane resolutions from 0.57 to 0.67mm/pixel, slice thickness of 1.25mm with 0.25mm overlap. The image sizes are 512*512 within slice, with 280 to 300 slices in Z direction.

Three chest radiologists evaluated the patient studies separately on 7mm hard copies separately. Meanwhile, the automatic detection is applied to thin slice multi-slice HR CT data. Finally, two experienced chest radiologists examined all the marks detected by both radiologists and computer, and determined ground truth by consensus.

In the previous work, we have reported a comprehensive knowledge-based automatic lung nodule detection system, which consists of CWPA and other modules [6]. Here, we report the preliminary result of the CWPA. The overall statistics are listed in Table 1. Analysis has shown that there were in total 50 nodules detected and confirmed by radiologists and the proposed lung nodule detection method together, of which 2 were ground glass nodules (GGNs). The three radiologists detected 21, 17, and 14 nodules, representing sensitivities of 42.0%, 34.0% and 28.0%, respectively. The automatic detection algorithm detected 37 nodules, achieving a sensitivity of 74.0%, with a mean false positive rate of 6.5 per patient study. The computer detection result had significant overlap with that of the individual radiologist, ranging from 64.3% to 71.4%. With the help of the proposed automatic detection system, radiologists would detect an average of 147% more nodules than alone, and reach sensitivities of 86.0%, 80.0% and 84.0%, respectively.

Since it is very hard for radiologists to detect nodules smaller than 3 mm on 7mm thickness sections, we excluded all confirmed nodules that were smaller than 3mm, and computed the statistics again. Table 1 shows that radiologists' performance increased. Also, since the proposed nodule detection algorithm based on cartwheel projection analysis does not yet possess the ability to detect ground glass nodules (GGNs), we then excluded GGNs. The statistics can be seen in Table 1.

If excluding GGNs and nodules smaller than 3mm, there were in total 31 confirmed nodules. Radiologists detected 17, 14, and 11 nodules, achieving sensitivities of 54.8%, 45.2% and 35.5%, respectively. The computer detected 27 non-GGN nodules that are greater than or equal to 3mm in diameter, achieving a sensitivity of 87.1%. The computer detection result overlap with that of individual radiologist ranged from 81.8% to 88.2%, and can help radiologists detect an average of 114% more nodules and reach sensitivities of 93.5%, 93.5% and 93.5%, respectively.

The size distribution of the detected nodules is illustrated in Figure 3. It can be observed that for nodules smaller than 3mm in diameter, the automatic detection algorithm performs significantly better than the radiologists. The reasons lie in two aspects. First, it is harder for radiologists to pick them up on thick sections. Secondly, analysis has shown that most of the small nodules missed by radiologists are located in central area of the lungs, which has many more anatomical structures than the peripheral area. In such situation, it is very difficult for radiologists to identify the small opacities using only 2D information. It can also be observed that even for middle-sized nodules up to 6 mm, the proposed automatic detection approach can detect more than radiologists. This is mainly because radiologists are sensitive to peripherally located nodules, yet less sensitive to

774

centrally located ones. In addition, some middle-sized nodules are also attached to vessels on 2D slices, which makes them less eye-catching to radiologists. However, as the nodule sizes go up and the nodules become more eye-catching, radiologists' performances increase.

All nodules confirmed: 50					
	Nodules detected	*Sensitivity %*	*Sensitivity with CWPA * %*	*Overlap with computer*	*Overlap rate %*
Radiologist 1	21	42.0	86.0	15	71.4
Radiologist 2	17	34.0	80.0	14	82.4
Radiologist 3	14	28.0	84.0	9	64.3
Automatic detection	37	74.0	-	*FPs/patient study:* 6.5	

All nodules ≥ 3mm: 33					
	Nodules detected	*Sensitivity %*	*Sensitivity with CWPA * %*	*Overlap with computer*	*Overlap rate %*
Radiologist 1	19	57.6	93.9	15	78.9
Radiologist 2	15	45.5	90.9	12	80.0
Radiologist 3	13	39.4	93.9	9	69.2
Automatic detection	27	81.8	-		

All non-GGN nodules: 48					
	Nodules detected	*Sensitivity %*	*Sensitivity with CWPA * %*	*Overlap with computer*	*Overlap rate %*
Radiologist 1	19	39.6	85.4	15	78.9
Radiologist 2	16	33.3	81.3	14	87.5
Radiologist 3	12	25.0	83.3	9	75.0
Automatic detection	37	77.1	-		

All non-GGN nodules ≥ 3mm: 31					
	Nodules detected	*Sensitivity %*	*Sensitivity with CWPA * %*	*Overlap with computer*	*Overlap rate %*
Radiologist 1	17	54.8	93.5	15	88.2
Radiologist 2	14	45.2	93.5	12	85.7
Radiologist 3	11	35.5	93.5	9	81.8
Automatic detection	27	87.1	-		

*: *Sensitivity with CWPA* refers to the sensitivities that radiologists can achieve with the help of the proposed automatic nodule detection algorithm based on cartwheel projection analysis.

Table 1. Experimental results of the proposed cartwheel projection analysis detection method.

CARS 2002 – H.U. Lemke, M.W. Vannier; K. Inamura, A.G. Farman, K. Doi & J.H.C. Reiber (Editors)
ᶜCARS/Springer. All rights reserved.

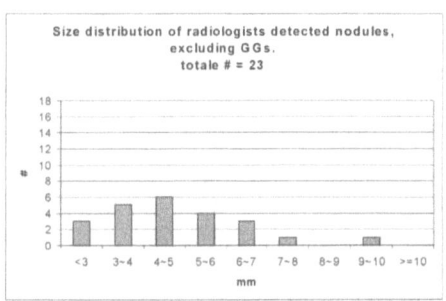 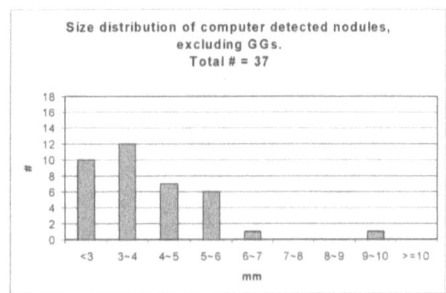

Figure 4. Size distribution of nodules detected by radiologists (left) and computer (right).

4. Conclusion

The proposed lung nodule detection method makes full use of the intensity and shape information of anatomical structures of interest. Preliminary results have shown that the method can achieve high sensitivity of detection while generating acceptably low false positives. Also, the automatic detection results have high overlap rate with radiologists, which could help radiologists to build confidence in the proposed automatic detection method. Finally, preliminary results have shown that with the proposed automatic detection, radiologists can detect substantially more nodules than alone and their detection sensitivity can be dramatically increased.

Acknowledgements

The authors would like to thank Dr. Jane P. Ko, Dr. Ami N. Rubinowitz, and Dr. Georgeann McGuinness of New York University Medical Center for clinical evaluations.

References

1. "Cancer Facts & Figures 2001", Atlanta: American Cancer Society (2001).
2. B.J. Flehinger, M. Kimmel and M.R. Melamed, "The effect of surgical treatment on survival from early lung cancer", *Chest*, vol.101, pp. 1013-1018, 1992.
3. L. Fan, J. Qian, G.Q. Wei, "Automatic Generation of Vessel-feeding Pulmonary Nodule Candidates from High-resolution Thin-slice CT Data", *US Patent,* pending, 2001.
4. L. Fan, C.L. Novak, J. Qian, G. Kohl, and D.P. Naidich, "Automatic detection of lung nodules from multi-slice low-dose CT images", *Proceedings of SPIE Medical Imaging 2001, Image Processing*, vol 4322, pp. 1828-1835, 2001.
5. C.L. Novak, L. Fan, J. Qian, G. Kohl, D.P. Naidich, "An Interactive System for CT Lung Nodule Identification and Evaluation", CARS 2001, pp. 599-604.
6. J. Qian, L Fan, G.Q. Wei, C.L. Novak, B. Odry, H. Shen, L. Zhang, D.P. Naidich, J.P. Ko, A.N. Rubinowitz, G. McGuinness, G. Kohl, E. Klotz, "Knowledge-based Automatic Detection of Multi-type Lung Nodules from Multi-detector CT Studies", Proceedings of SPIE Medical Imaging, vol 4684, 2002.

CARS 2002 – H.U. Lemke, M.W. Vannier; K. Inamura, A.G. Farman, K. Doi & J.H.C. Reiber (Editors)

776

Extraction and recognition of the thoracic organs based on 3D CT images and its application

Xiangrong Zhou, PhD [a], Takeshi Hara, PhD [b], Hiroshi Fujita, PhD [b], Yoshihiro Ida, RT [c], Kazuhiro Katada, MD [c], Kazuhiko Matsumoto, MS [d]

[a] Virtual System Laboratory, Gifu University, Gifu-shi, 501-1193, Japan
[b] Department of Information Science, Gifu University, Gifu-shi, 501-1193, Japan
[c] Department of Radiology, Fujita Health University Hospital, Toyoake-shi, 470-1192, Japan
[d] Ziosoft, Inc., Tokyo, 108-0073, Japan, Email: zxr@vsl.gifu-u.ac.jp

Abstract

A method for extracting and recognizing thoracic organ regions from three-dimensional (3D) CT chest images has been proposed in this paper. This method can be simply described as a pixel-labelling process, that is, each pixel in a chest CT image is attached with a predefined label that indicates a special organ or tissue of human body. The density distribution and strength of connectivity of different organ regions have been investigated and used for the recognition process. We developed a system to visualize the 3D CT images based on volume rendering technique and intergraded this method into it. We found that with the recognition results we can view the shape of a special organ without any overlap and can understand the relationship of human organs more clearly and easily.

Keywords: 3D CT images, image segmentation, thoracic organ recognition

1. Introduction

With the development of high-speed and high-quality radiological imaging devices such as multi-slice CT scanner, three-dimensional (3D) digital images have been becoming more and more popular in medical diagnosis since they can provide three dimensional information of the human body for physicians as well as patients directly and precisely in few seconds. However, in order to find out the suspicious regions and understand the 3D structure of the human body, medical doctors always have to spend much time and energy to view a lot of individual slices of 3D images on screen. Therefore, computer-aided diagnosis (CAD) and visualization of 3D images are strongly desired to reduce this burden.

The CAD systems are always required to provide an automatic detection of suspicious regions and a 3D view of the interesting regions based on CT images. As the first step of such a process, a reliable extraction of the human organs and recognition of the normal structure of the human body from CT images are necessary. Although a number of techniques have been proposed for extracting a special organ and detecting its abnormality, few of them put emphasis on identifying all the organs and recognizing the normal structure of the human body.

CARS 2002 – H.U. Lemke, M.W. Vannier; K. Inamura, A.G. Farman, K. Doi & J.H.C. Reiber (Editors)

We have developed an image processing system that can recognize the different organs from chest CT images. The identifying process of this system can be simply described as a pixel-labelling process, that is, each pixel of the CT image is attached with a label that represents a special region or organ of the human body. In this paper, a framework of image processing procedures for organ identification used in this system is described firstly, then, this method is applied to identify the thoracic organs from real chest CT images, and the result images are shown finally.

2. Methods

The input of the system is a 3D chest CT image as shown in Fig.1 (a). The output is a labelled image in which each target region has been identified with a predefined label that appears as a density value as shown in Fig.1 (b). A framework of image processing procedures is used to split the whole region of the original CT image into several target regions which are predefined as shown in Fig.1 (c).

2.1 Target organs and tissues
Each target region which should be recognized from an original CT image is defined in Fig.1 (c). Each label has been attached with a special intensity value used to distinguish regions from each other as shown in Fig.1 (b).

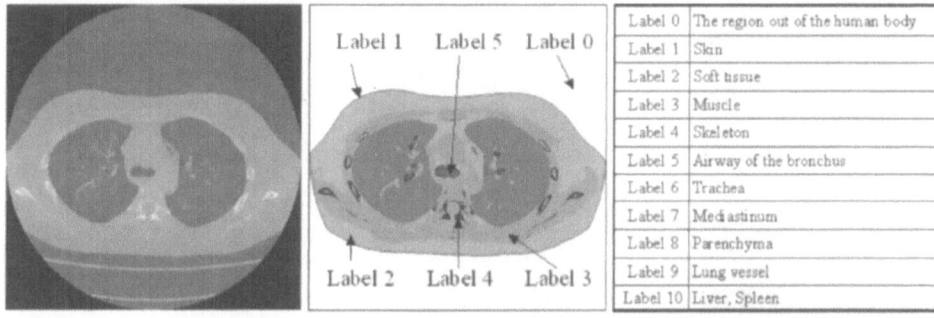

Label 0	The region out of the human body
Label 1	Skin
Label 2	Soft tissue
Label 3	Muscle
Label 4	Skeleton
Label 5	Airway of the bronchus
Label 6	Trachea
Label 7	Mediastinum
Label 8	Parenchyma
Label 9	Lung vessel
Label 10	Liver, Spleen

(a) 1 slice of a CT image   (b) Recognition result   (c) Labels definition
Fig. 1: Target regions which should be recognized from the CT images.

2.2 Extraction and recognition
The flow of the recognition process is shown in Fig.2. The air around the human body has a unique gray-level in CT image, so that the air region is extracted at first using a gray-level thresholding based on a histogram analysis. The extracted air regions are divided into 2 parts by the human body. The air region inside the human body is used to get the initial lung region and extract airway of the bronchus[1]. The air region outside of the human body is used to extract the contour of the body surface. As the next step, a combination of border following and filling process is used to extract the skin and segment the human body form the CT image. Based on the histogram of the region of human body, the soft tissue and initial skeleton regions are separated from the other organs sequentially using a gray-level thresholding process.

CARS 2002 – H.U. Lemke, M.W. Vannier; K. Inamura, A.G. Farman, K. Doi & J.H.C. Reiber (Editors)
ᶜCARS/Springer. All rights reserved.

778

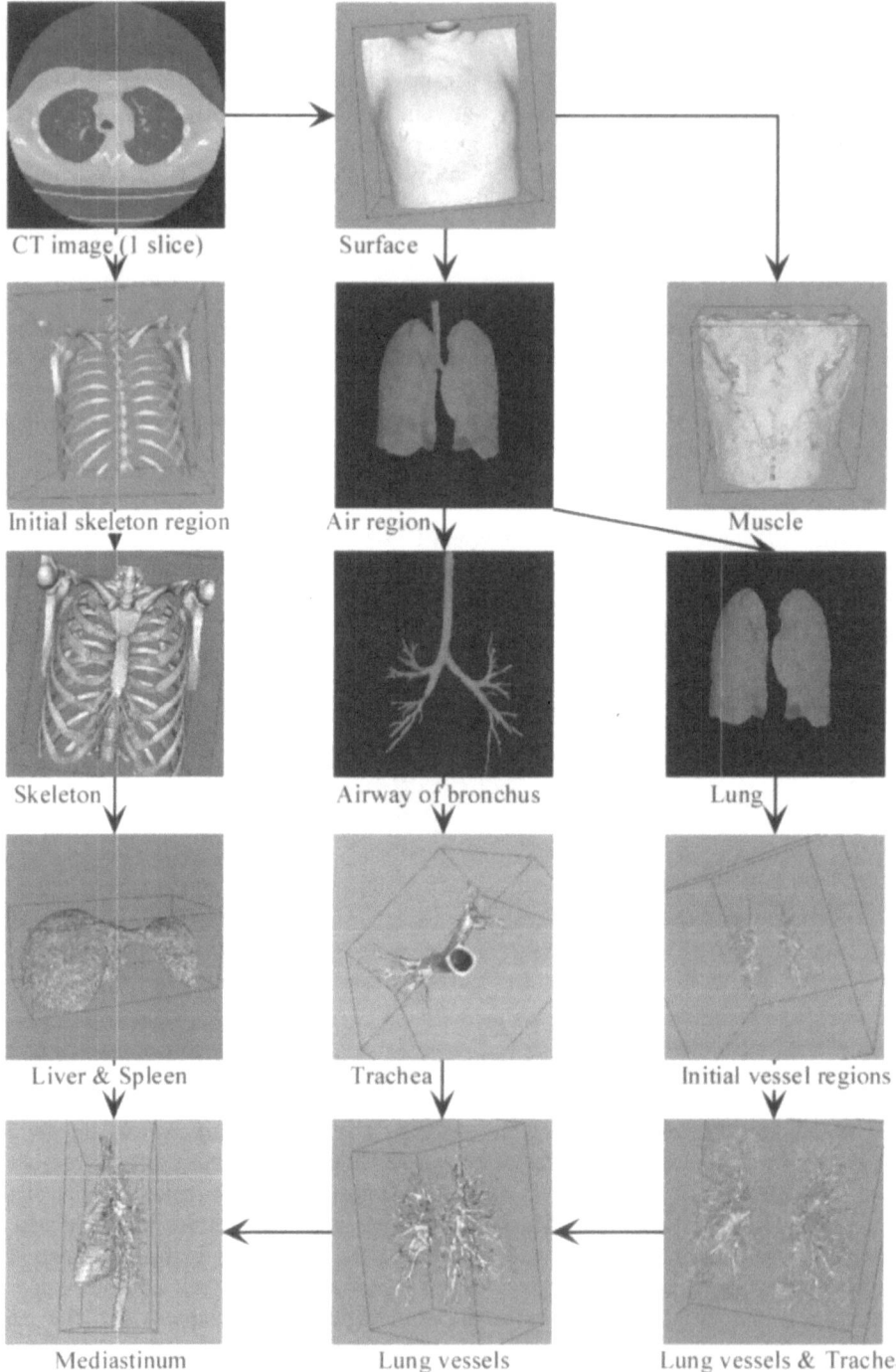

Fig. 2: The flow of the recognition process.

CARS 2002 – H.U. Lemke, M.W. Vannier; K. Inamura, A.G. Farman, K. Doi & J.H.C. Reiber (Editors)

The density distributions of the other organs (such as liver, mediastinum, vessels, etc) are overlapped together, so that we cannot separate those organs by only using gray-level thresholding. We noticed that each organ seemed to be constructed by a set of pixels which have similar density values and hang together closely with each other. Due to this property, strength of connectivity of each pixel has been defined and used to identify skeleton, liver, and mediastinum regions. In fact, a 3D region growing process has been applied to extract bone, liver and mediastinum regions sequentially using the initial skeleton regions as the seed points.

The trachea region is extracted using the information of the density value and Euclidean distance[2] from the surface of the airway of bronchus. In pulmonary hilum region, a 2D snakes method has been used to separate the connection between mediastinum and lung vessels. A combination of gray-level thresholding and 3D region growing process has been applied to separate lung vessels from parenchyma region. The threshold values and parameters of region growing used above are optimized automatically during the recognition process.

2.3 Visualization of CT images

A friendly user interface has been developed for visualization of 3D CT images (Fig.3). A 3D CT image can be viewed slice-by-slice from 3-directions at the same time under an intensity mode or a maximum-intensity projection (MIP) mode. A 3D view is also provided based on volume rendering and surface rendering techniques. With the recognition results stated above, we can select and view a special organ region or a set of them freely and easily.

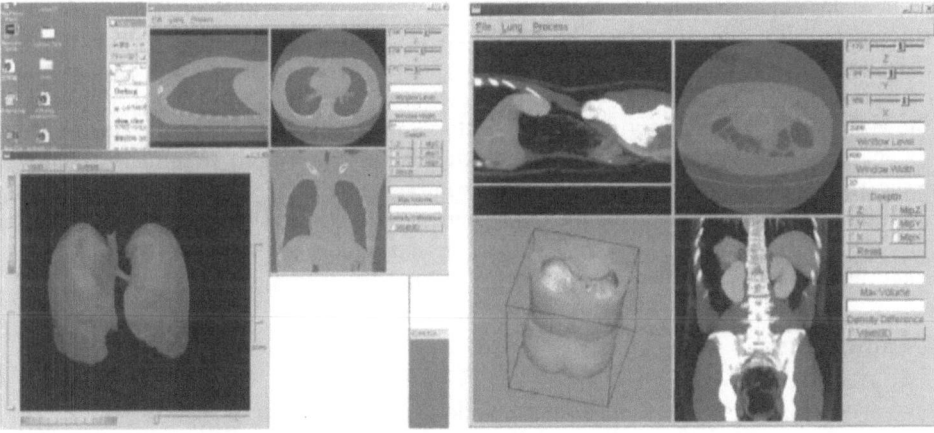

Fig. 3: A user interface for 3D CT image visualization.

3. Experimental results

We applied this framework to identify the thoracic organs from real 3D chest CT images. Two patient cases of multi-slice CT images were used in the experiment and each of them covers the entire human chest region. Every image is 512x512x500-600(pixel) digital image with 12 bits gray-level and high-resolution of 0.625x0.625x0.5(mm³), and is

780

obtained by a half-second Realtime Helical CT scanner "Aquilion" of Toshiba Medical Systems Corporation. With the recognition results, shown in Fig.1 (b), a series of 3D views has been obtained, as shown in Fig.4, to present the human body details from the outside to the inside.

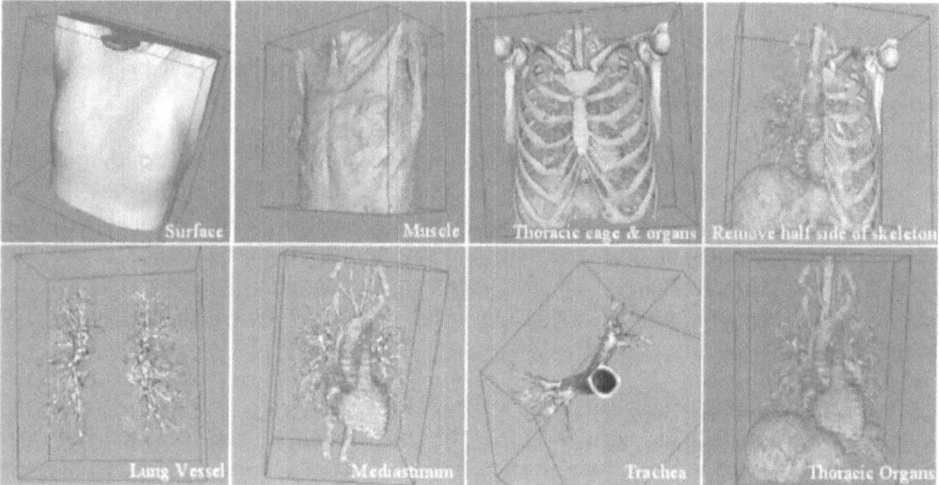

Fig. 4: 3D views of the human body from outside to inside based on recognition results.

Using the recognition results, we integrated CT values of pixels along rays casting through an entire volume to produce a 2D image resembling conventional chest radiography. By adjusting the projection coefficient of each organ before the 2D projection process, we can easily estimate or emphasize the influence of a special organ through reducing the obscurity caused by the overlap of organs and tissues in a volume (shown in Fig.5). It is helpful for trainee doctors to understand the human structure from 2D chest radiography images in image-diagnosis (interpretation) training. As another application, the storage space of CT images can be reduced based on recognition results. A multi-slice CT image covering the entire human chest region will need 200-300MB. In our experiment, we can simply delete the external region of the human body in a CT image and can save about 30% storage space without any information loss.

4. Conclusion

Several conclusions can be summarized as follows from the experimental results.
(a) The framework presented in section 2 can extract the thoracic organ regions successfully from multi-slice chest CT images. From the preliminary results, we confirmed that each target region defined in Fig.1(c) has been recognized and attached with a correct label.
(b) Because the human organs and tissues hang together and construct the human body, the policy of separating the human body into several detailed organ regions sequentially seemed more effective and easier to do than segmenting each special organ individually.
(c) The recognition results would be beneficial to the design of abnormal region detection by CAD system. Based on the recognition results, the detecting algorithm can be designed

CARS 2002 – H.U. Lemke, M.W. Vannier; K. Inamura, A.G. Farman, K. Doi & J.H.C. Reiber (Editors)

781

more specially and accurately. For example, instead of using one image-processing algorithm to scan the whole lung region and detect the lung cancer regions, using three algorithms for scanning blood vessel, trachea, and parenchyma regions seems to be more effective.

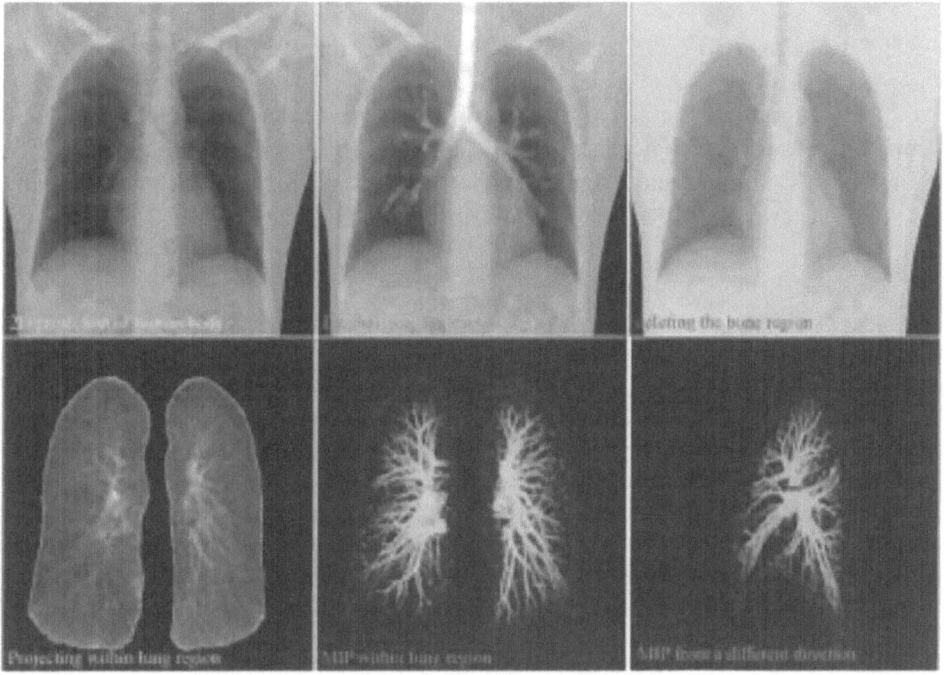

Fig. 5: Projection images based on 3D CT image.

Acknowledgements

Authors thank to Mr. Kobayashi, Mr. Hayashi and other members of Fujita's Laboratory and Visual System Laboratory (VSL) in Gifu University for their collaboration. This research was supported by a research grant from the VSL of Gifu University, in part by the Ministry of Health, Labour, and Welfare under a Grand-In-Aid for Cancer Research and in part by the Ministry of Education, Culture, Sports, Science and Technology under a Grand-In-Aid for Scientific Research, Japanese Government.

References

1. Kensaku MORI, Jun-ichi HASEGAWA, Jun-ichiro TORIWAKI, Hirofumi ANNO, Kazuhiro KATADA, "Automated Extraction of Bronchus Area from Three Dimensional X-ray CT Images", *Technical Report of IEICE*, PRU93-149, pp.49-55, Tokyo, 1994.
2. Toyofumi SAITO, Jun-ichiro TORIWAKI, "Euclidean Distance Transformation for Three Dimensional Digital Images", *Trans. IEICE*, Vol. J76-D-II, No.3, pp.445-453, 1993.

CARS 2002 – H.U. Lemke, M.W. Vannier; K. Inamura, A.G. Farman, K. Doi & J.H.C. Reiber (Editors)

782

A preliminary study for automated recognition of branches of pulmonary artery and vein using anatomical positional relations from a 3-D chest X-ray CT image

T.Yamaguchi[a], T.Kitasaka[a], K.Mori[a,b], Y.Mekada[a], J.Hasegawa[c], J.Toriwaki[a], H.Otsuji[d]

[a] Graduate School of Engineering, Nagoya University, Japan
[b] Image Guidance Laboratories, Dep of Neurosurgery, Stanford University, U.S.A.
[c] School of Computer and Cognitive Sciences, Chukyo University, Aichi, Japan
[d] Department of Radiology, Saiseikai Suita Hospital, Osaka, Japan

Abstract

This paper describes a method for recognition of branches of pulmonary artery (BPA) and vein (BPV) in 3-D chest X-ray CT images by using anatomical positional relations of pulmonary vessels. BPA and BPV should be recognized separately, because each BPA or BPV distributes from the hilar part to the peripheral part keeping connectivity. This paper tries to demonstrate potential possibility of automated recognition of BPA and BPV. Basically the proposed method extracts BPA and BPV separately by region growing from the hilar part. Seed points for growing are calculated by using two features: (a) specific BPA, BPV and bronchi (BR) keep steady positional relations on the particular slices (*key slices*) and (b) the BPA run along with the BR. The seed points for growing are calculated based on these features. The BPA and BPV are extracted by region growing with special growing kernels, which are designed to prevent misextraction. We applied the proposed method to chest X-ray CT images. The experimental result shows the method can extract the BPA and BPV satisfactorily.

Keywords: Pulmonary vessel, region growing, chest X-ray CT image

1. Introduction

Recent progress of 3-D imaging devices in the medical field, especially multi-detector row CT scanners, enables us to depict precise 3-D images of the inside of a human body. However, it also forces medical doctors to diagnose huge number of slice images for a patient. A computer aided diagnosis system (CAD) is expected to be developed for reducing the diagnostic load of clinicians. In the case of the CAD system for the lung, the system should have the following functions: (a) detection of suspicious regions such as tumors and (b) discrimination of benignancy or malignancy of suspicious regions. For both functions, anatomical information is very important in the recognition process of the CAD system. For example, the system requires the following information in benign/malignant discrimination process of tumors: (i) convergence of blood vessels toward the tumor, (ii) the type (artery or vein) of pulmonary vessels contacting to the tumor, and (iii) the running direction of vessel branches. Thus the recognition of branches of pulmonary artery (BPA) and vein (BPV) is an indispensable function for the CAD system of the lung. The classification method of BPA or BPV has been already reported in

CARS 2002 – H.U. Lemke, M.W. Vannier; K. Inamura, A.G. Farman, K. Doi & J.H.C. Reiber (Editors)

the reference [1]. This method classified BPA and BPV using only anatomical knowledge that BPA runs along with bronchi (BR). However, classification accuracy of pulmonary vessels has depended on extraction accuracy of BR significantly. This paper tries to recognize each BPA and BPV in the whole lung by the region growing method. The problems in discrimination of BPA and BPV are that they may contact with each other and that their borders are very indistinct.

In this paper, we show potential possibility of automated discrimination of the BPA and BPV in Section 2. Here complete separation of the BPA and BPV is demonstrated with several manual inputs. This demonstration makes technical problems of automated separation clear. In Section 3, we propose a method for reducing manual operations in the separation process of the BPA and BPV. The proposed method uses the knowledge that particular BPA, BPV and BR keep steady positional relations on particular slices, which are called *key slices*. We also use the knowledge that the BPA run along with the BR. The seed points for growing are calculated based on these features. The BPA and BPV are extracted by region growing with special growing kernels, which are used to limit the growing direction and to prevent misextraction. Experimental results are shown in Section 4 with brief discussion.

2. Potential possibility of recognition of BPA and BPV

The BPA and BPV run radially toward peripherals of the lung with branching off. Basically we can extract the BPA and BPV by expanding regions from the seed points allocated inside the pulmonary artery (PA) and vein (PV) in the hilum of the lung. In the region growing process, the contacts of BPA with BPV or with BR may cause errors in expansion so that the whole of BPA and BPV are recognized as only one region. Therefore these contacting parts are separated manually prior to the growing. Figure 1 illustrates separation of contacting parts. We mark contacting parts as *levees* which make the growing stop.

Six seed points should be specified to extract the BPA and BPV: (1) left PA, (2) right PA, (3) left superior PV, (4) right superior PV, (5) left inferior PV, and (6) right inferior PV. Region growing is started from these seed points. Figure 2 shows the extraction result of the BPA with manual specification of seed points and levees. This result exploits that automated extraction of BPA and BPV is possible if we can specify seed points and levees automatically by using some anatomical knowledge.

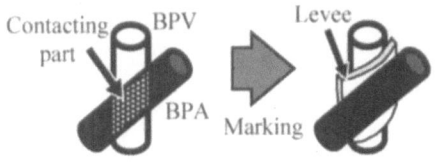

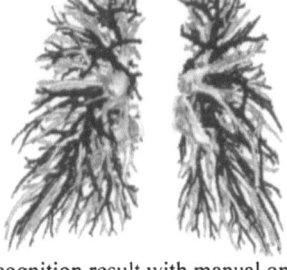

Figure 1. Removal of a contacting part. Levee is marked on the contacting part between BPA and BPV.

Figure 2. Recognition result with manual operation. (Dark gray region) BPA. (Light gray) BPV.

3. Proposed method

For the automated extraction of the BPA and BPV, seed points and contacting parts are determined automatically. Generally, there exist seven key slices (three in the left lung and four in the right lung) where steady positional relations among BPA, BPV, and BR are kept (Fig. 3 and 4). Seed points for growing can be found by recognizing specific BPA and BPV on key slices. Some of BPA and BPV between key slices, which may contact with each other, can be extracted separately by using region growing with a capsule type mask. In addition, BPAs running along with BR are extracted by using region growing with a half-capsule type mask. Remaining BPAs and BPVs are also extracted by region growing with a sphere type mask. The BPAs and BPVs extracted above are used as levees to prevent misgrowing. The whole procedure consists of five parts: (1) pre-processing, (2) recognition of particular pulmonary vessels on key slices, (3) recognition of pulmonary vessels between key slices, (4) recognition of BPAs running along with BR, and (5) recognition of remaining pulmonary vessels.

(1) Pre-processing

Lung and bronchus regions are extracted by the methods described in the references [2] and [3], respectively. Anatomical names of bronchial branches are recognized by the method shown in [4]. Bronchus region including the bronchus wall is obtained by applying a dilation operation to the extracted bronchus region.

(2) Extraction of particular pulmonary vessels on key slices

Key slices are determined using the positions of particular bronchial branches. Due to the space limitation, we explain a recognition procedure for A^8 here (Fig. 3(b)). Recognition of other pulmonary vessels is done by the similar way. The key slice shown in Fig. 3(b) is selected from input slices based on the positions of B^8 and B^{9+10}. The key slice is selected as the middle slice among the slices where both B^8 and B^{9+10} can be seen. The artery A^8 is searched in three areas defined around B^8. The size of each area is 25 x 25 (pixels) on the slice. If A^8 is not found in one area, the search process moves to another area. The artery A^8 is detected by finding a circle region in which all pixel values are between –300 H.U. and 200 H.U. The center of the circle moves inside the area in the search for each area. The initial radius is 20 pixels (12mm). If we cannot find a circle region in any of the defined area, we shrink the size of the circle by one pixel in the radius and continue the same search process.

(3) Extraction of pulmonary vessels between key slices

Several pulmonary vessels are connected each other between two key slices. For example,

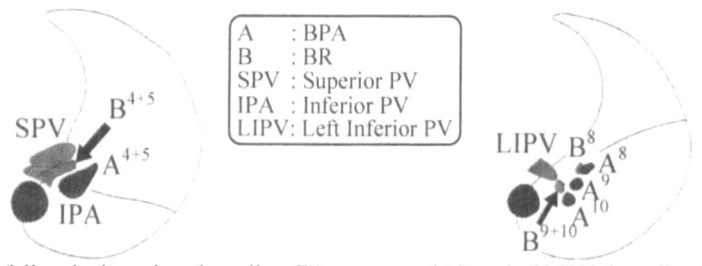

(a) Level of left lingular bronchus (key slice (F)).   (b) Level of LIPV (key slice (G)).

Figure 3. Examples of key slices (quotation from [5]). LIPV locates at the mediastinal part of BR B^8 and B^{9+10}. BPA A^8, A^9, and A^{10} locate lateral to the corresponding B^8 and B^{9+10}.

CARS 2002 – H.U. Lemke, M.W. Vannier; K. Inamura, A.G. Farman, K. Doi & J.H.C. Reiber (Editors)
°CARS/Springer. All rights reserved.

IPA shown in Fig. 3(a) and A^8, A^9, and A^{10} shown in Fig. 3(b) are connected. These pulmonary vessels are extracted by using region growing with a capsule type mask (Fig. 6). The direction of the capsule is the same direction which connects pulmonary vessels located on two key slices. The seed points are located at the center of gravity of the PV of the top key slice. The region is expanded if all of the CT value x inside the capsule satisfy the condition of -700 H.U. $\leq x \leq 200$ H.U..

(4) Extraction of BPAs running along with BR

BPAs which run along with BR are extracted from BPAs obtained in Section 3 (3). Region growing using a half-capsule type mask is employed here (Fig. 7). The direction of half-capsule is the same direction of the bronchial branch which is nearest to a BPA. A seed point is searched in extracted BPA existing inside a box defined by the location of the bifurcation point of BR. The region is expanded when all of the CT value x inside the half-capsule satisfy the condition of -700 H.U. $\leq x \leq 200$ H.U.. This region growing process is applied for all bifurcation points of BR.

(5) Extraction of remaining pulmonary vessels

The remaining BPAs and BPVs still contact with each other. A region growing method with a sphere-type mask is employed for preventing misextraction (Fig. 8). BPAs and BPVs extracted in the previous parts also used as levees in the growing process.

Step 1 We perform a region growing process with a sphere-type mask from the seed point located in BPV on the key slices. The radius of the sphere is one voxel. The growing is performed when voxel values inside the spherical neighbouring region of the target point are between -600 H.U. and 200 H.U. and all voxels inside the sphere are not marked as BPA. This growing process extracts BPV regions, which include several contact parts and parts of BPAs in peripherals.

Step 2 Regions growing is also performed from the seed point specified in BPA found on the key slice of Step 1. The same region growing method mentioned in the above step is used. Here growing is executed when no voxels of the sphere are marked as BPV region. In this extraction, we obtain BPAs that are not contacting to BPV regions, since BPV regions that are already extracted in the previous step work as levees.

Step 3 We execute region growing process for BPA and BPV regions from the seed points used in Steps 1 and 2. In this extraction, growing is performed if a voxel is connected to the target voxel by six-neighbourhood connectivity. This growing enables us to extract thin blood vessels existing in peripherals.

4. Result and discussion

We applied the proposed method to a chest X-ray CT image. The acquisition parameters of the CT image are: 512x512 pixels in slice, 355 slices, 0.625x0.625mm pixel size, 1.0mm reconstruction, and 2mm X-ray beam width. Figure 9 shows an example of recognition results. The experimental result showed that the proposed method can recognize BPA and BPV fairly automatically without manual operations. All of seed points are also automatically computed. Table 1 shows the number of voxels of extracted BPA or BPV by the proposed method. Misclassification of BPA and BPV of the left lung is much less than that of the right lung. This is because the contrast between PA and PV in the right hilar part is much lower than that of the left side. Pulmonary vessels cannot be discriminated by the capsule type mask appropriately. The proposed method does not use information of vessels that are not connected between key slices, such as superior

CARS 2002 – H.U. Lemke, M.W. Vannier; K. Inamura, A.G. Farman, K. Doi & J.H.C. Reiber (Editors)

786

pulmonary trunk. We consider that utilizing information of such vessels much improves recognition accuracy.

5. Conclusion

This paper proposed a method to recognize BPA and BPV from 3-D chest X-ray CT images. This method extracted each region by using anatomical knowledge with BPA and

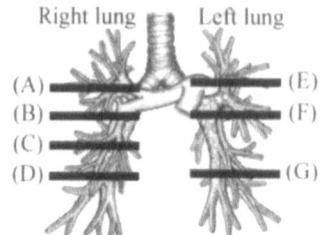

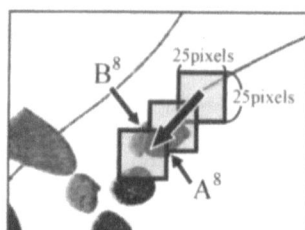

Figure 4. Positional relation between key slices (quotation from [6]).

Figure 5. Searching range of A^8 on the key slice (G).

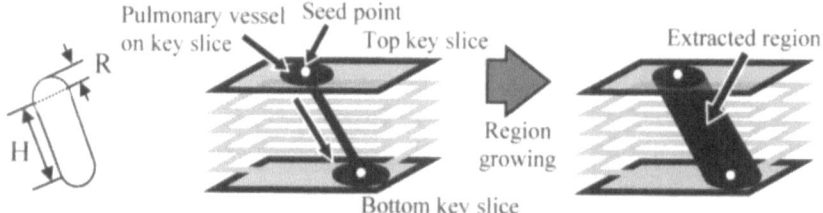

(a) Capsule type mask.　　(b) Region growing with capsule type mask.

Figure 6. Recognition of vessels between two key slices. Values of R and H are determined experimentally for each pulmonary vessel.

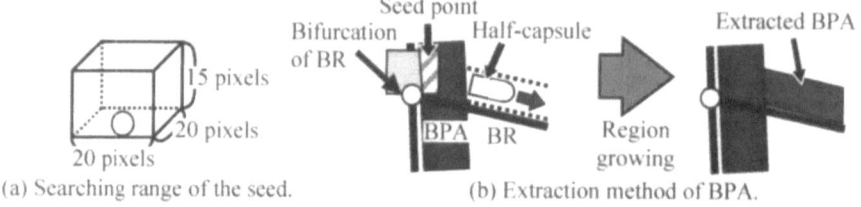

(a) Searching range of the seed.　　(b) Extraction method of BPA.

Figure 7. Extraction of BPAs running along with BR.

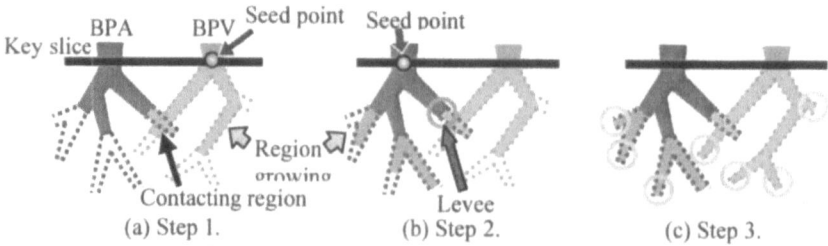

(a) Step 1.　　(b) Step 2.　　(c) Step 3.

Figure 8. Extraction of remaining pulmonary vessels.

CARS 2002 – H.U. Lemke, M.W. Vannier, K. Inamura, A.G. Farman, K. Doi & J.H.C. Reiber (Editors)
ᶜCARS/Springer. All rights reserved.

BPV, and by executing region growing. This paper showed the potential possibility of automated recognition of BPA and BPV which is indispensable in the CAD system for the lung. The future work includes: (a) improvement of classification accuracy of pulmonary vessels in the hilar part or in peripheral part, (b) evaluation of extracted BPA and BPV by a medical doctor, (c) application to large number of cases.

Acknowledgements

Authors thank to Dr. Shigeru Nawano of National Cancer Center Hospital East for providing CT image and thank to Mr. Tomoaki Tanaka of a member of our laboratory for assisting experiments and thank to our colleagues for useful suggestion and discussion. K.Mori thanks Dr. Ramin Shahidi and Dr. Calvin Maurer, Jr., of Stanford University for providing him an opportunity to write this paper. Parts of this research were supported by the Grant-In-Aid for Scientific Research from Japan Society for Promotion of Science, the Grant-In-Aid for Cancer Research from the Ministry of Health, Labour and Welfare, and the Grant-In-Aid for Scientific Research for Private University High-Tech Research Center provided by the Ministry of Education, Culture, Sports, Science and Technology of the Japanese government.

References

1. A.Tanaka, T.Tozaki, Y.Kawata, N.Niki, H.Ohmatsu, R.Kakinuma, M.Kaneko, K.Eguchi, and N.Moriyama, "Pulmonary Organs Analysis Method and Its Evaluation based on Thoracic Thin-section CT Images," Proc. SPIE, Vol.3661, pp.1299-1306, 1999.
2. J.Hasegawa, K.Mori, J.Toriwaki, H.Anno, and K.Katada, "Automated extraction of lung cancer legions from multi-slice chest CT images by using three-dimensional image processing," Systems and Computers in Japan, Scripta, Vol.25, No.11, 1994, translated from Denshi Joho Tsushin Gakkai Ronbunshi, Vol.J-76-D-II, No.8, August 1993, pp.1578-1594.
3. K.Mori, J.Hasegawa, J.Toriwaki, H.Anno, and K.Katada, "Automated extraction and visualization of bronchus from 3D images of lung," Proc.1st Computer vision, Virtual Reality and Robotics in Medicine, pp.542-548, 1995.
4. K.Mori, J.Hasegawa, Y.Suenaga, and J.Toriwaki, "Automated Anatomical Labeling of the Bronchial Branch and Its Application to the Virtual Bronchoscopy System," IEEE Trans. on Med. Img. Vol.9, No.2, pp.103-114, 2000.
5. H.Otsuji, "Analyzing procedure for dissection of hilar part segment, CT of the chest, J.Ikezoe and K.Murata, pp.68-74, Medical Science International, Tokyo, 1999. (in Japanese)
6. S.Ikeda, Photograph of the chest and its reading method, p.14, Shinnihonhouki, Tokyo, 1990. (in Japanese)

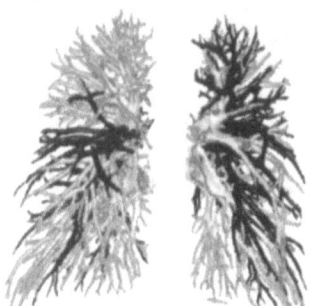

Figure 9. Automated recognition result.

Table 1. The number of voxels of extracted region. Correct BPA and BPV are extracted regions in Section 2. Although the border of each pulmonary vessel is not rigid, Correctness of each branch is assured by a medical doctor. Extracted BPA and BPV are recognition result by proposed method.

	Correct BPA	Correct BPV	Extracted BPA	Extracted BPV
Left lung	125079	102168	108552	91338
Right lung	114046	113797	64710	98070

CARS 2002 – H.U. Lemke, M.W. Vannier; K. Inamura, A.G. Farman, K. Doi & J.H.C. Reiber (Editors)
ᶜCARS/Springer. All rights reserved.

788

Development of a computer aided diagnosis system for three dimensional breast CT images

Y. Hanzawa[a], A. Shimizu[a], H. Kobatake[a], K. Miyakawa[b]

[a] Graduate School of Bio-Applications and Systems Engineering,
Tokyo University of Agriculture and Technology
2-24-16 Naka-cho, Koganei-shi, Tokyo 184-8588, Japan
[b] Department of Radiology, National Cancer Center Hospital
5-1-1 Tsukiji, Chuou-ku, Tokyo 104-0045, Japan

Abstract

We aim to develop a computer aided diagnosis system for automated detection of tumors in three-dimensional (3-D) breast CT images. This system consists of five steps. First the breast region is extracted from a 3-D breast CT image. Second, breast tumors are enhanced by a 3-D adaptive convergence index filter. Third, candidates of tumors are detected. Then, we measure two features, or the degree of sphericity of the candidates and average CT value in the candidate. Finally each of the candidates is classified as a tumor or a part of normal tissues. We applied the proposed system to twelve real 3-D breast CT images which have fourteen tumors in total. In the enhancement and extraction steps, all cancers were enhanced and detected, while 34 false positives which correspond to normal tissues were extracted. After the classification step, our system achieved 100% sensitivity with an average of 1.08 false positive detection per image.

Keywords: Computer-aided diagnosis system, 3D breast CT image, detection of tumor

1. Introduction

Breast cancer is a major cause of cancer deaths for women in the world. Mammography breast cancer screening has become popular and it has been shown that mammogram is effective to detect breast cancers in early stage. Currently 3-D images, such as 3-D ultrasound images, MR images or CT images are used for confirmed diagnosis and surgical planning of breast cancers. However, it is a great deal of labor for radiologists to interpret several hundreds slices with reconstructing the 3-D shape of cancers or other tissues in their mind. Therefore computer aided diagnosis (CAD) systems are required by radiologists and clinicians. Although CAD systems for 3-D ultrasound images [1] and MR images have been developed [2], the systems for 3-D CT images have not been proposed. In this paper, we present a CAD system for automated detection of tumors in 3-D breast CT images obtained with a multi-slice CT scanner [3].

2. Computer Aided Diagnosis system for 3-D breast CT images

The proposed CAD system consists of five steps; breast region segmentation, tumor enhancement, candidate extraction, measurement of features and classification of the candidates (Fig. 1).

CARS 2002 – H.U. Lemke, M.W. Vannier; K. Inamura, A.G. Farman, K. Doi & J.H.C. Reiber (Editors)
°CARS/Springer. All rights reserved.

2.1 Breast region segmentation

Since 3-D breast CT images contain several organs, it is necessary to extract breast regions. This process has two steps; rough extraction of the breast region and removal of unnecessary parts.

In the first step, the center of spine, top, center and bottom of sternum are estimated by a 3-D template matching (SSDA) [4]. After the bottom of sternum is refined by a threshold based method, slice images whose positions range between top and bottom of sternum are selected. Finally, the 3-D image is divided into four parts by using two planes and region 1 of Fig.2 is extracted as the coarse region. Here, one plane includes the estimated centers of sternum and spine and is perpendicular to axial planes of CT images, which are parallel to slice images. The other plane is perpendicular to the above-mentioned plane and includes the midpoint between the estimated centers of sternum and spine.

In the second step, to remove unnecessary parts which correspond to lung field, bones and heart, the system generates a 3-D mask image which contains all unnecessary parts. First lung field is extracted by thresholding at -400(H.U.) followed by a connected component analysis, such as small component removal. Then morphological dilation is used to extract rib and muscle around the lung field. Then, an original CT image is binarized at 80(H.U.) to decide the regions of spine, sternum and heart, and only the connected components whose volume is larger than 10,000 voxels are extracted and added to the mask image. Finally we apply a morphological closing operator to remove cave and cavity of the 3-D mask. The voxels contained in the 3-D mask are deleted from the region extracted at the first step.

2.2 Tumor enhancement

A 3-D adaptive convergence index filter is applied to the breast regions for the enhancement of spherical regions, such as tumors. This filter is the extension of 2-D convergence index filter which has been used for enhancement of breast tumors in 2-D mammograms [5]. It calculates a convergence index of the gradient vectors in the spherical region called support region and outputs it to the center P, or voxel of interest (Fig.3). The output of the filter is defined by

$$C = \max_{0 \leq r < l-d} \frac{1}{Md} \sum_{i=0}^{M-1} \sum_{j=r+1}^{r+d} \cos\theta_{ij} \tag{1}$$

where θ_{ij} is the angle between gradient vector g and half-line PQ. M is the number of the half-line, d and l are the width and the maximum radius of the support region, respectively.

Size of this filter r is adaptively changed in the calculation process and a maximum value is outputted. The output value of this filter ranges between 1 and -1. If all gradient vectors point to the center, the output is equal to 1. When all directions are the opposite to those mentioned above, the output is -1. And if the directions of all gradient vectors are perpendicular to the half-lines, the output is equal to 0. This filter has several advantages [5]. First, it can enhance the tumors even though the contrast to its background is low and it includes necrotic region. Second, it can be applied to various sizes of tumors because this filter changes its size adaptively.

CARS 2002 – H.U. Lemke, M.W. Vannier; K. Inamura, A.G. Farman, K. Doi & J.H.C. Reiber (Editors)

790

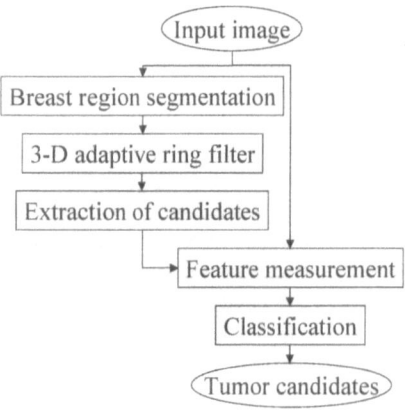

Fig. 1 Flow chart of the CAD system

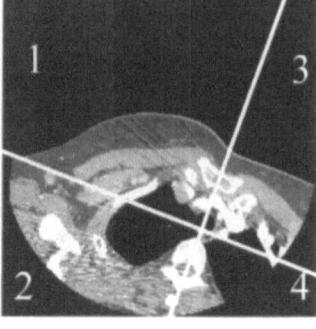

Fig. 2 Definition of the breast region

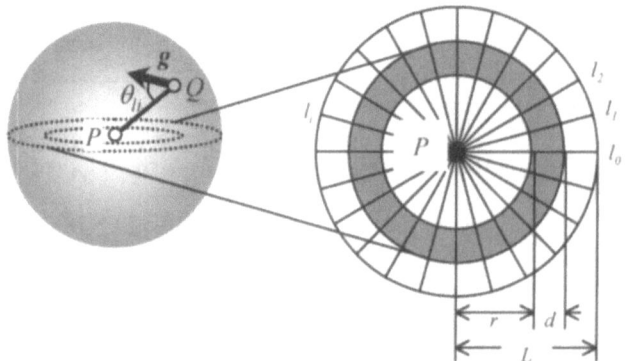

Fig.3 3-D adaptive convergence index filter (*left*) and cross section of the support region (*right*)

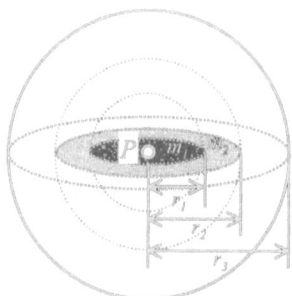

Fig.4 Three neighborhood regions for detecting local maximum points

CARS 2002 – H.U. Lemke, M.W. Vannier; K. Inamura, A.G. Farman, K. Doi & J.H.C. Reiber (Editors)

2.3 Candidate extraction

First, the system detects local maximum points from the enhanced image because the voxels in the tumors are expected to have higher values than those in normal tissues. To decrease the effect of noise to this process, we calculate mean values m_1 and m_2 in two neighborhood region of a point P (Fig.4). If $m_1 > m_2$, and the value of point P is maximum among the values of all voxels in the largest spherical region (radius $= r_3$), the point P is detected as a local maximum point. Then a region growing method is applied to the original CT image. Here the extracted maximum points are used as seed points. This process automatically decide the threshold value t as the minimum of the values which satisfy the following equation.

$$Tr > \frac{V(t-1)-V(t)}{V(t)-V(t+1)} \qquad (2)$$

where $V(t)$ is volume of the extracted region at threshold value t and Tr is a constant value predefined by a user.

2.4 Feature measurement

In this step, the proposed CAD system measures two features of the detected candidates, average CT values and degree of sphericity which can be calculated numerically from the surface area S and the volume V (Eq. 3). The surface area is approximated by the number of voxels on the surface and the volume is computed by counting the number of voxels in the region. The degree of sphericity ranges from 1 to infinity. The more complex the shape of the extracted region is, the larger the value is.

$$[\text{degree of sphericity}] = S^3 / 36\pi V^2 . \qquad (3)$$

2.5 Classification

The purpose of this process is classification between the candidates correspond to tumors and those correspond to normal tissues. The classification is based on Maharanobis distances between a feature vector of the candidate and mean feature vectors of two classes and each of the candidates is classified according to the following decision rule.

$$D_{normal} / D_{tumor} \geq Tc \quad then \quad Tumor. \qquad (4)$$

$$else \qquad\qquad Normal.$$

where D_{normal} and D_{tumor} are Maharanobis distances concerning normal class and tumor class, respectively. Tc is a threshold value.

3. Experiments

3-D breast CT images used in our experiments were obtained from twelve patients by a multi-slice helical CT scanner (Fig.5 (left)). These images were taken at 40 seconds after injection of contrast medium and include only one side of breasts that have tumors. Each CT image has about three hundreds slice images of 512 x 512 pixels. Spatial resolution of the pixel is 0.481 x 0.481mm, slice thickness is 0.5mm, slice interval is 0.5mm and

CARS 2002 – H.U. Lemke, M.W. Vannier; K. Inamura, A.G. Farman, K. Doi & J.H.C. Reiber (Editors)
ᶜCARS/Springer. All rights reserved.

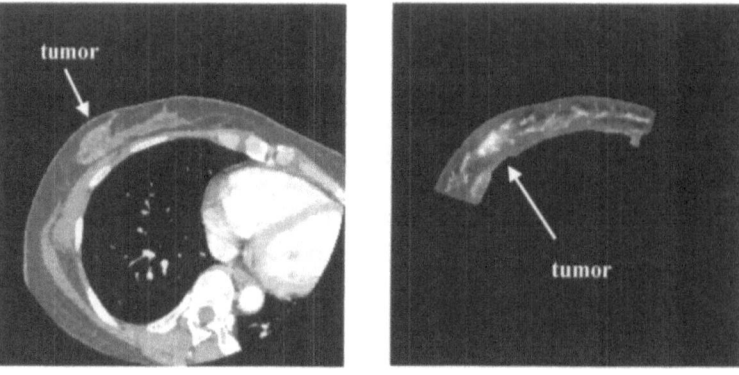

Fig.5 A slice of original 3-D CT (*left*) and enhancement result of the breast region (*right*)

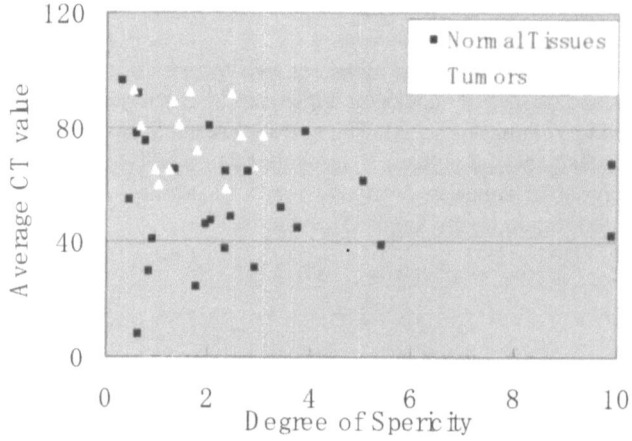

Fig.6 Scatter graph of the two features

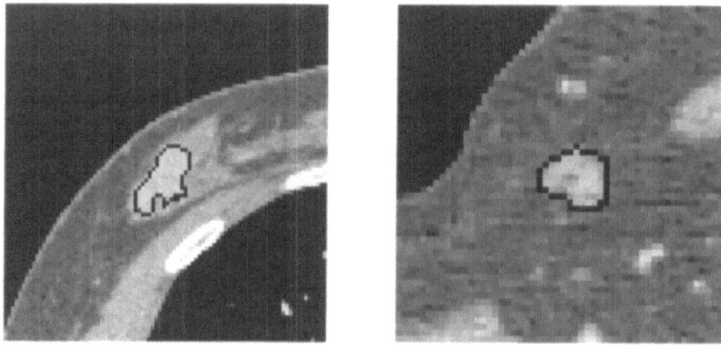

Fig.7 A detected tumor (*left*) and a false positive (lymph gland) (*right*)

CARS 2002 – H.U. Lemke, M.W. Vannier; K. Inamura, A.G. Farman, K. Doi & J.H.C. Reiber (Editors)

density resolution is twelve bits. Each image has at least one tumor and there are fourteen tumors in total. The sizes of tumors range approximately from 10mm to 45mm. Parameter values d, l, M, Tr and Tc are 5(voxels), 20(voxels), 26, 6 and 0.123, respectively.

An example of the segmented breast regions and the enhancement results is show in Fig.5 (right). 48 candidates are detected from the twelve CT images. Fourteen out of 48 correspond to the true tumors and 34 are false positives. Fig.6 shows the scatter graph of the two features. The classification results indicated a sensitivity of 100% with 13 false positives; seven lymph glands, four mammary glands and two greater pectoral muscles. Fig.7 shows examples of detected tumors and false positives.

4. Conclusions

This paper proposes a computer aided diagnosis system for automated detection of tumors in 3-D breast CT images obtained with a multi-slice helical CT scanner. We applied the system to twelve 3-D CT images of breasts and the experimental results showed that an average number of false positives was 1.08 per 3D image at a detection rate of 100%, which is quite promising results. In the future, we plan to increase the number of 3-D CT images for the performance evaluation and develop new features.

Acknowledgements

We are grateful to the members of Kobatake & Shimizu laboratory, Tokyo University of Agriculture & Technology, for their valuable advice and discussions. This study was supported in part by the Grant-in-Aid for Scientific Research from Ministry of Education, Culture, Sports, Science and Technology, Japan, the Grant-in-Aid for Cancer Research from Ministry of Health, Labour and Welfare, Japan.

References

1. Berkman Sahiner, Gerald L. LeCarpenttier, at.al: Computerized Characterization of Breast Masses Using Three-Dimensional Ultrasound Images, Proc. SPIE Medical Imaging, 3338: pp.301-312, 1998
2. K.G.A.Gilhuijs, M.L.Giger and U.Bick:A method for computerized assessment of tumor extent in contrast-enhanced MR images of the breast, Proc. of the First International Workshop on Computer-Aided Diagnosis, pp.305-310, 1999
3. Y. Hanzawa, A. Shimizu, H. Kobatake and K. Miyakawa Automated extraction of tumor tumors in three dimensional breast CT images and measurement of the features, IEICE Technical Report MI2001-72, pp.83-88, 2002 (in Japanese)
4. D.I.Barnea and H.F.Silverman: A class of algorithms for fast digital image registration, IEEE Trans. Computers, Vol.21, pp.179-186, 1972
5. H.Kobatake, W.Jun, Y.Yoshinaga, Y.Hagihara and A.Shimizu: Nonlinear adaptive convergence index filters and their characteristics. Proc. of ICPR, pp.526-529, 2000

CARS 2002 – H.U. Lemke, M.W. Vannier; K. Inamura, A.G. Farman, K. Doi & J.H.C. Reiber (Editors)

794

Development of automated detection and classification methods of masses on 3D breast ultrasound images

Takeshi Hara [a], Daisuke Fukuoka [b], Hiroshi Fujita [a]
Tokiko Endo [c], and Woo Kyung Moon [d]
[a] Department of Information Science, Gifu University
Yanagido 1-1, Gifu, Gifu 501-1193, Japan.
[b] Department of Electrical Information, Gifu National College, Japan.
[c] Department of Radiology, National Hospital of Nagoya, Japan.
[d] Department of Radiology, College of Medicine, Seoul National University
Hospital, Seoul, South Korea.

Abstract

We have developed a CAD system for masses on 3D breast ultrasound images and estimated the preliminary performance with about 200 cases. The detection and classification methods were based on edge detection and active balloon models to segment the mass regions. Volume rendering technique was also applied to prepare the 3D images to readers. It showed a good classification performance as an initial result. Especially, the classification performance showed a good rate because the cases employed in classifications scheme were difficult ones to discriminate by the ultrasound images in a physician's opinion, however the number of the case we used was not so large at this time.

Keywords: Breast, ultrasound, computer-aided diagnosis

1. Introduction

The technology of ultrasound devices for breast imaging significantly improved the resolutions of lesions of breast diseases. The usefulness is widely recognized not only for the detection of small masses but also for the classification of the lesions. We have developed a 3D breast imaging computer-aided diagnostic system by using 3D ultrasound breast images, although we have been developing a mammogram CAD system for detecting clustered microcalcifications and masses, because the diagnosis by using ultrasound images is strongly recommended for some younger people whose breasts tend to be dense one. Recently, mass screening with ultrasound devices for young women has proposed and has already started in some region in Japan. One of those examination employed Octson mechanism device, not handy-probe, to store stable regions of whole breast. By using the mechanism, patients have to lie prone on the examination equipment, because large four ultrasound probes move mechanically between adequate length below the breast. The device can archive over 50 scans with 3mm intervals per breast and can stores the image data on optical video disc. The reproducibility and ease-of-store of the breast image data is very useful to read them after the examination, because physicians can read the images of whole breast by slice-by-slice as 3D imaging data, although the device is too large to visualize lesions like magnification radiography.

CARS 2002 – H.U. Lemke, M.W. Vannier; K. Inamura, A.G. Farman, K. Doi & J.H.C. Reiber (Editors)
CARS/Springer. All rights reserved.

The new technology for the 3D imaging devices for breast diagnosis has been introduced by Medison Co. South Korea. The device bases on hand-probe mechanism that store the three-dimensional images corresponding to almost 5cm x 5cm area. The 3D images are created by moving a tiny probe set in the handy case.

The purpose of this work is to develop a computer-aided diagnosis system to detect and classify mass signals on the 3D breast ultrasound images, and to estimate the classification performance with over hundred images with biopsy proven. This paper mainly describes the classification scheme of masses indicated within 3D images from the equipment by Medison Co.

2. Materials and methods

2.1. Image dataset
The 3D images we employed were archived by the equipment by Medison Co.. There was a single prove that could scan within approximately 5cm x 5cm area on surface of a breast. This Medison device was mainly applied to classify the breast masses previously detected by other modality such as mammography or palpable examinations because of the narrow area of the scanning. The pixel size of images was within 256x256x256, and the scanning was examined in a few seconds moving the probe mechanically.

2.2. Segmentation of mass areas
The segmentation of masses region on ultrasound image was generally difficult tasks because the signal was week and noisy. Moreover, the posterior echo was eliminated by the nature of masses. Some approximation techniques were required to compensate the boundary to extract the feature values from the shape and/or the regions of masses.

We applied the active balloon models (ABM), a kind of active contour models [1] in three dimensional spaces, to determine the boundaries around masses. Fig.1 show an example of ABM in cubic area. This example illustrates the initial balloon (left) of polyhedron (1,280 triangle polygons) set inside of the cube, and the final shape of the balloon (right).

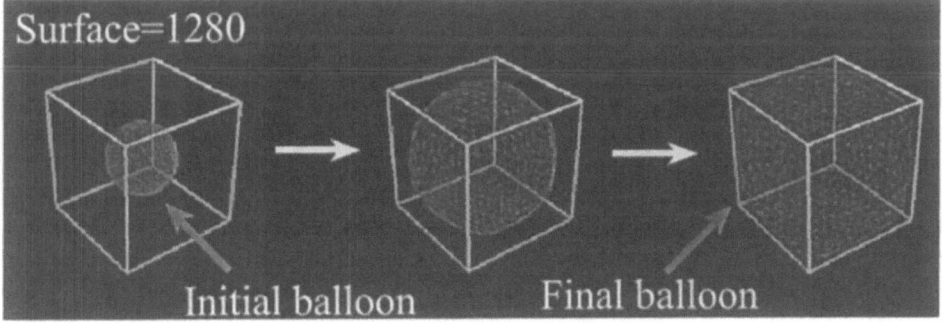

Fig.1 Extension of balloon shape in a cube

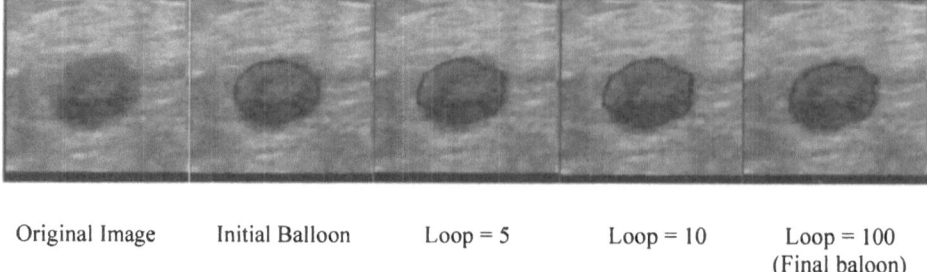

| Original Image | Initial Balloon | Loop = 5 | Loop = 10 | Loop = 100 (Final baloon) |

Fig.2 Example of extracted region by active balloon model

This balloon has 1,280 nodes as apexies of triangle polygons. All of nodes were moved by the energy functions defined as internal and external energies. The energy was based on the intensity and directions among the normal vectors connecting the apex.

Fig. 2 shows the example of extracting the mass region by this method. The initial balloon and the size was set automatically based on the concentrating point of boundaries roughly determined by voting approach from the edge [2]. The number of node was 1,280 points. The iteration of minimizing the energy was 100 times at this example. The fine area surrounding the edge was determined precisely. The feature extraction approaches from the shape and boundaries of masses were applied to this determined area.

2.3. Feature extractions

The features to classify masses were consisted of eight components as follows: (1) Depth-width ratio in 3D. This feature was calculated by dividing the mass area [pixels] on x-z plain by on y-z plain. (2) Ratio between Min-max length. Each of the length was determined by measuring the maximum and minimum distance within the mass region. (3) Volume of mass. The volume was defined by the regions indicated by the ABM. (4) Variance of density within anterior echo area. The anterior area was automatically determined based on the expanded region by the ABM. Fig. 3 shows the three divided surrounding the mass region. The regions were determined automatically by expanding the mass region in 20 pixels by using three dimensional morphological processing. The anterior echo area was indicated the bottom region on the figure. (5) Variance of density in internal area. The internal area also determined by the ABM as shown in the center region in Fig.3. (6) Variance of length from center of gravity to boundary. All of the length was calculated by measuring from the center of gravity to the nodes of the ABM. (7) Circularity of the region. This feature was determined by the ratio of the volume and surface area. (8) Density ratio between anterior and posterior echo area. The posterior and anterior regions were determined by the ABM such as the region of feature (4). The intensity of anterior echo tends to be attenuated when the mass was malignant one.

CARS 2002 – H.U. Lemke, M.W. Vannier; K. Inamura, A.G. Farman, K. Doi & J.H.C. Reiber (Editors)
ᶜCARS/Springer. All rights reserved.

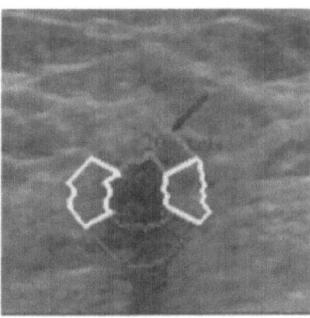

Fig. 3 Divided regions surrounding the mass area. Posterior echo area (above) and Anterior echo area (below).

2.4. Classification by artificial neural networks

The artificial neural network (ANN) technique was employed to classify the masses by using those eight features. The ANN we applied consisted of three layers with eight input units, twelve hidden units, and an output unit to express the malignancy of the input feature. The ANN structure was determined experimentally and was trained based on back-propagate algorithm by using some typical cases. The features were standardized between 0.0 and 1.0 to enter into the ANN.

2.5. Image display

The display of the 3D images is very important to recognize the mass shape and distribution of echo signals. We have tried to visualize the mass regions by using volume rendering and surface rendering approaches.

Fig. 4 shows the example of three dimensional display by using volume rendering technique clipping at the mass region. The scan images in any directions were shown by moving mouse to indicate the angle of view.

Fig. 5 and Fig. 6 show an example of surface rendering of benign and malignant masses, respectively. Rough surface of mass was well recognized as compared with the benign one. Emphasizing the shadows created by artificial lights in the space was very effective to tell the shape of the mass.

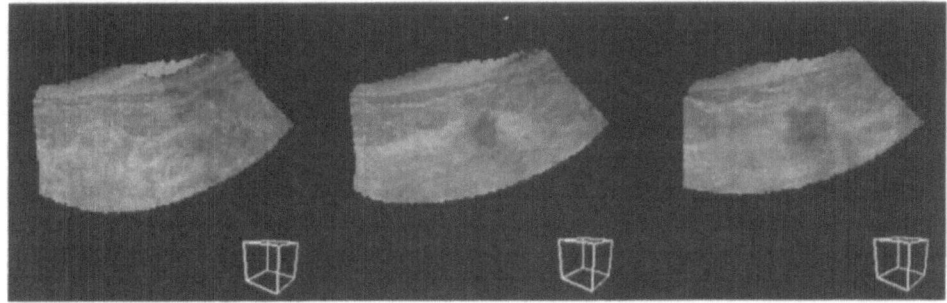

Fig.4 Examples of volume rendering images around a mass region.

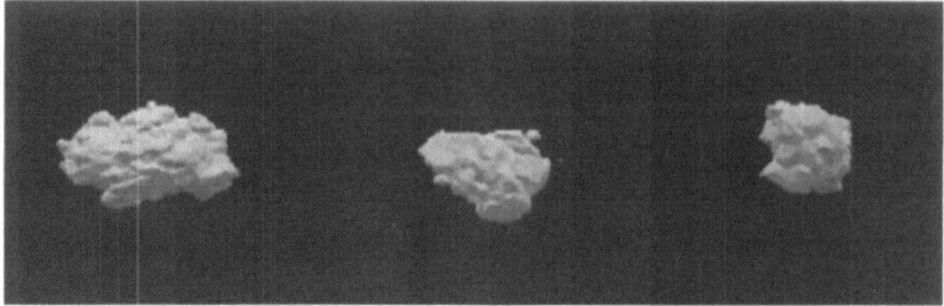

Fig.5 Examples of surface rendering images of a typical malignant mass

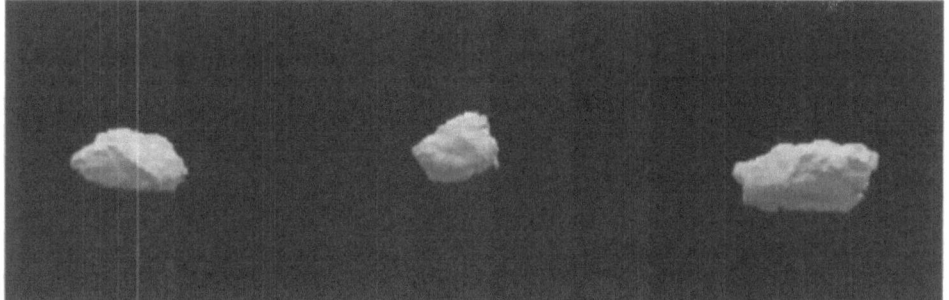

Fig.6 Examples of surface rendering images of a typical benign mass

3. Results and discussions

By employing 227 cases (147 benign, 80 malignant) with biopsy proven, the classification performance was 76%(61/80) sensitivity at 71% (104/147) specificity, although the consistency test approach was applied. The cases we tested were difficult to classify by well-experienced physicians by using only ultrasound images, so that this result may be adequate performance as an initial experiment. Figure 7 shows the user interface of our CAD system. Volume rendering images and patients list were shown on the same window. The volume images were rotated by moving mouse at the desired degree of view, and the position of clipping plain was determined by the same procedure of mouse movements.

4. Conclusions

We have developed a CAD system for masses on 3D breast ultrasound images and estimated the preliminary performance with about 200 cases. The detection and classification methods were based on edge detection and active balloon models to segment the mass regions. Volume rendering technique was also applied to prepare the 3D images to readers. It showed a good classification performance of 76% sensitivity at 71% specificity as an initial result. It was concluded that this scheme would be effective for the diagnostic aid of ultrasound images for breast diseases.

CARS 2002 – H.U. Lemke, M.W. Vannier; K. Inamura, A.G. Farman, K. Doi & J.H.C. Reiber (Editors)
ᶜCARS/Springer. All rights reserved.

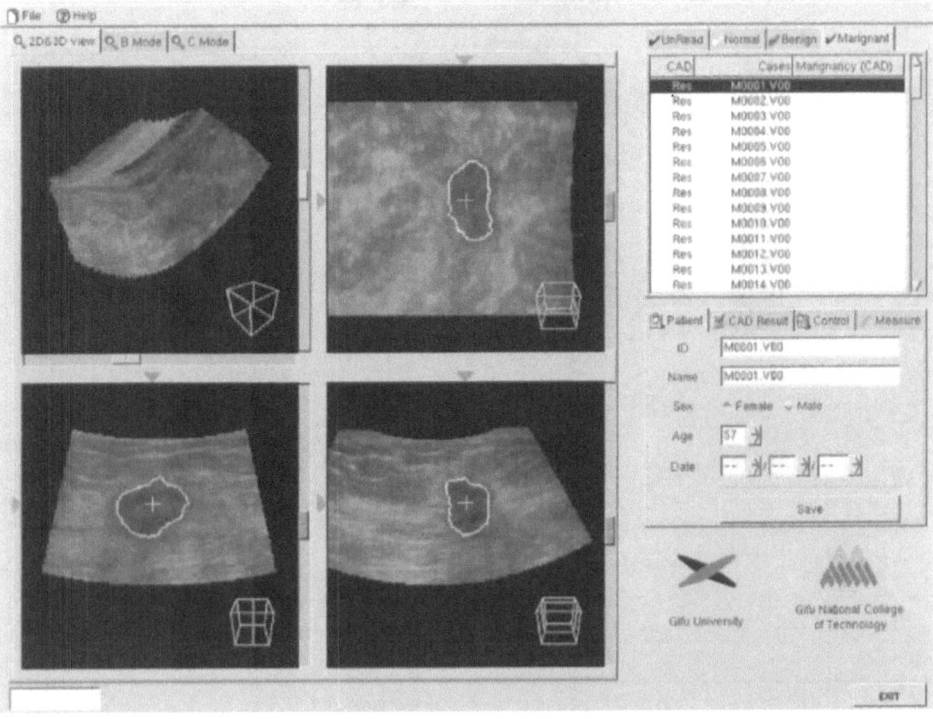

Fig.7 Overview of graphical user interface of our CAD system

Acknowledgements

This work was partly supported by a Grant-In-Aid for Cancer Research from the Ministry of Health, Labour, and Welfare, and by a Grant-In-Aid for Scientific Research, from the Ministry of Education, Culture, Sports, Science and Technology.

References

1. M. Kass, A. Witkin, and D. Terzopoulos: "Snakes: Active contour models", Int. J. Comput. Vision, 1, 1, 321-331, 1988.
2. D. Fukuoka, T. Hara, H. Fujita, et al.: "Dynamic Region-contour-extraction method with automated initial-contour production and unification of contours", the transactions of the institute of electronics, infomartion and communication engineering, J81-D-II, 6, 1448-1451, 1998.

2002 International Symposium on Cardiovascular Imaging
Chairman: Johan H.C. Reiber, PhD (NL)

Invasive Coronary Imaging

CARS 2002 – H.U. Lemke, M.W. Vannier; K. Inamura, A.G. Farman, K. Doi & J.H.C. Reiber (Editors)

Coronary atherosclerosis: from pathophysiology to imaging in clinical practice.

Francois Ledru MD
Department of Cardiology and Cardiovascular Radiology,
Hôpital Européen Georges Pompidou,
75015 Paris, France

Abstract

Many new ideas in the pathophysiology and clinical presentation of coronary atherosclerosis have emerged over the last decade including the concept of plaque vulnerability and the acknowledgement of the crucial role played by platelets and thrombosis in the occurrence of acute coronary events such as unstable angina, myocardial infarction and many sudden cardiac deaths. Epidemiology and large follow up trials have taught physicians and scientists that coronary atherosclerosis often has surprising and unexpected outcomes. Currently available imaging techniques of the coronary vasculature – from X-ray angiography to intravascular ultrasound or angioscopy - have helped identifying the players of the drama. However, considerable work remains to be done before physicians could expect to defeat the coronary heart disease pandemy in the future. Physicians expect imaging techniques to be less invasive but even more accurate than current technologies and to help them prospectively identify those patients with the higher risk coronary lesions.

Keywords: Coronary artery disease, coronary angiography, atherosclerosis

1. Introduction

Atherosclerosis remains the second cause of deaths in the world (after infectious diseases) and the first cause in the most developed countries. Fifteen million people (equivalent to the population of Chili) pay the death toll every year. Despite well-known preventive and cost-effective strategies and treatments aiming at reducing risk factors such as tobacco use, dyslipidemia, diabetes, sedentarity and hypertension, this rate is still growing overtime in most countries. On the other hand, our knowledge of the natural history of atherosclerosis has never been so accurate and subtle today. These recent pathophysiological concepts will be reviewed, the value and limitations of currently available imaging techniques will be discussed and new directions in the development of future imaging modalities will be suggested.

2. Atherosclerosis, the mysterious disease

Atherosclerosis chronically affects the vessel wall of the large arteries. It may be conceived as the accelerated process of vessel wall ageing, although the first indices of this process may appear as early as in the first decade of life. It exposes to two different kinds of complications : chronic ischemia due to flow-limiting stenoses and acute ischemia responsible for acute symptoms from refractory ischemia to infarction and sudden death. This latter complication is the most threatening and as such has received the greatest interest over the last 20 years.

The first new concept in atherosclerosis was that disruption or even erosion of the endothelium that covers the atheromatous cap was recognised as the key event precipitating intraluminal thrombosis with resulting blood flow interruption either due to total occlusion of a large artery (carotid or coronary arteries ...) or due to distal embolization and obstruction of the microcirculation (brain, myocardium...).

At the beginning of the 80's, it was thought that disruption and thrombosis were closely related to severe obstructions, and that the risk of acute events could be simply predicted by the atheromatous burden and stress-induced ischemia. Many studies, however, contradicted this initial and basic thought. At least in the coronary arteries, it was shown that acute thrombosis and occlusion could complicate mild or minimally severe lesions. This may be due to compensatory vascular remodelling that initially accommodates the atheromatous plaque without lumen deformation. Compensatory remodelling has indeed been correlated to unstable plaques while vessel skrinkage or failure to compensate for the plaque has been associated with stable plaques[1]. Thus, it is not the severity of the obstruction that determines risk. This emerged as the second new concept in atherosclerosis. Since these non-obstructive plaques are far more numerous than obstructive lesion, they happen to account for the majority of lesions resulting in acute myocardial infarction (AMI) [2-4]. This finding likely explains why as many as 70% of patients victim of an AMI were previously free of any symptom and why any coronary artery disease (CAD) had not been detected. Besides, when more severe coronary lesions lead to thrombosis, the resulting occlusion is more likely to result in limited myocardial injury (non-Q-wave AMI[5]) or in no injury at all[6] (due to development of a collateral circulation or preconditioning).

These surprising findings prompted closer analyses of the atheromatous plaque structure and composition and its relation with the occurrence of acute thrombosis. It was discovered that the major determinants of the plaque's susceptibility to rupture (also called vulnerability) were the size and consistency of the lipid-rich atheromatous core, the thickness of the fibrous cap covering the core, and inflammation and collagen depletion in the vicinity of the cap[7 8]. In contrast, collagen and smooth muscle cell repair processes yield stability. Thus, the risk of plaque disruption depends more on plaque composition than on plaque size. This became the third new concept. The elevation of fibrinogen and C-reactive protein in patients with unstable angina may be markers of ongoing plaque inflammation and may serve as additional global markers of risk in asymptomatic patients.

Rupture triggers are far less well-known and may depend more upon local triggers (geometry of plaque deformation, mechanical resistance of the cap to high shear rates, fatigue...) than upon systemic factors (adrenergic tonus...).

CARS 2002 – H.U. Lemke, M.W. Vannier; K. Inamura, A.G. Farman, K. Doi & J.H.C. Reiber (Editors)
°CARS/Springer. All rights reserved.

Once the endothelium is eroded or disrupted, platelets adhere to the sub-endothelium and may promote thrombosis. Not all ruptured plaques do initiate thrombosis. Since plaque rupture is silent, the proportion of plaques that heal without further complication is unknown. The thrombotic response, which is important for the clinical presentation and outcome, appears also poorly determined by systemic factors such as platelet hyper-reactivity and the balance between the fibrinolytic and coagulation systems whether they are acquired or genetically-determined. Local factors may be more prominent as suggested by the high thrombogenicity of the lipid core and inflammatory zones and the release of thrombogenic substances by macrophages and inflammatory cells (tissue factor, PAI-1...)[8]. Thus, these local factors may also relate to the plaque composition and structure. Much remains to be known in this setting.

Once thrombotic occlusion or distal embolization has occurred, it may not be too late for the patients. Since, these patients have become symptomatic, they most benefit from the considerable information collected during angiography studies and intervention trials with anti-thombotic and platelet blocking agents or interventional procedures. Invasive management strategies to resolve thrombus and seal the plaque and potent treatments to stabilise the plaque (oral antiplatelet and cholesterol-lowering agents) and prevent new lesion formation (statins...) have proved effective to alter the natural evolution of atherosclerosis and to prevent recurrent acute cardiovascular events.

3. New challenges in cardiovascular imaging from a physician point-of-view

Increasing further our knowledge of the pathophysiology, natural history and consequences of coronary atherosclerosis will be highly dependant upon our ability to image the various above-mentioned processes. Available imaging techniques will need to be improved and new modalities developed.

Coronary angiography is useful to predict outcome in already symptomatic patients. Quantitative Coronary Arteriography (QCA) may help identify vulnerable plaques but the predictive value of quantitative markers of stenosis geometry remains insufficient to be useful to the patient[4]. In the early phase of acute coronary syndromes (ACS), culprit lesions are often characterised by various degrees of eccentricity, irregularity, ulceration, filling defects or haziness. These so-called complex lesions have been related to complicated plaques at histology (ruptured plaques, plaque haemorrhage, plaques covered by mural thrombus or recanalized thrombus)[9]. Presence of complex culprit lesions not only characterises ACS but has been associated with poor prognosis. Prognosis is even worse when there are multiple such plaques. However, sensitivity of X-ray angiography to detect and quantify lesion complexity and accuracy to quantify stenosis dimensions remain low as compared to other imaging modalities such as intravascular ultrasound (IVUS) or angioscopy. 3-dimensional angiography may partly improve such inaccuracy. However, one of the major challenges in coronary angiography is the improvement in image acquisition techniques and image resolution and the development of quantitative tools and relevant and reproducible indexes to facilitate more accurate detection and quantification of small irregularities of the endoluminal boundaries that indicate surface erosion, endothelial tears or thrombotic plaques.

As demonstrated above, however, luminography yields limited information on a pathologic process that mainly affects the vessel wall. The ability to get an insight to the components of the plaque and its dynamic and stepwise evolution would greatly improve our knowledge of the mechanisms and triggers of plaque rupture and thrombosis, considerably influence detection of high-risk patients and completely change preventive strategies. IVUS already provides very interesting information about wall pathology. New technologies in vascular applications such as optical coherence tomography, Raman spectroscopy, thermography ... are also extremely promising. Their invasiveness and costs will likely restrict their use to a fraction of CAD patients, those undergoing percutaneous interventions or participating in atherosclerosis-regression trials[10]. As suggested previously, and from a public health point-of-view, non-invasive imaging by multislice spiral computed tomography coronary angiography and magnetic resonance angiography are even more promising. The latter technology has the potential to describe the lumen dimensions and quantify vessel wall thickness, analyse its structure and composition, and study flow reserve and intra-arterial hemodynamics, all in a single study. Efforts should be made in the future to continue reducing acquisition time and improving both temporal and spatial resolution as well as vessel wall contrast.

4. Conclusion

Atherosclerosis has become the New Frontier in cardiovascular imaging. Less invasive and even more accurate imaging technologies and modalities of coronary arteries would, and likely will, markedly change the way physicians care of their patients and reduce the death toll millions of people pay to CAD every year, as much in the same magnitude as coronary angiography in the 80's has changed the care of millions of patients with ACS or AMI and has reduced hospital mortality rate from 30% to less than 8%.

References

1. 1 Varnava AM, Mills PG, Davies MJ, "Relationship between coronary artery remodeling and plaque vulnerability". *Circulation*, 105. 8., 939-43., 2002.
2. 2 Little WC, Constantinescu M, Applegate RJ, Kutcher M, Santamore WP, "Can coronary angiography predict the site of a subsequent myocardial infarction in patients with mild-to-moderate coronary artery disease?". *Circulation*, 78. 1157-66, 1988.
3. 3 Alderman EL, Corley SD, Fisher LD, Chaitman BR, Faxon DP, Foster ED, et al., "Five-year angiographic follow-up of factors associated with progression of coronary artery disease in the Coronary Artery Surgery Study (CASS). CASS Participating Investigators and Staff". *J Am Coll Cardiol*, 22. 4., 1141-54, 1993.
4. 4 Ledru F, Théroux T, Lespérance J, Laurier J, Ducimetière P, Guermonprez J, et al., "Geometric features of coronary artery lesions favoring acute occlusion and myocardial infarction : a quantitative angiographic study". *J Am Coll Cardiol*, 33. 5., 1353-61, 1999.
5. 5 Ambrose JA, Tannenbaum MA, Alexopoulos D, Hjemdahl-Monsen CE, Leavy J, Weiss M, et al., "Angiographic progression of coronary artery disease and the development of myocardial infarction". *J Am Coll Cardiol*, 12. 1., 56-62, 1988.

CARS 2002 – H.U. Lemke, M.W. Vannier; K. Inamura, A.G. Farman, K. Doi & J.H.C. Reiber (Editors)

6.   6   Lichtlen PR, Nikutta P, Jost S, Deckers J, Wiese B,   Rafflenbeul W, "Anatomical progression of coronary artery disease in humans as seen by prospective, repeated, quantitated coronary angiography. Relation to clinical events and risk factors. The INTACT Study Group". *Circulation,* 86. 3., 828-38, 1992.

7.   7 Davies MJ, Woolf N, Rowles P, Richardson PD, "Lipid and cellular constituents of unstable human aortic plaques". *Basic Res Cardiol,* 1. 33-9, 1994.

8.   8   Kullo IJ, Edwards WD,   Schwartz RS, "Vulnerable plaque: pathobiology and clinical implications". *Ann Intern Med,* 129. 12., 1050-60., 1998.

9.   9 Levin DC, Fallon JT, "Significance of the angiographic morphology of localized coronary stenoses: histopathologic correlations.". *Circulation,* 66. 2., 316-20, 1982.

10. 10   De Franco AC,   Nissen SE, "Coronary intravascular ultrasound: implications for understanding the development and potential regression of atherosclerosis". *Am J Cardiol,* 88. 10A., 7M-20M., 2001.

CARS 2002 – H.U. Lemke, M.W. Vannier; K. Inamura, A.G. Farman, K. Doi & J.H.C. Reiber (Editors)

A novel approach for the detection of pathlines in X-ray angiograms: the wavefront propagation algorithm

Jasper Janssen, Gerhard Koning, Patrick J.H. de Koning, Joan C. Tuinenburg, Johan H.C. Reiber

Leiden University Medical Center, Department of Radiology, Division of Image Processing, PO Box 9600, 2300 RC Leiden, The Netherlands

Abstract

This paper presents a new pathline approach, based on the wavefront propagation principle, and developed in order to reduce the variability in the outcomes of the Quantitative Coronary Artery analysis. This novel approach, called wavepath, reduces the influence of the user-defined start- and endpoints of the vessel segment and is therefore more robust and improves the reproducibility of the lesion quantification substantially. The validation study shows that the wavepath method is totally constant in the middle part of the pathline, even when using the method for constructing a bifurcation- or side-branch pathline. Furthermore, the number of corrections needed to guide the wavepath through the correct vessel is decreased from an average of 0.44 corrections per pathline for the old algorithm, to an average of 0.12 per pathline. Therefore, it can be concluded that the wavepath algorithm improves the overall analysis substantially.

Keywords: Automatic pathline detection, quantitative coronary arteriography, wavefront propagation

1. Introduction

Quantitative coronary arteriography (QCA) has been widely accepted as the method for the accurate assessment of the morphology of coronary vessels and the location and severity of coronary obstructions from X-ray arteriograms [1]. The accurate derivation of clinically relevant variables, such as the obstruction diameter, interpolated reference diameter, percent diameter stenosis and plaque area, not only facilitates the objective evaluation of clinical research trials, but has also proved to be useful for the selection of the appropriate recanalization devices in interventional cardiology [2, 3]. Over the years, we have developed analytical software packages for both cinefilm [4] and on-line digital applications [5]. The high accuracy and precision of these packages have been established and described elsewhere [1-5].

In spite of the demonstrated accuracy and precision of the packages, there is still some variability demonstrated in the outcomes of the coronary lesion quantification parameters, when analyzing the same segment repeatedly. This variability is partly caused by different start- and endpoint positioning and different corrections of the detected contours. The analysis results are computed on the basis of the arterial contours of the segment under study, which have been detected automatically using a method based on the minimal cost

CARS 2002 – H.U. Lemke, M.W. Vannier; K. Inamura, A.G. Farman, K. Doi & J.H.C. Reiber (Editors)
^cCARS/Springer. All rights reserved.

algorithm [6] and/or the Gradient Field Transform [7]. These methods require a pathline as input [8], which is a rough approximation of the centerline of the vessel segment to be analyzed. The image is resampled along scanlines that are perpendicular to and evenly distributed along the pathline. The resulting contours depend therefore on the resampling of the image data along the scanlines and thus on the pathline that is found. The pathline itself depends on the start- and endpoints that are defined by the user. Therefore, a small variation in the start- and endpoints may result in a significant variation in the coronary lesion parameters due to the pathline-algorithm. In an attempt to minimize the influence of the user-defined start- and endpoints of the vessel segment, we have developed a new pathline-algorithm, based on a wavefront propagation. This method, that is called the wavepath, is (within a certain range) independent of the start- and endpoint positions and consequently improves the reproducibility of the lesion quantification substantially.

More research has been performed by other people that also aimed at reducing the variability in QCA measurements, introduced by the analyst. One approach aimed at detecting the entire coronary tree using a skeletonization process [9] and another approach used the wavefront propagation in order to perform a coronary segmentation (contour detection) without the use of a pathline [10]. We chose to use the wavefront propagation for the detection of the pathline of the vessels. In our opinion the wavefront is not precise enough to perform a contour detection

2. Methods

To be applicable in the environment of the QCA system, the algorithm must satisfy the following criteria: 1) the resulting pathline must remain within the vessel boundaries over its entire length; 2) its course must be insensitive to small variations in the user-defined start- and endpoints, which have to be located inside the artery under study; 3) it should be fast enough for on-line applications; and, 4) it should also be suitable for functioning as a model for the contour detection of more complex morphology, such as a bifurcation or side-branch.

The new algorithm that we have developed is based on the wavefront propagation principle [11]. A wavefront is initiated in the image and expands using a local speed that depends on the local intensity-value of the image. Our approach of pathline detection consists of the following steps: 1) an appropriate preprocessing that consists of a smart subsampling [8] and a filtering to reduce the influence of background shading; and 2) the wavefront algorithm. The nonlinear subsampling is applied mainly to decrease the processing time of the algorithm and results in an image that is 3 times smaller in its dimensions. A grey level morphology filter is applied in this low-resolution image. The filter enhances the structures with a size in a predefined range (the coronary arteries) that are present in the image and reduces the shading in the background caused by overlaying structures. Therefore, it provides an appropriate input for the wavefront algorithm.

The purpose of the wavefront algorithm is to find the fastest path from the user-defined startpoint to the endpoint. In the filtered low-resolution image an eight-connected wave is initialized from the startpoint, after defining a speedfunction for the wave, which connects to every possible grey level in the image a value that represents the velocity of the

810

wavefront. After the wave has been propagated (Fig. 1) and reached the endpoint(s), the backtrack algorithm finds the fastest way back through the wave using the arrival time image, resulting in a low-resolution pathline that is subsequently transformed back into the high-resolution image and smoothed to obtain the final resulting pathline.

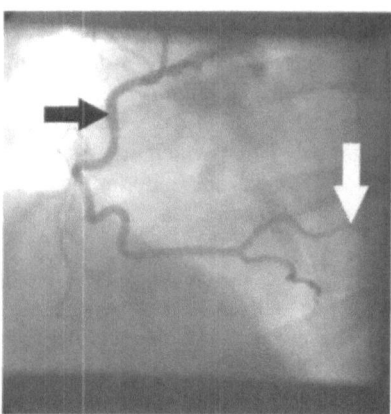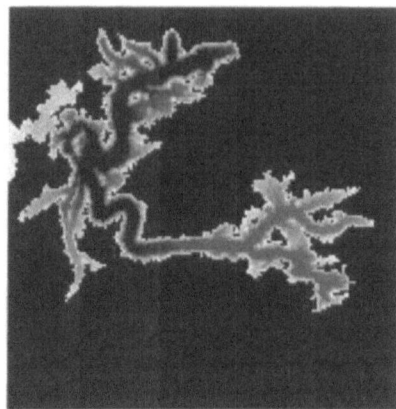

Fig. 1: Wavefront propagation: Initial image (left) with startpoint (black) and endpoint (white), and resulting image (right).

In case the pathline follows an erroneous path, for example when two arteries overlap, the user has the option to add an additional point to force the path through a certain part of the image. Another option has been developed, denoted the 'live-wire', where the user sets the startpoint and can move the endpoint over the entire image and immediately find the pathline between the fixed startpoint and the variable endpoint.

In the analysis of an artery, either being a coronary or a peripheral artery, three different situations can be distinguished that require different protocols. The first case is the analysis of a single segment that is supported by the known quantitative coronary artery packages. The second case is the analysis and quantification of a vessel bifurcation, such as occurs in a carotid artery or major vessels in the coronary tree, and the third case is the sidebranch analysis, which applies to e.g. renal artery analysis, but also to a diagonal branch of an LAD-artery. The first case requires just a single pathline from start- to endpoint as discussed above. The other two situations require a more sophisticated pathline in order to appropriately detect all arterial boundaries. In the case of a bifurcation, we need the pathline algorithm to provide an initial model for the detection of three contours. To achieve this, one proximal point and two distal points are needed, one in each branch of the bifurcation. Basically, we are constructing two different pathlines to connect those three points (Fig. 2). Since the startpoint for both waves is identical, we can use solely one single wave and let it propagate until it has reached both endpoints. Subsequently the backtracking from both endpoints back to the startpoint is carried out. The procedure for constructing a pathline in the situation of a sidebranch is slightly different. In this case we are interested in two contours and we need two different proximal points and one distal point. We use the distal point as the startpoint for the propagation and the proximal points as endpoints and achieve the two necessary pathlines.

CARS 2002 – H.U. Lemke, M.W. Vannier; K. Inamura, A.G. Farman, K. Doi & J.H.C. Reiber (Editors)
ᶜCARS/Springer. All rights reserved.

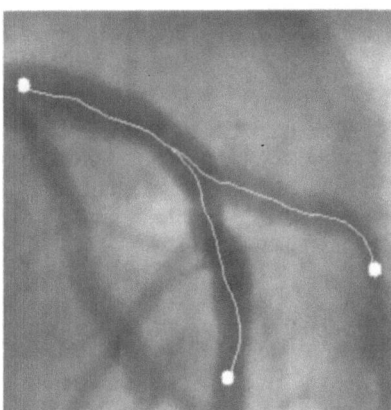 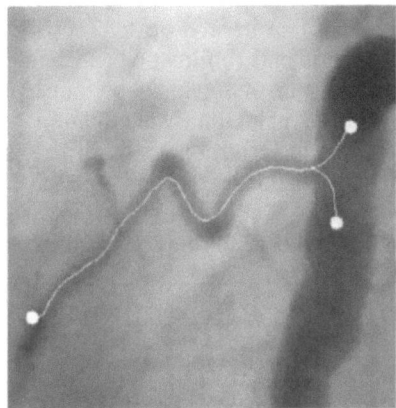

Fig. 2: Pathlines for bifurcation (left) and pathlines for sidebranch (right)

3. Results

Since the goal of this research is to achieve a reliable and reproducible method for pathline detection, the performance of our wavepath algorithm can be determined relative to the existing pathline, by moving the start- and endpoints in small areas and calculating the variabilities in the pathline positions. We used 25 locations for the start- and endpoints, resulting in 625 pathlines. Using these pathlines, we compute the variation in local position of the pathlines per scanline. We also calculate the number of corrections needed for the pathline to be acceptable (i.e. it must lie within the assumed arterial bounds over its entire length). This is performed for our new pathline-method as well as the existing method.

For the first validation experiment a set of 49 coronary segments was used, selected from 33 digital coronary arteriograms (512^2 x 8 bits) from the Philips Digital Cardiac Imaging system. The results, averaged over all 49 segments show that the existing pathline method shows variations over its entire length, due to the fact that small changes in start- and endpoints lead to different pathlines. The new method, however, shows variability only at the start and end of the pathline, whereas the essential middle part of each pathline (approximately 72 percent of its length) is exactly the same for all 625 pathlines (Fig. 3). The average number of corrections needed per pathline is much lower for the new algorithm compared to the old, 0.12 against 0.44 (see Table 1).

	number of corrections per pathline
Existing pathline	0.44
Wavepath (Straight Segments)	0.12
Wavepath (Bifurcation)	0.18
Wavepath (Sidebranch)	0.12

Table 1: Average number of corrections per pathline for all pathline methods

812

Note that using our new method, at maximum 1 correction point was necessary, whereas the old algorithm needed up to 6, 7 or even 8 correction points in a few cases. In the further experiments (bifurcation and side-branch) we use 9 different locations for the start- and endpoints, resulting in 729 pathlines. For the validation, we used 43 segments from 38 arteriograms. Again, it turns out that the pathlines contain some variability at the start and end, whereas the central parts of all 729 pathlines are exactly identical (Fig. 4). Note that this includes that the separation point is at the exact same location for all pathlines in each segment! The average number of corrections needed per pathline is 0.18 for the bifurcation and 0.12 for the sidebranch (see Table 1).

```
Title:
variation.eps
Creator:
gnuplot 3.7 patchlevel 0
Preview:
This EPS picture was not saved
with a preview included in it.
Comment:
This EPS picture will print to a
PostScript printer, but not to
other types of printers.
```

Fig. 3: Local variations of the wavepath approach and the existing pathline in single vessel segments

```
Title:
variation_bifurcation.eps
Creator:
gnuplot 3.7 patchlevel 0
Preview:
This EPS picture was not saved
with a preview included in it.
Comment:
This EPS picture will print to a
PostScript printer, but not to
other types of printers.
```

```
Title:
variation_sidebranch.eps
Creator:
gnuplot 3.7 patchlevel 0
Preview:
This EPS picture was not saved
with a preview included in it.
Comment:
This EPS picture will print to a
PostScript printer, but not to
other types of printers.
```

Fig. 4: Local variations of the wavepath approach in bifurcation (left) and sidebranch (right) version

4. Discussion

Although in the validation study the wavepath was only tested on digital images (512^2 x 8 bits) from the Philips Digital Cardiac Imaging system in one single resolution, pilot experiments show that the principles can be generalized towards other types of images and even to other vascular applications. Minor changes in the filtering and tuning of the wavepath, make the algorithm suitable for these other applications, which will be tested in the future.

The overall goal of our research is to make the entire QCA-analysis more reproducible, and the new pathline method is one part of it. That does not mean that a robust pathline algorithm in itself makes the total analysis more reproducible. As indicated, the image is resampled along scanlines, perpendicular to and evenly distributed along the pathline. Obviously, the total length of the pathline will change when the start- and endpoint change, in spite of the robustness of the pathline in the important area. Therefore, since

CARS 2002 – H.U. Lemke, M.W. Vannier, K. Inamura, A.G. Farman, K. Doi & J.H.C. Reiber (Editors)
ⒸCARS/Springer. All rights reserved.

the resampling of the pathline for the contour detection is dependent upon the position of the start- and endpoint as well as the length of the pathline, this last mentioned dependency must be solved as well, in order to make the entire QCA-analysis more reproducible.

5. Conclusions

The new approach for the automated detection of pathlines (wavepath) in digital coronary arteriograms has proven to outperform the existing pathline algorithm. Validation results of the wavepath algorithm have demonstrated that it is very reproducible and the need for user interaction has been minimized. The algorithm is also suitable for application in bifurcation or sidebranch analysis in coronary vessels.

References

1. J.H.C. Reiber, P.W. Serruys, C.J. Kooijman, W. Wijns, C.J. Slager, J.J. Gerbrands, J.H.C. Schuurbiers, A. de Boer, and P.G. Hugenholtz, "Assessment of short-, mediumand long-term variations in arterial dimensions from computer-assisted quantitation of coronary cineangiograms", *Circulation*, Vol 71, 280–288, 1985.
2. J.H.C. Reiber, and P.W. Serruys, *Quantitative coronary arteriograph*, Kluwer Academic Publishers, Dordrecht, 1991a.
3. J.H.C. Reiber, and P.W. Serruys, *Cardiac Imaging*, Chapt. Quantitative coronary arteriography, pp. 211–281, Saunders, Philidelphia, 1991b.
4. J.H.C. Reiber, P.M.J. v. d. Zwet, and C.D. v. Land, *Advances in Quantitative coronary arteriography*, Chapt. Quantitative coronary arteriography: equipment and technical requirements, pp. 75–111,Kluwer Academic Publishers, Dordrecht, 1992.
5. J.H.C. Reiber, P.M.J. v. d. Zwet, G. Koning, C.D. v. Land, B. v. Meurs, J.J. Gerbrands, B. Buis, and A.E. v. Voorthuisen, "Accuracy and precision of quantitative digital coronary arteriography: observer-, short- and medium-term variabilities", *Cath Cardiovasc Diagn*, Vol 28, 187–198, 1993.
6. P.M.J. v.d. Zwet, C.D. v. Land, G. Loois, J.J. Gerbrands, and J.H.C. Reiber, "An on-line system for the quantitative analysis of coronary arterial segments", *Computers and Cardiology*, pp. 157–160, 1990.
7. P.M.J. v.d. Zwet and J.H.C. Reiber, "A new approach for the quantification of complex lesion morphology: the gradient field transForm; basic principles and validation results", *J Am Coll Cardiology*, Vol 24(1), 216–224, 1994.
8. P.M.J. v.d. Zwet, I.M.F. Pinto, P.W. Serruys, and J.H.C. Reiber, "A new approach for the automated definition of path lines in digitized coronary angiograms", *Int J Cardiac Imaging*, Vol 5, 75–83, 1990.
9. G. Tommasini, P. Rubartelli, and M. Piaggio, "A deterministic approach to automated stenosis quantifcation", *Catheterization and Cardiovascular Interventions*, Vol 48, 435–445, 1999.
10. F.K. Quek and C. Kirbas, "Vessel extraction in medical images by wavepropagation and traceback", IEEE Transactions on Medical Imaging, Vol 20, 117–131, 2001.D. Adalsteinsson and J.A. Sethian, "A fast level set method for propagating interfaces", J. Comp. Physics, Vol 118, 269–277, 1995.
11. W.A. Barrett and E.N. Mortensen, "Interactive live-wire boundary extraction", *Medical Image Analysis*, Vol 1, 331–341, 1997.

CARS 2002 – H.U. Lemke, M.W. Vannier; K. Inamura, A.G. Farman, K. Doi & J.H.C. Reiber (Editors)

814

A numerical 3D coronary tree model

Denis Sherknies[a], Jean Meunier[b]

[a]University of Montreal, sherknie@iro.umontreal.ca,
[b]University of Montreal

Abstract

We present a method that defines a numerical 3D model of the main coronary arteries of the human heart at end-diastole. The data used in this article are a subset of the data used in two articles by Dodge et al. [1, 2]. 26 subjects with normal hearts, having measures for the 3 main arteries (right coronary artery, left anterior descending artery and left circumflex artery), were chosen. The method used to obtain the heart model can be summarized as follows: A well-formed subject is chosen as the reference. Subsequently, each of the other subjects is fitted to the reference with affine transformations (translation, rotation and scaling). The model is obtained by applying the mean of the inverse affine transformations back on the reference coronary tree. This model is the first step for the 3D construction of an atlas of the structure and motion of coronary arteries for cardiac contraction analysis.

Keyword: 3D, coronary, model

1. Introduction

When confronted with the task of recovering 3D information of the coronary arteries from angiographic images, one can use multiple views [3, 4], but due to the structure of the coronary tree, there exist a large number of possible ambiguities. The use of a priori knowledge in the form of a qualitative model [5], quantitative model [6], or a combination of both [7], helps alleviate these ambiguities. The use of a model can also help in the reconstruction of coronary arteries from a single view cineangiogram [8, 7]. Qualitative models can contain information in the form of a graph structure used for labeling purpose, quantitative models can be expressed with global shape descriptors as in a parametrically deformable model [9] or with more local attributes, like the location and variation of branching points [1]. It is an accepted fact that the location of the coronary arteries is variable, nonetheless certain constancy exists. And even if numerical models do not capture all the subtleties of the coronary tree, they offer certain advantages over the qualitative models, would it only be for anatomical visualization purpose.

In 1988 Dodge et al. published an article in which they describe the 3D location of branching points, among others, of the coronary tree [1]. An article published in 1992, added information about the lumen diameter at the different reference points [2].

Dodge's articles are often cited in the literature (32, 54 respectively [10]) and a phantom called *Coronix* [11], used in various simulation studies, has also been constructed based on Dodge's data.

CARS 2002 – H.U. Lemke, M.W. Vannier; K. Inamura, A.G. Farman, K. Doi & J.H.C. Reiber (Editors)
ᶜCARS/Springer. All rights reserved.

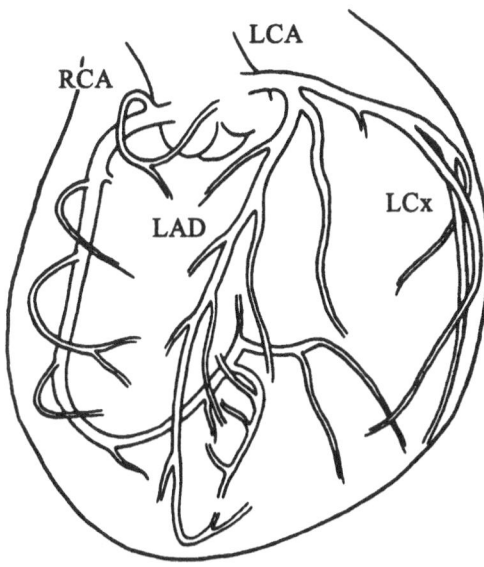

Figure 1. Right coronary artery dominance anatomy. RCA: Right coronary artery; LCA: Left coronary artery; LAD: Left anterior descending; LCx: Left circumflex. *From Dodge [1]*

Starting with Dodge's data we made some transformations in order to obtain a model less dependent on certain parameters like the absolute position of the coronary tree or the relative heart size. We are interested in the spatial location of reference points along the coronary tree in order to construct a model that will be used for tracking the motion of coronary arteries.

2. Data

The coronary tree present itself as a hierarchical structure divided in 3 main sections according to the heart region irrigated. We use here a nomenclature devised by Dodge et al. [1], see Figure 1. The left coronary artery (LCA) starts at the left of the aorta as the left main artery (LM) and divides itself into the left anterior descending artery (LAD) and the left circumflex artery (LCx). The right coronary artery (RCA) starts at the right of the aorta and irrigates the right side of the heart. Each of these main arteries divides themselves into smaller ramifications. The artery that irrigates the heart's anterior wall is said to define the dominance anatomy. There are three dominance anatomies: the right dominance, left dominance and the balanced anatomy.

The original data comes from the 3D location of 102 points along the coronary tree of 37 normal subjects. The measurements were taken at the end diastole by a biplane angiographic apparatus and were corrected for optical magnification and X-ray beam divergence, see Dodge's et al. articles for more details [1, 2].

For the elaboration of our model, a subset of the original data was selected, based on certain criteria. We kept only the subjects where the three main arteries were present. Also, the reference points from secondary branches and those having sporadic presence were dropped. We ended up with 26 subjects having a coronary tree composed of 36 reference points. See Table 1 for the demographic description of the subjects.

Age	Gender		Coronary dominance		
	M	F	Left	Balanced	Right
26 to 77 (mean, 48)	23	3	2	22	2

Table 1. Demographic summary

CARS 2002 – H.U. Lemke, M.W. Vannier; K. Inamura, A.G. Farman, K. Doi & J.H.C. Reiber (Editors)

816

3. Methodology

In order to construct a *coronary tree model* that is immune to certain influences, we allow some transformations of the selected subset data. For example, scaling attenuate the inter-subject variation of the overall size of the coronary tree, translation and rotation bring the coronary tree in a reference space that is less dependant on the relative position between the body and the measuring apparatus.

In a way similar to Guimond et al. [12], the method used for obtaining the heart model can be summarize as follow:

- First, a well-formed subject is chosen as a reference, the *reference subject*;
- Subsequently, the reference subject is fitted to each of the other subjects with affine transformations (translation, rotation and scaling);
- An average of the affine transformations is then computed;
- Finally, the *coronary tree model* is obtained by applying the average transformation on the *reference subject*.

The choice of the well-formed subject is based ... on its well-form! Without large variations to what could be described as an ideal normal subject.

Next, to find the affine transformations we consider this problem as a classic computer vision problem known, among various aliases, as *model-based object location*. It can be stated as follow: knowing the correspondence between two 3D points sets and their locations, find the best geometric transformation that minimize a cost function with respect to some constraints. Different analytical and numerical techniques exist that solve such problems. Closed form solutions solved by singular value decomposition [13] or represented by orthonormal matrices [14] or unit quaternions [15] exist and they all give similar results [16].

The problem can be formulated as follow: given the relation between two points sets $\{m_i\}$ and $\{d_i\}$, $i = 1..N$ as $d_i = s\mathbf{R}m_i + \mathbf{T} + \mathbf{V}_i$ where s is a scaling factor, $\mathbf{R}$ is a 3×3 rotation matrix, $\mathbf{T}$ is a translation vector and $\mathbf{V}_i$ is a noise vector. We want to find $\hat{s}$, $\hat{\mathbf{R}}$ and $\hat{\mathbf{T}}$ that minimize the sum of the Euclidean distances between corresponding points $\sum_{i=1}^{N} \left\| d_i - \left(\hat{s}\hat{\mathbf{R}}m_i + \hat{\mathbf{T}} \right) \right\|^2$. We solve the scaling factor using Horn method [15] and the translation and rotation using Arun method [13]. The three transformation components can be solved independently. By expressing the points sets by their respective centroids $\overline{m} = 1/N \sum_{i=1}^{N} m_i$ and $\overline{d} = 1/N \sum_{i=1}^{N} d_i$ as $m_i' = m_i - \overline{m}$ and $d_i' = d_i - \overline{d}$, the translation component is simplified and we are left with the scaling and rotation components only. The scaling is independent from the rotation and can be define as $\hat{s} = \sqrt{\sum_{i=1}^{N} \left\| d_i' \right\|^2 / \sum_{i=1}^{N} \left\| m_i' \right\|^2}$. The solution to the rotation matrix is $\hat{\mathbf{R}} = \mathbf{VU}^t$ where the singular value decomposition of the correlation matrix $\mathbf{H} = \sum_{i=1}^{N} m_i' d_i''$ is $\mathbf{H} = \mathbf{ULV}'$.

CARS 2002 – H.U. Lemke, M.W. Vannier; K. Inamura, A.G. Farman, K. Doi & J.H.C. Reiber (Editors)
°CARS/Springer. All rights reserved.

The translation component can then be found by using the rotation matrix on the centroids $\hat{\mathbf{T}} = \bar{d} - \hat{\mathbf{R}}\bar{m}$.

Like previously stated, the *coronary tree model* results from the application of the average transformations on the *reference subject*.

4. Results

After applying the outlined method on the 26 coronary trees, we obtain the *coronary tree model*, see Figure 2. The average coefficients of transformation found after fitting the *reference subject* to the other subjects are:

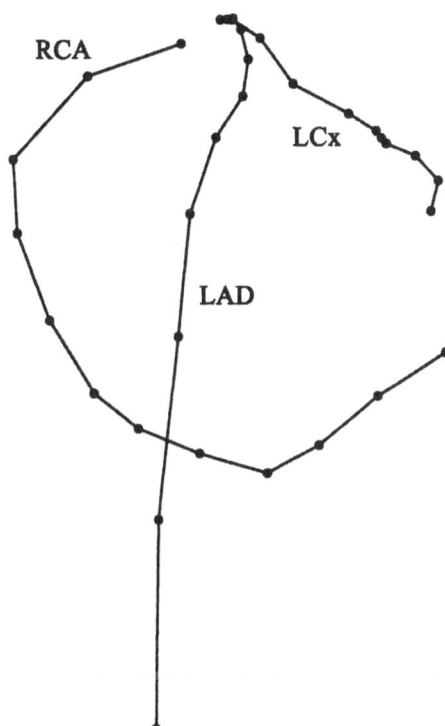

Figure 2. Wire-frame of the *coronary tree model* with an angle of view similar to Figure 1. *See Figure 1 for definitions.*

- for the scaling factor, $s = 1.08$;
- for the rotation expressed as the angles of rotation about the x, y, and z axes respectively, $\alpha = -0.04$, $\beta = 0.09$, $\gamma = -0.31$ and
- for the translation component, $\mathbf{T}_x = 0.59$, $\mathbf{T}_y = 0.18$ and $\mathbf{T}_z = -0.04$, corresponding to the translation on the specific axes.

The average distance between the matching points of the *coronary tree model* and the other subjects is 0.84 cm (0.15 SD). This average distance was 1.42 cm (0.45 SD) before applying the mean transformation.

5. Conclusions

We have presented a method that composes a model of the main coronary arteries of the human heart based on 3D reconstructions of 26 normal hearts. Although the reference system used by Dodge et al. was adequate for their study, the proposed method focuses on the morphological variations and considerably reduces the variability observed by their group by eliminating heart size, orientation and position variations. This model is the first step for a more general 3D atlas of the structure and motion of coronary arteries that will help cardiac contraction analysis and understanding.

CARS 2002 – H.U. Lemke, M.W. Vannier; K. Inamura, A.G. Farman, K. Doi & J.H.C. Reiber (Editors)
°CARS/Springer. All rights reserved.

818

Acknowledgements

The authors express their gratitude to Dr J. Theodore Dodge Jr. for having so generously shared his data.

References

1. Dodge JT, Brown BG, Bolson EL, Dodge HT: "Intrathoracic spatial location of specified coronary segments on the normal human heart." *Circulation* 78: 1167-1180, 1988.
2. Dodge JT, Brown BG, Bolson EL, Dodge HT: "Lumen diameter of normal human coronary arteries: influence of age, gender, anatomic variation and left ventricular hypertrophy or dilation." *Circulation* 86: 232-246, 1992.
3. MacKay, SA and Potel, MJ and Rubin, JM. "Graphics methods for tracking three-dimensional heart wall motion." *Computers & Biomedical Research*, 15(5), pp. 455-73, Oct 1982.
4. Saito T. and Misaki M. and Shirato K. and Takishima T. "Three-dimensional quantitative coronary angiography." *IEEE Transactions on Biomedical Engineering*, 37(8), pp. 768-77, Aug 1990.
5. P. Windyga, M. Garreau, M. Shah, H. Le Breton, and J.L. Coatrieux. "Three-dimensional reconstruction of the coronary arteries using a priori knowledge." *Medical & Biological & Computing*, 36:158–64, 1998.
6. Sarwal, A. and Dhawan, A. P. "Three dimensional reconstruction of coronary arteries from two views." *Comput Methods Programs Biomed*, 65(1), pp. 25-43, Apr 2001.
7. Chalopin, C. and Finet, G. and Magnin, I. E.. "Modeling the 3D coronary tree for labeling purposes." *Medical image analysis*, 5(4), pp. 301-315, Dec 2001.
8. Nguyen, T.V. and Sklansky, J. "Reconstructing the 3-D medial axes of coronary arteries in single-view cineangiograms." *IEEE Transactions on Medical Imaging*, 13, pp. 61-73, 1994.
9. Sarry, L. and Boire, J.-Y. "Three-dimensional tracking of coronary arteries from biplane angiographic sequences using parametrically deformable models. " *IEEE Transactions on Medical Imaging*, 20, pp. 1341-51, 2001.
10. ISI Web of Knowledge. http://woscanada.isihost.com/. 2002
11. Renaudin CP, Barbier B, Roriz R, Revel D, and Amiel M. "Coronary arteries : new design for three-dimensional arterial phantoms." *Radiology*, 190(2) :579–82, February 1994.
12. Guimond, A., Meunier, J. and Thirion, J.-P. "Average brain models : a convergence study." *Computer Vision and Image Understanding* (77) : 192-210. 2000.
13. Arun, K.S. and Huang, T.S. and Blostein, S.D. "Least-squares fitting of two 3-D point sets." *IEEE Transactions on Pattern Analysis and Machine Intelligence*, PAMI-9, pp. 698-700, 1987
14. Horn B.K.P., H.M. Hilden, and S. Negahdaripour. "Closed-form solution of absolute orientation using orthonormal matrices." *Journal of the Optical Society of America* A, 5 :1127-35, 1988.
15. Horn, B.K.P. "Closed-form solution of absolute orientation unit quaternions." *Journal of the Optical Society of A*, 4 :629–42, 1987.
16. Eggert, D.W. and Lorusso, A. and Fisher, R.B. "Estimating 3-D rigid body transformations: a comparison of four major algorithms." *Machine Vision and Applications*, 9, pp. 272-90, 1997.

CARS 2002 – H.U. Lemke, M.W. Vannier; K. Inamura, A.G. Farman, K. Doi & J.H.C. Reiber (Editors)

Automatic stent border detection in IntraVascular UltraSound images for quantitative measurements of the stent parameters

Jouke Dijkstra[a], Gerhard Koning[a], Joan C. Tuinenburg[a], Pranobe V. Oemrawsingh[b], Clemens von Birgelen[c], Johan H.C. Reiber[a,b]

[a] Department of Radiology, Leiden University Medical Center, P.O. Box 9600, 2300 RC Leiden, the Netherlands

[b] Department of Cardiology, Leiden University Medical Center, P.O. Box 9600, 2300 RC Leiden, the Netherlands

[c] Department of Cardiology, University Hospital Essen, Hufelandstraße 55, 45122 Essen, Germany

Abstract

This paper describes a knowledge and model guided system for the automatic contour detection of the vessel, lumen and stent borders in IntraVascular UltraSound (IVUS) images. The different steps of a complete analysis of an IVUS pullback sequence are carried out such, that the different components each other. The stent detection assists the vessel detection and both detections assist the lumen detection.

Keywords: IntraVascular UltraSound, quantitative analysis, border detection

1. Introduction

IntraVascular UltraSound (IVUS) is a catheter-based technique, which provides real-time high-resolution tomographic images of both the lumen and the arterial wall. Nowadays the IVUS imaging technique is used very often to assess the results of the stent placement, to assess the plaque symmetry for directional atherectomy or brachytherapy, or to assess the in-stent restenosis or neo-intimal hyperplasia in follow-up after the placement of a drug coated stent [1, 2]. In the current clinical use of IVUS, the wall of a particular coronary segment is inspected visually by manually moving the ultrasound catheter through the vessel. The global positioning of the catheter is guided by X-ray angiography. In this way the section with the narrowest lumen can be selected and analyzed quantitatively by using a manual caliper in its simplest approach or by outlining the lumen, vessel, or stent borders in a more accurate approach. This will result in the calculation of the percent cross-sectional area narrowing at that particular cross-section, and the minimum and maximum diameters. The inter- and intra-observer variability for these measurements has been studied widely and is high [3, 4]. Furthermore, manual analysis of the images is tedious and time consuming. As a result, only a few images are analyzed from the entire image sequence. Nowadays the creation of pullback series using a motorized pullback device, resulting in image runs of several hundreds of images to be analyzed, becomes more common.

820

With the continuing improvement in IVUS imaging and increasing computing power, it is now feasible to develop and clinically apply automated methods for the quantitative analysis of the coronary arterial wall, stent and plaque burden, both in single transversal slices and in three-dimensional pullback runs [5, 6, 7]. The automated segmentation of lumen, vessel and stent boundaries will reduce the required analysis time and the subjectivity of the manual tracings. The use of the motorized pullback devices allows creating meaningful longitudinal cross-sections, which provide a fast and comprehensive overview of the entire pull back sequence. Newer acquisition devices already support this option on-line.

Modern computer equipment allows the visualization and analysis of more than one pullback image series at the same time, which is very useful for the definition and comparison of the corresponding vessel segment at different acquisition moments e.g. at pre-intervention, post-intervention and follow-up. For the selection of the identical vessel segments in the different runs, the three-dimensional reconstruction is very useful. It also makes it easier to compare the runs to angiograms, because the anatomical landmarks can be found easily by reviewing the longitudinal cross-sections.

2. Methods

To perform the border detection, we have developed a method, which uses a three-dimensional model of the vessel and incorporates knowledge about the morphologic structures, the ultrasound catheter properties and ultrasound specific artifacts. The (semi-) automated method is based on the combination of transversal and longitudinal contour detection techniques. From the pullback series, a user-defined number of longitudinal cross-sections (usually 8 or 16) are created. In these cross-sections the user defines the different segments for the analysis, e.g. a stent segment, a distal segment, and a proximal segment as reference.

2.1. Stent detection
The procedure starts with the stent detection in the transversal slices in a defined segment. The stent contour detection is performed only in the transversal images since the struts are not always visible in each longitudinal image making the border definition much more difficult. In the transversal images, normally enough stent struts are visible to define the stent border. The stent detection is done in three steps. The first step is the global estimation of the location of the struts in the polar transformed image based on the intensity of the struts and their distance towards the catheter. The weight factors for the intensity are based on the fact that the stent struts generally have a higher intensity than the surrounding tissue and it is more likely that bright stent struts are located closer to the catheter than calcified spots. This distance compensation depends on the depth and gain settings of the acquisitions system and the presence of in-stent restenosis. As a next step, the candidate points to create a model for the second more local detection of the strut location are selected by a minimum cost algorithm (MCA). This second detection uses the approximately circular shape of the stent and image gradient information. In the third step, the results of the stent detection in the entire target segment are checked for their consistency with a three-dimensional model. This model is calculated based on all the contours. In case a contour does not fit in the overall model, the detection is re-performed

CARS 2002 – H.U. Lemke, M.W. Vannier; K. Inamura, A.G. Farman, K. Doi & J.H.C. Reiber (Editors)
©CARS/Springer. All rights reserved.

using information whether the detected contour was too far away or too close to the catheter. Fig. 1a shows the 3D stent contours before correction and fig. 1b after correction. This final check is quite useful in regions where the stent struts are quite difficult to distinguish from calcified spots or the definition of the struts is very weak. It should be noted that in situations such as direct stenting, large differences in diameter might occur

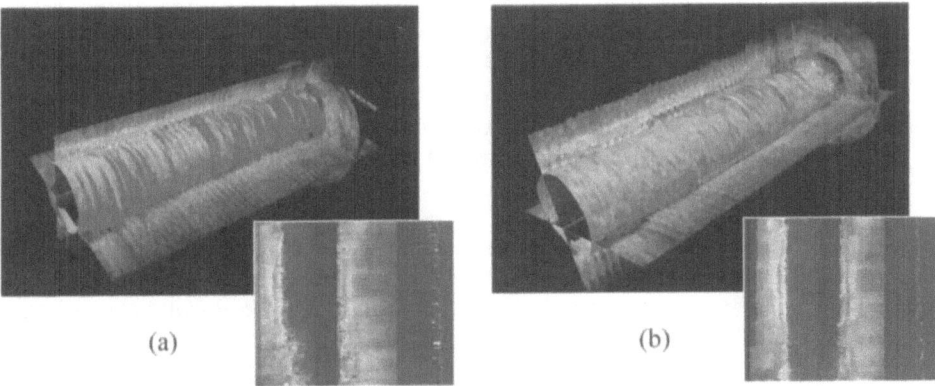

(a)   (b)

over the entire length of the stent.

Fig. 1: Stent border detection (a) without 3D correction, (b) with 3D correction.

2.2. Longitudinal contour detection
In a number of the longitudinal cross-sections (usually 4, a factor which has been determined experimentally), the vessel contours are detected *simultaneously*, which means that they have knowledge about each other's position. For example, the following situation may occur. At one side of the vessel in the longitudinal image, a clear vessel transition is present which would force the vessel contour detection to the left. On the other side of the vessel, multiple potentially vague vessel transitions in different directions are present. The simultaneous technique will now select the combination of the strong transition at one side, and a transition on the other side, which matches best with the morphologic continuity of the vessel and the shape and size of the vessel. This technique is especially useful for regions behind calcified plaque and in side branches where no or sparse image information is available to support the contour detection.

The lumen contours are detected in the same longitudinal images as the vessel contours. The detection is based on the location of the catheter, the already detected vessel contour, and gradient information from the image. The lumen-intima border is the first more or less continuous edge seen from the catheter. A simultaneous detection for the lumen is not meaningful since the shape can be much more irregular. A rough tissue classification based on gray value and texture, supports the contour detection in areas where the catheter is located against the wall and no lumen can be distinguished.

2.3. Transversal contour detection
For each longitudinal contour, the corresponding points in the transversal images are calculated, resulting in attraction points for the transversal contour detection. The contour detection in the transversal images is guided by these attraction points, but not forced,

CARS 2002 – H.U. Lemke, M.W. Vannier; K. Inamura, A.G. Farman, K. Doi & J.H.C. Reiber (Editors)
CARS/Springer. All rights reserved.

822

which has the advantages that some errors in the longitudinal contour detection can be overruled by the transversal contour detection. If necessary, these attraction points can be selected by the user for correction. The corrections will be applied both in the transversal and the longitudinal images, which makes the user-interaction procedure more efficient.

The border detection in the stented pullback segment can be improved by first performing the stent detection. This transversal stent contour can then be transferred to the longitudinal images. By stating that the vessel contour should always be outside of the stent contour, the results of the vessel border detection both in the longitudinal as well as in the transversal images can be improved considerably because the stent struts attract the vessel border detection. The lumen border can optionally be forced inside the stent border. In case of in-complete stent expansion it should be possible to define the lumen contour outside the stent contour.

Based on all the contour data, the derived parameters are calculated over the defined segments. Fig. 2 shows an example how an output graph may look like. In this example also a distal and a proximal segment have been defined so that the vascular remodeling in the stented segment can be demonstrated.

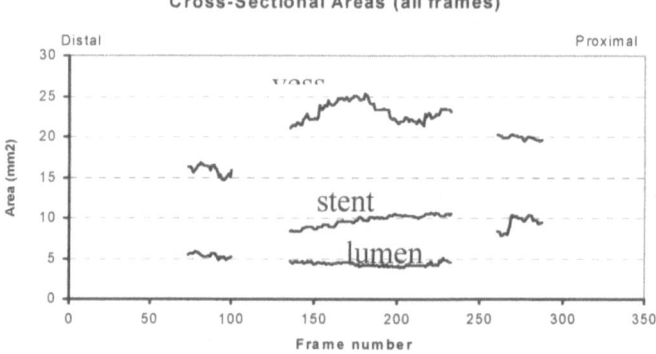

Fig. 2: Example of an output graph for quantitative IVUS measurements.

3. Results

To assess the accuracy of the contour detection techniques, experts manually did draw the vessel and lumen borders in a set of 240 randomly selected slices from different in-vivo pullback sequences acquired by different ultrasound systems (Boston Scientific and EndoSonics). In these series the different borders were also detected automatically by the quantitative software in the entire segment. The cross-sectional vessel and lumen areas circumscribed by the borders of both the manually traced and automatic detected borders in the corresponding slices were compared and resulted in correlation coefficients of 0.99 and 0.98, respectively. Most problems for the vessel contour still occur in areas behind calcified plaque due to different interpretations by experts. For the lumen contour very weak interfaces may result in a difference in interpretation between experts or between the experts and the software.

CARS 2002 – H.U. Lemke, M.W. Vannier; K. Inamura, A.G. Farman, K. Doi & J.H.C. Reiber (Editors)

In another set of in-vivo pullback runs, both post-intervention and follow-up, the automatically detected stent boundaries in 210 slices were compared to the manually drawn stent boundaries and resulted in a correlation coefficient of 0.99. It should be noted that for the automatic detection at least three struts have to be visible in the image, but this also holds for the expert. In some cases no struts were visible at all while they should be present based on the location in the segment and the type of stent. This may be caused by the catheter orientation.

Furthermore, we analyzed 14 pullback sequences of coronary vessels with obstructive coronary artery disease (acquired in-vivo). These pullback series were also analyzed with the validated analytical software on the TomTec system. The vessel and lumen areas in 877 slices determined by our system correlated well with the results of the TomTec system (r-values of 0.99 and 0.98, respectively).

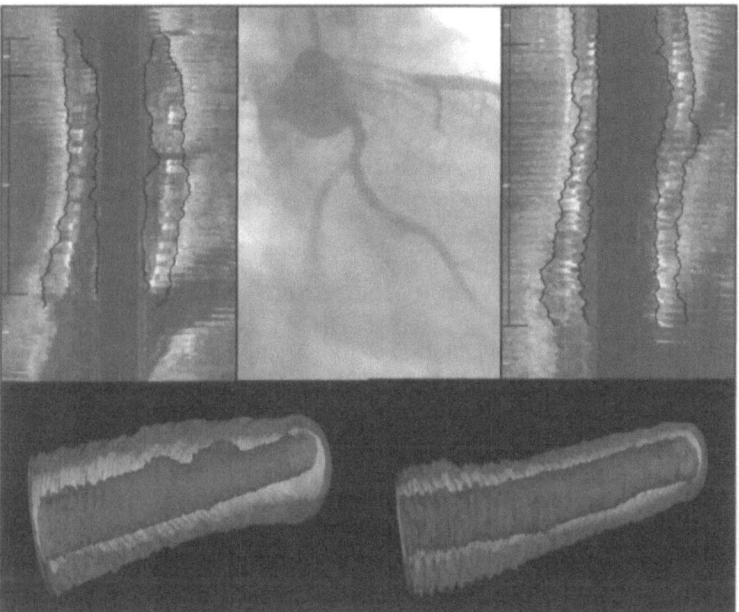

Fig. 3: Example of the use of three-dimensional quantitative IVUS to study the lumen gain in a DCA procedure. From the volumetric calculations it appeared that the amount of in-stent restenosis was redueed from 128.5 mm³ to 71.2 mm³. the MLD increased from 1.9 to 2.6 mm.

4. Discussion

In a set of 50 pullback runs (acquired with Endosonics equipment without ECG triggering which is quite common in clinical practice) the entire stented segment was analyzed automatically and the most distal and the most proximal slice in a continuous series of slices containing stent struts was selected to assess the stent length. The comparison of these distances with the original stent lengths resulted in an average overestimation of 0.35 +/- 1.42 mm by IVUS.

The catheter displacement during pullback can be affected by the cardiac motion. It has been reported that the catheter tip may move up to 5 mm during the cardiac cycle when it is placed on a single spot in the coronary vessel. This longitudinal movement can also be noticed when determining the start and end slice of a stent. In a number of slices the stent struts are visible, then they disappear and next they become visible again, both at the distal and proximal location of the stent. The length measurement of the stent may be affected by this. By using images from the same cardiac cycle, this problem should be less prominent. Another problem for the length measurements and thus the volume measurements can be the non-uniformity of the pullback speed, e.g. due to difference in resistance during the pullback through curved vessels. This can be noticed by stent lengths measurements resulting in different lengths than expected.

5. Conclusion

Due to the flexible use of more than two longitudinal cut planes and the advanced knowledge-guided contour detection approach, the new IVUS analysis system has proven to be suitable for clinical research studies. Due to the nature of the IVUS imaging technique, which results in image artifacts and drop-out regions, there is still a need for some user-interaction, but by using efficient user-interaction which apply corrections in a three-dimensional nature, the number of corrections is quite small. The inclusion of the automatically detected stent boundary will support in-stent restenosis studies, for instance to examine the effect of coated stents, or the effect of a DCA procedure as demonstrated in figure 3.

Acknowledgements

This project was supported by the Dutch Technolgy Foundation (NWO-Technologiestichting STW) under grant nr. LGN 3419.

References

1. Nissen SEY, P.G. "Intravascular Ultrasound: Novel pathophysiological insight and current clinical applications" *Circulation* 2001;103:604-616.
2. Reiber J, Koning G, Dijkstra J, et al. "Angiography and Intravascular Ultrasound" In: Sonka M, Fitzpatrick J, eds. *Handbook of Medical Imaging* - Volume 2: Medical Image Processing and Analysis. Belligham, WA.: SPIE, 2000:711-808.
3. Peters RJG, Kok WEM, Rijsterborgh H, et al. "Reproducibility of quantitative measurements from intracoronary ultrasound images" *European Heart Journal* 1996;17:1593-1599.
4. Blessing E, Hausmann D, Sturm M, Wolpers HG, Amende I, Mugge A. "Intravascular ultrasound and stent implantation: Intraobserver and interobserver variability" *Am Heart Journ.* Feb 1999;137(2):368-371.
5. Dijkstra J, Wahle A, Koning G, Reiber JHC, Sonka M. "Quantitative coronary ultrasound: state of the art". In: Reiber JHC, Wall EEvd, eds. *What's new in Cardiovascular Imaging.* Dordrecht: Kluwer Academic Publishers, 1998:79-94. Developments on Cardiovascular Medicine; vol 207.
6. Von Birgelen C, Mintz GS, de Feyter PJ, et al. "Reconstruction and quantification with three-dimensional intracoronary ultrasound : An update on techniques, challenges, and future directions" *Eur Heart Journ* 1997;18:1056-1067.
7. Dijkstra J, Koning G, Tuinenburg JC, Oemrawsingh PV, Reiber JHC. "Automated Border Detection in IntraVascular Ultrasound Images for Quantitative Measurements of the Vessel. Lumen and Stent Parameters" In: *Proc.Computers in Cardiology 2001*, Rotterdam, NL, IEEE Computer Society Press :25-28.

Invasive Coronary and Vascular Imaging

CARS 2002 – H.U. Lemke, M.W. Vannier; K. Inamura, A.G. Farman, K. Doi & J.H.C. Reiber (Editors)

ECG-gated 3D-rotational coronary angiography (3DRCA)

V. Rasche[1], A. Buecker[2], M. Grass[1], R. Koppe[1], J. Op de Beek[3], R. Bertrams[3], R. Suurmond[3], H. Kuehl[4], R.W. Guenther[2]

[1]Philips Research Laboratories,Hamburg, Röntgenstr. 24-26, D-22315 Hamburg
[2]Aachen University of Technology, Department of Diagnostic Radiology
[3]Philips Medical Systems, Best, The Netherlands
[4]Aachen University of Technology, Department of Internal Medicine

Abstract

To investigate the feasibility of 3D-RCA for high-spatially resolved 3D reconstruction and visualization of the coronary arteries in the pig model. Two-dimensional projections of the coronary artery tree were acquired during rotation of the X-ray fluoroscopy system (INTEGRIS V3000, Philips Medical Sytems, Best, The Netherlands) around a pig. The pigs were anaesthetized and under mechanical respiratory support with heart rates between 75 and 102 bpm. Data acquisition was performed over an angular range of 180° during continuous injection of Iodine (300mg/ml) through a catheter introduced to the ostium of either the left or the right coronary artery tree. To ensure constant filling of the artery tree, the injection of contrast was started slightly before starting the scan. After the data acquisition, a gated reconstruction was performed. Volume reconstructions at isotropic spatial resolution down to 250μm were performed using a gating window of 20 or 40ms length. By moving the gating window over the cardiac a multi-phase reconstruction of the coronary arteries could be provided, yielding a temporally resolved impression of the coronary artery tree. Volumes reconstructed from data obtained during diastole provide a clear visualization of the coronary artery tree including proximal, medial and distal parts. The feasibility of 3D-RCA could be shown in the animal model. The excellent results imply that data acquired over a single rotational run can provide high quality morphological three-dimensional information of the coronary arteries in the catheter laboratory.

Keywords: 3D coronary angiography, 3D-rotational angiography, X-ray angiography

1. Introduction

The use of two-dimensional X-ray projection data has recently been proven to allow three-dimensional reconstruction of high-contrast objects such as arteries selectively filled with contrast agents (CA) or bones [1-2]. This technique is based on the so-called rotational angiography in which the X-ray tube and detector are rotated around the patient while continuously injecting CA into the artery. This method has recently been introduced to the market as 3D Rotational Angiography (3D-RA) by several vendors of high-end vascular X-Ray systems. Due to the relatively slow rotation speed of these systems (<60°/s), the data acquisition times are relatively long, e.g. several seconds for the required 180° rotation. This has limited the application of 3D-RA to non-moving structures so far, and its clinical use almost exclusively to neurological indications. The generation of three-dimensional angiograms of the coronary arteries has been within the realm of the so-called modeling technique. In this approach, the coronary artery tree is generated from the knowledge of its two-dimensional projected centerlines and widths in at least two-projections [3] acquired under known projection geometry. Although the results of the modeling technique are impressive, its application has been limited by the required cumbersome user interaction for the definition of the two-dimensional centerlines and vessel widths. From the end-user point of view, either a significant reduction of the required user interaction or even the fully automatic generation of a three-dimensional coronary angiogram is highly appreciated.

The objective of this work is to investigate the feasibility of using an ECG-gated 3D-RA approach for the fully automated, geometrically accurate 3D reconstruction of the coronary arteries selectively filled with contrast agents on the beating heart in a pig model.

2. Method

All data were acquired on a standard vascular X-Ray C-arm system (Integris V3000, Philips Medical Systems, Best, The Netherlands, see Figure 1). Two-dimensional X-ray projections either of the right or the left selectively CA-filled coronary artery tree were acquired during continuous rotation of the system over an angle of 180° at a frame rate of 25 or 50fr/s.

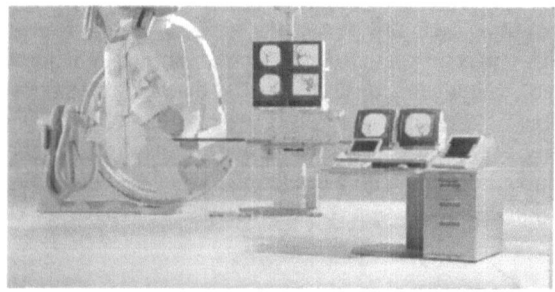

Figure 1: Integris BV3000, Philips Medical Systems, Best, The Netherlands

For the data acquisition, a 38cm image intensifier (II) and a 512^2 image matrix were used. Depending on the size of the pig's heart, the real imaging field of the II was set either to 25cm or to 21cm resulting in a pixel size on the detector of $480^2 \mu m^2$ or $410^2 \mu m^2$, respectively. Two different angular velocity of the system were used, optimized according to the maximal tolerable length of the CA-bolus (see Table 1). The start point of the data acquisition was synchronized with the R-peak of the pig's ECG using a freely selectable trigger delay.

Protocol	fr/s	T_{acq} [s]	T_{pulse} [ms]	ω [°/s]	# proj
I	25	8	10	30	200
II	50		7		400
III	25	11	10	19	275
IV	50		7		550

Table 1: Overview of the acquisition protocols used.

CARS 2002 – H.U. Lemke, M.W. Vannier; K. Inamura, A.G. Farman, K. Doi & J.H.C. Reiber (Editors)

For different runs of the same anatomy, the trigger delay was chosen differently to ensure proper angular inter-leaving of the acquired projection data. For assessing the minimally required number of projections, two or four rotational runs were performed for each of the coronary artery trees with different trigger delays at 0%, 25%, 50%, and 75% (0% and 50% in case of two runs) of the duration of the average RR interval. The pigs were anaesthetized and under mechanical respiratory support, which was suspended during the data acquisition. CA was injected continuously (Iodine, 300mg/ml) at flow rates between 1 and 2ml/s through a catheter introduced through the femoral artery to the ostium of either the left or the right coronary artery tree. To ensure proper filling of the entire arterial tree, the injection of the CA was started slightly before starting the scan. The overall amount of contrast administered varied between 9ml (Protocol I/II single branch) and 24 ml (Protocol III/IV injection in the left main coronary artery).

For reconstruction of each of the triggered data sets, the gating window was positioned in late diastole for the left coronary artery tree (LCA), and 50ms earlier for the right coronary artery tree (RCA). The gating window was chosen as short as possible to ensure minimal residual motion over the entire arterial tree. Depending on the frame rate used during the acquisition, the minimal gating window was 40 ms (25fr/s) or 20ms (50fr/s), if only a single projection per heart phase was selected for reconstruction. The selected projections were corrected for II distortions and then three-dimensionally back-projected using a slightly modified Feldkamp algorithm that considers the real projection geometry and compensates for the non-equidistant angular sampling of the projection data. For the assessment of the impact of the number of projections on the resulting image quality, the volume data sets were reconstructed separately from the projection data acquired with different trigger delays, and were combined in a stepwise manner. The reconstructed volume data were visualized either using maximum intensity projections (MIP) or volume rendering (VR).

3. Results

So far, the gated 3D Rotational Coronary Angiography approach has been applied to five pigs, the heart rate of which varied from 75bpm to 102 bpm. Depending on the heart rate and the rotation speed, each of the acquired data sets yielded between 12 and 17 gated projections for the chosen gating window. For all pigs, both coronary artery trees could be reconstructed at a high isotropic spatial resolution of $400^3 \mu m^3$ from the gated data of a single rotational run. The course of the RCA, the LCA and the LCX could be visualized almost entirely, including proximal, medial and distal

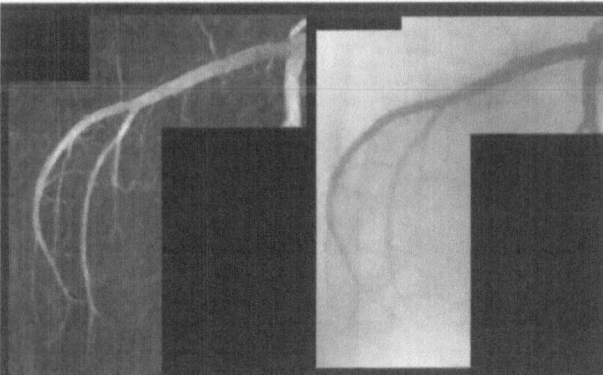

Figure 2: Comparison of a maximum intensity projection (MIP) of the reconstructed LAD (left) to the original CathLab projection. The reconstructions were performed at a spatial resolution of $250^3 \mu m^3$.

830

parts as well as first and second order branches. The comparison of the resulting MIPs of the reconstructed data to the original projection data showed no significant loss of image information. All main vessels could be clearly visualized without noticeable blur, including the first, second, and partly third order branches. Tiny arteries were partly hidden behind background artifacts caused by the severe angular under-sampling. Figure 2 shows the comparison of the original LR X-ray projection to the MIP of the data set reconstructed at high isotropic spatial resolution of $250^3 \mu m^3$ from 13projections obtained during a single rotational run (Protocol III). The heart rate of the pig was 78 bpm. Figure 3 summarizes the obtainable image quality in the left and right coronary artery tree. The volumes were reconstructed from 14 projections selected out of a single rotational run (Protocol IV). The heart rate of the pig was 93bpm.

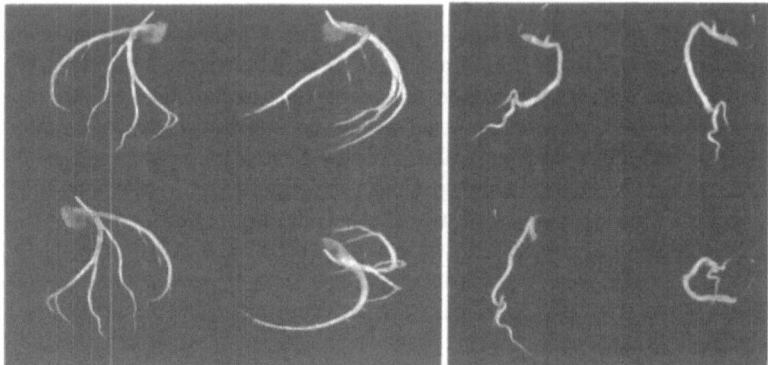

Figure 3: Volume-rendered views of the entire course of the LCA (left) and the RCA (right). Each of the images show a double-angulated view (upper left), an AP view (upper right), a LR view (lower left), and a FH view (lower right). Spatial resolution $0.4^3 mm^3$.

The combination of several data sets further improved the resulting image quality and especially the visual impression of the vessel contours, predominantly by an improved suppression of background artefacts (see Figures 4,5). In case of the RCA, however, this did not improve the depiction of tiny vessels (see Figure 4). In case of the LCA, the

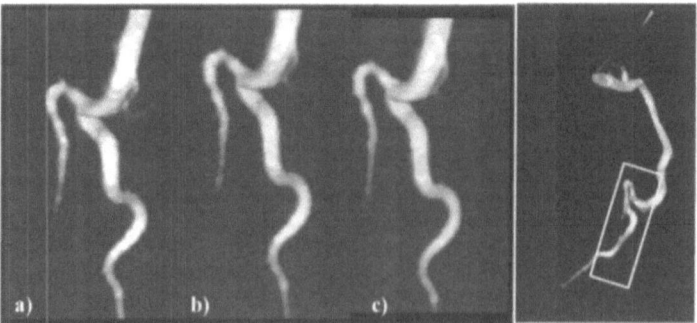

Figure 4: Comparison of reconstructions of the RCA using a single run a), two runs b), and four runs c). The position of the reconstruction window is indicated in the right image.

depiction of tiny vessels (see Figure 5) could be improved by using data of two rotational runs. In all experiments, the almost entire course of the major left and right coronary arteries including 1st and very often 2nd order branches could be assessed.

4. Conclusion

It is shown that gated-3D Rotational Coronary Angiography is feasible in the pig model. The data demonstrate that geometrically accurate, isotropic, high-spatially resolved volume reconstructions of the coronary arteries are feasible from a single rotational run and with a single injection of contrast agent. Since data of single runs yield already high quality images, there is a big potential of keeping the necessary radiation and contrast dose to a well acceptable range. The obtained image quality indicates that the data might be used for accurate volumetric measurements such as vessel diameters, lengths and eccentricity, bifurcation angles, and, of course, for the assessment of the optimal projection angle for the intervention.

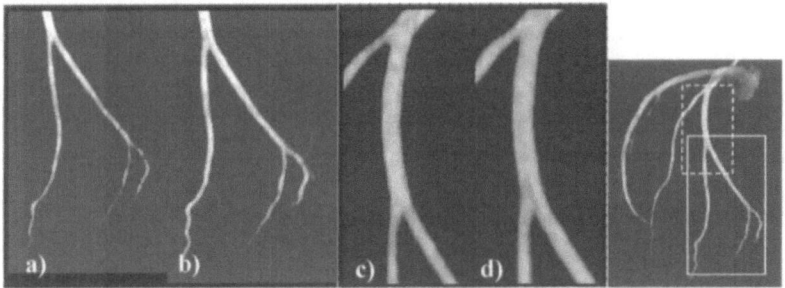

Figure 5: Comparison of reconstructions of the distal a,b) and the proximal c,d) parts of the LAD. a,c) are single run reconstructions, where b,d) were reconstructed from data obtained during two rotations. The location of the reconstruction windows is indicated in the right image.

Compared with the so-called modeling approaches presented earlier, gated 3D Rotational Coronary Angiography offers the big advantage that the volume information is provided fully automated without any time-consuming user interaction. The technique does not substantially increase the overall procedure time, since reconstruction and visualization can be performed almost in real-time.

References

1. M. Grass, R. Koppe, et al., Three-dimensional reconstruction of high-contrast objects using C-arm image intensifier projection data, Comp Med Imag and Graphics, 23:311-321 (1999)
2. M. El-Sheik, J. T. Heverhagen, et al., Multiplanar reconstructions and three-dimensional imaging (computed rotational osteography) of complex fractures by using C-arm systems: initial results, Radiology, 221: 843-849 (2001)
3. S.J. Chen and J.D. Carroll, 3-D reconstruction of coronary arterial tree to optimize angiographic visualization, IEEE Trans Med Imag, 19:318-336 (2000)

CARS 2002 – H.U. Lemke, M.W. Vannier; K. Inamura, A.G. Farman, K. Doi & J.H.C. Reiber (Editors)

Automatic trinocular 3D reconstruction of coronary artery centerlines from rotational X-ray angiography

C. Blondel[a], R. Vaillant[b], F. Devernay[a], G. Malandain[a], N. Ayache[a]

[a] INRIA, 2004 rte des Lucioles, BP 93, 06902 Sophia Antipolis, France
[b] GEMSE, 283 rue de la Minière, 78530 Buc, France

Abstract

We present a method for fully automatic 3D reconstruction of coronary artery centerlines using three X-ray angiogram projections from a single rotating monoplane acquisition. The reconstruction method consists of three steps: (1) filtering and segmenting the images using a multiscale analysis, (2) matching points in two of the segmented images using the information from the third image, and (3) reconstructing in 3D the matched points. This method needs good calibration of the system geometry and requires breatheld acquisitions. The final algorithm is formulated as an energy minimization problem that we solve using dynamic programming optimization. This method provides a fast and automatic way to compute 3D models of vessels centerlines. It has been applied to both phantoms, for validation purposes, and patient data sets.

Keywords: Coronary angiography, 3D reconstruction, matching

1. Introduction

X-ray angiography is the most frequently used imaging modality to diagnose coronary artery diseases and to assess their severity. Traditionally, this assessment is performed directly from the angiograms, and thus, can suffer from viewpoint orientation dependence and from lack of precision of quantitative measures due to magnification factor uncertainty. Three dimensional (3D) reconstruction of the coronary arteries from the angiograms would lead to higher accuracy and reproducibility in the diagnosis and to better precision in the quantification of the severity of the diseases ([1], [2]). Reconstructing the coronary artery centerlines provides geometrical and topological information that is necessary to compute the optimal orientation of the imager for stenosis characterization ([3]) or to give an initial point to the computation of the deformation field of the vessels along the cardiac cycle ([4], [5]).

2. Methodology

2.1 Images acquisition and segmentation

Automatic reconstruction methods using only two images ([2], [5]) have not been shown to be sufficiently reliable for a wide clinical application. Because we are interested in an automatic procedure, we have chosen to use three images. The acquisition routine we used provides a way to obtain them, performing one run with a monoplane system. An angiogram sequence is acquired with a single C-arm, which rotates around the patient. We

CARS 2002 – H.U. Lemke, M.W. Vannier; K. Inamura, A.G. Farman, K. Doi & J.H.C. Reiber (Editors)
^cCARS/Springer. All rights reserved.

determine the acquisition geometry from system calibration using a helical phantom. The rotational acquisition is performed with a zero Cranial/Caudal angle and with the Left Anterior Oblique (LAO)/Right Anterior Oblique (RAO) angle varying from 90 degrees RAO to 90 degrees LAO. Three images of the same cardiac phase are selected from the angiogram sequence. Depending on the rotation speed and on the heart rate of the patient, the LAO/RAO angle between two successive selected images varies between 25 degrees and 40 degrees.

The images are segmented using multiscale analysis and local maxima extraction ([6]). A set of scales is selected, taking into account the diameters of the coronary arteries we want to extract. For each of the selected scales, the image is convoluted by a gaussian kernel with size corresponding to the scale. At each image point, we compute the intensity and the direction of the response of a rectilinear structure detector based on the eigenvalues of the Hessian matrix of the image greyscale values. For a given point, the intensity encodes the likelihood of belonging to a rectilinear structure and the direction encodes a tangent vector to this rectilinear structure. After iterating at each scale, we compile a multiscale analysis that summarizes, for each image point, the scale that corresponds to the largest response, and the corresponding response value and tangent angle ([7]). We store these values as scale, response, and tangent maps.

To segment the vessels, we then apply a hysteresis thresholding to the response maps. Hysteresis thresholding of a map retains connected components with all points that have values above a low threshold and with at least one point with a value above a high threshold. The two thresholds are computed as constant quantile values (at 90% and 98%) of the histogram of response maps generated from the three images. Finally, local maxima extraction of the thresholded response maps leads to a segmentation of the coronary artery centerlines in the angiograms. The segmentation's output is a list of linked points we call "chains". This process is fully automatic. Although the general quality of the segmentation is pretty good, some discrepancies between the segmentation and the real vessel tree may occur. A first difficulty is that vessels can be broken into several disconnected components and that discontinuities may occur at bifurcation points. A second difficulty is that two distinct vessels can superimpose in the angiogram and be detected as one single vessel. Consequently, the matching process has to be robust with respect to the segmentation it uses as input.

2.2 Potential matching points computation

Potential matching points are determined in the following manner: for each point p^1, we compute the corresponding epipolar line l^{12} in the second image and compute its intersections with the second image's segmentation. We note $\{p^{12}_k\}_k$ this set of all points that potentially match with p^1. We call these points "candidates". Typically, in the experiments we conduced, the number of candidates was about 5 in average and ranged from 0 to 15.

Once all the candidate matching points are determined, we assign them a score based on the intensity and direction information the multiscale analysis provides. For each value of k, we can compute, using stereoscopic reconstruction, r^{12}_k the corresponding reconstructed 3D point and p^{123}_k the corresponding reprojected point in the third image (see figure 1).

834

We now can assign a score s^{123}_k to any choice of a k value, using the values of multiscale analysis at position p^{123}_k in the third image. Natural choices for this score can be the multiscale intensity at these positions or the angular closeness between computed and predicted tangents ([8], [9]). Finally, we use a multiplicative combination of these scores because the correct matching points should give simultaneously large multiscale intensity values and good correspondences between computed and predicted tangents.

We iterate this process for every point of every chain of the first image's segmentation. We now index chains numbers by i and points numbers by j (for instance, $p^{12}_{i,j,k}$ denotes the kth candidate of the jth point of the ith chain in the first image's segmentation).

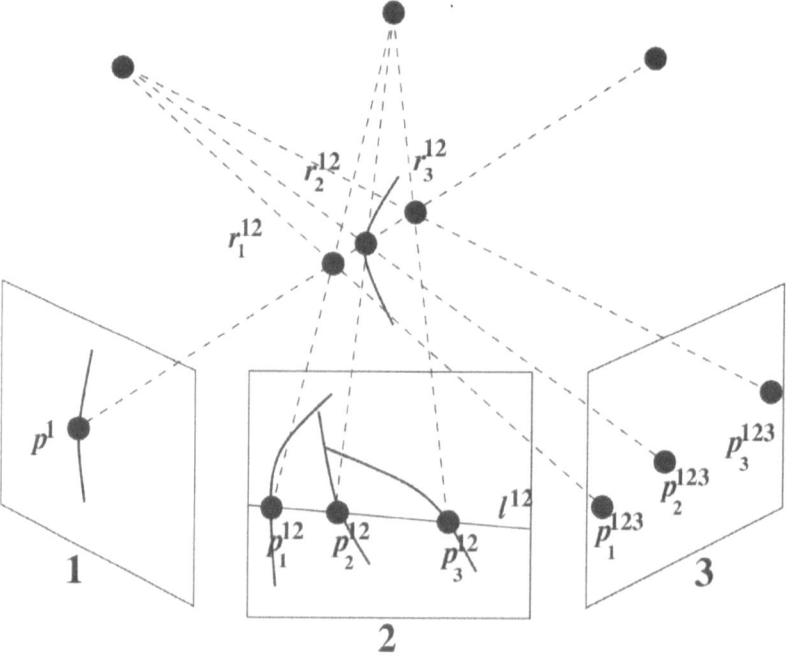

Figure 1: p^1 is in the segmentation of image 1, $\{p^{12}_k\}_k$ are its matching candidates in image 2, $\{r^{12}_k\}_k$ are the associated reconstructed points, and $\{p^{123}_k\}_k$ are the associated reprojected points in image 3

2.3 Selection algorithm
When attempting to match the points, two approaches are possible: point to point matching and chain to chain matching. For fixed given values of i and j, point to point matching would consist in selecting the value k, and thus the point $p^{12}_{i,j,k}$, that gives the best score $s^{123}_{i,j,k}$. For a fixed given value of i, chain to chain matching would consist in selecting the values $\{k_j\}_j$ that produce the connected set of candidates among the set $\{p^{12}_{i,j,k}\}_{j,k}$, with the best sum of scores $\Sigma_j s^{123}_{i,j,k}$. We do not retain these two approaches because of the following arguments. The point to point matching algorithm does not take into account the consistent geometrical behaviour of neighbouring points and thus gives noisy and geometrically incoherent reconstructions. The chain to chain matching algorithm assumes implicitly that the segmentations have no cuts and that a chain in the first image represents only one artery. These hypotheses are necessary to ensure connexity

CARS 2002 – H.U. Lemke, M.W. Vannier; K. Inamura, A.G. Farman, K. Doi & J.H.C. Reiber (Editors)
ᶜCARS/Springer. All rights reserved.

of the matched chain in the second image and of the reprojected chain in the third image. Violating these hypotheses makes the algorithm produce false reconstructed vessels.

We observe that, in *most cases* (except when vessels are superimposed), two neighbouring points in an angiogram are real neighbours in 3D, and thus should be matched and reprojected as neighbours in the other angiograms. We see that, relatively to the former remark, point to point matching is underconstrained and chain to chain matching is overconstrained. We also want to allow a point not to be matched if it has no candidate or if all the candidates infer only a small score positive contribution compared to the geometrical incoherence they induce. Taking all of this into account, we build a semi-local energy formulation of the matching problem. For a given value of i, we compute the sequence of candidates indices $K^{123}{}_i = (k^{123}{}_{i,1}, ..., k^{123}{}_{i,J})$ that minimizes:

$$E^{123}{}_i (K) = - \Sigma_j \, s^{123}{}_{i,j,k_j} + \alpha \, \Sigma_j \, T \, (p^{12}{}_{i,j,k_j}, \, p^{12}{}_{i,j,k_{j-1}}) \text{ where } T \, (p^{12}{}_{i,j,k_j}, \, p^{12}{}_{i,j,k_{j-1}}) \text{ denotes the}$$

geometrical penalty between two successive matched points. We now allow the case $k = 0$, which encodes the fact that we choose not to match the point with any candidate. We take as a convention $s^{123}{}_{i,j,0} = 0$ and $T \, (p^{12}{}_{i,j,k_j}, \, p^{12}{}_{i,j,k_{j+1}}) = 0$ if $k_j = 0$ or $k_{j+1} = 0$. This implicitly means that a point that is not matched has no positive score contribution nor negative geometrical penalty contribution. T can be, for instance, the 2D distance in the second image between the matched points of two successive points in the first image:

$$T \, (p^{12}{}_{i,j,k_j}, p^{12}{}_{i,j,k_{j+1}}) = \| \, p^{12}{}_{i,j,k_j} \, p^{12}{}_{i,j,k_{j+1}} \, \|.$$

We remark that if the geometrical penalty is above a threshold, it indicates a change in the 3D connected component we match. As soon as we have identified a 3D discontinuity in the matching, the penalty must remain constant. Thus, we give a high threshold to the penalty T, to make it more robust and not to privilege close disconnected 3D components with respect to far disconnected 3D components. We solve this global recursively-defined minimization problem using a dynamic programming method.

2.4 Reconstruction algorithm symmetrization
The former algorithm is asymmetric: it depends fundamentally on the ordering of the three images. We can symmetrize the algorithm by applying it to the six possible orderings and gathering the six different reconstructions. It also allows recovering vessel parts that could not correctly be reconstructed using only one specific ordering because of the occlusion and depth effects.

To produce the algorithm output, we gather, for each ordering, the matched points from all the chains and then gather the six reconstructions obtained by reordering the images.

3. Results

We applied the algorithm to a physical coronary artery tree phantom and to data sets acquired from patients who held their breath. We show projected views of the resulting 3D reconstructed centerlines for a patient data set in figure 2. The images are 512^2x8bpp. Typical running time of our method on a 333MHz Sun Ultra 10 workstation is 14 seconds for thesegmentation process and 6 seconds for the matching process.

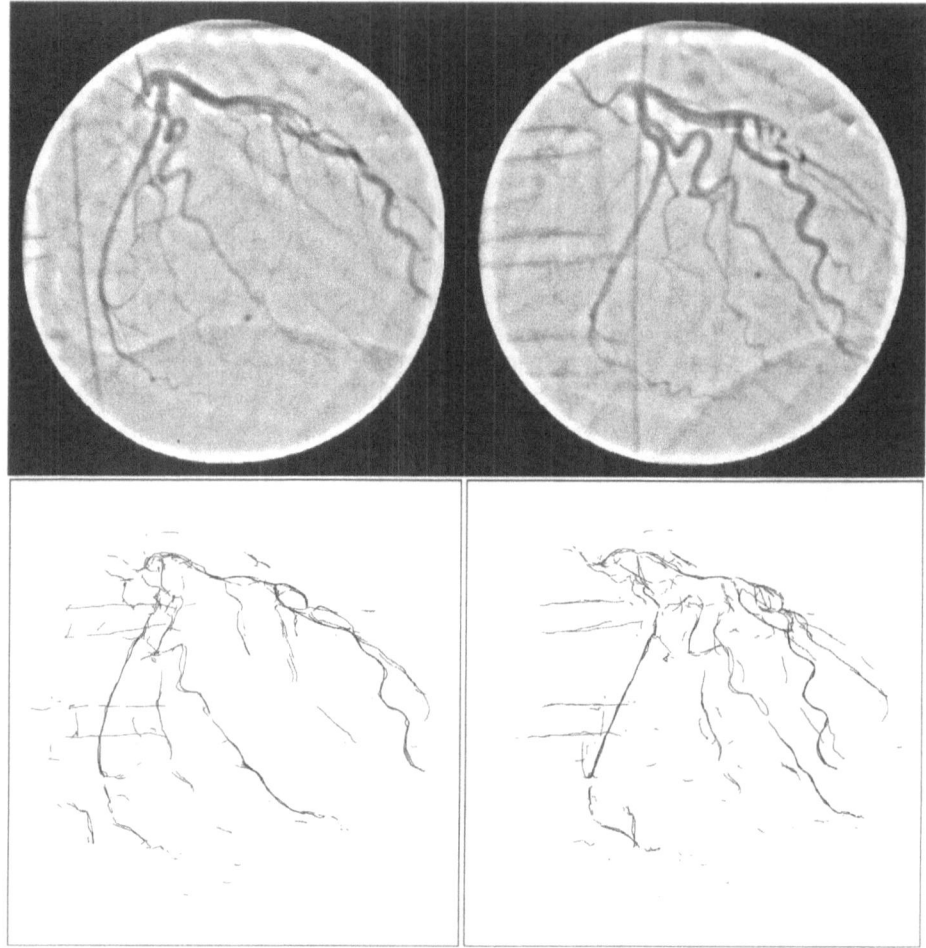

Figure 2: top images show two views, from a patient data set, bottom images show the corresponding reprojection of the 3D centerlines (the views are distinct from those we match)

4. Conclusions

We have developed a fully automatic algorithm to perform the 3D reconstruction of coronary artery centerlines from three angiograms, taken from a single rotational acquisition. As demonstrated in the previous section, this approach can be used to recover the geometry of the main arteries. This is useful for determining geometrically exact 3D reconstructions of IVUS volumes ([10]). A limitation of the current algorithm is the need for breath-hold acquisitions. Approaches derived from computer vision ([11]) may help to solve this issue. The idea is to simultaneously apply the matching strategy described above and to optimize a criterion, which depends on the quality of the geometric model of the acquisitions. Another extension of this work is the application of temporal tracking algorithms ([4]) to the other frames of the rotational acquisition. The obtained results will

CARS 2002 – H.U. Lemke, M.W. Vannier; K. Inamura, A.G. Farman, K. Doi & J.H.C. Reiber (Editors)
©CARS/Springer. All rights reserved.

then be a 4D description of the vessels as used in [5]. This model will be obtained with a single injection of contrast media and on a single plane acquisition system.

Acknowledgements

We would like to thank Guy Shechter for very helpful and enriching discussions. Our gratitude also goes to the ChIR team members (http://www-sop.inria.fr/chir/) for their everyday scientific support and friendship.

References

1.   Messenger J.C., Chen S.Y., Carroll J.D., Burchenal J.E., Kioussopoulos K. and Groves B.M., "3D coronary reconstruction from routine single-plane coronary angiograms: clinical validation and quantitative analysis of the right coronary artery in 100 patients", The International Journal of Cardiac Imaging 16(6): 413-427, December 2000.

2.   Chen S.Y. and Carroll J.D., "3-D reconstruction of coronary arterial tree to optimize angiographic visualization", IEEE Transactions in Medical Imaging 19(4), April 2000.

3.   Chen S.Y. and Carroll J.D., "Computer Assisted Coronary Intervention by Use of On-line 3D Reconstruction and Optimal View Strategy"', Medical Image Computing and Computer-Assisted Intervention Proceedings, Lecture Notes in Computer Science Vol. 1496: 377-385, Springer, Cambridge, October 1998.

4.   Shechter G., Devernay F., Coste-Manière E. and McVeigh E., "Temporal tracking of 3D coronary arteries in projection angiograms", Proceedings of SPIE Medical Imaging 4684, San Diego, February 2002.

5.   Ding Z. and Friedman M.H., "Quantification of 3-D coronary arterial motion using clinical biplane cineangiograms", The International Journal of Cardiac Imaging 16(5): 331-346, October 2000.

6.   Krissian K., Malandain G., Ayache, N., Vaillant R. and Trousset Y., "Model-Based Multiscale Detection of 3D Vessels", Proceedings of the IEEE Conference on Computer Vision and Pattern Recognition: 722-727, Santa Barbara, 1998

7.   Mourgues F., Devernay F., Malandain G. and Coste-Manière E., "3D+t Modeling of Coronary Artery Tree from Standard Non Simultaneous Angiograms", Medical Image Computing and Computer-Assisted Intervention Proceedings, Lecture Notes in Computer Science Vol. 2208:, Springer, Utrecht, 2001.

8.   Faugeras O. and Robert L., "What can two images tell us about a third one?", European Conference on Computer Vision, 485-492, 1994.

9.   Ayache N., "Artificial Vision for Mobile Robots: Stereo Vision and Multisensory Perception", 135-154, The MIT Press, Cambridge, 1991.

10. Reiber J., Koning G., Dijkstra J., Wahle A., Goedhart B., Sheehan F.H. etal., "Angiography and Intravascular Ultrasound", in: Sonka M., Fitzpatrick J.M., editors. Handbook of Medical Imaging - Volume 2: Medical Image Processing and Analysis. Belligham, W.A.: SPIE, 2000: 711-808.

11. Triggs B., McLauchlan P., Hartley R., Fitzgibbon A., "Bundle Adjustment - A Modern Synthesis" in "Vision Algorithms: Theory and Practice": 298-375, Springer Verlag, Lectures Notes in Computer Science, 2000.

CARS 2002 – H.U. Lemke, M.W. Vannier; K. Inamura, A.G. Farman, K. Doi & J.H.C. Reiber (Editors)

838

Improved endpoint localization in guide wire tracking during endovascular interventions

Shirley A.M. Baert, Wiro J. Niessen
Image Sciences Institute, University Medical Center Utrecht, Rm E 01.334,
P.O.Box 85500, 3508 GA Utrecht, The Netherlands
{shirley,wiro}@isi.uu.nl

Abstract

A method is presented which improves endpoint localization in guide wire tracking during endovascular interventions under X-ray fluoroscopy. Accurate guide wire tracking can be used to improve guide wire visualization in the low quality fluoroscopic images, and to estimate the guide wire position in world coordinates. Guide wire tracking is performed using a two-step approach: first, the position of the guide wire is obtained by fitting a spline using a feature image. Subsequently, the spline is iteratively moved towards the tip of the guide wire for more accurate tip localization. For both steps a feature image is calculated in which line-like structures are enhanced. The method is validated using a golden standard, obtained by manual tracings of three observers. By comparing the results to guide wire tracking without explicit endpoint detection, we found that accurate tip localization significantly improved localization accuracy.

Keywords: Interventional radiology, X-ray fluoroscopy, endpoint detection

1. Introduction

Endovascular interventions are increasingly replacing more invasive open surgical procedures. During these interventions, guide wire and catheter position are monitored under fluoroscopic control. In previous work [1], a method was presented which could track J-tipped guide wires in 96% of the frames, with a similar accuracy as manual operators. However, the endpoint position was estimated less accurately, and the method was limited to guide wires with a shaped tip. Accurately localizing the tip of the guide wire is important, e.g. in biplanar imaging to reconstruct the position in 3D, or to determine spatial correspondence with 3D rotational angiography data which may have been obtained prior to the intervention.

There has been a considerable amount of work on the enhancement and extraction of curved line structures. In medical imaging, it is used to extract anatomical structures, such as (centerlines of) blood vessels [2-6]. In this paper a method is proposed which improves endpoint localization in guide wire tracking and extends the previously presented method [1] to straight guide wire tracking.

CARS 2002 – H.U. Lemke, M.W. Vannier; K. Inamura, A.G. Farman, K. Doi & J.H.C. Reiber (Editors)
ᶜCARS/Springer. All rights reserved.

2. Methods

To represent the guide wire, a third order spline parameterization is used. The tracking method essentially consists of a two-step approach; in the first step (i) the spline is positioned on the guide wire and subsequently (ii) the spline is moved towards the tip of the guide wire for more accurate tip localization.

(i)
We assume that the position in frame N is known. To determine the position of the guide wire in the next frame, first the rough displacement of the guide wire is estimated. Hereto a template is constructed which is rigidly registered to a feature image using cross-correlation. In the feature image line-like structures are enhanced by determining the eigenvalues of the Hessian matrix at scale σ. The Hessian matrix is defined as:

$$H = \begin{pmatrix} I_{xx} & I_{xy} \\ I_{xy} & I_{yy} \end{pmatrix}$$

where I_{xy} represents a scaled Gaussian derivative operator:

$$I_{xy} = \frac{\partial^2}{\partial x \partial y} G(x,\sigma) * I$$

Let $|\lambda_1| > |\lambda_2|$ denote the absolute eigenvalues of the Hessian matrix with corresponding eigenvectors $\vec{e}_1, \vec{e}_2$. On line-like structures λ_1 has a high output; the sign of this eigenvalue determines whether it concerns a dark (positive) or bright (negative) line. Therefore the feature image is set to λ_1 if positive and to zero otherwise.

Subsequently, the spline is fitted on the feature image using an energy minimizing approach (Powell's direction set method), where the energy term consists of an internal part related to the geometry of the guide wire (curvedness) and an external energy term which depends on greyvalue and directional information contained in the feature image. In this step the inner product between the spline and the orientation of the feature is used given by

$$O(\vec{x}_i) = \lambda_1 (\vec{e}_2 \cdot \vec{x}_i)$$

This assures that the spline achieves a similar orientation as the guide wire in the image.

(ii)
After this first step in the fitting procedure, the endpoint of the spline is not necessarily positioned on the endpoint of the guide wire, especially in case of guide wires with a straight tip. In order to determine the endpoint, the length of the guide

CARS 2002 – H.U. Lemke, M.W. Vannier; K. Inamura, A.G. Farman, K. Doi & J.H.C. Reiber (Editors)

840

wire is increased at the tip, while fixing the tail position. This procedure is carried out iteratively such that the endpoint of the spline is advanced beyond the endpoint of the guide wire. A graph is constructed which represents the value of the feature image along the spline. Tip localization is now achieved by determining the maximum gradient of the graph within a spatial window of the previous guide wire position. This maximum gradient position most likely represents the endpoint of the guide wire. In order to be robust to noise a coarse-to-fine approach is used. First at a large scale the gradient maximum is determined whereas precise localization is achieved at smaller scales see Figure 1.

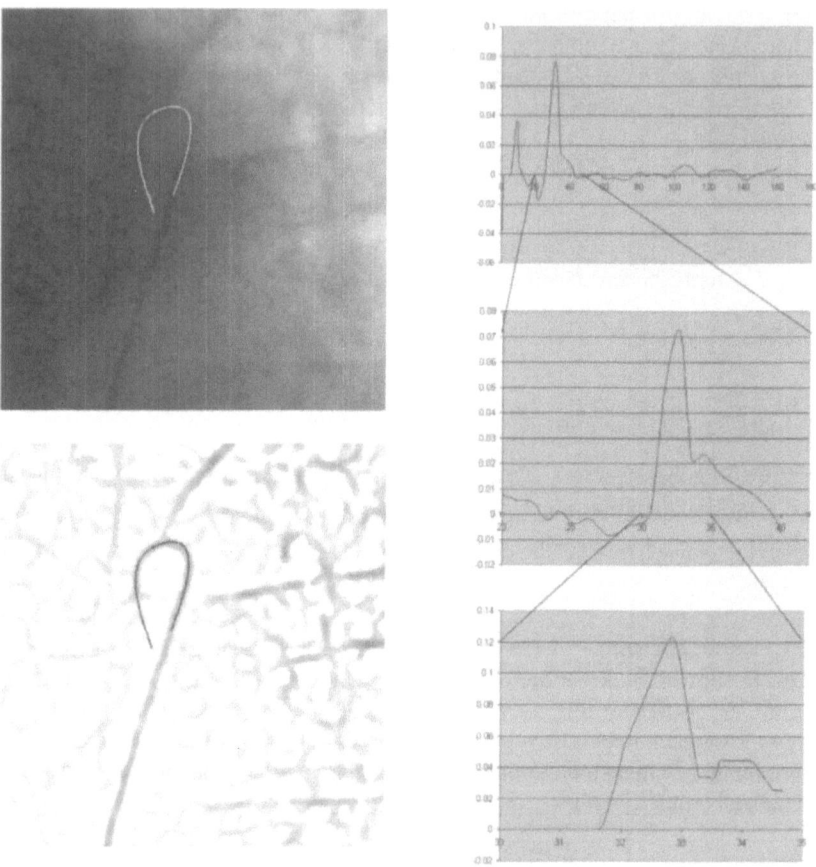

Figure 1: Left: Image which shows that the spline is advanced beyond the endpoint of the guide wire in the original image (upper left) and in the feature image (lower left). Right: Gradient along the spline at multiple scale ($\sigma = 4$ upper right, $\sigma = 2\sqrt{2}$ middle right and $\sigma = 2$ lower right) which are used to accurately determine the endpoint. Along the x-axis, the length of the spline is plotted, where 0 represents the endpoint of the spline. The y-axis represents the gradient of the greyvalue of the feature image along the spline. A first estimate of the endpoint position (maximum gradient of feature along spline) is obtained at a large scale, whereas precise localization is achieved within a small window from this position at the smaller scale.

CARS 2002 – H.U. Lemke, M.W. Vannier; K. Inamura, A.G. Farman, K. Doi & J.H.C. Reiber (Editors)
©CARS/Springer. All rights reserved.

3. Results

In a previous study tracking success and endpoint localization were evaluated versus a golden standard obtained as the average manual tracing of three observers [1]. For the tip distance the inter-observer variability was 1.46 pixels. In that study no explicit endpoint detection was incorporated and for the automatic tracking method, a mean tip distance error of 4.38 pixels was found.

To determine whether the endpoint detection scheme proposed here improves results we randomly selected images in three categories: (i) images in which the guide wire endpoint was accurately tracked (error < 2 pixels (pixelsize approximately 0.4 mm)) with the previous method, (ii) images in which the guide wire endpoint was reasonably tracked (2 pixels < error < 6 pixels) and (iii) images in which the guide wire was not tracked accurately (error > 6 pixels).

A total of 21 frames have been tested, 7 frames in each of the categories. Table 1 shows the tip distance error in pixel units for the three different categories, without and with specific endpoint localization. It can be observed that for the first category (i), a mean error value of 1.15 pixels for the tip distance is obtained if the automatic method was used without endpoint detection. Using the method with endpoint detection, the mean error value increased to 1.84 pixels, which is larger than inter-observer variability (1.46 pixels) but still smaller than one millimeter, since the pixelsize is approximately 0.4 mm.

[pixels]	Without endpoint detection	With endpoint detection
Cat. (i) error<2	1.15	1.84
Cat. (ii) 2<error<6	5.06	2.67
Cat. (iii) error>6	11.15	3.01

Table 1. Tip error distance in pixel units for three different categories of images, without and with explicit error detection.

In the second category (ii), a mean error of 5.06 pixels was found using the method without tip detection. If explicit endpoint detection is added, the mean error for the tip distance decreased to 2.67 pixels. Finally, in the last category (iii), the mean error for the tip distance decreased from 11.15 pixels to 3.01 pixels if endpoint detection is incorporated, which is an error reduction of 73 %.

4. Conclusion

Accurate endpoint localization is an important prerequisite for e.g. reconstructing guide wire position in 3D or providing virtual endoscopic views at the tip of the guide wire. An approach has been presented which accurately determines the end position of a guide wire during endovascular interventions. In the method, first a spline is positioned on the guide wire, and subsequently this spline is advanced beyond the endpoint. By inspecting a feature image along the spline, the endpoint of the guide wire is localized. The approach is carried out in a coarse-to-fine fashion, since a first estimate at a higher scale is less prone

CARS 2002 – H.U. Lemke, M.W. Vannier; K. Inamura, A.G. Farman, K. Doi & J.H.C. Reiber (Editors)

842

to noise, while accurate localization is achieved at low scale. By validating the results with respect to a golden standard obtained by averaging manual tracings of three observers, we found that this explicit endpoint detection scheme significantly improved localization accuracy. In cases where the error was medium to large, the error reduced with 47 % and 73 % respectively. Thus the proposed method is an important prerequisite for e.g. localizing the guide wire tip in 3D.

The results presented in the study concerned J-tipped guide wires since for these images ground truth was available from manual tracings from a previous evaluation study. In experiments with the explicit endpoint localization we found that guide wire tracking could also successfully be applied to guide wires with a straight tip. In order to quantify tracking success in case of straight guide wires, an evaluation study will be carried out.

References

1. S.A.M. Baert, W.J. Niessen, M.A. Viergever, *Guide wire tracking during endovascular interventions,* submitted.
2. Th. Koller, G. Gerig, G. Székely, D. Dettwiller, *Multiscale Detection of Curvilinear Structures in 2-D and 3-D Image Data,* European Conference on Computer Vision 1995, IEEE Computer Society Press, pp. 864-869.
3. R. Kutka, S. Stier, *Extraction of Line Properties Based on Direction Fields,* IEEE Transactions on Medical Imaging 1996, Vol. 15, No. 1: pp. 51-58.
4. C. Lorenz, I.-C. Carlsen, T.M. Buzug, C. Fassnacht, J. Weese, *Multi-scale Line Segmentation with Automatic Estimation of Width, Contrast and Tangential Direction in 2D and 3D Medical Images,* Proceedings CVRMed-MRCAS 1997, J. Troccaz, E. Grimson, R. Mosges (eds.), Lecture Notes in Computer Science, Vol. 1205, Springer-Verlag, pp. 233-242
5. R. Poli, G. Valli, *An Algorithm for Real-time Vessel Enhancement and Detection,* Computer Methods and Programs in Biomedicine 1997 No. 52: pp.1-22.
6. Y. Sato, S. Nakajima, H. Atsumi, S. Yoshida, Th. Koller, G. Gerig, R. Kikinis, *Three-dimensional Multi-scale Line Filter for Segmentation and Visualization of Curvilinear Structures in Medical Images,* Medical Image Analysis 1998, Vol.2, No.2: pp. 143-168.

CARS 2002 – H.U. Lemke, M.W. Vannier; K. Inamura, A.G. Farman, K. Doi & J.H.C. Reiber (Editors)

Improved radiological control of endovascular prothesis positioning, using a region-contour cooperation approach

A. Raji, J. Lemoine, Y. Lahfi, J.C Bossu [a], F. Boudghene [b]

[a] Laboratoire d' Etude et de Recherche en Instrumentation Signaux et Systèmes
Université Paris 12 Val de Marne, 94010 Créteil, France
[b] Hôpital TENON, Paris, France

Abstract

In this paper, we present an image processing aid system to assist the surgeon in the task of positioning endovascular prothesis in the framework of aneurysm treatment applications. It consists in improving the quality of radiological control images used by the operator in two steps. A pre-processing step allows to compute an enhanced image from which the area of interest is segmented. The important informations such as the regions and contours of the artery are then extracted and superposed to the control images used during the surgical operation.

Keywords: Segmentation, contours, matching

1. Introduction

Recent developments in medical imaging, especially in data acquisition and processing, are giving new methods to explore the human body in order to enhance diagnostic and pathology treatment. For example, data fusion techniques based on combining different data types such as radiography, scanner, rmn, ... are used to improve the real time assistance during a surgical intervention. Several solutions are proposed in different other areas like the 3D image reconstruction and the image matching. In the framework of the abdominal aneurysm pathology treatment, we have developed an image processing system to assist the endovascular prothesis positioning. We present in this paper a description of this system components and related work.

2. Clinical process, drawbacks and solutions

2.1 The pathology

The aneurysm is defined by the loss of an artery borders alignment consequently to a local deterioration of the artery tissue [1,2]. The most frequent aneurysm is the abdominal one. It affects the artery situated at the kidneys level. According to the Laplace rule, the force applied to the artery wall is proportional to its radius. This implies a continuous growth of the aneurysm size. A surgical intervention becomes necessary when the dimension of the aneurysm reaches a certain threshold. It consists in replacing the affected portion of the artery by an artificial tube made up of synthetic material: the endovascular prothesis.

2.2 The treatment

The classical process used for prothesis positioning is heavy, complicated and not entirely safe. The first step consists in collecting data such as radiographic, scanner and irm images which are used to construct a 3D profile of the aneurysm. Between the time these measures are made and the time the synthetic prothesis is acquired some characteristics of the aneurysm such as its dimension and shape may change due to biological and physiological factors. Such changes must be detected and updated in the saved data prior to performing the surgical operation, which is not the case in the classical procedure used at present.

The prothesis is introduced in the femoral artery and guided until the aneurysm position under radiological images control. The principal difficulty of this system is the poor quality of such images. In fact, a contrast product is injected to the patient, prior to the operation, in order to obtain some relatively good images from which the surgeon estimates visually informations like the path to be followed by the prothesis. But the effect of the contrast product disappears straight away in few seconds while the hole operation takes about twenty minutes. Furthermore, the system used at present is unidirectional and does not allow a backward step, e.g. the prothesis can not be moved back. And finally, the prothesis must be positioned with high precision because of the probable presence, in the vicinity of the prothesis cast region, of critical vessels that risk to get blocked up.

2.3 An image processing aid system

In order to attenuate the drawbacks of the classical clinical procedure and to improve the visual and semantic information that can be usefull during the surgical operation, we propose an image matching technique between the well contrasted images taken at the beginning of the operation and the poor quality images which serve to control the operation progress. Our method is based on image segmentation by deformable contours approach, and a gray-level transformation method to enhance both of the contrasted and non-contrasted images. Then, the two types of images are combined to obtain throughout the surgical operation a good control image constituted of the segmented area of interest, e.g. the arterial section and its vicinity, superposed to the detected contours in the same region, giving to the operator an improved visual way to control the operation.

3. Methods

3.1 Pre-operation processing

As mentioned in the precedent section, the major difficulty of the system is the poor quality of the control images which makes very hard the localization of the prothesis with regard to the artery borders and the aneurysmal section during the prothesis displacement. Fig.1 shows an example of such images.

In a pre-operation preparation step, the patient is subject to a contrast liquid injection. This let the surgeon visually localize the position of the aneurysm, the path to be followed when introducing the prothesis and the position of the sensible vessels that require high attention because of the blocking up risk when positioning the prothesis. These informations are noted relatively to a ruler fixed on the operation table. However, on the one hand, the effect of the contrast liquid is very brief and disappears within few seconds,

CARS 2002 – H.U. Lemke, M.W. Vannier; K. Inamura, A.G. Farman, K. Doi & J.H.C. Reiber (Editors)
CARS/Springer. All rights reserved.

and on the other hand, this liquid is propulsed with the blood in the vessels in a progressive manner such that it does not cover all of the area of interest at the same time, as illustrated in Fig.2. And obviously, the quantity of injections is limited for medical reasons.

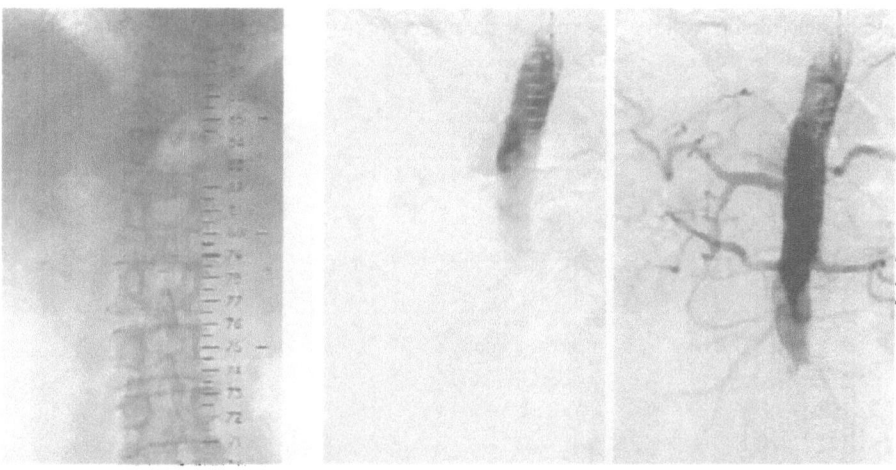

Fig.1 Radiological image control   Fig.2 The effect of the contrast liquid

In order to exploit the contrast information allowed by the injected liquid, we can remark that this information is present only at a certain time which marks the passage of the liquid. So, if we note **I** (t) the image sequence, the passage of the contrast liquid at any position in the image can be found by examining the derivative function:

$$\mathbf{I}\,(t) = d\,\mathbf{I}\,/\,dt$$

Moreover, since we are more interested in the magnitude of the contrast than in its occurrence time, we can retrieve this information by simply computing the well contrasted image by:

$$\mathbf{I}_c = max[\mathbf{I}(t)] - min[\mathbf{I}(t)]$$

The result of such an operation is shown in Fig.3. It reveals very clearly the regions where the contrast liquid has transited, e.g. the blood circuit, while it suppresses from the image all of the regions that remain grey-level constant except some artifacts due to the noise characteristics of the used imagery system. Furthermore, the obtained image highlights better than in any single image of the sequence the sensible regions such as the secondary vessels that fork from the principal artery.

Hence, we can see that this simple pre-processing step can improve significantly the quality of the visual information used before the surgical operation start. The idea then is to further enhance this information and make it permanently available in the radiological image control throughout the hole operation progress.

846

3.2. Image enhancement and contour detection

The borders of the artery represent the most useful information during the prothesis introduction process. Simple gradient operators can generally be used to determine the contour information. However, these operators work well only on high contrasted and noiseless images which is not the case here. We have used rather a deformable contour model, such methods have proved to be more robust than derivative methods in the presence of noise [3].

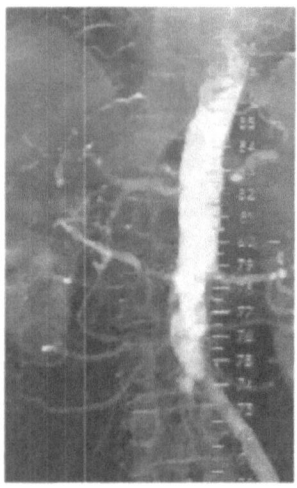   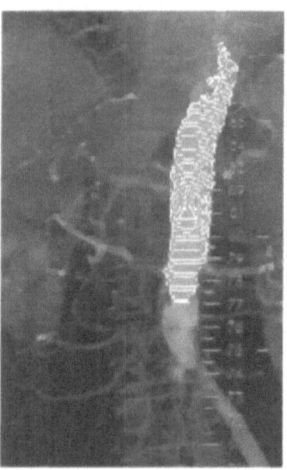

Fig.3 The pre-processing enhancement   Fig.4 The artery contour detection by deformable model

The model we used [4] is implemented as a geometrically deformation of a discrete closed curve which is iteratively expanded to detect the contour of the region constituted by similar grey-level pixels. The region of interest corresponds in our case to the artery. The first closed curve initialized by the operator determines a reference region whose attributes such as grey level mean and standard deviation are calculated. Then, the closed contour is iteratively deformed by moving its vertices toward the outside of the reference region in a radial direction. This deformation process is controlled by a similarity measure. Each vertex of the deformable contour is blocked when it attempts to expand to a region which does not present the same features as the reference region. Fig.4 illustrates the contour detection by this method.

However, as shown in this figure the obtained final contour does not delineate all of the arterial section. Furthermore, the connections of the secondary vessels to the artery, which represent high important information at the prothesis placement phase because of the blocking up risk of these vessels, are not detected. This is due to the heterogeneity of this region which, in this image, can be segmented in several different regions from the grey-level distribution point of view. In order to successfully apply the deformable contour method to compute the accurate contour of the artery, a pre-segmentation step is needed to improve the homogeneity of the arterial region. We have developed in the framework of another work a grey-level transformation based method [5] that allows to segment the image in a given number of classes while it increases the homogeneity of each of these

CARS 2002 – H.U. Lemke, M.W. Vannier; K. Inamura, A.G. Farman, K. Doi & J.H.C. Reiber (Editors)
ⓒCARS/Springer. All rights reserved.

classes. The method is based on an optimal classification of grey levels with respect to the probability density function of the image, followed by a local parametric grey level transformation applied to the obtained classes in such a way that the homogeneity of each class is improved and the global image contrast is increased at the same time. The segmentation is controlled by mean of two parameters representing the desired number of classes and an homogeneity coefficient.

In the radiological enhanced image it is clear that the grey levels are to be classified into two classes: the artery and vessels connected to it and the image background. Fig.5 shows the classification obtained by the presented method applied inside an area of interest containing the main portion of the artery and its bifurcations toward the secondary vessels. The arterial region is described in the segmented image by an homogeneous grey-level distribution which makes the contour detection by the deformable model easier and more accurate.

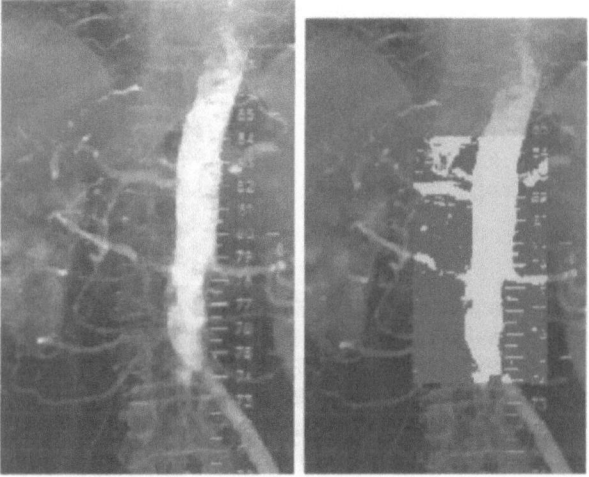

Fig.5 Segmentation example applied in a reduced are of interest

3.3. Image matching
The last stage in the presented work is the matching of the previously processed image with the radiological control images during the surgical operation as illustrated in fig.6. At present, this is made by a simple superposition of the two types of images, without any consideration of the possible displacement of anatomical elements or the imagery system components. This estimation is still made visually by the operator. But, in the framework of a future work, we plan to use fixed marks, such as vertebra or metallic elements, to establish a rigorous matching scheme between the pre-processing results and the control images in real time during the surgical operation progress.

4. Results

We have obtained satisfactory results with respect to the visual control of the operation. Indeed, the success of the operation in classical conditions relies on the skill and experience of the operator, for whom the proposed method gives an efficient tool to improve the control conditions

848

and to increase consequently the success rate of such operations. Furthermore, this method can be used to estimate quantitative informations for other purposes like mathematically establishing an approximate model of the aneurysm and simulating the operation on computer for training.

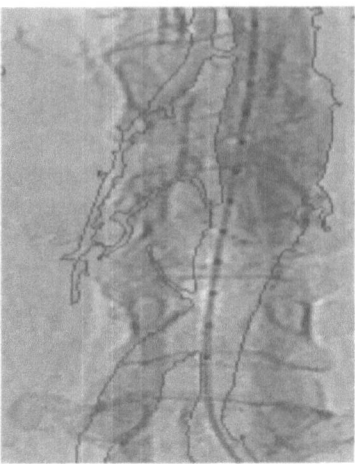

Fig.6 Superposition of the pre-processed and control images

5. Conclusion

We present an image segmentation system aiming to give a satisfactory visual control of the endovascular prothesis positioning in the framework of the aneurysm pathology treatment. The method has been successfully applied in experimental environment, and will be implemented in clinical process. The pre-processing step have been emphasized leading to significant improvement of the used images. We plan to achieve this work by implementing a matching technique between the obtained results and the real time images used for the operation control. The final aim will be to obtain a 3D image control system.

References

1. May J, White GH, Waugh R, Stephen MS, Chaufour X, Yu W, Harris JP. Adverse events after endoluminal repair of abdominal aortic aneurysms: a comparison during two successive periods of time. J Vasc Surg 1999;29:32-7
2. Blum U, Voshage G, Lammer J, et al. Endoluminal stent-grafts for infrarenal abdominal aortic aneurysms. N Engl J Med 1997;336:13-20
3. C. Kervrann and F. Heitz, Statistical Deformable Model-Based Segmentation of Image Motion, IEEE Transactions on Image Processing, vol. 8, no. 4, 1999, 583-588.
4. A. Raji, E. Petit, J. Lemoine, S. Djeziri A geometrically deformable contour model. 9th international conference on image analysis and processing -Vol. I, pp. 510-518, Florence, Italy, 17-19 september 1997
5. A. Raji, A. Thaïbaoui, E. Petit, P. Bunel, G. Mimoun, A gray-level transformation-based method for image enhancement. Pattern Recognition Letters, Vol.19, n° 13, pp 1207-1212, 1998.

CARS 2002 – H.U. Lemke, M.W. Vannier; K. Inamura, A.G. Farman, K. Doi & J.H.C. Reiber (Editors)

Modeling and process design of a new type of catheter for special endovascular treatments of abdominal aortic aneurysms

P. Joli[a], Ch. François [b], T. Gagarina [a], F.Boudghène[c]

[a] Laboratoire Systèmes Complexes, Evry, France
[b] Laboratoire d'informatique Industrielle et d'Automatique, Vitry, France
[c] Service de radiologie Hopital Tenon, Paris, France

Abstract

A consortium of laboratories named MATEO (directed by Professor Frank Boudghène) has been created in response to a national call in Health Technologies, and we have focused our project on the risks related to the endoluminal method (endovascular) stent placement in aorta with a flexible catheter. In order to improve the actual surgical method, it is necesary to dispose a catheter with an actuated distal part. In this paper, we define the mechanical design and the modeling of a new actuator based on the deformation of three cylindrical nickel bellows due to internal hydraulic pressure of physiological water. This device produces bending movement as an elastic continuum without the need for an additional skeletal structure. Two actuators are implemented in the distal part of the catheter, one into the tip and one just before the part where is localized the endoprosthesis. The first actuator allows a control to open the way through the vessels and the second actuator allows a control of the orientation of the distal part just before the dropping phase of the endoprosthesis. The geometrical constraints due to a severe reduction are satisfied and a real scale prototype has been carried out (fig.1).

Keywords: Endovascular treatment, microactuators, mechanical design

1. Introduction

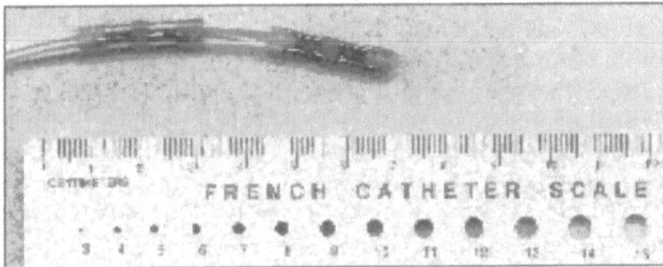

Fig. 1: Distal part of the catheter (real scale).

The actual process consists of introducing a long flexible catheter inside an iliac artery until it reaches the damaged area (aneurysm) of the abdominal aorta just under the ostium of the renal arteries, or of the thoracic aorta just after the origin of the supra-aortic vessels

CARS 2002 – H.U. Lemke, M.W. Vannier; K. Inamura, A.G. Farman, K. Doi & J.H.C. Reiber (Editors)

850

[2]. Inside the distal part of the catheter, a very flexible endoprosthesis is inserted between the inner and outer flexible sheaths of the catheter. When the distal part of the catheter is inside the aortic aneurysm, the endovascular operator removes the outer sheath of the catheter by manipulating the proximal part of the catheter which is outside the patient. The flexible endoprosthesis is thus released, and by extensional force the stents of the endoprosthesis hook the artery wall. The blood flows through the endoprosthesis and thus the progress of the arterial pressure injury on the aneurysm wall is stopped and the aneurysm is healed. This process is quite ingenious but it has some drawbacks which leave room for improvements. The reproducibility of this method is not satisfied for two main reasons [3]:

- The first reason is related to the lack of vision feedback for the endovascular operator due to the absence of internal vision. The surgeon only has external indirect vision projected in 2D by using instantaneous X-Ray Radio after having injected a contrast material (chemical dye) to highlight the vessels (2D X-Ray fluoroscopy projection). Because an x ray is a two dimensional image of three dimensional structure, this leave the surgeon unsure which way to move the catheter. Moreover the amount of chemical dye injected must be limited, so the contrast material is not used continuously and the surgeon must work at times without any vision.

- The second reason is related to the lack of force feedback for the endovascular operator due to the friction force all along the catheter and the inherent flexibility (passive compliance) of the catheter which looks like a long plastic tube. There is a very low risk of puncturing the artery, causing internal bleeding, if the pushing force is too high at the same time as the tip of the catheter pinches the artery wall. But the higher risk is a bad positioning of the endoprosthesis in the aneurysm because of the difficulty for the endovascular operator to control the orientation of the distal part of the catheter, where the endoprosthesis is located, just before dropping it. This can lead to a post-operative shock, if the endoprosthesis blocks the passage of the blood in vital arteries, or the failure of the operation if blood leaks between the endoprosthesis and arterial wall.

The problem of lack of vision could be resolved by a virtual 3D reconstruction from a database of preoperative images provided by an external vision system like computed tomography angiography (CTA) or magnetic resonance angiography (MRA). The limit of these conventional external vision systems is the considerable time required for image reconstruction, so it is not possible to use them at this moment as a navigation system working in real time. An intermediate solution is the use of appropriate techniques for « matching » preoperative and operative images [3]. But in near future, we think, with new better adapted algorithms of image reconstruction and the constant workstation developments, that it will be possible to track the moving of the catheter and so give the surgeon access to high-resolution 3D video image of surgical field in real time [4]. This concept of a virtual surgical field is the basis of the current success of minimally invasive procedure with assisted computing surgery [5], [6]. A team of the MATEO consortium is working on this problem area.

The inherent friction contact force along the catheter, between the distal part and the proximal part manipulated by the endovascular operator, can not be reduced but it is possible to work around it if the distal part of the catheter is actuated. With a remote control system, the endovascular operator can control its orientation and thus improves the

CARS 2002 – H.U. Lemke, M.W. Vannier; K. Inamura, A.G. Farman, K. Doi & J.H.C. Reiber (Editors)

positioning and the reproducibility of the process just before dropping the endoprosthesis. Two types of remote control are possible and can be or not used together:

- Using a force feedback control connected to a haptic system, a sense of touch can be restored to the surgeon in order to prevent excessive contact force of the tip of the catheter against the artery wall. This type of remote control needs force and slip contact sensing.
- Using an internal vision feedback control. It is possible to embed optical fibers in the catheter and use infrared light to image through highly scattering media such as blood.

The surgeon has to keep the control of the catheter, but during the insertion phase of the catheter, we can imagine an intelligent control [11] which drives coherently the different actuators inside the steerable tip-catheter to prevent excessive contact force and to open the way through the complex path of the vessels. Another team of the MATEO consortium is working on this problem area.

2. Technical background of the invention

Recently, a new generation of endoscope and catheter have been developed by using wires or springs made into shape memory alloy (SMA) [5], [7], [8], [9]. These are widely used in the design of micro robotic system [13] because, they have some advantages like fitting in a very small volume, providing large forces. It is not necessary to pull the wires, they produce a contraction force and a reasonable amount of deformation when they are heated by an electric current applied to them. However there have drawbacks like a large bandwidth which can not be compatible to control a dynamic system and a highly non-linear behavior. But the most inconvenient for us, principally for the safety of the patient is to introduce an electrical current inside the catheter, and so in the vessels (wet surrounding). But another reason is to avoid any electromagnetic interference in order to preserve the possibility of using a RMA as we have seen in the introduction. A wire with inside an ionic polymer conducting film is an alternative actuator (quick response and low driving voltage) already used for a design of a micro-catheter [12].

Another approach that we have followed is the utilization of hydraulic actuators. They have the main advantage to be suited to wet surrounding and they do not produce electromagnetic interference. Moreover they keep at milimetric scale a high power mass/ratio and they are very safe if we use physiological water. The main drawback is the many connecting tubes necessary for the remote control, which can significant increase the rigidity of the catheter. However the lateral compliance is very important for moving inside an artery that is why the shaft of the actuator itself must be lateral flexible without it being necessary to introduce an articulated endoskeleton. We did not find any paper, only international published patents, presenting a flexible catheter or endoscope with a hydraulic actuator. In [13] [14] the basic principle of these hydraulic actuators consists of 3 or 4 tubular elastomeric bladder disposed in parallel and connected between two disks. A tubular braid of inextensible filaments is fitted around each tubular bladder. When a fluid is supplied into the tubular bladder, it expands in the radial direction (fig.2), and thus contracts in the longitudinal direction. As a result when the pressure is increased only in one tubular bladder, the hydraulic actuator produces a bending movement in the direction

CARS 2002 – H.U. Lemke, M.W. Vannier; K. Inamura, A.G. Farman, K. Doi & J.H.C. Reiber (Editors)
°CARS/Springer. All rights reserved.

of the tubular bladder. The main problem of these hydraulic actuators is the volume occupied by the expanded tubular bladders, which can strongly press some other structural components inside the distal part of the catheter. To resolve this problem, we have advantageously replaced each tubular bladder and its associated braid by a metallic bellow.

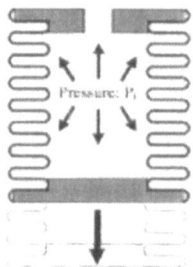   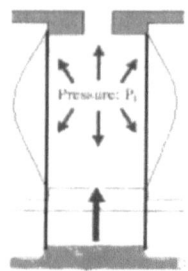

Fig 2: a) Longitudinal extension of a bellow   b) Radial expanding of a braid

The metallic bellows which are produced by microelectrodischarge machining, can have very small diameter (9/10 mm). Moreover, they can have very thin convolution wall (8/1000 mm) in this manner they keep theirs lateral compliance. The convolutions ensure that a bellow is significantly stiffer radially than longitudinally and that longitudinal extension is therefor much greater   than radial expansion   when subjected to internal pression.. So even with high internal pressure they fit in a small volume (fig. 2). These bellows can support very high internal pressure without damage for the bellow, the major risk is the buckling which increases with the length of the bellow and with the feedback force at the ends of the bellow. Another advantage of the metallic bellow is that they have a longitudinal rigidity and they can support themselves without any internal pressure and without any other rigid components. There is no moving part inside the actuator itself, which means it is easier to miniaturize it. No endoskeleton has to be considered, so we keep the lateral compliance. The metal used in our prototype is the nickel, but it is possible to use copper, which has the advantage of not being ferromagnetic. We have found recently a paper presenting a similar system of bellow actuator but in a completely different application for designing a finger of a subsea robot manipulator [1].

3. Design of the distal part of the catheter

The bellow actuator consists of three bellows placed in a parallel arrangement forming the vertices of an equilateral triangle (diameter of surrounding circle is 3,5 mm). These three bellows are constrained between two cylindrical supports (diameter 5,3 mm).

Two actuators are used in the distal part of the catheter, one just before the location of the endoprosthesis and one just after in the tip of the catheter (fig.3). The first actuator helps the endovascular manipulator to control the orientation of the distal part just before dropping the endoprosthesis and the second actuator helps the endovascular manipulator to open the way for the rest of the catheter in the case of a complex surgical path (bend artery, arterial bifurcation).

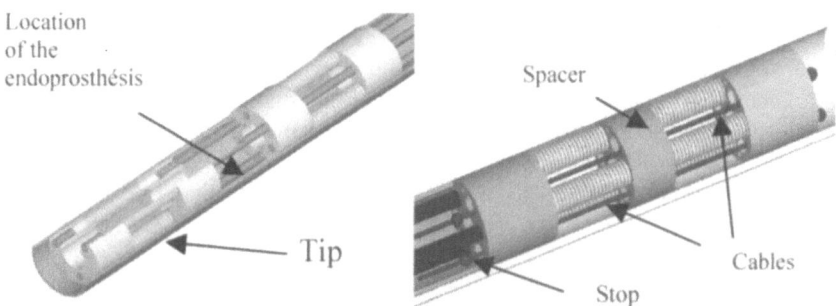

Fig.3: Design of the distal part   Fig.4: Design of the modified bellow actuator

As we can see in the Figure 4, the bellow actuator has been modified by an intermediate cylinder called « spacer » placed between the two cylinder supports in order to reduce the risk of buckling . Moreover we have introduce security cables with stops at each end to avoid large deformation of the nickel bellow. All the tubular holes in the different cylinders are made by conventional micromachining . Some of these holes have only 0,4 mm. In the middle of each cylinders   there is a tubular hole of 1,5 mm in order to introduce surgical tools. All the cylinders are made in Plexiglas to facilitate the assembly task. Indeed the ends of the bellows are fixed inside the cylinders with a photosensitive glue.

4. Modeling of the bellow actuator

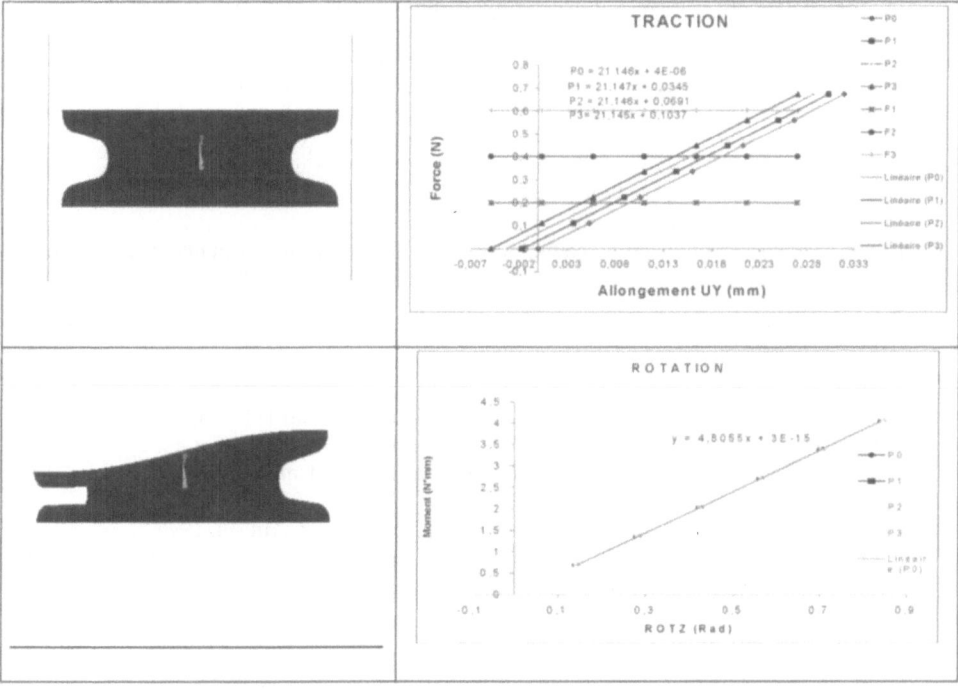

Fig.5: Modelling of one convolution of the bellow (shell 3D)

CARS 2002 – H.U. Lemke, M.W. Vannier; K. Inamura, A.G. Farman, K. Doi & J.H.C. Reiber (Editors)
©CARS/Springer. All rights reserved.

854

Figure 5 shows different numerical results, which define the deformations of one convolution of a below for two types of loading: axial force and lateral torque. By changing geometrical characteristics like internal or external diameter, we have made an optimal choice between resistance and compliance of the bellow. A Finite Elements Modeling of the bellow actuator has been made and we have obtained a bending rotation of 40 degree with 3 bars in one bellow and 1 bar in the two others. The length of the actuator is 16,3 mm.

5. Conclusion

We have presented in this paper a new design of actuator for flexible catheters in order to decrease the risks inherent to endovascular stent placement. A prototype has been carried out and the next step is to test it on a endotrainer . In parallel, a work of modelling has been made on the actuator in order to optimise the parameter of the bellows.

Acknowledgements

We wish to thank the French National Research and Education ministry

References

1. D. M.Lane and al "The AMADEUS Dextrous Subsea Hand: Design, Modeling, and Sensor Processing" IEEE J. of oceanic engineering, Vol 24, N°1, January 1999.
2. F. Boudghene-Stambouli « Traitement endovasculaire des maladies aortiques par endoprothèses », Doctorat de l'Université René Descartes de Paris, 1996.
3. P.Dario, M.C.Carrozza, B. Allotta, E. Guglielmelli " Micromechatronics in Medecine" IEE/ASME Transactions on mechatronics. Vol.1. No.2. June 1996
4. R.Sebben, J.Hall, "Aortobifemoral Angiography: Initial Experience with the Toshiba Aquilion Multislice CT Scanner" eMedical Review [Originaly pubished in the japanese edition of the Toshiba Medical Review, Issue 80]
5. P. Dario and all. « A miniature steerable end-effector for application in an integrated system for computer assisted artroscopy» International Conference on Robotics and Automation, Proceedings of the IEEE, Albuquerque, New Mexico, April 1997.
6. L.Versweyveld, "Intuitive's da Vinci robot and Estech's RAP catheter used in USA's first closed-chest heart bypass operation" Virtual Medical World Fev 2002 (www.hoise.com/vmw)
7. Fukuda and al. «Active catheter system with multi degrees of freedom. Mechanism and experimental results of active catheter with multi units and multi D.O.F. ». Proc. of the 4 Int. Symp. on Micro Machine and Human Science, Nagoya (1993).
8. Ph. Bidaud, N. Troisfontaine, M Larnical. Optimal design of micro-actuators based on sma wires
9. Lim G.and al. "Multi-link active catheter snake motion" Robotica,Vol. 14, 1996
10. S. Fatikow, U. Rembold "Microsystem Technologie and Microrobotics" Springer-Verlag editor
11. D.Duhaut. "Using a multy-agent approach to solve the inverse kinematics". In Intelligent Robot and System Conference, IROS, p.2002-2007
12. Guo Sh. and al: "Micro Catheter System with Active Guide Wire", Proc. of Int. Conf. On Robotics and Automation, Nagoya, 1995, pp.79-84.
13. Nagayoshi and al. "endoscope" United States Patent N°5,179,934 Jan. 19, 1993
14. Ueda Y. "Endoscope with elastic actuator comprising a synthetic rubber tube with only radial expansion controlled by a mesh-like tube" United Patent N°4,832,473 May 23 1989

Left and Right Ventricular Function

CARS 2002 – H.U. Lemke, M.W. Vannier; K. Inamura, A.G. Farman, K. Doi & J.H.C. Reiber (Editors)

Quantitative biplane angiography for right and left ventricular volume determination

F. K. Schmiel, D. G. W. Onnasch, K. Moldenhauer, H. H. Kramer

Klinik für Kinderkardiologie der Christian-Albrechts-Universität zu Kiel,
Abt. Biomed. Technik, Schwanenweg 20, D-24105 Kiel, Germany

Abstract

A computer program is presented, which is suitable for both enddiastolic and endsystolic and semi-automated biplane frame-by-frame volume determination of the right (RV) and left (LV) ventricle. Compared to other programs an important features is presenting the biplane images side by side after optimal pairing. That means the images are rotated in such a way that the epipolar lines in both planes represent the same cross sectional planes. Additionally, the magnifications of the frontal and lateral projection are fitted resulting in identical scales. The paired images are necessary for a reliable assignment of the anatomical structures of the heart to their X-ray projections. Especially in evaluations of the RV this is useful for correctly tracing the pulmonary valve in the frontal projection as this structure is superimposed by the pulmonary artery and parts of the RV. Furthermore the fitting of the magnifications in both projection planes can be used for detecting faulty geometric calibrations, which become obvious, when the corresponding distances in the planes do not agree. As a result of optimal image pairing the mean percent difference of the calibrated vertical extent of the lateral and frontal projection is significantly ($p<0.01$) reduced as compared to the unpaired biplane ventricular analysis.

Keywords: Quantitative biplane angiography, ventricular analysis, border detection

1. Introduction

Since the early beginning of the clinical application of ventricular angiography the angiograms had not only been evaluated qualitatively e. g. for getting dynamic morphological information, but also quantitatively for the determination of the left and right ventricle, e. g. volumes and contraction patterns. All methods of ventricular volume determination from angiographic image sequences are based upon the delineations of the ventricular borders. Depending upon the X-ray equipment (gantry) the volumes had been determined form single as well as from biplane angiograms using an ellipsoid as a geometric model of the ventricle. Two different methods for calculating the volumes of the ellipsoids had been applied: the area-length method and the multiple slice method [1,2]. From the ellipsoidal volumes the real volumes of the ventricle are determined by using correction equations with different correction parameters. There is no doubt that the biplane evaluation is superior concerning the reliability of the ventricular volumes. This applies especially for the right ventricle and for left ventricles with abnormal geometry (e. g. left ventricular aneurisms or HOCM). Taking all these considerations into account it is recommendable to perform biplane evaluations whenever it is possible.

858

One of the main problems in quantitative biplane angiography (QBA) is the correct tracing of the ventricular contours, i. e. the tracings in both planes must correctly correspond to the border of the three-dimensional geometry of the ventricle. Especially the delineation of the right ventricular valve planes is very complicated, as these structures are superimposed by parts of the opacified right ventricle. Until now all computer assisted biplane evaluation programs have the lack that it cannot easily be seen whether the biplane tracings of the ventricle are compatible or not. Therefore we developed a computer program for biplane evaluation of angiographic image sequences with image pairing of both projection planes allowing an easy judgement of the compatibility of biplane ventricular contour tracings [3].

2. Description of the software program

2.1 Program structure

The QBA program consists of a modular structure (Fig. 1) with linked files used for data exchange with our cardiac information system (CIS). I. e. the program can run as a stand-alone version as well as in combination with CIS. The structure of the linked files is independent from the specific database (e. g. Microsoft Access®) thus it can be used with different CIS. The program consists of two parts: (a) contour tracing and (b) contour evaluation. The data exchange between both parts is performed by a contour file ('contour.ctr') which contains the contour coordinates and some other data (header) necessary for the evaluation of the contours.

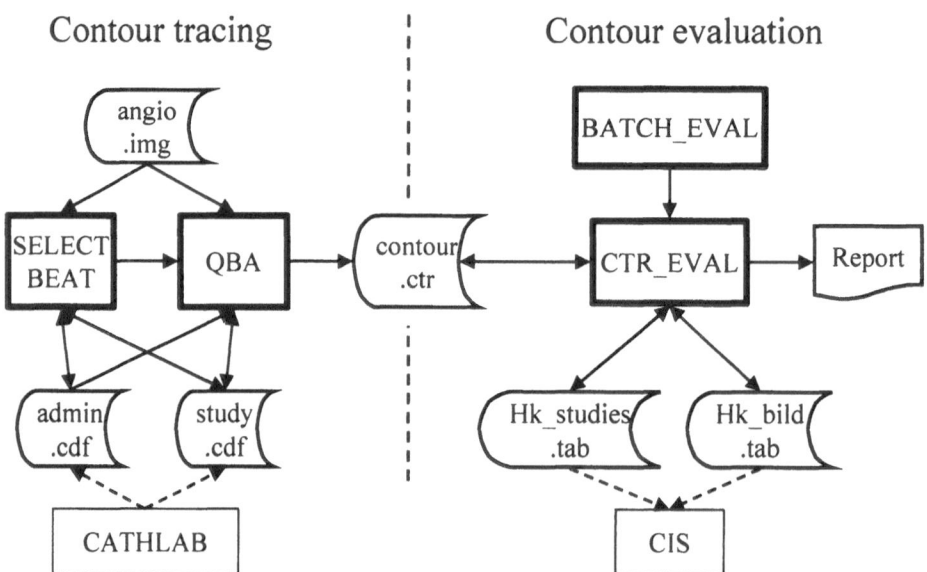

Fig. 1: Program structure.

After selecting the frames of the cardiac beat to be evaluated 'SELECT_BEAT' the main input file of the contour tracing module 'QBA' is the image file which contains the angiographic image sequences of both projection planes. Additionally two more input files

CARS 2002 – H.U. Lemke, M.W. Vannier; K. Inamura, A.G. Farman, K. Doi & J.H.C. Reiber (Editors)
©CARS/Springer. All rights reserved.

('admin.cdf', 'study.cdf') are used. The format of the files is netcdf. The contents are data from our cathlab program: (a) 'admin.cdf' contains the data being specific for the examination including the body weight and height of the patient, which are necessary for calculating normal values of ventricular volumes and (b) 'study.cdf' contains the technical data of the single angiography, e. g. heart rate, projection angles of the gantry, image intensifier distances and image intensifier formats. These data are used for calculating the magnification factors and for image rotation, both necessary for the optimal image pairing. Today the data of the netcdf-files are entered manually from the cathlab protocol, but we have planed to get these data automatically from our cathlab program. The output file of the contour tracing module ('contour.ctr') contains not only the coordinates of the contours but also as a header all other technical and patient data that are necessary for the evaluation of the contours (calculation of ventricular volumes etc.). Thus the contour evaluation module can evaluate the contour file ('contour.ctr') independently from the netcdf files, i. e. the examination can be evaluated even if both netcdf files are lost.

The contour file ('contour.ctr') is the main input file of the contour evaluation module 'CTR_EVAL'. Additionally the data of both netcdf-files or contour header are used for the evaluation of the contour data. The following parameters are calculated for each pair of frontal and lateral contours corresponding to the frames of the biplane image sequence: (a) areas of the ventricular outlines (biplane), (b) longest diameters of the ventricular outlines (biplane), (c) biplane multiple slice volume of the ventricle, ordinate of the (d) upper (biplane) and (e) lower border of the ventricular outlines (biplane). The results are printed as an angiographic report of the patient. Furthermore the results are stored in the files 'Hk_studies.tab' and 'Hk_bild.tab' respectively. These two files are used for interfacing the results with the database of our CIS. The file 'Hk_studies.tab' contains the data that are specific for the single angiography (projection angles, image intensifier distances, size of the image matrix, geometric calibration factors, site of contrast injection etc.), whereas the file 'Hk_bild.tab' contains those data that are assigned to the single frame of the biplane image sequence (volumes, areas, longest diameters, heart phase [endiastole, endsystole, diastole or systole], mode of contour determination [automatic, splines, manual etc.], traced heart chamber, name of the evaluator, date of the evaluation etc.)

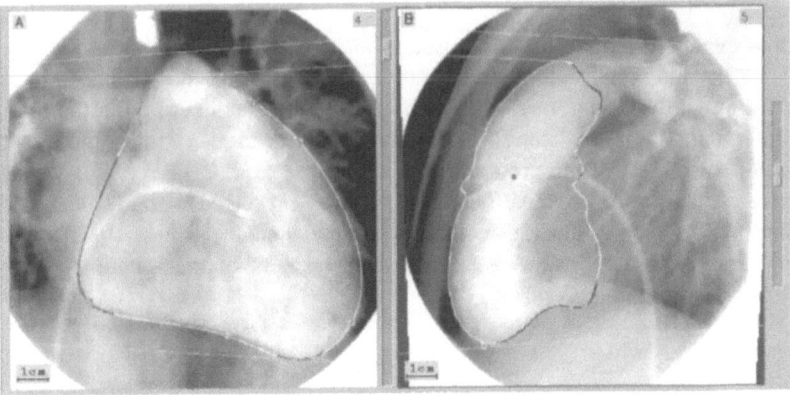

Fig. 2: A biplane enddiastolic RV angiogram after optimal image pairing.

CARS 2002 – H.U. Lemke, M.W. Vannier; K. Inamura, A.G. Farman, K. Doi & J.H.C. Reiber (Editors)

2.2 Program features

After selecting appropriate enddiastolic and endsystolic images the contour tracing part is started. First of all the position of four opaque markers, which are fixed in a square on the image intensifier input screen, are determined (automated or manually corrected) [4,5]. In combination with the image intensifier distances and the rotation angles of the gantry the marker positions are used for dewarping, rotating, and fitting of the geometric magnification of the images of the frontal and lateral projection. This results in biplane images with optimal pairing, i. e. the epipolar lines in both planes represent the same cross sectional planes (Fig. 2). The position of the epipolar lines can be moved simultaneously in both planes by a slider. Thus it is easily possible to check whether the vertical positions in the frontal and lateral projection corresponds to each other or not [3]. This is one of the most important feature of our program as erroneous tracings of the ventricular contours, concerning their vertical extent, are recognised by the user instantly.

There are three different algorithms used for ventricular border detection: (a) fully automated, (b) manually, and (c) semi-automated. For the fully automated version it is necessary to define a circular region of interest around the ventricle. The ventricular border is determined by image segmentation using the principle of minimal radial inertia [6]. Satisfactory results of this algorithm are achieved only in adequately opacified left ventricles. The manually performed contour tracing uses the manual positioning of a spline curve on the ventricular contour. If the spline curve is only roughly positioned over the ventricular border as a first approximation; a stripe of 20 pixels around the spline is used as a region of interest for the segmentation algorithm (applying the principle of minimal radial inertia). This method is utilized for the semi-automated detection of the ventricular contours. It results in satisfactory results not only in left but also in right ventricles (Fig. 4). This feature is remarkable because the geometric variability of the right ventricle is more pronounced compared to the left ventricle. Concerning the saving of time automated border recognition is not superior to manually contour tracing , if only enddiastolic and endsystolic images are evaluated. But if the ventricular borders of all images of a total cardiac cycle have to be traced, the (semi-)automatic detection of ventricular borders is an essential advantage concerning the saving of time as well as the reproducibility of the results.

The contour evaluation module can be used in an interactive as well in a non-interactive mode. Using the interactive mode, the contour files ('contour.ctr') can be selected by a browser. Additionally it must be decided whether the results are stored in the output files used for interfacing with the database. The non-interactive mode of the contour evaluation module can be used to call the program in a batch run ('BATCH_EVAL'). We used this mode for re-evaluation of contour files that had been produced with an older version of the tracing module having not the feature of optimal image pairing. The results of this evaluation are used as comparative values for assessment of the reliability of our new program using optimal image pairing.

CARS 2002 – H.U. Lemke, M.W. Vannier; K. Inamura, A.G. Farman, K. Doi & J.H.C. Reiber (Editors)
ᶜCARS/Springer. All rights reserved.

3. Results

A measure of the reliability of optimal image pairing is the difference of the vertical extent of the traced ventricular contours between the frontal (A) and lateral (B) projection of right ventriculograms of infants, children and adolescents of various cardiac diseases. The superiority of optimal image pairing can be seen when the percent differences [100*(B-A)/B] are compared (Table 1 and Fig. 3). The standard deviations of enddiastolic and endsystolic evaluations are both significantly reduced (p<0.01). This proves that the reliability of ventricular contour tracing can be improved by using the method of optimal image pairing.

RV- Evaluation	paired			unpaired		
	Mean	SD	N	Mean	SD	N
Enddiastole	2.78	5.37	39	-3.78	8.43	131
Endsystole	2.91	6.88	20	-5.91	10.02	127

Table 1: Mean values and standard deviations (SD) of the percent differences of the vertical extents.

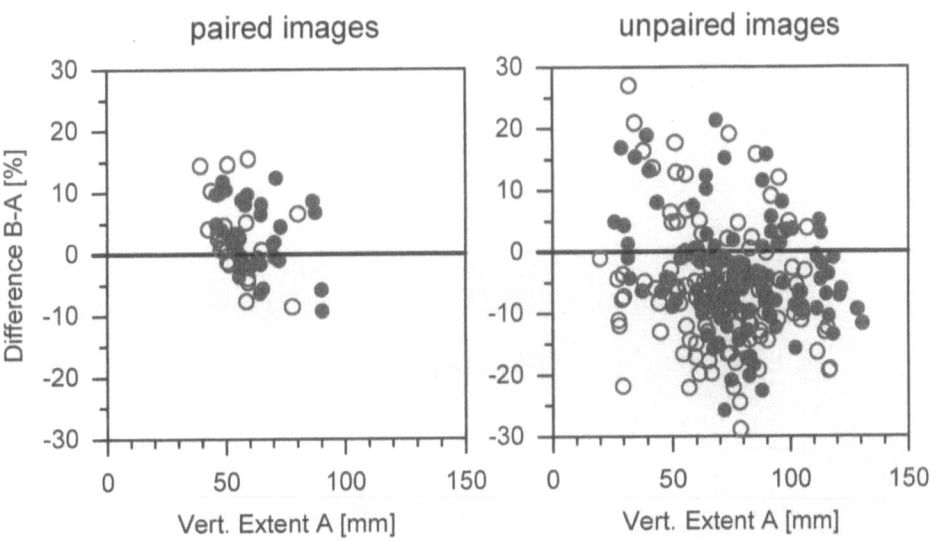

Fig. 3: Percent differences of the right ventricular vertical extents for enddiastolic (•) and endsystolic (o) contours with paired and unpaired biplane images.

For a subset of our evaluations we determined the ventricular contours of the enddiastolic and endsystolic frames of the same digital angiogram with and without optimal image pairing. The resulting ventricular volumes show a significant scatter but no essential systematic error (Fig. 4).

CARS 2002 – H.U. Lemke, M.W. Vannier; K. Inamura, A.G. Farman, K. Doi & J.H.C. Reiber (Editors)
©CARS/Springer. All rights reserved.

4. Conclusions

The presented computer program for the determination of left and right ventricular volumes is characterized by an essential improvement of the accuracy of ventricular contour tracing. It uses the redundant information on the vertical extend of the ventricular silhouette as given by the calibrated biplane gantry system to improve and facilitate contour tracing. The semi-automated mode for ventricular border recognition makes the frame-by-frame analysis of total cardiac cycles possible with an acceptable amount of time and allows routine pressure volume analyses.

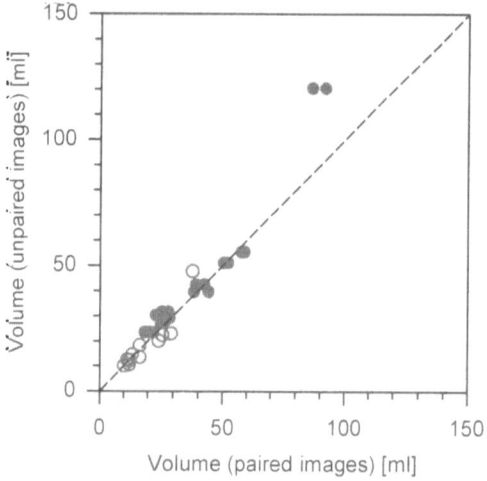

Fig. 4: Biplane right ventricular analysis (area-length method) for 23 endsdiastolic (•) and 12 endsystolic(o) contours traced biplane with and without optimal image pairing.

References

1. D.G.W. Onnasch, Computerized geometric evaluation of angio- and echocardiographic images. Herz 10, 228-237, 1985.
2. J.H.C. Reiber, G. Koning, J. Dijkstra et al., Angiography and intravascular ultrasound. In: Handbook of Medical Imaging, eds: M. Sonka and J. M. Fitzpatrick, Vol. 2, 711-808, SPIE Press Bellingham, Washington, 2000.
3. D.G.W. Onnasch, F.K. Schmiel, H.H. Kramer, Problems in quantitative evaluations of biplane X-ray angiocardiograms. In: Computer Assited Radiology and Surgery , eds: U.U. Lemke et al., 967-972 Elsevier, Amsterdam, 2001.
4. D.G.W. Onnasch and G.P.M. Prause, Geometric image correction and iso-center calibration at oblique biplane angiographic views. Computers in Cardiology, IEEE Comp. Soc. Los Alamitos, 647-650, 1992
5. D.G.W. Onnasch, G.P.M. Prause and J.D.F. Redmer, Automatic correction of variable image distortion for accurate geometric measurements in digital angiographic systems. Medizinische Physik 95, 84-85, 1995.
6. M. Kralemann, D.G.W. Onnasch, Entwicklung eines halbautomatischen Verfahrens zur Segmentierung des Ventrikels in Angiographien. Biomed. Technik 41 (Ergänzungsband), 646-647, 1996.

CARS 2002 – H.U. Lemke, M.W. Vannier; K. Inamura, A.G. Farman, K. Doi & J.H.C. Reiber (Editors)

Development and evaluation of a software package for right ventricular analysis

J.J.H. Hensgens, B. Weijers, J-P.M.M. Aben, A.P.G. Kroes
Pie Medical Imaging, Maastricht, The Netherlands

Abstract

The increasing demand for quantitative analyses of the heart encouraged us to develop a software program for the analysis of the right ventricle (RV). The currently available software programs for analysis of the left ventricle (LV) are not suitable for RV analysis mainly because of two reasons:

1. The automatic segmentation algorithm developed for LV analysis cannot be applied to RV analysis because of a different shape and poor local contrast quality;

2. The volume and regression models, developed for LV analysis, are not appropriate for RV analysis.

Based on literature and discussions with several experts in the field, these difficulties can be overcome with our newly developed Right Ventricle Analysis (RVA) software by using:

1. A very fast and easy manual segmentation method based on splines;

2. 7 different volume models designed for the determination of the RV volume.

At present, preparations are made for the evaluation of the first version of the CAAS II RVA software package. The purpose of this evaluation is to establish the reproducibility and accuracy of the newly developed software. At the conference, the features of the CAAS II RVA will be presented and the outline of the evaluation study will be discussed.

Keywords: Right ventricle, analysis, volume

1. Introduction

The right ventricle (RV) volume estimation has always had less attention than the left ventricle (LV) volume estimation. This is partly due to the fact that the LV was considered to be the more important chamber of the heart and partly because the complex shape of the RV.

Currently, the interest in quantitative right ventricular volume estimation is growing, especially in pediatric cardiology. However, the currently available software programs for left ventricle analysis (CAAS II LVA) are not suitable for the RV. Therefore, Pie Medical Imaging developed CAAS II RVA, a software package for the quantitative analysis of RV X-ray images.

An important feature of quantitative analysis of heart and vessels is contour detection. The following characteristics of the RV prevent the possibility of implementing the fast and easy automatic contour detection that we use for the quantitative LV analysis:

- The outline of the contrast in the RV is less clear than in the left ventricle;
- A diseased RV shape differs significantly from a non-diseased RV shape;
- The right ventricular wall is less smooth than the left ventricular wall;
- Multiple projection angles are used, which results in a large variability in RV shape.

Due to these properties, it is not possible to fully automatically detect the RV contour, after indicating the valve and apex, within acceptable accuracy. Therefore, to define the RV contour, the following methods are implemented in the CAAS II RVA software:
Semi-automatic contour detection based on splines;
Manual contour detection.

Additionally, the more complex internal geometry of the RV compared to the left ventricle hampers the volume calculation. To overcome this, several research groups have developed volume models especially for the analysis of the RV. Seven of these models have been implemented in our CAAS II RVA software. This report describes the applications of the developed CAAS II RVA software package and the outline of the evaluation study.

2. RVA software applications

The CAAS II RVA software for the analysis of right ventricles of the heart was developed because of the increasing demand for objective quantification of right ventricular volumes. Especially in pediatric cardiology, the interest in determining RV volumes is increasing.

It appeared that the software already in use for the quantification of left ventricular volumes is not suitable for the correct analysis of right ventricles. To overcome this Pie Medical Imaging developed a new CAAS II program that meets the requirements for a correct RV analysis. In the next paragraphs, the most important features of the CAAS II RVA software are presented.

2.1. Contour detection
Contours of the ventricle can be found either semi-automatically or manually. The semi-automatic contour detection method is very easy to use. By indicating some control points the computer fits the right ventricle contour by using a mathematic curve definition known as splines. The first two control points indicate the position of the pulmonic valve. Hereafter, the user can optimize the contour detection by adding a number of control points [1]. Additionally, it is possible to further improve the results. This optimization method is based on the gray values of the RV image.

Alternatively, the manual detection method can be used. With this method the user defines the contour of the RV by drawing the contour of the ventricle manually. As mentioned for the semi-automatic method it is possible to improve the outcome of your contour by using the optimization method based on the gray values of the RV image.

CARS 2002 – H.U. Lemke, M.W. Vannier; K. Inamura, A.G. Farman, K. Doi & J.H.C. Reiber (Editors)
©CARS/Springer. All rights reserved.

2.2. Volume calculation

Seven different models for the calculation of the RV volume have been implemented in the RVA software. Five of these models are used for biplane analysis, one model can be used for biplane and monoplane analysis, and one model can only be used for monoplane analysis. Each model has at least one regression formula that will correct for the assumed mathematical shape and the muscles.

1. Simpson model
The Simpson model uses the anterior-posterior view and the lateral view of the RV. The images are divided into 100 equal slices. The cross section of the RV when viewed from above is assumed to be an ellipse. [2] [3]

2. Parallelepiped model
The biplane Parallelepiped volume model is based on the premise that the planar surface areas of an object, observed in two projections perpendicular to each other, are directly proportional to the size of that object irrespective of its precise shape. [4]

3. Boak model
The Boak model uses biplane images and assumes the ventricle to be a series of hemi-elliptical cylinders, and predicts the RV volume and surface area based on dimensions of the cross sections. [5]

4. Area Length model
The biplane Area Length model is based on the premise that the RV is an ellipsoid of revolution. [4]

5. Multiple Slices model
The biplane Multiple Slices model is comparable to the Simpson method. The ventricle is modeled as an ellipsoid and the image is divided into 100 slices. [6] [7]

6. Three Sided Pyramid model
The Three Sided Pyramid volume model is based on the assumption that the right ventricular chamber resembles a pyramid with a triangular base. This model can be used with monoplane and biplane projection images. [8] [9] [10]

7. Two-chamber model
The Two-chamber model uses only the lateral view of the RV. In this view, there is a clear separation at the superior aspect of the tricuspid valve between outflow tract or infundibulum above and inflow tract or RV body below. The outflow tract is assumed to be cylindrical whereas the RV body is assumed to be more ellipsoidal. [2]

Based on these models stroke volume, cardiac output, cardiac index, end-diastolic volume, end-systolic volume, indexed volumes and the ejection fraction are determined.

2.3. Wall motion

The centerline wall motion model is implemented in the RVA software to characterize regional ventricular function. This method allows the user to estimate the ventricular wall motion by measuring the motion of 100 cords drawn perpendicular to a centerline constructed in the middle of the end-diastolic and end-systolic contours. [11]

3. Clinical evaluation

At present, preparations are made for the clinical evaluation of the first version of the CAAS II RVA software package. The purpose of this evaluation is to establish the reproducibility and accuracy of the newly developed software.

Quantitative data derived from the CAAS II RVA software for X-ray angiography will be compared to the volume data derived from images obtained by magnetic resonance imaging (MRI). Every volume model and its regression formula will be studied concerning its applicability in right ventricular volume estimation.

Patients (adults and children) with normal right ventricular volumes and function as well as patients with diseased right ventricular volumes will be included in the study.

References

1. van Dam, A., Foley , J. D. & Hughes, J. *Computer graphics, Principles and Practice in C,* 1995.
2. Graham, T. P., Jr., Jarmakani, J. M., Atwood, G. F. & Canent, R. V., Jr. Right ventricular volume determinations in children. Normal values and observations with volume or pressure overload. *Circulation* **47**, 144-53, 1973.
3. Gentzler, R. D., 2nd, Briselli, M. F. & Gault, J. H. Angiographic estimation o f right ventricular volume in man. *Circulation* **50**, 324-30, 1974.
4. Arcilla, R. A., Tsai, P., Thilenius, O. & Ranniger, K. Angiographic method for volume estimation of right and left ventricles. *Chest* **60**, 446-54, 1971.
5. Boak, J. G., Bove, A. A., Kreulen, T. & Spann, J. F. A geometric basis for calculation of right ventricular volume in man. *Cathet Cardiovasc Diagn* **3**, 217-30, 1977.
6. Lange, P. E., Onnasch, D., Farr, F. L., Malerczyk, V. & Heintzen, P. H. Analysis of left and right ventricular size and shape, as determined from human casts. Description of the method and its validation. *Eur J Cardiol* **8**, 431-48, 1978.
7. Lange, P. E., Onnasch, D., Farr, F. L. & Heintzen, P. H. Angiocardiographic right ventricular volume determination. Accuracy, as determined from human casts, and clinical application. *Eur J Cardiol* **8**, 477-501, 1978.
8. Ferlinz, J. Measurements of right ventricular volumes in man from single plane cineangiograms. A comparison to the biplane approach. *Am Heart J* **94**, 87-90, 1977.
9. Ferlinz, J., Gorlin, R., Cohn, P. F. & Herman, M. V. Right ventricular performance in patients with coronary artery disease. *Circulation* **52**, 608-15, 1975.
10. Wellnhofer, E., Krulls-Munch, J., Sauer, U., Oswald, H. & Fleck, E. [A new methodologic approach for determining right ventricular volumes from transesophageal echocardiography]. *Z Kardiol* **83**, 482-94, 1994.
11. Sheehan, F. H. et al. Advantages and applications of the centerline method for characterizing regional ventricular function. *Circulation* **74**, 293-305, 1986.

CARS 2002 – H.U. Lemke, M.W. Vannier; K. Inamura, A.G. Farman, K. Doi & J.H.C. Reiber (Editors)

Integration of tools for the estimation of heart vitality by tissue Doppler and myocardial velocity gradients into a clinically useable software environment

M. Hastenteufel[a], I. Wolf[a], R. de Simone[b], S. Mottl-Link[b], H.-P. Meinzer[a]

[a] Div. Medical and Biological Informatics
Deutsches Krebsforschungszentrum,
Im Neuenheimer Feld 280, 69120 Heidelberg, Germany
[b] Div. of Cardiac Surgery, University of Heidelberg
Im Neuenheimer Feld 110, 69120 Heidelberg, Germany

Abstract

Due to the very frequent cause of death by sudden cardiac infarct, cardiac motion analysis is of high clinical interest. The knowledge about the complex three-dimensional (3D) heart wall motion pattern, particular in the left ventricle, provides valuable information about potential malfunctions. Echocardiography is the predominant technique for evaluation of cardiac function. Beside morphology, tissue velocities can be obtained by Doppler techniques. Strain rate data provides additional information about the contraction ability of the myocardium and can be estimated as myocardial velocity gradients. This is known as strain rate imaging. We have developed methods for the assessment, visualization and quantification of tissue movement and contraction by means of 3D tissue Doppler echocardiography. The tissue Doppler and strain rate images can be visualized and quantified by different methods. The methods are integrated into an interactively usable software environment, which is a first step to make them available in routine clinical medicine.

Keywords: Three-dimensional echocardiography, tissue Doppler, cardiac motion analysis

1. Introduction

Sudden cardiac death is one of the most frequent causes of death in industrial nations. The stenosis of a coronary artery results in a disturbed heart wall motion. Therefore cardiac motion analysis is of high clinical interest. Nowadays, echocardiography is the predominant technique for the evaluation of left ventricular function and the assessment and quantification of valvular heart lesions. Using tissue Doppler techniques it has also become feasible in the last years for the diagnosis of wall motion disorders. Echocardiography has the advantage over MRI based methods for cardiac motion analysis to be less expensive, to be feasible intra-operatively as well as at the bedside and to be more widely-used. Reliable information can only be obtained from three-dimensional data plus - as the heart is a moving organ - time. The knowledge of the motion and contraction pattern inside the myocardium, particular in the left ventricle, provides valuable information about potential malfunctions of the heart, for example myocardial ischemia.

CARS 2002 – H.U. Lemke, M.W. Vannier; K. Inamura, A.G. Farman, K. Doi & J.H.C. Reiber (Editors)

868

Velocities of the myocardium can be obtained by tissue Doppler echocardiography (TDI), also called tissue velocity imaging (TVI) or Doppler myocardial imaging (DMI), respectively [1]. In addition to pure velocity information of the myocardium, the contraction behavior of the heart muscle can be assessed by means of strain rate calculation. Strain rates can be computed from tissue velocities as myocardial velocity gradients. This is known as strain rate imaging (SRI). In the following we describe methods for the assessment, quantification and visualization of cardiac motion and contraction by means of myocardial velocities and strain rates obtained by tissue Doppler echocardiography. The usage of not only those described methods for cardiac motion analysis but also general medical image processing techniques by physicians in routine clinical medicine relies on integrated, easily and interactively usable software tools. Thus the described methods are integrated into an interactively useable software environment, which is already in clinical use for the assessment of heart valve disease and the quantification of regurgitant jets. This software provides the physician with a valuable and clinically useable tool for diagnosis of cardiac motion and is a step towards establishing cardiac motion analysis in routine clinical medicine.

2. Material and Methods

2.1 Data acquisition
Transesophageal as well as transthoracical Doppler echocardiography is used for data acquisition. We use a Sonos 5500 DSR ultrasound system (Philips Medical Systems, Andover, Mass, USA), that allows digital data storage. The multiplane technology allows for the rotation of the two-dimensional acquisition sector around its bisection line. Four-dimensional data sets are acquired by the built-in rotational controller of the system triggered by ECG and respiratory gating. The backscatter (i.e. morphology data) and Doppler data are stored separately, each with 8 bits per pixel. After acquisition, the data are either stored on a magneto-optical disc for transfering to our off-line processing system or transferred directly using the optional LAN interface.

2.2 Estimation of strain rate by myocardial velocity gradients
The velocities inside the myocardium, measured by tissue Doppler, provide valuable information about heart wall motion. However, with the knowledge of velocities inside the myocardium one can not distinguish between actively and passively moving tissue and the overall translation of the heart is not taken into account. Strain rate provides additional information to pure tissue velocities. Strain (here, for simplicity, explained in one dimension) is the relative change in length of two points and thus a measure for the contraction of the myocardium. Strain rate is the rate, at which this contraction occurs and can be computed along the ultrasound beam as the myocardial velocity gradient (MVG) by

$$\dot{\varepsilon}_N = sr = \frac{v_1 - v_2}{x}$$

where v_1 and v_2 are given velocities at two points inside the myocardium and x is the distance between these two points [2,3,4,5]. We have developed methods for the estimation of strain rate for two-dimensional (B-Mode) cine-loop acquisitions or, slice by slice, for dynamic 3D volumetric acquisitions [6].

CARS 2002 – H.U. Lemke, M.W. Vannier; K. Inamura, A.G. Farman, K. Doi & J.H.C. Reiber (Editors)
ᶜCARS/Springer. All rights reserved.

2.3 The EchoAnalyzer™ System

For the analysis of the echocardiographic data sets an echocardiographic analysis system called EchoAnalyzer™ [7] has been developed by our group and integrates several up-to-date visualization and quantification methods. Figure 1 shows a screenshot of the user interface of EchoAnalyzer™. It is designed to speed up the use of three-dimensional echocardiographic techniques and it integrates leading-edge methods in a user-friendly environment, making them available for routine clinical medicine. For example, color-coded, interactive 4D volume visualization, measurements of cavity volumes, ejection fraction and cardiac output, regurgitation quantification and display of flow profiles is provided. Furthermore, visualization methods for improved orientation in three-dimensional echocardiographic data sets [8] as well as a new segmentation algorithm especially designed for cardiac ultrasound images [9] are integrated.

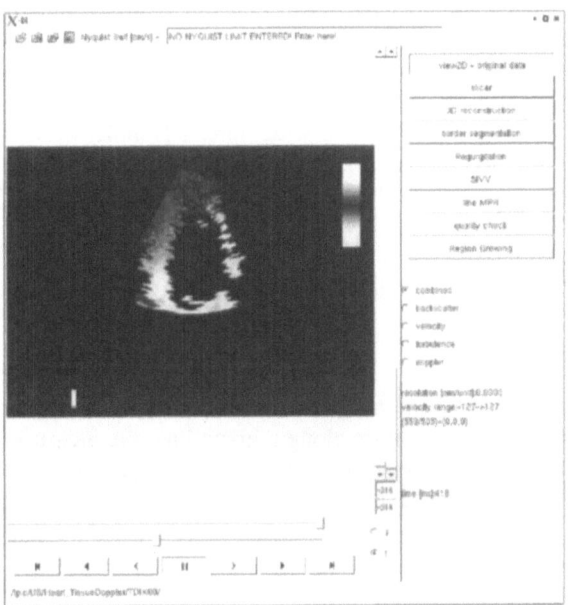

Fig. 1: The user interface of EchoAnalyzer ™. On the left handside a slice of a three-dimensional tissue Doppler data set is shown. On the right handside the user can easily switch between the integrated functions.

The software is developed in C++ using the GUI library Qt (Trolltech, Oslo, Norway) and the visualization library vtk and runs on all 32-bit Windows systems and on all major Unix derivatives including Linux. Due to its object-orientated and component-based design, new visualization and quantification methods can be easily integrated into the EchoAnalyzer™ software framework. Up to now, EchoAnalyzer™ is used by our institution for the assessment, quantification and visualization of heart valve diseases and regurgitant jets [10]. After completion of internal evaluation the software will be available for multicenter evaluation.

CARS 2002 – H.U. Lemke, M.W. Vannier; K. Inamura, A.G. Farman, K. Doi & J.H.C. Reiber (Editors)

In the following section we describe methods for visualization and quantification of heart wall vitality which have been integrated into the EchoAnalyzer™ software and therefore be made available for routine clinical medicine.

3. Results

In addition to the methods described in [7] the following visualization and quantification methods have been integrated into the EchoAnalyzer ™ software. Between the functions can be easily switched for mutual benefit.

3.1 Visualization
The grey-scale data (morphology), the tissue Doppler data as well as the strain rate data can be displayed as cine-loops with different look-up tables. With the curved M-mode the user can draw a line along, e.g. the outer wall of the left ventricle and the velocities, or the strain rates, respectively, of the points at the given line are displayed like a conventional M-mode. This can be done on the original slices or after a multiplanar reconstruction. Curved M-mode requires a reasonably high frame-rate, which is difficult to achieve for three-dimensional data acquisition with a wide spread Doppler sector. Moreover, color volume rendering of the 3D (over time) tissue Doppler data, strain rate data or grey-scale data can be performed by means of the heidelberg raytracing model [11]. Tissue Doppler data can be rendered in the same color encoding that is used during conventional two-dimensional echocardiography for displaying the velocity values on the screen of the echocardiographic device. For visualization of strain rate data an adapted look-up table is used.

3.2 Quantification
For the quantification of heart wall motion and contraction the software provides plotting of velocities and strain rate distribution along a given line, the measuring of peak as well as mean velocities and strain rates during a heartbeat and the calculation of velocity and strain rate distributions inside a user specified region of interest (ROI).

4. Limitations and perspective

Current echocardiographic devices do not measure the true velocity vector but the projection of the true velocity vector onto the ultrasonic beam direction. Thus an estimation of just one strain rate component of the true 3D strain rate tensor is possible. Furthermore this leads to a high angle dependency of the measured velocities and the computed strain rates [12]. Having a complete 3D velocity field one can extract more valuable information about tissue movement and the computation of the complete 3D strain rate tensors including all principles and shear strain rates becomes possible. Therewith the above mentioned angle dependency of tissue Doppler and strain rate methods for the assessment of cardiac motion could be solved. Thus our further research effort is concentrated on the reconstruction of a true 3D velocity field inside the myocardium. We are working on two approaches. In a mathematical approach we are aiming at the reconstruction of the velocity field by using variational principles. The velocity field can be reconstructed by minimizing an energy functional which includes the

CARS 2002 – H.U. Lemke, M.W. Vannier; K. Inamura, A.G. Farman, K. Doi & J.H.C. Reiber (Editors)
©CARS/Springer. All rights reserved.

measured velocities as well as an assumption about the three-dimensional velocity field. These assumption can be a smoothness constraint or some physical properties and act as a regularization of the mathematically ill-posed reconstruction problem. Using for example a spatial and temporal smoothness constraint, the energy functional can be written as

$$E = \left\| v_m - P_n(\vec{v}) \right\|^2 + \lambda \sum_{i,j} \left(\frac{\partial v_i}{\partial x_j} \right)^2 + \mu \sum_i \left(\frac{\partial v_i}{\partial t} \right)^2$$

where v_m is the measured velocity by tissue Doppler, $P_n(\vec{v})$ is the projection of the real velocity vector onto the ultrasound beam direction, $\dfrac{\partial v_i}{\partial x_j}$ and $\dfrac{\partial v_i}{\partial t}$ are spatial and temporal, respectively, derivates and λ and μ are weighting factors.

In a second approach methods for measuring velocities from different position are presently being developed and investigated. Thereby the ultrasound probe is tracked with a magnetic position system. Furthermore the two described approaches can be combined.

5. Conclusion

We have developed methods for the assessment, quantification and visualization of myocardial motion and contraction by means of tissue Doppler echocardiography. The methods are integrated into an interactively useable software environment, called EchoAnalyzer™, which is already in clinical use for the assessment of heart valve diseases.

The integration of the described methods into a user friendly, clinically useable software tool can be a step towards establishing (three-dimensional) cardiac motion analysis by means of tissue Doppler and strain rate imaging in day-to-day clinical medicine. The limitation of one-dimensional estimation of myocardial velocities has to be solved in the future.

Acknowledgements

This work is supported by the Deutsche Forschungsgemeinschaft (DFG) within the SFB 414 "Information Technology in Medicine - Computer and Sensor Supported Surgery".

References

1. W.N.McDicken, G.R.Sutherland, C.M.Moran, L.N.Gordan, "Color Doppler velocity imaging of the myocardium", Ultrasound Med Biol, Vol. 18, pp.651-654, 1992
2. A.D.Fleming, X.Xia, W.N.McDicken, G.R.Sutherland, L.Fenn, "Myocardial velocity gradients detected by Doppler imaging", Br J Radiology, Vol. 67, No. 799, pp.679-688, 1994
3. A.Heimdal, A.Støylen, H.Torp, T.Skaerpje, "Real-time strain rate imaging of the left ventricle by ultrasound", J Am Soc Echocardio, Vol. 11, pp.1013-1019, 1998

4. M.Uematsu, K.Miyatake, N.Tanaka, H.Matsuda, A.Sano, N.Yamazaki, M.Hirama, M.Yamagashi, "Myocardial velocity gradients as a new indicator of regional left ventricular contraction: detection by a two-dimensional tissue Doppler imaging technique", J Am Coll Cardio, Vol. 26, pp.217-223, 1995

5. J.D'hooge, A.Heimdal, F.Jamal, T.Kukulski, B.Bijnens, F.Rademakers, L.Hatle, P.Suetens, G.R.Sutherland. "Regional strain and strain rate measurements by cardiac ultrasound: Principles, implementation and limitation", Eur J Echocardio, Vol. 1, pp.154-170, 2001

6. M.Hastenteufel, I.Wolf, R.de Simone, H.P.Meinzer, "Heart wall motion analysis by dynamic strain rate imaging from tissue Doppler echocardiography", Proc. SPIE Medical Imaging, Physiology and Function from Multidimensional Images, A.V.Clough, C.T.Chen (eds), Vol. 4682, 2002, in print

7. I.Wolf, R.de Simone, G.Glombitza, H.P.Meinzer, "EchoAnalyzer – A System for Three-Dimensional Echocardiographic Visualization and Quantification", Proc. Computer Assisted Radiology and Surgery, 902-907, Elsevier, Berlin, 2001

8. I.Wolf, R.de Simone, M.Hastenteufel, S.Mottl-Link, H.P.Meinzer, "Visualization techniques for improved orientation in three-dimensional echocardiography", Proc. SPIE Medical Imaging, Visualization, Image-Guided Procedures, and Display, S.K.Mun (ed), Vol. 4681, 2002, in print

9. I.Wolf, G.Glombitza, R.de Simone, H.P.Meinzer, "Automatic segmentation of heart cavities in multidimensional ultrasound images", Proc. SPIE Medical Imaging, Image Processing, K.Hanson et al (eds), Vol. 3979, pp. 273-283, 2000

10. R.de Simone, G.Glombitza, C.Vahl, H.P.Meinzer, S.Hagl, "Three-dimensional Doppler: Techniques and clinical applications", Eur Heart J, Vol. 20, pp. 619-627, 1999

11. H.P.Meinzer, K.Meetz, D.Scheppelmann, U.Engelmann, H.J.Baur, "The heidelberg raytracing model", IEEE Computer Graphics and Applications, Vol. 11, No. 6, pp.34-43, 1991

12. P.L.Castro, N.L.Greenberg, J.Drinko, M.J.Garcia, J.D.Thomas, "Potential pitfalls os strain rate imaging: angle dependency", Biomedical Scienes Intrumentation, Vol. 36, pp.197-202, 2000

CARS 2002 – H.U. Lemke, M.W. Vannier; K. Inamura, A.G. Farman, K. Doi & J.H.C. Reiber (Editors)

3D Stress echocardiography: a novel application based on registration of real-time 3D ultrasound images

Raj Shekhar[a], Vladimir Zagrodsky[a], Mario Garcia[b], James D. Thomas[b]

[a]Department of Biomedical Engineering, Lerner Research Institute
[b]Department of Cardiovascular Medicine
The Cleveland Clinic Foundation, Cleveland, Ohio 44195, USA

Abstract

Stress echocardiography is a common clinical procedure to diagnose myocardial ishemia by comparing myocardial wall motion in pre- and post-stress ultrasound images. Complicated imaging protocol, incomplete data, and misaligned pre- and post-stress images, however, are known limitations of conventional stress echocardiography. We have proposed here a new stress testing procedure that uses real-time three-dimensional (3D) ultrasound in place of conventional ultrasound and termed the new procedure "3D stress echocardiography." Real-time 3D ultrasound is an emerging modality capable of imaging a beating heart in its entirety in the time of one cardiac cycle without requiring gating. The proposed 3D stress echocardiography addresses the limitations of complicated imaging protocol and incomplete data by collecting volumetric data rapidly. The problem of misaligned image sectors is solved by registering pre- and post-stress 3D images. We have described here our mutual information-based image registration and interactive 3D image visualization methods that are key engineering developments to enable performing 3D stress echocardiography. These methods were customized to meet the specific needs of 3D stress echocardiography. The preliminary results of the study are encouraging. Image registration used in conjunction with real-time 3D ultrasound offers the potential to simplify stress echocardiography and improve its diagnostic accuracy.

Keywords: Image registration, three-dimensional ultrasound, stress echocardiography

1. Introduction

Stress echocardiography is a frequently used clinical procedure to diagnose myocardial ischemia (imbalance between blood flow supply and demand in the heart muscle) by comparing the wall motion information in pre- and post-stress ultrasound images of the left ventricle (LV). Complicated imaging protocol, incomplete data and misaligned pre- and post-stress images, however, are known limitations of conventional stress echocardiography, performed using two-dimensional (2D) ultrasound.

Using real-time three-dimensional (3D) ultrasound in conjunction with stress testing, a combination we call 3D stress echocardiography, addresses the aforementioned limitations and has the potential to increase the diagnostic power of stress echocardiography. Real-time 3D imaging, a new development in ultrasound image acquisition, has the ability to image a beating LV in its entirety without gating, thus

CARS 2002 – H.U. Lemke, M.W. Vannier, K. Inamura, A.G. Farman, K. Doi & J.H.C. Reiber (Editors)
ᶜCARS/Springer. All rights reserved.

874

reducing image acquisition duration to the time of a single cardiac cycle. 3D stress echocardiography addresses the problems of complicated imaging protocol and limited views through rapid volumetric acquisition. In conventional stress echocardiography, a sonographer must collect images from multiple viewing directions and locations on the chest. This task becomes especially challenging upon stress because image collection must be completed within approximately a minute of the termination of stress (achievement of peak stress) while closely monitoring the patient's vital signs. Volumetric acquisition obviates the need for imaging the heart from multiple viewing directions, thus greatly simplifying the imaging protocol. Since the imaging lasts less than a second, it is easier to capture any transient wall motion activity that cannot be captured by all cine loops in conventional stress echocardiography. Additionally, volumetric acquisition provides complete wall motion data for every part of the LV for a given stress level. Real-time 3D ultrasound thus collects complete and accurate wall motion information.

3D Stress echocardiography can also address the limitation of misaligned image planes in the conventional method. By registering pre- and post-stress volumetric images retrospectively, identical anatomical planes of the heart, before and after stress, can be presented to a reviewing physician for making an accurate diagnosis. Conventional stress echocardiography cannot provide this capability because it does not collect enough data to permit image registration. Furthermore, the availability of volumetric data in 3D stress echocardiography allows visualization of any cross-section (i.e., all regions) of the LV and, therefore, a more comprehensive wall motion analysis than is currently possible.

The long-term objective of our research is to develop necessary post-processing methods including image registration, image segmentation and image visualization to enable performing 3D stress echocardiography accurately and objectively, and to demonstrate its diagnostic superiority to conventional method. In this paper, we describe image registration and image visualization methods and our preliminary results.

2. Methods

Automatic 3D ultrasound image registration and interactive visualization of real-time 3D images are prerequisites for performing 3D stress echocardiography. Image registration must be automatic because 20-30 image pairs must be registered in each case. Any manual approach will make the exercise tedious, besides being subjective and operator dependent. The characteristically poor quality of ultrasound images, the lack of clearly identifiable landmarks, and the need for nonrigid 3D registration make manual or feature-based registration less feasible. Interactive visualization is necessary because conventional mechanisms of reviewing echocardiographic images saved on videotapes or in the form of digital movies are fundamentally limited to 2D images. The strength of having 3D data is that any arbitrary cross-section of the heart, not just a few standard planes, can be viewed. Interactive oblique slicing of real-time 3D data is both computationally and memory intensive, especially in the proposed 3D stress echocardiography because properly aligned pre- and post-stress images must be displayed simultaneously.

We perform registration of 3D ultrasound images using a voxel similarity-based algorithm, which meets the requirements developed above. The specific voxel similarity

CARS 2002 – H.U. Lemke, M.W. Vannier; K. Inamura, A.G. Farman, K. Doi & J.H.C. Reiber (Editors)

measure used is mutual information (MI) that is defined as a function of two volumetric images and a given orientation between them. MI-based registration is an iterative method in which an optimization algorithm seeks the maximum of the MI measure. Successful convergence relies on having the MI function free of ripples and local maxima. To minimize ripples and local maxima, we employ 3 x 3 x 3 median filtering of the original resolution data and intensity quantization (discarding 1-3 least significant bits). Further smoothness of the MI function is achieved by using partial volume (PV) interpolation for resampling one 3D image on the grid points of the other. We use downhill simplex optimization algorithm that provides a good trade-off between robustness and computation. To enhance its robustness further, we have developed a multi-function extension that uses the consensus of three MI functions computed at three different levels of intensity quantization. The net effect of the preprocessing steps and the PV interpolation is a smooth MI surface despite the characteristic low signal-to-noise ratio of ultrasound images and the presence of speckle noise, which leads to robust and reliable registration. The details of our method have been previously published [1].

Our visualization technology allows interactive display of up to three arbitrary cross-sections of the time-varying volumetric ultrasound data. Throughout the visualization, the frames of the time-varying data are animated at the original rate of 25 frames/sec, which must be maintained so that the underlying heart motion is not altered. Displaying an oblique cross-section involves generating new samples on the cut plane. Overall, this visualization requires approximately 25 million trilinear interpolations per second (MTRIPS) that translate to 525 million floating-point operations per second (MFLOPS) and 225 million memory accesses per second (MMAPS). While most modern microprocessors meet the floating-point operation requirement, at 80 nsec/memory access, only 12.5 MMAPS are currently possible. A CPU-only implementation, even on most modern computers, therefore, does not provide the necessary speed. To make visualization interactive, we take advantage of the hardware acceleration provided by commercially available, advanced 3D texture mapping graphics boards rated at over 300 MTRIPS. To obtain the board's specified performance, the 3D image data must fit the available 64-128 MB texture memory. We have developed novel data bricking and caching concepts to (1) reduce data requirement and (2) minimize the amount of data transfer between the texture and system memories during an interactive visualization session. Additional details on the visualization of time-varying 3D ultrasound images have been reported [2].

Using the developed registration and visualization methods, we have performed 3D stress echocardiography in two subjects. 3D ultrasound images were first recorded at the resting (pre-stress) state and then at the peak-stress (post-stress) state following exercise on a bicycle. A 2.5 MHz real-time 3D ultrasound scanner (Volumetrics, Inc., Durham, North Carolina, USA) was used for all imaging. This scanner produced a sequence of volumetric images, shaped approximately like a truncated pyramid, with 60 degrees azimuth and elevation angular spans, at a frame rate of 25 Hz. The scan depth was 140 mm. The actual number of frames in pre- and post-stress data sets depended on the heart rate, and it was 20 and 12 respectively in the first subject, and 18 and 9 respectively in the second subject.

Pre- and post-stress images were first temporally aligned. For each post-stress image, a pre-stress image having approximately the same cardiac phase was determined. Each pair was then registered using a nonrigid, 7-parameter transformation model. The seven parameters included six rigid-body transformation parameters and global scaling. Rigid-body transformation represented misalignment due to sonographer's inability to duplicate the ultrasound probe's location and angle between two imaging sessions (probe placement error), whereas the global scaling represented stress-induced physiologic changes. During the registration process, it is crucial to separate the two registration errors and correct only for the probe placement error. Using a special scheme, we transformed post-stress images to align with their corresponding pre-stress images to eliminate the probe placement error while preserving diagnostically critical stress-induced changes. Pre- and post-stress images were viewed side-by-side by extending the developed visualization method to handle two data sets simultaneously. As described earlier, reviewing physicians had the ability to vary the anatomical plane interactively to visualize all regions of the LV. Two clinical experts evaluated the registration accuracy visually. For each subject, they were each given registered and nonregistered pre- and post-stress images in a random order, and asked to pick the pair that was better aligned. This constituted a preliminary, qualitative validation of our evolving 3D stress echocardiography procedure.

3. Results

We have performed extensive investigation of the accuracy and the capture range of our MI-based registration technique before applying it to the 3D stress echocardiography application. Any deviation from the perfect solution was used to define the accuracy. Capture range was defined as the largest starting misalignment below which registration was expected to succeed in 95% cases. Both parameters were measured in terms of a metric, called average distance error, which represented the average misalignment (in Euclidean distance) at the eight vertices of a 10 cm cube. The accuracy and the capture range for the rigid-body + global scaling transformation mode used in the current application were 1.7 mm and 44.0 mm, respectively. PV interpolation, in principle, permits subvoxel accuracy that was indeed achieved because the measured accuracy (1.7 mm) was smaller than the voxel dimension (2.19 mm x 2.19 mm x 0.55 mm). Comparing capture range (44 mm) to the overall volume dimension (140 mm x 140 mm x 140 mm) revealed that grossly misaligned volume pairs could also be successfully registered. Furthermore, if the starting misalignment happened to be outside the capture range, it was possible to perform an approximate registration either manually or using an existing automatic method before refining the result using the MI-based method.

We have also shown that a sequence of twenty 128 x 128 x 512 sized 3D images (160 Mb) can be visualized at a maximum frame rate of 50 Hz when displaying three intersecting planes through the data. This performance was achieved with Wildcat 5110 graphics adapter (3DLabs, Inc., Sunnyvale, California, USA). The maximum frame rate achieved was twice the desired frame rate of 25 Hz, the original acquisition frame rate for all images used in this study. Consequently, the visualization was slowed down to 25 Hz to maintain the original heart motion. In the current 3D stress echocardiography application that required visualization of two data sets (160 MB pre-stress data and 96 MB post-stress data) side-by-side, the maximum frame achieved was between 40-50 Hz; the exact frame rate depended on the imaging plane being displayed. As before, the frame rate was slowed down to the desired 25 Hz by introducing delays. While the registration ensured that the

CARS 2002 – H.U. Lemke, M.W. Vannier; K. Inamura, A.G. Farman, K. Doi & J.H.C. Reiber (Editors)
©CARS/Springer. All rights reserved.

displayed pre- and post-stress images showed the identical anatomy, replaying the images at their acquisition frame rates showed, as expected, the stressed heart to beat faster. A feedback we received from the clinical experts was that synchronizing the cardiac phases of pre- and post-stress images facilitates making diagnosis. We provided this additional capability by slowing down the display of post-stress images to a frame rate equal to the product of the acquisition frame rate and the ratio of resting to peak-stress heart rates.

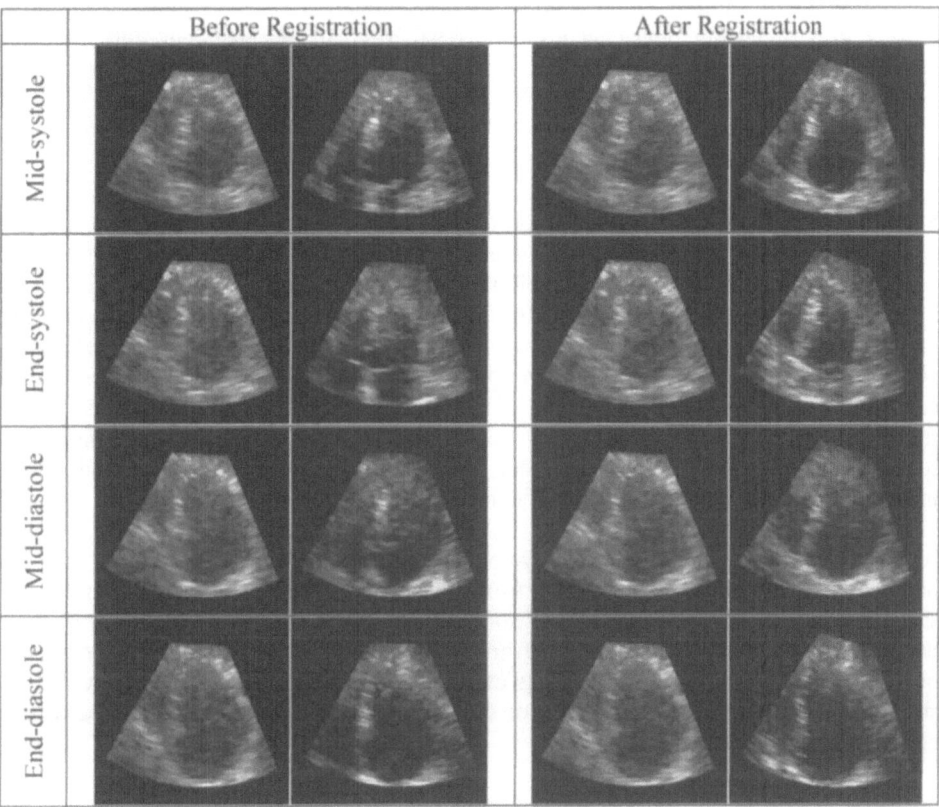

Fig.1. Comparison of pre- and post-stress images before and after image registration in four phases. Note a better alignment of the LV cavity following image registration.

The results of 3D stress echocardiography are presented in Fig. 1, in which rows of images correspond to mid-systolic, end-systolic, mid-diastolic and end-diastolic phases of the heart. Shown in each row are the pre- and post-stress images in the first subject, before and after registration, respectively. A better spatially matching of the LV regions can be seen following registration. Both clinical experts correctly identified the registered data set in the first subject. In the second subject, one expert correctly identified the registered data set, whereas the second expert called the two sets equivalent. The starting misalignment in the second case was smaller than the smallest misalignment that a human eye can discern. Consequently, minimal alignment correction was needed in the second subject, a case indicating that the sonographer was reasonably successful in duplicating the probe location and orientation. Such a coincidence is rare, but not unexpected.

CARS 2002 – H.U. Lemke, M.W. Vannier; K. Inamura, A.G. Farman, K. Doi & J.H.C. Reiber (Editors)
©CARS/Springer. All rights reserved.

878

4. Discussion and conclusions

3D Stress echocardiography is one of many emerging applications made possible by the advent of real-time 3D ultrasound imaging capability. These advanced applications are helping overcome the limitations of existing procedures as well as provide novel capabilities. 3D Stress echocardiography, in particular, has the potential to simplify the imaging protocol, shorten the duration of stress testing procedure, and, most importantly, present to a reviewing physician pre- and post-stress images that represent the same anatomy. It is extremely important that the same regions of the LV are compared for an accurate diagnosis, a condition that conventional stress echocardiography cannot fulfill. Moreover, the availability of registered 3D images allows visualizing any region of the pre- and post-stress LV, thus performing a comprehensive wall motion analysis.

Registration and interactive visualization of real-time 3D ultrasound images are two key engineering methods that enable 3D stress echocardiography. We have demonstrated accurate and reliable automated registration of 3D ultrasound images [1]. Furthermore, we have implemented interactive visualization using commercially available graphics hardware for standard desktop computers and demonstrated that the necessary performance could be achieved [2]. In addition to these general capabilities, 3D stress echocardiography requires the ability to temporally align pre- and post-stress image sequences, an understanding of the sources and nature of misalignment, and a method to separate the undesired probe placement misalignment error from the desired stress-induced changes. We have developed the necessary understandings and methods.

As part of our ongoing research and development, we are applying the developed methods on a larger patient population recruited from the pool of patients undergoing conventional stress echocardiography as part of their normal treatment at our institution. Many of these patients will also have angiography performed on them. A more rigorous validation will be performed by comparing the findings of conventional stress echocardiography and 3D stress echocardiography against those of the angiography, a gold standard for detecting coronary artery disease.

Acknowledgements

The development of 3D stress echocardiography is supported by a research grant (RG-01-0071, Principal Investigator – Raj Shekhar) from The Whitaker Foundation. We also acknowledge the assistance of the staff of the Echocardiology laboratory in the collection of 3D ultrasound images.

References

1. R. Shekhar and V. Zagrodsky, "Mutual information-based rigid and nonrigid registration of ultrasound volumes," *IEEE Trans. Med. Imag.*, vol.21, pp. 9-22, 2002.
2. R. Shekhar and V. Zagrodsky, "Interactive Visualization of Four-Dimensional Ultrasound Data," *Medicine Meets Virtual Reality*, J. D. Westwood *et al.*, vol. 85, pp. 485-487, IOS Press, Amsterdam, 2002.

CARS 2002 – H.U. Lemke, M.W. Vannier; K. Inamura, A.G. Farman, K. Doi & J.H.C. Reiber (Editors)
©CARS/Springer. All rights reserved.

Detecting changes in myocardial perfusion

Tracy L. Faber[a], James R. Galt[a], Ji Chen[a],
Benjamin M.W. Tsui[b], Ernest V. Garcia[a]
[a]Department of Radiology, Emory University;
[b]Department of Biomedical Engineering, Univ. of North Carolina at Chapel Hill

Abstract

Existing and new algorithms were evaluated for their efficacy in detecting and quantifying serial changes in myocardial perfusion from SPECT. Measures generated from standard perfusion quantification methods, i.e., summed stress score (SSS) and stress total severity score (STSS), and new methods using t-scores were investigated for their usefulness in finding perfusion changes. We generated 36 simulations with various perfusion defect sizes and severities using the NURBs-based CArdiac Torso (NCAT) phantom. We compared the methods' abilities to detect perfusion differences within a given defect size, or lesion mass changes within a given defect severity. For a 10% change in defect severity, SSS and STSS changes averaged 0.07 ± 0.1 and 0.17 ± 0.1, respectively. The STSS and SSS values correlated with the true change of mass as $y=8.4x - 1.33$, $r=0.97$, and $y= 0.44x + 0.23$, $r=0.86$, respectively. Regional t-scores detected all 10% perfusion changes and most 5% perfusion changes. Measured changes in defect masses correlated with true mass changes as $y=0.55x-0.25g$, $r=0.93$. Even in this limited study, it is evident that currently available techniques, such as SSS and STSS are not sufficient for detecting small changes in perfusion severity and size. New methods, such as t-scores, are needed.

Keywords: SPECT, myocardial perfusion, automatic quantification

1. Introduction

The goal of this study was to investigate existing and new algorithms for their efficacy in detecting and quantifying serial changes in myocardial perfusion from SPECT. It is widely recognized that computer quantification of myocardial perfusion images improves not only the overall diagnostic yield but also enhances reliability, accuracy, confidence and reproducibility of interpretation. These quantitative approaches are well established for assessing abnormalities in myocardial perfusion, usually by comparison to a normal data base [1,2]; however, they *have not* been developed to quantify changes between one study and another, such as is needed in assessing the effect of interventions or medical therapy or the progression or regression of CAD [3,4]. Nevertheless, there is an increasing use of comparing changes in perfusion to assess therapy, but in most of these studies the changes observed are only significant between groups and not in individual cases, such as is needed to manage patients [3,5-6]

We evaluated two existing quantitative approaches for assessing normality in SPECT perfusion studies for their adaptability in assessing changes in myocardial perfusion. We also developed and tested two additional approaches using Students' t-statistic. To

CARS 2002 – H.U. Lemke, M.W. Vannier; K. Inamura, A.G. Farman, K. Doi & J.H.C. Reiber (Editors)

880

perform this analysis we used a sophisticated software phantom to simulate real-world acquisitions of patient studies with completely characterized perfusion defects.

2. Methodology

Standard perfusion quantification methods that determine whether or not a perfusion study is normal typically compare the test case to a normal database and judge where the distribution falls below a lower limit of normal. A single score can be generated from these analyses and used to judge overall severity of cardiac disease. These measures are often compared in serial studies of the same patient to determine whether perfusion has improved or worsened.

For example, the stress total severity score (STSS) [7] is a well-known approach for analyzing overall perfusion normality. It is obtained by summing the number of standard deviations below normal of each abnormally perfused myocardial sample. Thus, this score increases when the number of abnormal myocardial pixels increases; that is, when the defect gets larger. It also increases when the defect gets more severe and the myocardial perfusion values fall even further from the normal limit. We analyzed the accuracy of STSS changes for detecting changes in defect size and severity.

The summed stress score (SSS) [8] is similar to the stress total severity score in that it provides a single number indicating severity of LV disease. The SSS is computed by dividing the LV into 20 sectors, using six walls at three depths (6 x 3 = 18 segments) plus two apical regions. The six myocardial walls are the anterior, inferior, anterolateral, inferolateral, anteroseptal and inferoseptal wall. Each sector is scored according to the severity of the perfusion abnormality, where 0=normal, 1=equivocal, 2=mildly reduced, 3=severely reduced, and 4=no perfusion. The sector scores are summed to provide the SSS. These values can be assigned qualitatively or quantitatively; we used a method also based on perfusion quantification to assign them quantitatively. Changes in SSS were also evaluated for their ability to assess changes in size and severity of perfusion defects.

We also investigated a new approach using segmental t-scores to detect changes in myocardial perfusion. We looked at differences in the means of perfusion samples in each of the twenty segments. A significant difference in any of the sectors was defined with an alpha value of less than or equal to .05. Changes in the number of affected sectors were used to determine changes in the defect size.

Finally, we defined a region-of-interest (ROI) as the abnormally perfused area in one of the studies for comparison. Then, we compared means in that ROI between two serial studies using the t-test [9]. Significant differences in the means were used to assess changes in defect severity. Changes in mass of the defects, as measured by the perfusion quantification program, were compared to the true changes in mass.

To generate test data we used the 4-D NURBs-based CArdiac Torso (NCAT) phantom from the University of North Carolina [10-11]. This phantom includes a model of the heart with many options for varying the simulations, including addition of cardiac and respiratory motions, inclusion of perfusion abnormalities, variations in radioactivity concentration in non-cardiac structures, and creation of differing numbers of output gates. We used the phantom with the addition of a single perfusion defect of exactly known size

CARS 2002 – H.U. Lemke, M.W. Vannier; K. Inamura, A.G. Farman, K. Doi & J.H.C. Reiber (Editors)

and severity.   The NCAT phantom software creates "gold standard" activity and attenuation maps, which we used to create simulated projections containing both noise and detector response. Projections were reconstructed using filtered backprojection.

A total of 36 simulations were used. The differences in the simulations were entirely in perfusion defect size and severity, where severity was measured as a percentage below normal perfusion. In all cases, normal perfusion was set to 100. The defect size ranged from an angular extent of $30°$ to $60°$, in steps of $15°$, and from an axial extent of 30% to 50%, in steps of 10%, of the long-axis length. The defect severity ranged from 45% to 60% of normal perfusion, in steps of 5%. Thus, we had $3*3*4 = 36$ simulations from which we could generate thousands of two-way comparisons to investigate. However, we were interested in the abilities of these algorithms to detect small changes. Therefore, we compared the methods for their abilities to detect either a 5 or 10% absolute (e.g., 55% to 60% or 50% to 60%) difference in perfusion within a given defect size. Within a given defect severity, we looked at the abilities of the methods to detect size changes while holding the angular extent steady but randomly varying the axial length. This resulted in true mass changes of -11 to –6 gram.

3. Results

Results for two of the simulations are shown in Figure 1. This illustrates the difficulty in visually assessing changes in perfusion defect severity from serial slices, as well as inconsistencies in current quantitative methods.

Changes in STSS correlated with absolute changes in defect severity as y=4.7x - 0.61, r=0.77. Changes in SSS correlated less well with absolute changes in defect severity: y= -0.26x - 0.50, r=0.56. For a 10% *relative* change in defect severity, SSS changes averaged 0.07 ± 0.1; SSS changes averaged 0.17 ± 0.1. For a 20% *relative* change in severity, SSS changes averaged 0.12 ± 0.08; STSS changes averaged 0.31 ± 0.13. When there was no change in defect severity, STSS correlated with the true change of mass as y=8.4x – 1.33, r=0.97. SSS correlated with the true change in mass as y= 0.44x + 0.23, r=0.86.

Segmental *t*-scores were unable to detect any change in severity with perfusion changes of 5%, and were only able to detect 10% perfusion changes when the defect had a $45°$ or greater angular extent. However, changes in size of 20% of the axial extent when angular extent did not change, or a change in 15% of angular extent with a 10% difference in axial extent caused a significant difference in *t*-scores.

Regional t-scores could be used to detect all 10% perfusion changes and most 5% perfusion changes; however, they failed to find the 55-60% changes in lesions less than $60°$ in angular extent.   Changes in perfusion defect masses computed from images correlated with the true lesion mass changes as y=0.55x-0.25, r=0.93.

882

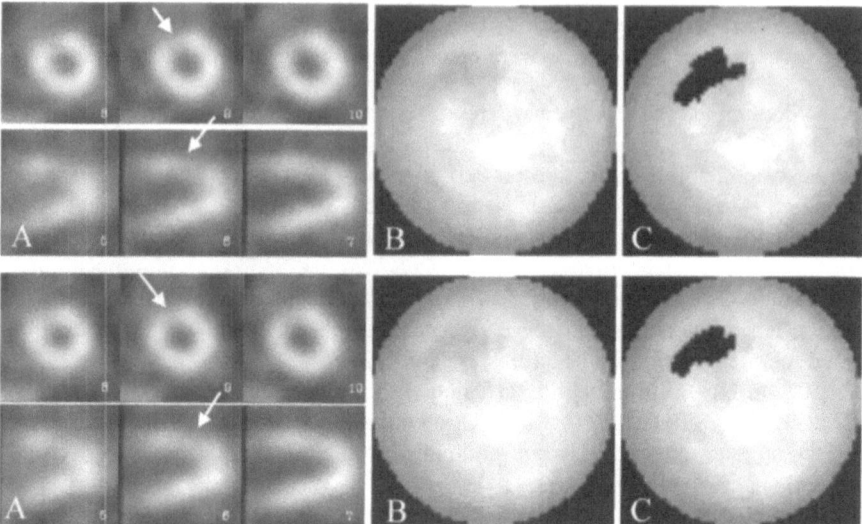

Figure 1. Top and bottom rows show two different simulations with perfusion defects of the same size but different severity. A. Short-axis (top) and vertical-long axis sections of the reconstructed slices are shown, with arrows marking the location of the defects. B. Polar maps indicating the results of normal perfusion quantification. This is a two-dimensional representation of maximal myocardial counts sampled from the short-axis slices shown in A. C. Polar maps with regions of abnormal perfusion (when compared to a normal database) displayed in black. Additional analysis showed that the study shown in the top row had a STSS=107, SSS=9. The study shown in the bottom row had a STSS=104, SSS=10. (Higher scores indicate more abnormality.) Which study is more abnormal? T-scores showed that perfusion in the defect in the top study is significantly lower than that in the bottom study with $p<0.05$. In fact, defect perfusion is 55% of maximum in the top study and 60% of maximum in the bottom study. Thus, perfusion is more abnormal in the top study.

4. Discussion

Both SSS and STSS ranged widely about their means for 5% changes and could not be reliably used to detect these changes. SSS underestimated changes so much that this measure could not be reliably used to detect 10% changes, either. STSS changes did not correlate very will with changes in perfusion severity; although, they did correlate surprisingly well with changes in perfusion mass. However, this disparity in accuracy for detecting size changes as compared to severity changes is probably due to the test population, since we only looked at two possible perfusion severity changes (5% and 10% change) over a wide range of defect sizes, while there was a wider range of perfusion defect mass changes (-11 to 6 gm) over only 4 defect severities. In general, it is expected that segmental evaluations of perfusion differences are not very sensitive to perfusion severity differences, since they rely on an average of regional perfusion values. This was true for SSS as well as for segmental t-scores. Conversely, regional t-scores were the best at detecting defect severity changes, since this method allowed us to generate a more specific hypothesis to test. Mass changes as measured by perfusion quantification methods correlated quite well with real lesion mass changes; although, we did we underestimate these changes. This is probably a result of the partial volume effect [12].

CARS 2002 – H.U. Lemke, M.W. Vannier, K. Inamura, A.G. Farman, K. Doi & J.H.C. Reiber (Editors)
CARS/Springer. All rights reserved.

Since size and severity of perfusion defects are inextricably linked in SPECT due to the partial volume effect [12], we did not attempt to determine whether or not any of these methods could distinguish between the two.

5. Conclusion

Currently available techniques for perfusion quantification are not sufficient for detecting small changes in perfusion severity and size. New methods, specifically designed for detecting those changes, are needed. T-scores may be one possible solution.

Acknowledgements

This research was funded in part by research grant NIH R01 HL68904.

References

1. Van Belle E, Abolmaali K, Bauters C, et al, "Restenosis, late vessel occlusion and left ventricular function six months after balloon angioplasty in diabetic patients", *J Am Coll Cardiol*, 34, 476-485, 1999.
2. Garcia E, DePuey EG, Sonnemaker RE, et al., "Quantification of the Reversibility of Stress Induced SPECT Thallium-201 Myocardial Perfusion Defects: A multicenter trial using Bull's-eye polar maps and standard normal limits", *J Nucl Med*, 31, 1761-1765, 1990.
3. deKemp RA, Ruddy TD, Hewitt T, et al., "Detection of Serial Changes in Absolute Myocardial Perfusion with Rb-82 PET", *J Nucl Med*, 41, 1426-1435, 2000.
4. Watson DD, Germano G, DePuey EG, "Panel on instrumentation and quantification", *J Nucl Cardiol*, 6, 93-155, 1999.
5. Dakik KA. Kleiman NS, Farmer JA, et al., "Intensive medical therapy vesus coronary angioplasty for suppression of myocardial ischemia in survivors of acute myocardial infarction: a prospective, randomized pilot study", *Circulation,* 98, 2017-23, 1998.
6. Guethin M, Kasel AM, Coppenrah K, "Delayed response of myocardial flow reserve to lipid-lowering therapy with fluvastatin", *Circulation*, 99, 475-481, 1999.
7. Garcia EV, DePuey EG, DePasquale EE, "Quantitative Planar and Tomographic Tl-201 Myocardial Perfusion Imaging", *Cardiovasc Intervent Radiol*, 10, 374-383, 1987.
8. Berman DS, Kiat H, Friedman JD, et al., "Separate acquisition rest Tl-201/stress Tc-99m sestamibi dual-isotope myocardial perfusion single-photon emission computed tomography: A clinical validation study", J *Am Coll Cardiol*, 22, 1455-1464, 1993.
9. Neter J, Kutner MH, Nachtsheim CJ, Wasserman W, Applied Linear Statistical Models, chapter 16, Richard D. Irwin, Inc., Chicago, 1996.
10. Terry JA, Tsui BMW, Perry JR, Hendricks JL, Gullberg GT, "The design of a mathematical phantom of the upper human torso for use in 3-D SPECT imaging research", in *Biomedical Engineering: Opening New Doors,* D.C. Mikulecky and A.M. Clarke eds., pp 185-190, New York University Press, New York, 1990.
11. Segars WP, Lalush DS, Tsui BMW, "A realistic spline-based dynamic heart phantom", *IEEE Trans Nucl Sci*, 46, 503-506, 1999.
12. Hoffman E, Huang SC, Phelps ME, "Quantitation in positron computed emission tomography: 1. Effect of object size", *J Comput Assist Tomog,* 3, 299-308, 1979.

Non-Invasive Cardiovascular Imaging - Clinical Approach - An ESCR Symposium

CARS 2002 – H.U. Lemke, M.W. Vannier; K. Inamura, A.G. Farman, K. Doi & J.H.C. Reiber (Editors)

Non-invasive approach to coronary heart disease

R. Rienmüller, B. Schröttner, U. Reiter, G. Reiter
Interdisciplinary Cardiac Imaging Center
University of Graz, Austria

Abstract

Based on more than 2000 cardiac EBT studies using the above mentioned protocol it is possible like in an "One-Stop-Shop" to assess the extent of coronary atherosclerosis as Coronary Calcium Score (first part of the definition of coronary heart disease) to evaluate the degree, location and number of stenotic lesions in the proximal 5-6cm of the coronary arteries , to determine the severity of coronary heart disease by measuring the global and regional myocardial blood flow (second part of the definition of coronary heart disease) and to measure the functional left ventricular parameters giving the information if they are still in normal range or changed either as a sequel of the coronary heart disease or as a compensatory mechanism to keep myocardial blood flow as adequate as possible with respect to the balance of oxygen supply and demand.

Keywords: Coronary heart disease, magnetic resonance, electron beam tomography

1. Introduction

„Coronary heart disease is defined as manifestation of atherosclerosis in the coronary arteries. As the disease is a multifactorial process leading to myocardial ischemia it may appear as angina pectoris, myocardial infarction, cardiac dysrhythmia, sudden death or cardiac insufficiency" (J. Meyer; 1996).

Coronary atherosclerosis is a complex process affecting all three layers of the arterial wall causing thickening of the intima and adventitia mainly by extensive fibrosis often with calcification and causing thinning of the media mainly by lost of smooth muscle. Myocardial ischemia in coronary atherosclerosis is defined as imbalance between myocardial oxygen supply and demand. The inadequate coronary blood flow results in changes of the biochemical, electrical and mechanical function of the cardiac structures. In this situation the essential physiological mechanism to compensate reduced coronary blood flow is an increase of cardiac output and /or reduction of the vascular resistance.

Atherosclerosis of the coronary vasculature is the leading cause of death among men and women worldwide. 60% of men and 42% of women presenting with acute myocardial infarction or sudden death has no prior history of disease.

From clinical point of view there is a need to detect and to quantify the amount of atherosclerosis as well as to measure myocardial blood flow quantitatively before the onset of clinical symptoms of coronary heart disease. However there is no reliable noninvasive screening method to evaluate the presence, severity and progression of coronary heart disease. The present and future aspects of EBT will be evaluated with respect to following questions:

- Does the patient have coronary atherosclerosis?
- If positive: What is the stage of coronary atherosclerosis?
- Is this coronary atherosclerosis of haemodynamic effect?
- Does the patient have myocardial ischemia? (infarction?)
- If positive: What are the physiological and pathophysiological compensatory mechanisms
- to prevent myocardial damage?
- If positive: What are the mechanisms to keep the heart in the present function?

2. Method

2.1 Electron Beam Tomography (EBT)

Using EBT with short exposure time of 100 or 50ms and the availability of acquiring up to 2x17 images/s it is possible to study most of the important morphological and functional determinants of the heart. A four steps diagnostic approach was developed at the University of Graz, to study patients with suspected or known coronary heart disease.

1. Native single slice scan, 100ms exposure time to identify and to measure the extent of coronary calcification .
2. Multi slice scan, 50ms exposure time and intravenous contrast agent application to measure myocardial blood flow.
3. Multi slice scan, 50ms exposure time and intravenous contrast agent application to measure functional determinants as enddiastolic and endsystolic volumes, ejection fraction, left ventricular muscle mass and global and regional wall thickness changes over the cardiac cycles.
4. Single slice scan, 100ms exposure time and intravenous contrast agent application to evaluate the morphological state of the proximal 4-6cm of the subepicardial coronary arteries.

The EBT study of the individual patient to measure coronary calcification last approximately 5min. The complete protocol of the EBT study lasts up to 30min with an effective radiation dose of approximately 9mSV and a need for up to 200ml of intravenously applied contrast agent.

3. EBT results

3.1 Coronary atherosclerosis

In several studies was shown that coronary artery calcification as seen by EBT is always associated with coronary wall atheroma. Several studies demonstrated that the increasing amount of coronary calcification (Coronary Calcium Score) is accompanied by an parallel increase of the amount of "soft" atherosclerotic plaques.

In our and in other studies was shown that independently of patient´s age,with increasing coronary calcification score the probability having coronary artery stenotic lesions above 50% is continuously increasing.

CARS 2002 – H.U. Lemke, M.W. Vannier; K. Inamura, A.G. Farman, K. Doi & J.H.C. Reiber (Editors)
©CARS/Springer. All rights reserved.

In patients after dilatation of coronary stenotic lesions the coronary calcium score predisposes to higher restenosis rate.

3.2 Myocardial blood flow

In experimental study it was shown that there is a linear relationship between the myocardial blood flow measured with the bubble method vs EBT after intravenous contrast agent application. In clinical studies (n > 2000) we could show:

- that it is possible to measure myocardial blood flow in a daily routine work
- the mean value of the "normal" myocardial blood flow at rest is $75 \pm 10\text{ml}/100\text{g}/\text{min}$
- by doubling the heart rate using treadmill test in "healthy" patients there is an increase of myocardial blood flow of about 100%
- in presence of just one coronary stenotic lesion above 50% (i.e. LAD) regional reduction of myocardial blood flow is frequently seen
- in patient with several diffuse stenotic lesions above 50% the myocardial blood flow may be in normal range if there is tachycardia and/or increase of cardiac output and/or increase of blood pressure
- in patients with bradycardia and/or low cardiac output and/or low blood pressure, reduced myocardial blood flow at rest may be found even with normal coronary arteries
- in patients after successful dilatation of significant LAD stenosis there may be increase or decrease or no change of myocardial blood flow

The proximal 5-6 cm of the coronary arteries maybe routinely evaluated by EBT after contrast agent application with respect to stenotic lesions above or below 50 % or occlusion with an accuracy comparable to coronary angiography.

3.3 Functional parameters

The left ventricular functional parameters as EDV, ESV, SV, EF, LVMM, global and regional wall thickness may be also determinate on daily routine basis.

4. Present experience using MR in patients with suspected or not known coronary heart disease

In contrast to EBT using MRI this approach is more time consuming and it requires more patients cooperation to image the coronary arteries. The evaluation of the functional-parameters is possible with higher degree of accuracy than by EBT because of the higher contrast resolution of MR. There are encouraging results and approaches to evaluate myocardial perfusion after intravenous contrast agent applications. The continuous progress in MR technology is very promising that in the near future MR will be used in clinical routine in patients with known or suspected coronary heart disease. Especially there are very interesting results in blood flow measurements not only in the great cardiac vessèls but also intraventriculary and in the proximal coronary arteries. These flow measurements will increase our understanding of the determinants of myocardial blood flow and perfusion.

CARS 2002 – H.U. Lemke, M.W. Vannier; K. Inamura, A.G. Farman, K. Doi & J.H.C. Reiber (Editors)

The use of imaging in chest pain

Michael Rees[a]. Timothy Cripps[b]
[a]University of Bristol UK
[b]Bristol Royal Infirmary UK

Abstract

556 patients from an open access chest pain clinic were assessed by exercise ECG as a preliminary step to stratify those patients who should undergo coronary angiography. 21% of patients selected by this means had normal coronary angiography. Those patients who had positive coronary angiography had predominantly 3 vessel disease. Patients selected by gated perfusion scanning had 88% concordance with coronary angiography

Keywords: Chest pain, coronary disease, coronary angiography

1. Introduction

Rapid access chest pain clinics are a new development in the UK in order to increase the accessibility of patients with suspected cardiac disease to hospital. At present the UK has a problem with its immediacy of treatment of patients with cardiac disease. Long waiting lists for coronary angiography and revascularisation procedures are normal. There is therefore a need to target patients accurately who would benefit from this treatment and combine this with an investigation methodology which will insure rapid treatment for those that require it. Coronary angiography has long been accepted as the definitive investigation for determining if a patient requires revascularisation however it is not possible to perform coronary angiography on every patient with chest pain and so strategies have been devised to select patients for this investigation. The approach to this varies from country to country in the UK patients tend to be selected on the basis of clinical examination and exercise stress testing without the use of non invasive imaging. It is known that this approach has a relatively low sensitivity and predictive value for the diagnosis of coronary disease particularly in some groups of patients i.e. middle aged females however in many countries a high incidence of normal coronary arteriograms is acceptable particularly if this results in early detection of treatable disease and a low incidence of missing significant disease. This approach however has a low cost effectiveness and also a known incidence of mortality and morbidity from angiography. overall risk of mortality from coronary arteriography should be less than 0.2% and the risk of major adverse effects less than 0.5%, however certain groups are at higher risk, those with three vessel disease, left main stem disease and aortic valve disease. Other groups at high risk include the elderly and those with multivessel cardiovascular disease [1].

The interest in the use of non-invasive cardiac imaging as a means of selection of patients for coronary arteriography is growing. Recent developments in echocardiography, magnetic resonance imaging computed tomography and nuclear imaging have made it

CARS 2002 – H.U. Lemke, M.W. Vannier; K. Inamura, A.G. Farman, K. Doi & J.H.C. Reiber (Editors)
©CARS/Springer. All rights reserved.

possible for these modalities to be used for non-invasive diagnosis of coronary disease. What has not been investigated is the use of these modalities in the selection of patients for arteriography or use of these modalities in an investigation regimen for selection of patients from an open access population of patients with chest pain.

We decided to audit the use of non-invasive imaging in a population of 556 patients who were referred to an open access chest pain clinic and investigate the possible effects that increased use of imaging would have on the treatment of this group of patients

2. Patients and methods

556 patients were referred to the clinic in the first year via the open access route. These patients were screened and following this initial process 236 patients were sent back the referring source with a non-cardiac chest pain diagnosis. The remaining patients went on to be investigated for cardiac chest pain. The majority of these patients underwent exercise tolerance testing; those patients that could not be exercised were referred for perfusion scanning (n=38). Patients with positive exercise tests or positive perfusion scans were referred for coronary angiography. Patients with indeterminate or negative exercise test or negative perfusion scans were either followed up with further investigations or referred back to the referral source. As a result of these investigations 134 patients underwent coronary arteriography.

3. Results

Of the patients referred to angiography 125 of the patients had positive exercise tests and 9 positive perfusion scans. Of the 9 patients with perfusion scans all 9 had evidence of coronary disease on angiography, with concordance of severity of disease with angiography in 8/9 cases. 2 patients with normal scans but symptoms strongly suggestive of angina had normal coronary angiograms. Of the patients with positive exercise tests 89% of male patients had coronary disease on angiography but only 56 % of the female patients had coronary disease on angiography. 21.5% of the total number of patients (n=27) had normal coronary angiograms.

Of the patients with positive coronary angiograms 76% were three vessel disease, 18% had double vessel disease and 6% had single vessel disease. Results of follow up of the patients with indeterminate exercise tests are awaited.

3.1 Revascularisation
Of the total number of patients referred to the clinic 43 patients underwent coronary by pass surgery an 12 patients underwent percutaneous coronary angioplasty

3.2 Time of patient processing
Initial consultation and exercise testing take place at the same patient visit. After this time to perform further investigations vary dependant on urgency and investigation type. A non-urgent patient may wait up to 15 months for an angiogram and up to 9 months for a perfusion scan. If both of these tests are required the patient may then wait over two years,

CARS 2002 – H.U. Lemke, M.W. Vannier; K. Inamura, A.G. Farman, K. Doi & J.H.C. Reiber (Editors)

892

with a further wait for surgery, giving a maximum potential time from referral to final treatment of up to three years. The average time taken for a patient with a positive exercise test to angiography is 3 months; the average time taken for a patient with an equivocal exercise test is 15 months.

3.3 Cost effectiveness

Coronary angiography can be carried out either as an inpatient or outpatient. Perfusion scanning can be carried out as a one-day protocol or a two-day protocol. The costs of angiography are approximately 3-5 times that of perfusion scanning which are in turn 3-5 times that of exercise tolerance testing. The costs of work days lost and other expenses including drugs doctor time resulting from diagnostic and treatment delays cannot easily be calculated but are substantial

4. Discussion

The audit demonstrates that combining exercise ECG with perfusion imaging results in a significant t improvement in sensitivity and specificity of diagnosis of patients with angiographic coronary artery disease. Performing these two investigations sequentially in the UK environment however results in considerable delays in achieving final diagnosis and treatment. It is possible to combine the tests by performing a single stress exercise ECG and perfusion scan which would avoid these delays.

The second issue is that in view of the substantial number of normal coronary arteriograms(>20%) there will be a significant number of people who will have major adverse events at angiography with normal coronary arteries. Although the risk for angiographic mortality is related in part to severity of coronary disease the major adverse events are more generalised risks for angiography. With approximately 5,000-7000 patients per annum undergoing coronary angiography as a result of chest pain clinic referral in the next few years there will be 25-30 major adverse events of which 5-6 will occur in patients with normal coronary arteries who in all probability should not be undergoing the examination.

Perfusions scans have been proven to be a strong predictor of adverse cardiac events [2] and a normal perfusion scan is also a powerful predictor of freedom from adverse cardiac events. Perfusion scanning may have a greater predictive value of prognosis than coronary arteriography [3] in certain groups of patients particularly those at low risk of infarction. Many authors have demonstrated the relatively low sensitivity and specificity of exercise ECG testing as a discriminator of coronary disease, this is particularly true in the group of patients who have mild to moderate perfusion impairment [4]. Exercise ECG is also a poor localiser of ischaemic territory in comparison to perfusion scanning [5]. This is also demonstrated in our study which shows that the majority of patients who underwent coronary angiography had three vessel disease, with a relatively low yield of single and double vessel disease.

Gated SPECT scanning has the facility of providing information on left ventricular function [6] as well as perfusion. It is clear that a combination of myocardial perfusion

CARS 2002 – H.U. Lemke, M.W. Vannier; K. Inamura, A.G. Farman, K. Doi & J.H.C. Reiber (Editors)

893

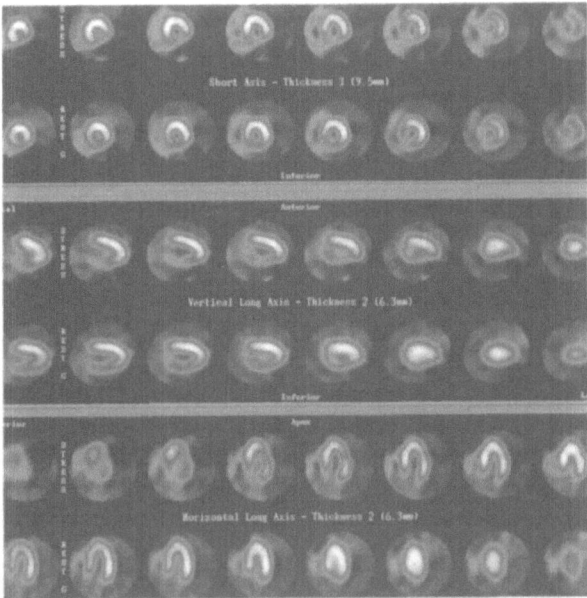

Fig 1 Abnormal perfusion scan showing fixed and reversible defects

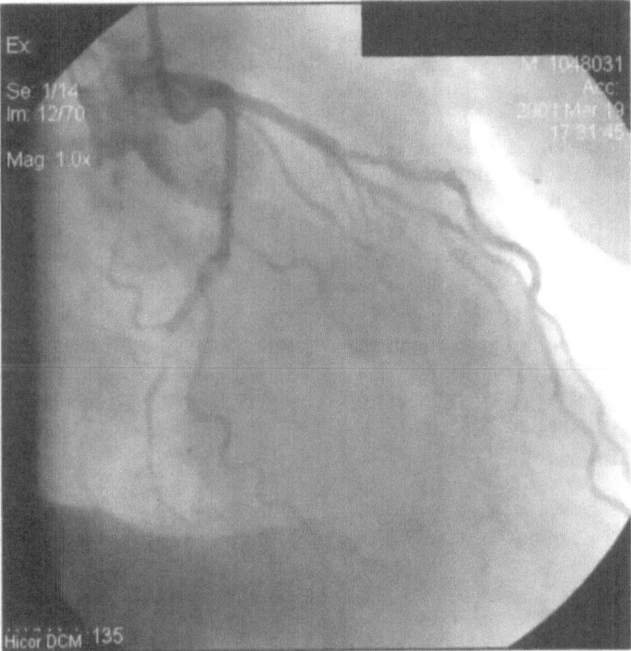

Fig 2 Abnormal coronary arteriogram showing two vessel disease

CARS 2002 – H.U. Lemke, M.W. Vannier; K. Inamura, A.G. Farman, K. Doi & J.H.C. Reiber (Editors)
ᶜCARS/Springer. All rights reserved.

894

information combined with information on left ventricular function provides improved prognostic and risk stratification information.

There must be a concern that exercise ECG testing as a sole method of screening patients will reduce the likelihood of detecting disease which is treatable by coronary angioplasty. In our study we found few patients who were suitable for undergoing coronary angioplasty which would have resulted in an improvement in speed of definitive treatment. Of the 556 patients initially referred to the clinic to date only 55 have undergone coronary artery revascularisation, which is 10% of the initial patient group.

5. Conclusions

The audit of 556 patients demonstrated that exercise ECG assessment of patients as a screening test prior to coronary angiography is a poor discriminator of patients with coronary disease in a population of patients referred to an open access chest pain clinic. The test is relatively sensitive for detecting patients with three vessel disease in male patients but is not sensitive as a method of determining coronary artery severity in female patients and has a low detection rate for single vessel disease and patients who would benefit from angioplasty. Patients who underwent perfusion scanning had a higher concordance with angiographic results.

References

1   J. Ross Jr et. Al. for the American College of Cardiology/American Heart Association Task Force on the Assessment of Diagnostic and Therapeutic Cardiovascular Procedures (Subcommittee on Coronary Angiography) JACC vol 10. No4; 935-49 1987

2   Machecourt J Longere P Fagrat D et.al. Prognostic value of Thallium 201 single photon emission computed tomographic myocardial perfusion imaging according to extent of myocardial defect. Study in 6926 patients with follow up at 33 months. J.Am College Cardiol 23:1096-1106. 1994

3   Chiamvimonvat V Goodman SG Langer A Barr A Freeman MR Prognostic value of dipyridamole SPECT imaging in low-risk pateints after myocardial infarction. J OF Nuc Card Vol 8(2) pp136-143,2001.

4   Galassi AR ,Azzarelli S,Lupo L,Mammana C,Foti R, Tamburino C Musumeci S Giuffrida G. J of Nuc .Card. Vol 76(6) 575-583, 2000

5   Kang X Berman DS Lewin HC Miranda R Agafitei R Cohen I Friedman JD Germano G. Comparative localisation of myocardial ischaemia by exercise electrocardiography and myocardial perfusion SPECT. J Nuc. Card vol 7;pp.140-145,2000

6   Rees MR, Parkin V, Wilde P. The use of gated perfusion scanning in the assessment of left ventricular volume. Eur J. radiol. Vol 38(3)pp.200-204 ,200

Advances in Cardiovascular MRI and CT
– A NASCI Symposium

CARS 2002 – H.U. Lemke, M.W. Vannier; K. Inamura, A.G. Farman, K. Doi & J.H.C. Reiber (Editors)

3D active appearance models: application to cardiac MR and ultrasound image segmentation

B.P.F. Lelieveldt[a], S.C. Mitchell[b], J.G. Bosch[a], R.J. van der Geest[a],
M. Sonka[b], J.H.C. Reiber[a]

[a]Division of Image Processing, Dept. Radiology, Leiden University Medical Center, P.O. Box 9600, 2300 RC Leiden, The Netherlands
[b]Dept. Electrical and Computer Engineering, University of Iowa, Iowa City, USA

Abstract

This paper presents a novel, 3D model-based method for three-dimensional image segmentation: A 3-D Active Appearance Model (AAM) is reported as an extension of the 2D AAM framework introduced by Cootes and Taylor. The model's behavior is learned from manually-traced segmentation examples during an automated training stage. Information about shape and image appearance of the cardiac structures is contained in a single model. This ensures a spatially- and/or temporally consistent segmentation of three-dimensional cardiac images. The clinical potential of the 3-D Active Appearance Model is demonstrated in short-axis cardiac magnetic resonance (MR) images and four-chamber echocardiographic sequences. The method's performance was assessed by comparison with manually-identified independent standards in 56 clinical MR and 64 clinical echo image sequences. The AAM method showed good agreement with the independent standard using quantitative indices of border positioning errors, endo- and epicardial volumes, and left ventricular mass. The 3D AAM shows high promise for successful application to MR and echocardiographic image analysis in a clinical setting.

Keywords: Model based segmentation, cardiac MRI, echocardiography.

1. Introduction

Nowadays, a variety of 2D and 3D image modalities enable the cardiologist to examine cardiac function quantitatively in a non-invasive manner. However, to retrieve quantitative indices of cardiac function from these images, typically the contours of the left ventricle are required. Due to the large amount of image data to be analyzed, robust automatic methods to detect the LV contours are highly desired. In previous work [2,3], Active Appearance Models (AAMs)[1] have shown great potential for segmentation of cardiac images, mainly because AAMs exploit prior knowledge about the cardiac shape and image appearance in a generic way. So far, AAMs have been applied to 2D and 2D + time (cardiac MR [2] and echocardiography[3]). In this paper, a novel, truly 3D Active Appearance Model is presented that models the intrinsically 3D shape and image appearance of the left ventricle in cardiac image data. The method is applied to contour detection in two substantially different modalities: cardiac MR imaging and echocardiography.

CARS 2002 – H.U. Lemke, M.W. Vannier; K. Inamura, A.G. Farman, K. Doi & J.H.C. Reiber (Editors)

898

2. Methods

Active Appearance Models (AAMs), as introduced by Cootes et al.[1], describe the shape of objects and their grey level appearance in a set of example images as a statistical model. An AAM is created from user-placed contours defining the shape of the objects of interest in each training image. The shape and intensity changes observed in the training are modeled by applying a Principle Component Analysis (PCA) to the shape and gray level variations observed in the training set. The resulting AAM describes an object as a linear combination of an average image and a set of eigenvariations.

In the 3D AAM presented here, the shape and appearance of the entire Left Ventricle (LV) is modeled from a set of expert drawn left ventricular contours in a volumetric 3D data set. Each training sample consists of a stack of manually drawn contours and the corresponding image data. In the MR application, the 3D training shapes are resampled using a manually defined characteristic landmark point on the LV surface representing the attachment of the right ventricle to the left ventricle, and defining a regularly spaced grid of corresponding surface points. For echocardiographic sequences, corresponding shape points on the endocardial contour are defined for each frame of one complete cardiac cycle (ED to ED) based on expert drawn contours and represented as a surface of 3D points. The resampled 3D LV point sets are aligned using Besl's closed form 3D registration method [4] for corresponding point sets, and a mean LV shape is calculated. Subsequently a Principal Component Analysis (PCA) is applied to the shape sample point distributions, yielding the most characteristic shape eigenvariations.

The image appearance of the LV in the MR and echocardiographic image data is modeled by warping the 3D training image volumes to the mean shape, yielding a shape-free intensity voxel model. The average image appearance and the corresponding eigenvariations are calculated by applying a PCA on the intensity distributions around the average intensity volume. Finally, the intensity and shape models are combined by expressing each shape-intensity sample as a linear combination of eigenvectors, and subsequently applying a PCA to the combined shape-intensity parameter vectors. As a result, the 3D shape and image appearance of the heart are modeled, where the eigenvariations describe the most characteristic variations in the population.

The 3D AAM is fitted to an image volume in a true 3D manner. The intensity difference between the voxel model and the target volume is minimized using a least squares minimization by deforming the 3D model along the model eigenvariations, while optimizing for 3D translation, rotation and scale at the same time. In a separate training step, the derivatives required to steer the optimizition towards a minimum are pre-computed for all model parameters. When applied to cardiac MR volume data, the matching procedure results in a 3D segmentation for the complete left ventricle endo- and epicardium, with a typical calculation time of less than 30 seconds on a standard PC workstation. For echocardiographic time sequences, the matching yields a time-continuous segmentation for one complete cardiac cycle, located in both time and space.

CARS 2002 – H.U. Lemke, M.W. Vannier; K. Inamura, A.G. Farman, K. Doi & J.H.C. Reiber (Editors)
°CARS/Springer. All rights reserved.

3. Experimental validation

To assess the clinical potential of the 3D AAM method, it was evaluated on two modalities: cardiac MR imaging and echocardiography.

3.1 Cardiac MR

56 cardiac MR studies were collected from 18 patients (various common pathologies) and 38 normal subjects. Images were acquired with slice thickness 8-11mm at a resolution of 256x256 pixels, FOV 400-450 mm. LV ENDO and EPI contours were expert traced in ED for the complete LV. Validation and training was performed on the ED volumes using a leave-one-subject-out approach. The initial position for the model matching was fully automatically determined using a previously validated, Hough transform based approach. Due to the 3D nature of the model, we expected the model to sometimes miss a slice: manual contours might be present, where no automatic contours were found. Therefore for each study, the number of slices missed by the model was recorded, and volume measures for the LV (ENDO volume, EPI volume and LV wall mass) were compared for the slices with manual and automatic contours. In addition, mean signed and unsigned border positioning errors were computed.

The 3D AAM method showed correct contours in 53 out of 56 cases. In three cases, the matching did not converge to a correct solution, and these cases were excluded from further quantitative analysis. In a total of 391 manually defined MR slices, the 3D AAM fully automatically identified contours in 359 slices. In 28 out of 56 cases, the method detected contours in all slices, where manual contours were present. In 18 cases, computer determined borders were missing in one MR slice and in 7 cases, two slices were missed by the model. Global functional parameters such as ENDO and EPI volume and LV mass correlated well: $Y=0.88X + 8.4$ ($r^2=0.94$) for automated vs manual LV ENDO volume and $Y= 0.91X + 12.1$ ($r^2=0.97$) for automated vs manual EPI volume. LV wall mass correlated with $Y = 0.80X + 18$ ($r^2= 0.82$). Average signed ENDO and EPI border position errors were -0.46 ± 1.33 mm and -0.29 ± 1.16 mm, respectively. Average unsigned ENDO and EPI border position errors were 2.75 ± 0.86 mm and 2.63 ± 1.16 mm, respectively.

3.2 Echocardiography

129 sets of transthoracic echocardiographic four-chamber sequences were acquired at 25 frames/sec from unselected infarct patients participating in a clinical trial. These were single-beat (end-diastole to end-diastole) sequences with 15 to 33 image frames per heart beat artificially extended to three cardiac cycles. Images were digitized at a resolution of 768×76 pixels with different calibration factors (0.28 to 0.47 mm/pixel). An independent expert manually identified the LV contours in the image sequences. The total data set was split randomly into a training set of 65 patients and a testing set of 64 patients, on which segmentation performance was evaluated.

To compare the automatically detected contours with the observer-identified independent standard, the number of segmentation failures was determined. Failures were identified as segmentations in which the 3D AAM borders did not agree well with the independent standard (average unsigned spatial distance component > 7.5 mm). In the successfully

CARS 2002 – H.U. Lemke, M.W. Vannier; K. Inamura, A.G. Farman, K. Doi & J.H.C. Reiber (Editors)

900

segmented images, unsigned three-dimensional endocardial border positioning errors were defined as unsigned distances between matched model points and image-based 3D shape points extracted for the testing-set images in a same manner as the training set shape points. These distances were calculated in 3D and also split into a spatial (xy) and a temporal (z) component, where the temporal component can be converted to milliseconds. Furthermore, endocardial areas were determined for all time slices; regression analysis was used to compare the computer-determined areas with the independent standard.

In 57 of the 64 tested echocardiographic image sequences (success rate 89%), the 3D AAM-defined borders agreed well with the independent standard. In the successful 57 temporal sequences, three-dimensional absolute endocardial surface positioning errors were 3.90 ± 1.38 mm; the 2D spatial component was 3.35 ± 1.05 mm, which compares favorably with two-dimensionally determined (within the same image frame) inter-observer variability of 3.82 ± 1.44 mm. The intra-observer variability was 2.32 ± 0.75 mm. The result also compares reasonably well with the previously reported two-dimensional endocardial border positioning errors of 3.35 ± 1.22 mm (success rate 97%) achieved by our less-general 2-D + time Active Appearance Motion Model implementation. The temporal component of the border positioning error was 37.0 ± 29.6 ms, less than a single frame duration of 40 msec. Frame-based area regression over the 57 successful matches showed a good correlation (y =0.83x + 3.6, r^2= 0.79).

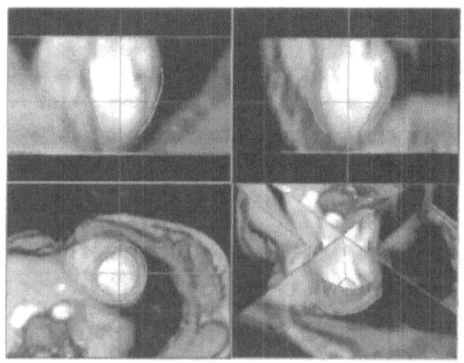 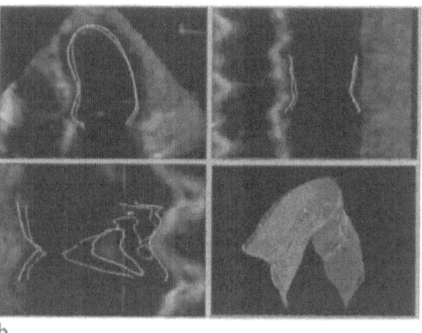

a   b

Figure 1. 3D AAM generated contours for cardiac short-axis cardiac MR data (a) and echocardio-graphic 2D + time volume data (b). For both applications: the bottom right subimages show the segmented surfaces, and the other subimages are orthogonal cross-sections through the volume data.

4. Discussion

The results of the study show a high robustness of our fully automated 3D AAM approach for both applications. In the MR application, the method demonstrated a clinically acceptable accuracy in 53 out of 56 cases both in border positioning errors and in ENDO and EPI volume and LV mass. However, the contours of the apex were slightly less accurately detected than the mid-ventricular contours, most likely due to the fact that the apex only asserts a small influence in the minimization criterion. The border positioning errors as well as the volume and mass measures revealed a slight but systematic bias

CARS 2002 – H.U. Lemke, M.W. Vannier; K. Inamura, A.G. Farman, K. Doi & J.H.C. Reiber (Editors)
°CARS/Springer. All rights reserved.

towards "too small" contours. This can be mainly attributed to shifts in heart position between slices due to the differences in respiration level during MR acquisition. However, given the fact that this method is fully automated, and detects ENDO- and EPI contours simultaneously, the 3D AAM demonstrated great potential to fully automate the analysis of routinely acquired short-axis cardiac MR image data sets. Extension to 3D + time, as well as to analysis of stress MR studies is ongoing.

For the ultrasound application, results were promising but less convincing than those achieved using our previously reported 2-D+time AAM approach. Area regression over the 57 successful matches exhibited a systematic area underestimation of 3.8% ($y = 0.83 x + 3.6$, $r^2 = 0.79$). Compared to the 2D+time AAM ($y = 0.91 x + 1.73$, $r^2 = 0.76$; area underestimation 2.9%), a slightly higher systematic area error and a flatter regression line were observed. In part, this can be attributed to the extra degree of freedom hat the 3D AAM has to cope with. The 2D + time AAM uses a priori knowledge of the phase/time aspect. However, the non-Gaussian distribution of intensity values in ultrasound is likely to be an even more important problem. Its indication is that model localization in the time dimension is much more accurate than in the spatial localization. For the 2D+time AAM approach in ultrasound, intensity distributions were normalized non-linearly to deal with ultrasound-specific intensity properties; this resulted in a substantially improved accuracy of the border localization. The non-linear normalization improved both the systematic area underestimation and the slope of the area regression. The 3D version of this correction has not yet been developed. After its implementation, further improvements of segmentation accuracy in the echocardiographic images are expected.

5. Conclusions

A three-dimensional Active Appearance Model method for analysis of volumetric cardiac images and temporal image sequences was presented. Its performance and flexibility were assessed in two substantially different cardiac imaging modality case studies, where the 3D AAM demonstrated the potential to reduce user interaction for quantitative cardiac image analysis to a minimum.

References

1. T. F. Cootes, C. Beeston. G. J. Edwards, and C. J. Taylor, "A Unified Framework for Atlas Matching Using Active Appearance Models.," *proc. IPMI, Lecture Notes in Computer Science*, vol. 1630, pp.322-333, 2001.
2. S. C. Mitchell, B. P. F. Lelieveldt, R. J. van der Geest, J. G. Bosch, J. H. C. Reiber, and M. Sonka, "Multistage Hybrid Active Appearance Model Matching: Segmentation of Left and Right Cardiac Ventricles in Cardiac MR Images," *IEEE TMI.*, vol. 20(5), pp 415-423, 2001.
3. J.G. Bosch. S.C. Mitchell. B.P.F. Lelieveldt, F. Nijland, O. Kamp. M. Sonka and J.H.C. Reiber. "Automatic Segmentation of Echocardiographic Sequences by Active Appearance Motion Models", *IEEE TMI (in press)*
4. P. J. Besl and N. D. McKay, "A Method for Registration of 3-D Shapes." *IEEE Trans. PAMI*, vol. 14, pp. 239-256, 1992.

CARS 2002 - H.U. Lemke, M.W. Vannier, K. Inamura, A.G. Farman, K. Doi & J.H.C. Reiber (Editors)

Automatic correction of myocardial boundaries in MR cardio perfusion analysis

Luuk Spreeuwers[a], Femke Wierda[a], Marcel Breeuwer[b]

[a] University Medical Center Utrecht, Image Sciences Institute,
Heidelberglaan 100, 3584 CX Utrecht, Netherlands
[b] Philips Medical Systems, Medical Imaging Information Technology
Building QV 162, P.O. Box 10000, 5680 DA Best, Netherlands

Abstract

Magnetic Resonance Imaging (MRI) has become an important technique for imaging cardiovascular diseases. Recent advances in MRI allow fast recording of contrast enhanced myocardial perfusion scans. These MR perfusion scans are made by recording, during a period of 20-40 seconds short axis slices of the heart. The scanning is triggered by the patient's ECG typically resulting in one set of slices per heart beat. For perfusion analysis, the myocardial boundaries must be traced in all images, dividing the heart into the left and right ventricle blood volumes and the myocardium of the left ventricle. Care must be taken not include part of the right or left ventricle blood volumes in the myocardium segment, because this may have a significant effect on the perfusion analysis. On the other hand, for accurate estimation of the perfusion parameters, all of the available myocardium area in the image should be used. In this paper a method is proposed to automatically correct for any inclusion of left and right ventricle into the myocardium segment and optimally place the myocardial boundaries.

Keywords: Perfusion, segmentation, myocardium

1. Introduction

Cardio vascular diseases are one of the major death causes in the western society. Reduced blood perfusion of the myocardium of the left ventricle is a direct result of cardio vascular diseases. The perfusion of the myocardium can be measured using contrast enhanced Magnetic Resonance cardio perfusion scans. These scans are made by recording a number of short-axis slices through the myocardium (see fig.1) during a period of 20-40 seconds.

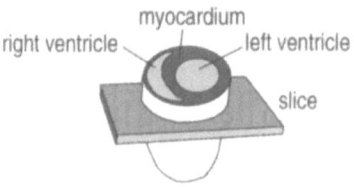

Fig.1 Short axis slice through the heart

The scanning is triggered by the patient's electro cardiogram (ECG), typically resulting in one set of slices per heart beat and each set of slices showing exactly the same phase in the contraction cycle of the heart. A contrast agent is injected in the patient and subsequently the heart is imaged. The contrast agent shows brightly in the MR images. In an image sequence, one can observe the contrast first entering the right ventricle, then the left ventricle and finally the perfusion in the myocardium. This is illustrated in fig.2.

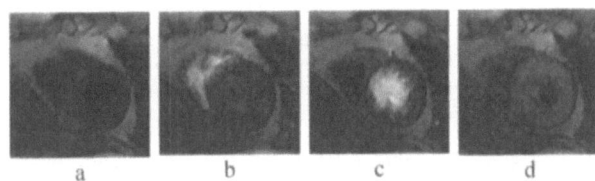

Fig.2 Four images of an MR cardio perfusion scan. a) before contrast; b) contrast in right ventricle; c) contrast in left ventricle; d) perfusion in myocardium

Recent research has shown a good correlation between MR myocardial perfusion measurements and the presence of a coronary-artery disease [1,2]. As a measure for perfusion in the myocardium, often the maximum upslope of the intensity-time curve of the myocardium is used. The intensity-time curve is the intensity of a single position in the myocardium (or in the left or right ventricle) plotted as a function of time. Intensity-time curves for the left and right ventricles and the myocardium are shown in fig.3 as well as the maximum upslope in the myocardium.

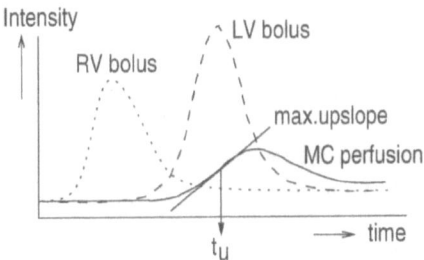

Fig.3 Intensity-time curves of the left and right ventricles and the myocardium. t_u is the maximum upslope time

Since the signal in the myocardium is very noisy, generally the myocardium is divided into segments [1,3,4] and the measurements are averaged over these segments. These segments coincide with areas of the myocardium which are supplied with blood from a certain coronary artery. In this way, if a reduced perfusion is observed in a myocardial segment, it can be traced back to the supplying artery. A division of the myocardium into 6 segments is shown in fig.4.

CARS 2002 - H.U. Lemke, M.W. Vannier; K. Inamura, A.G. Farman, K. Doi & J.H.C. Reiber (Editors)
°CARS/Springer. All rights reserved.

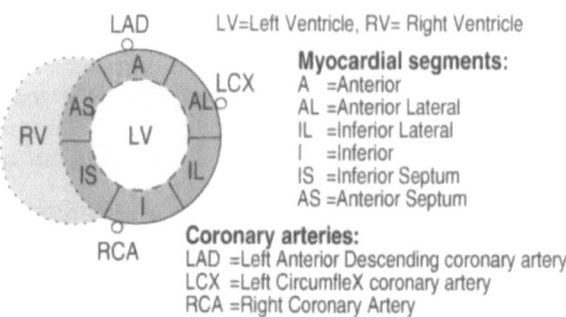

Fig.4 Division of the myocardium into 6 segments

Since the signal strengths in the left and right ventricles are much higher than in the myocardium, extreme care should be taken not to include any part of the left and right ventricles into the myocardial segments. This is not as easy as it seems, since the boundaries of the left and right ventricle blood volumes can be very irregular due to the presence of papillary muscles and trabeculae.

In literature on MR cardiac perfusion analysis, the effect of inclusion of the left and right ventricle blood volumes is hardly addressed at all, while it may have a significant effect on the outcome of the perfusion analysis. In this paper this effect is analysed and a method for correction of the myocardial boundaries is presented. This research is part of a larger project on MR cardio perfusion analysis in collaboration with Philips Medical Systems, the German Heart Institute, Berlin, Germany and the Cardiac MR Unit of the Leeds general Infirmary, United Kingdom (see e.g. [5,6]).

2. Sensitivity of perfusion analysis for boundary position

To investigate the influence of the exact position of the myocardial boundaries on the estimated maximum upslope, the sensitivity of the maximum upslope for the position of the boundaries was determined. For each myocardial segment the inner boundary was moved over small distances relative to the centre of the left ventricle and for each position the average of the maximum upslope for the segment was calculated (see fig.5).

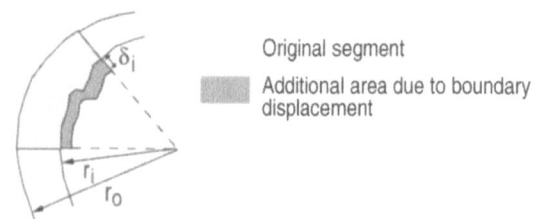

Fig.5 Displacement of the inner boundary over a small distance

CARS 2002 - H.U. Lemke, M.W. Vannier; K. Inamura, A.G. Farman, K. Doi & J.H.C. Reiber (Editors)
°CARS/Springer. All rights reserved.

Since the maximum upslope in the left (and right) ventricles is much higher than in the myocardium, one would expect the average maximum upslope in a segment to increase if more of the left ventricle is included into the segment due to the boundary displacement. If no pixels of the left ventricle are included into the segment, the average maximum upslope should remain constant. For the time on which the maximum upslope takes place exactly the opposite behaviour can be expected. Since in the left ventricle the upslope time is earlier than in the myocardium, including pixels of the left ventricle into the myocardial segment reduces the average of the upslope time in the segment. The boundary position for each segment can be corrected by starting with a displacement that deliberately includes part of the left ventricle and moving the boundary outward until the maximum upslope and upslope time become constant.

3. Experiments and results

For a set of 9 image sequences, the myocardial boundaries were manually traced and 6 segments were assigned. The inner boundary was displaced over a range of +/- 3 pixels by sub-sampling the curve with a one degree step and moving each point relative to the centre of gravity of the inner boundary over a distance defined by the displacement. For each pixel the maximum upslope was calculated by convolution with a derivative of a 1-dimensional Gaussian in time with standard deviation 1.0 and finding the maximum and the corresponding time. The resulting curves give the maximum upslopes and upslope times for each segment as a function of the displacement of the inner boundary of the myocardium. A typical result is given in fig.6.

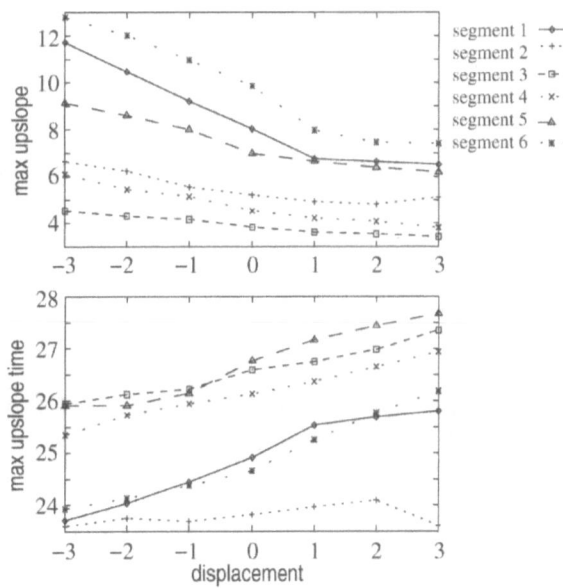

Fig.6 Maximum upslope and upslope time as function of the radial displacement
of the inner myocardial boundary

906

From these measurements it becomes clear that the exact position of the myocardial boundaries may have a large influence on perfusion measurements, just as we expected. Most of the obtained curves show the predicted behaviour, i.e. increased average maximum upslope and decreased upslope time when more pixels of the left ventricle are included into the segment. For some of the segments that bordered on the right ventricle, a deviation of this behaviour can be observed that is caused by including part of the right ventricle. Segments 1,2 and 3 in fig.7 show this deviating behaviour. The maximum upslope does not remain constant in this case, because if the number of myocardium pixels in the segment decreases (by moving the inner myocardial boundary outwards), the influence of the included right ventricle pixels becomes larger and, hence, the maximum upslope increases (the upslope in the right ventricle is much larger than in the myocardium). Likewise, when the inner myocardial boundary moves outward, the upslope time will not remain constant, but decrease, because the influence of the included right ventricle pixels in the segment increases and the upslope time in the right ventricle is lower.

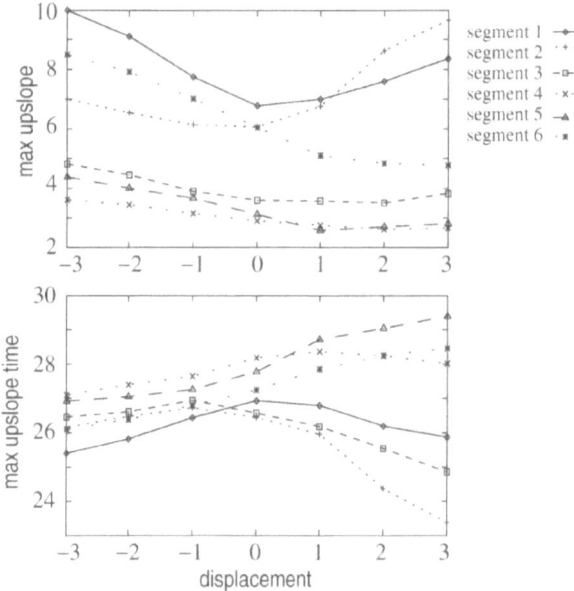

Fig.7 Maximum upslope and upslope time as function of the radial displacement of the inner myocardial boundary; deviating behaviour due to inclusion of right ventricle pixels (segments 1,2 and 3)

This means the position of the outer myocardial boundary must be corrected as well. The position of the outer myocardial boundary can be corrected in a similar way as described here for the inner boundary. We plan to extend the boundary correction procedure with the outer boundary correction.

CARS 2002 - H.U. Lemke, M.W. Vannier; K. Inamura, A.G. Farman, K. Doi & J.H.C. Reiber (Editors)
CARS/Springer. All rights reserved.

4. Conclusions

A method is proposed for analysis of the effect of the position of myocardial boundaries on myocardial perfusion analysis using contrast enhanced MR perfusion scans. The sensitivity analysis shows that the position of the myocardial boundaries is very important for accurate perfusion analysis. Using these sensitivity measurements, a correction for the boundary positions can be determined which results in more reliable perfusion analysis. Currently the correction is only implemented for the inner myocardial boundary. In the near future we plan to include a correction of the outer myocardial boundary as well.

Acknowledgements

We thank Dr. Ingo Paetch, Dr. Eike Nagel and Dr. Nidal Al-Saadi of the Cardiac MR Department of the Deutsches Herzzentrum Berlin and Dr. John Ridgway of the MR Department of the Leeds General Infermary for kindly supplying image material.

References

1. Wilke et al., "Myocardial perfusion reserve: assessment with multisection, quantitative, first-pass MR imaging", *Radiology*, Vol. 204, No. 2, pp. 373-384, 1997.
2. N. Al-Saadi et al., "Noninvasive detection of myocardial ischemia from perfusion reserve based on cardiovascular magnetic resonance", *Circulation*, Vol. 101, pp. 1379-1383, 2000.
3. J. Schwitter et al. "Echo-planar MR perfusion imaging is highly reliable in detection of coronary-artiry disease", in *Proceedings Int. Society of Magnetic Resonance in Medicine*, pp. 34, Denver, Colorado, USA, 1-7 April 2000
4. M. Schmitt et al., "Quantification of myocardial perfusion reserve with magnetic first-pass measurements on patients with known coronary artery disease", in *Proceedings Int. Society of Magnetic Resonance in Medicine*, pp. 531, Denver, Colorado, USA, 1-7 April 2000
5. L.J. Spreeuwers and M. Breeuwer, "Automatic detection of the myocardial boundaries of the right and left ventricle in MR cardio perfusion scans", in *Proceedings SPIE Medical Imaging*, Vol. 4322, pp. 1207-1217, San Diego, USA, 19-22 Febr. 2001
6. M. Breeuwer, M. Quist, L.J. Spreeuwers, I. Paetsch, N. Al-Saadi and E. Nagel, "Towards automatic quantitative analysis of cardiac MR perfusion images", in *Proceedings of the CARS conference*, Berlin, Germany, June 2001

CARS 2002 – H.U. Lemke, M.W. Vannier; K. Inamura, A.G. Farman, K. Doi & J.H.C. Reiber (Editors)

FAST analysis tool of global and local heart functions by MRI tagging

C. Dornier[a], M. K. Ivancevic[b], G. Lecoq[c], A. Righetti[c], J.P. Vallee[a,b]

[a] Unité d'Imagerie Numérique, Division d'Informatique Médicale, Département de Radiologie, HUG, CH-1211 Geneva, Switzerland
[b] Division de Radiodiagnostic et de Radiologie Interventionnelle, Département de Radiologie, HUG, CH-1211 Geneva, Switzerland
[c] Division de cardiologie, Département de médecine interne, HUG, 1211 Geneva, Switzerland

Abstract

This work presents a dedicated and powerful tool for assessing both global and local heart functions with only one Magnetic Resonance Imaging (MRI) tagging exam. The border between the left ventricle and the endocardium is frequently undefined on the first frame of a tagged MRI cine series, but not on the last frame. To measure the global heart function (such as end-diastolic volume, end-systolic volume and ejection fraction), we investigated the potential of HARP software to retrospectively track the end-diastolic contour from the end-systolic contour. The major parameters, which influence the tag analysis with HARP software, are the space between tags and the temporal resolution of the acquisition sequence. Simulated tagged images have been used to optimise these parameters in order to obtain an automatic analysis. For the LV-EF estimation, MRI tagging was compared to the standard cine in volunteers (n=20) and to contrast cine angiography in patients (n=7). The LV-EF derived from the MRI tagging is linearly correlated to the standard cardiac cine LV-EF (r=0.99, p<0.001) and to the contrast cine angiography LV-EF (r=0.95, p<0.002). For the same acquisition time, an accurate estimation of global heart function can be obtained in addition to quantitative regional function.

Keywords: Ejection fraction, MRI tagging, HARP

1. Introduction

MRI tagging spatially modulates the longitudinal magnetization of the subject to create saturated signal regions, called tags, in the myocardium. Tags appear as a succession of regularly spaced dark lines in the image and it is necessary to have at least two tag directions for performing a 2D heart analysis. FAST spoiled gradient echo imaging creates cine sequences that show deformation of the tag lines during cardiac contraction (End-Diastolic (ED) to End-Systolic (ES) states). Tag contrast decreases with time and tags rapidly disappear inside the cavity due to the blood flow.

MRI tagging is usually used to assess local strains inside the myocardium but has never been used to compute global parameters of the heart function such as ED volume, ES

CARS 2002 – H.U. Lemke, M.W. Vannier; K. Inamura, A.G. Farman, K. Doi & J.H.C. Reiber (Editors)

909

volume and Ejection Fraction (EF). This lack can be explained by the following reason: the border between the left ventricle and the endocardium is frequently undefined on the first frame of a tagged MRI cine series because both myocardium and blood in the left ventricle are tagged. To measure global parameters of the left ventricle function, we investigated the potential of HARP software [1] to retrospectively track the ED contour from the ES contour. HARP software is presented and was chosen because it does not require LV segmentation over all frames, which is a necessary stage in the concurrent software FindTags [2].

2. Methodology

2.1 HARP software
This software is based on the use of isolated spectral peaks in SPAMM-tagged magnetic resonance images, which contain information about cardiac motion. The inverse Fourier transform of a spectral peak is a complex image whose calculated angle is called a harmonic phase (HARP) image (Figure 1). HARP image sequences can be used to automatically track material points (markers) through time. The accuracy of the tracking process depends on two major parameters of the acquisition sequence, which are the space between two adjacent tag lines and the temporal resolution of the sequence.

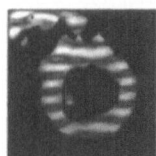 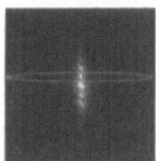 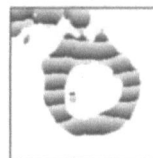

Figure 1: SPAMM-tagged images of the LV short-axis view (left), the magnitude of the corresponding Fourier transform (middle), and the corresponding HARP image (right). Ellipse in the Fourier domain correspond to the size of the bandpass filter.

2.2 Image analysis
All the tag analyses were based on the drawn of two regions of interest (ROI) on the short-axis images: one corresponding to the LV endocardium and the other corresponding to the LV epicardium. The two ROI were manually drawn by clicking on the frame corresponding to the ES state. The polygonal lines were replaced by a B-Spline curve in order to have smoother ROI. To provide a thin transmural analysis, five regularly spaced ROI between endocardial and epicardial ROI were added. For assessing local strains inside the myocardium, the different ROI were divided into 8 segments, each segment containing 2 markers. We used the definition of unit elongation or simple strain found in [1]:

$$e = \frac{\left\| q_i^t - q_j^t \right\|}{\left\| q_i^{t_0} - q_j^{t_0} \right\|} - 1$$
Eq. 1

where $q_i^{t_0}$ represents the position of the marker i in the first frame t_0 and q_i^t represents the position of the marker i in the frame t.

This quantity is zero if the distance between the points remains unchanged, negative if there is shortening, and positive if there is lengthening. To measure circumferential strains at any location within the LV wall, we simply use the points along a circle centered at the LV long axis. To measure radial strains we simply use the points along a ray emanating

CARS 2002 – H.U. Lemke, M.W. Vannier; K. Inamura, A.G. Farman, K. Doi & J.H.C. Reiber (Editors)
°CARS/Springer. All rights reserved.

910

from the long axis. In either case, the strains are measured by tracking the different points using HARP tracking and calculating *e*.

Global parameters such as ED, ES volumes and EF were computed only by the endocardial ROI. ED images were chosen as the first phase after triggering off the R-wave and ES images were defined as the images with the smallest cavity area. On volunteers short-axis tagged images, with a complete coverage of the heart, only the ES areas were drawn on the corresponding frame. The ED areas were retrospectively tracked from the ES area. The volume of each slice was determined from the area within the endocardial tracing (including papillary muscles) multiplied by the slice thickness. The ED Volume (EDV) and ES Volume (ESV) were calculated by summing the volumes of all short-axis slices. The EF was calculated as (EDV - ESV) / EDV. On patients short-axis tagged images, the ventricular volume was determined with the simplified Simpson's formula by using one long-axis view (Length) and two short-axis views (Mitral_Valve_Plane_Area and Papillary_Muscle_Plane_area):

$$Volume = \frac{Length}{2}\left(Mitral\_Valve\_Plane\_Area + \left(\frac{2\ Papillary\_Muscle\_Plane\_Area}{3} \right) \right) \quad \text{Eq. 2}$$

The EDV was computed using areas and length in the ED state. The ESV was computed using areas and length in the ES state. The EF was calculated as (EDV-ESV)/EDV.

3. Data

3.1 Simulations
Simulated short-axis tagged images have been used to present the two parameters influence on the analysis accuracy. In the first image (ED state), the myocardium had an annular shape ($r_{endo\_diastole}$=17 mm, $r_{epi\_diastole}$=34 mm). In the last image (ES state) the myocardium was deformed differently between vertical and horizontal directions: the endocardium preserved a circular shape ($r_{endo\_systole}$=6.8 mm) whereas the epicardium shape became elliptic ($rx_{epi\_systole}$=20.5 mm, $ry_{epi\_systole}$=27.3 mm) (Figure 2). Simulating tag spacing was realized by changing the spatial resolution of the applied patterns (applied patterns were realized by a succession of black and white lines in two perpendicular directions). Simulating the temporal resolution of the sequence was achieved by changing the frame number between the first frame and the last frame.

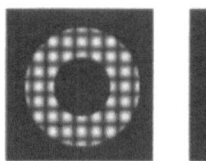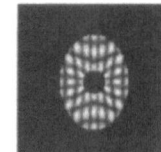

Figure 2: Simulated short-axis tagged images: ED state (left), ES state (right).

3.2 In-vivo studies
MRI exam were realized on a Marconi Eclipse 1.5T MR system. For the healthy volunteers (n=20), global parameters of the heart function obtained by MRI tagging were correlated to results obtained by the standard CINE MRI sequence. For the patients (n=7), only the tagging sequence has been realized. Global parameters of the heart function were

CARS 2002 – H.U. Lemke, M.W. Vannier; K. Inamura, A.G. Farman, K. Doi & J.H.C. Reiber (Editors)
'CARS/Springer. All rights reserved.

compared to values obtained by contrast cine angiography and local strains inside the myocardium were compared to results obtained by a SPECT Thallium Imaging.

The volunteer protocol consisted of one two-chamber view, one four-chamber view and coverage of the whole heart in the short axis. The images were first acquired with the tagged sequences (tag FA: 90°, tag spacing=12mm, read direction tags, TR/TE=7.6/2.6ms, FA:15°, bandwidth=31.25kHz, 8mm slice thickness, FOV nominally 35cm adapted to the volunteer's size, 64x256 matrix, RAM factor 2, ECG gating, Cardiac coil). The same views were repeated with a standard cine sequence (TR/TE=9.5/3.3ms, FA:35°, bandwidth =25kHz, 8mm slice thickness, 128x256 matrix, RAM factor 2, ECG gating.). Both image series were acquired during breath-holds. Multislice short-axis cine images were analysed using NIHimage (National Institutes of Health, Bethesda, Maryland, http://rsb.info.nih.gov/nih-image/). On cine images, both ED and ES endocardial areas were manually drawn with inclusion of the papillary muscles. The segmentation process was performed five times for each patient and the results averaged. The tagging method was applied to patients (n=7), with known coronary disease with a previous myocardium infarct, and correlated to the EF measured from contrast cine angiography. The patient protocol consisted of one four-chamber view, and four regularly spaced short axis views to cover the ventricle. Tagged images were acquired both at rest and during a 15-minute period of Dobutamine stress (7.5 µg/kg/min).

4. Results

4.1 Parameter influences
Bad tracks of markers occur when there is maladjustment between tag spacing and temporal resolution. When tracking markers along the last frame to the first frame, the ROI drawn on the last frame is then copied to the previous frame and the different markers are moved in the frame in order to recover equivalent positions regarding to the next frame. This stage is repeated until the first frame has been tracked.

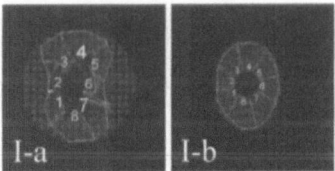 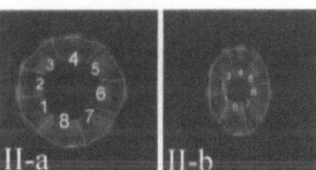

Figure 3: Influence of the tag spacing in the tracking stage. The endocardial and epicardial ROI are drawn on the ES frame (I-b and II-b) and retrospectively tracked to the ED frame (I-a and II-a). In these two simulations, we use 6 frames for the contraction stage. With a tag spacing equal to 4.5 mm (I-a and I-b), displacement of the tag lines between two frames is superior to the tag spacing and leads to a bad-tracking stage. With tag spacing equal to 18 mm (II-a and II-b), displacement of the tag lines between two frames is inferior to the tag spacing and leads to a good tracking stage and a complete automatic analysis could be performed.

When the tag spacing is too small or when the delay between two frames allows the myocardium to move more than the tag spacing, a tag jumping occurs and bad results will be obtained (Figure 3). By adapting acquisition sequence, it is possible to reduce considerably tag jumping. In the eventuality that bad tracks occurs we have added an option to manually correct bad tracked points, which allows obtaining accurate results.

Another problem that can occur when the endocardial contraction is very important is that when reporting the endocardial ROI on the previous frame, some points can be placed inside the cavity and will be bad tracked. To overcome this problem, an alternative is to place the endocardial ROI not exactly at the myocardium/cavity contour but 2 mm away from the cavity inside the myocardium.

4.2 In-vivo studies

Global function: by placing the contour 2 mm from the true cavity boundary, HARP software was able to track the contour on all the volunteers and patients. The results of the study on healthy volunteers are presented on table 1. A very good correlation ($y=0.86x+15.74$, $r=0.99$) is obtained between the standard cine and tagging methods (Figure 4). The LV-EF obtained by MRI tagging is about 8%±1% ($p<0.001$) less than the LV-EF obtained by cine MRI. This can be explained by the fact that the ES volume is overestimated in MRI tagging compared to CINE MRI because the endocardial border is place inside the myocardium and not at the myocardium/cavity contour.

In the patient's study, an excellent correlation was found between the LV-EF determined by MRI tagging and contrast cine angiography ($y=1.03x +8.02$, $r=0.95$, $p<0.002$). The patient's number needs to be increase in order to obtain more accurate statistics.

Table 1: Cine MRI versus MRI tagging (n=20)			
	EDV (ml)	ESV (ml)	EF (%)
cine MRI (mean ± sd)	56 ± 17	22 ± 9	61 ± 5
MRI tagging (mean ± sd)	50 ± 17	24 ± 10	53 ± 6
Difference (%)	-6 (-10.6%)*	2 (8.2%)**	-8 (-14.3%)★
95% CI of the difference	-9 ~ -2	0 ~ 3	-9 ~ -8
Limits of agreement	-20 ~ 9	-4 ~ 8	-10 ~ -6
EDV = end-diastolic volume; ESV = end-systolic volume; EF = ejection fraction; CI = confidence interval; MRI = magnetic resonance imaging			
* $P < 0.003$ ** $P < 0.02$ ★ $P < 0.001$			

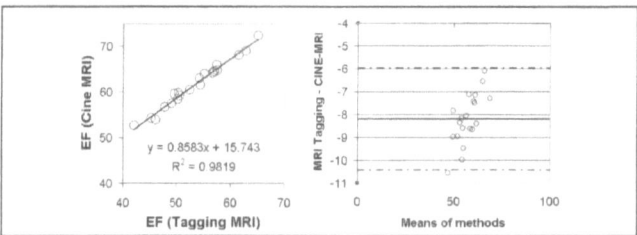

Figure 4: Ejection fraction: linear regression (left) and Bland Altman diagram (right) (solid line: mean; dashed line: mean ± 2 SD) between cine MRI and MRI tagging.

Local function: Strain analysis is presented and even with a tag spacing of about 12 mm, strain differences between endocardium and epicardium can be observed and absence of contraction in the infarct segments (segments 7-8) is clearly highlighted (Figure 5). In the patient's study, strain analysis has been correlated to SPECT Thallium Imaging and contraction problems have been measured by the two modalities in the same myocardium segments (infarct segment has a hypocaptation with a value <55-60%) (Figure 6).

CARS 2002 – H.U. Lemke, M.W. Vannier; K. Inamura, A.G. Farman, K. Doi & J.H.C. Reiber (Editors)
©CARS/Springer. All rights reserved.

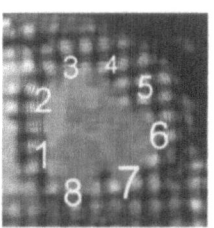 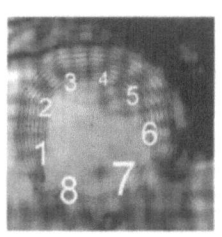 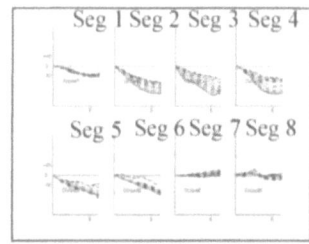

Figure 5: Strain analysis of a patient with a prior infarct in segments 7-8. Left: ED frame with the tracked ROI, middle: ES frame with the manually drawn ROI, right: time evolution of the circumferential strains for the eight segments. Contraction is less important at the epicardium (dashed black line) than at the endocardium (solid black line). Infarct segments have no contraction.

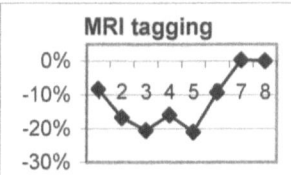 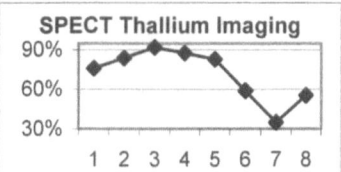

Figure 6: Correlation between MRI tagging and SPECT Thallium Imaging for classifying segments as normal or infarct. Segment is infracted if the maximum circumferential strain is comprise between 0% to –10% with MRI tagging and if the hypocaptation has a value inferior to 55-60% with SPECT Thallium Imaging.

5. Conclusions

This work demonstrates the ability of the cardiac tagging sequence to provide a good estimate of the left ventricular ejection fraction when compared with results obtained from standard cine MRI and contrast cine angiography. Indeed quick analysis can be realized because tracking the different markers (HARP software) is faster than segmenting the LV placing markers along tag lines and adjusting these markers along the different frames (FindTags). Cardiac tagging thus provides us information on both, regional and global cardiac function with high reliability without increasing the acquisition time.

Acknowledgements

Swiss National Science Foundation (grant 31-57020.99) for partial support, HUG Research and Development Funds 1999. Nael F. Osman, Department of Electrical and Computer Engineering, Center for Imaging Science, The Johns Hopkins University, Baltimore, Maryland. David Foxall, Philips Medical System, 595 MinerRd, Cleveland, OH4143.

References

1. N.F. Osman, W.S. Kerwin, E.R. McVeigh, and J.L. Prince, "Cardiac motion tracking using CINE harmonic phase (HARP) magnetic resonance imaging", *Magnetic Resonance in Medicine*, 42, 1048-1060, 1999.
2. Guttman MA, Zerhouni EA, McVeigh ER, "Analysis and visualization of cardiac function from MR images", *IEEE Comp. Graph Appl.*, 17(1): 30-38, 1997.

Advances in Cardiovascular MRI and MSCT
– A NASCI Symposium

CARS 2002 – H.U. Lemke, M.W. Vannier; K. Inamura, A.G. Farman, K. Doi & J.H.C. Reiber (Editors)

Correlation of quantitative MR-angiography of the carotid artery with in vivo measurement during carotid endarterectomy

R. Guzman [a], A. Barth [a], L Remonda [b], J.P.H. de Koning [c], R.J. van der Geest [c], H. Oswald [b] and G. Schroth [b]

[a]Department of Neurosurgery, University of Bern, Bern, Switzerland
[b]Department of Neuroradiology, University of Bern, Bern, Switzerland
Department of Radiology[3], University of Leiden, Leiden, The Netherlands

Abstract

Objectives: Continuous quality control of carotid endarterectomy (CEA) for atherothrombotic stenosis is mandatory to improve the safety and efficiency of this operation. Noninvasive quantitative measurement of vessel lumen enlargement would enable a systematic objective assessment of the operative results. For this purpose, we performed postoperative control of patients with high-grade carotid artery stenosis with magnetic resonance angiography (MRA). A new software to segment vessels in 3D-MRA data, based on the wavefront propagation algorithm, was used. The results of the automated measurements on MRA were correlated with direct intraoperative determination of the vessel diameter. *Method:* In a prospective series of 15 patients undergoing CEA, the diameter of the common and internal carotid arteries was measured at a distance of 1cm from the bifurcation. All patients had a radiological control with gadolinium-enhanced 3D-MRA within 4 days after surgery. A new software allowing automated segmentation and quantification of 3D-MRA data was used to measure the cross-sections of the common and internal carotid arteries. Based on the surface of the cross-sections the vessel diameter was calculated. A correlation of vessel diameters as determined intraoperatively and on 3D-MRA was performed. *Results:* Statistical analysis showed no significant difference between intraoperative and 3D-MRA diameter determination. The mean diameter ($\pm$SEM) of the common carotid artery was 10.1$\pm$0.4mm as measured intraoperatively and 10.0$\pm$0.5mm as calculated on 3D-MRA. For the internal carotid artery the mean diameter ($\pm$SEM) was 6.7$\pm$0.4mm vs. 7.0$\pm$0.4mm for intraoperative and 3D-MRA respectively. Intraoperative and 3D-MRA data were found to highly correlate with a correlation factor of r=0.90 for the common and r=0.96 for the internal carotid artery measurements. *Conclusions:* This new automated segmentation and quantification software for 3D-MRA analysis allows accurate measurements of vessel dimensions.

Keywords: Carotid artery; MRA; vessel segmentation

1. Introduction

Continuous control and assessment of surgical results are necessary to insure the quality of carotid endarterectomy (CEA) and to improve its efficacy for stroke prevention.

CARS 2002 – H.U. Lemke, M.W. Vannier; K. Inamura, A.G. Farman, K. Doi & J.H.C. Reiber (Editors)

918

Overall quality of CEA is not only determined by the perioperative occurrence of neurological complications, but also depends on the quality of the reconstruction of the stenosed bifurcation. Invasive methods such as digital subtraction angiography (DSA) are not appropriate to systematically assess the morphological results of carotid bifurcation reconstruction. However, magnetic resonance angiography (MRA) combined with Doppler ultrasonography offers a non-invasive possibility to assess the morphological results of CEA. In order to perform quantitative analysis we used a newly developed software (University of Leiden [1]), for automated segmentation and measurement of blood vessels based on 3D-MRA data. A clinical correlation analysis between vessel measurements performed on DSA and MRA in order to validate the results obtained with this new software was published earlier [2]. A statistically significant correlation could be demonstrated between DSA and automated MRA vessel measurements [2]. To further ascertain the value and accuracy of this new software we wanted to correlate intraoperative vessel measurements to quantitative analysis of MRA. In the present prospective study, we performed intraoperative measurements on the reconstructed carotid arteries in a consecutive series of 15 patients operated on for high grade carotid artery stenosis. All patients received a postoperative MRA which was analysed using the new segmentation software. Correlation of vessel diameter as obtained intraoperatively and on 3D-MRA was performed.

2. Methods

2.1 Patients and treatment characteristics

We prospectively analyzed 15 patients who underwent CEA for high-grade carotid artery stenosis. Mean age was 68 years, 11 male and 4 female. CEA was performed on the left side in 7 patients and on the right side in 8 patients. After removal of the plaque, the arteriotomy was closed with a running 6-0 Prolene suture without any venous or artificial patch [3]. The diameter of the common (CCA) and internal carotid artery (ICA) was measured at a distance of 1cm from the carotid bifurcation using a vernier caliper. All patients had a radiological control with gadolinium-enhanced 3D-MRA within 4 days after surgery.

2.2 MR angiographic techniques and image postprocessing

All MRA investigations were performed on a 1.5 T imaging system equipped with a gradient overdrive (Magnetom Vision, Siemens Medical System, Erlangen, Germany). The maximum achievable gradient amplitude was 25 mT/m and the slew rate was 180 T/m/sec. A spoiled 3D fast low-angle shot (FLASH) MR-angiography was performed by using a 4 x 2 circularly polarized phased array neck coil. The sequence was performed with 32-36 coronal partitions each 1.94-2.5mm thick, 2.84-3.15 ms repetition time T_R, 1.03-1.11 ms echo time T_E, 35-40° flip angle, 70x140x280 mm^3 FOV by a36 x 92 x 256 image matrix and a scan time of 9-9.5 sec [4]. Four consecutive 3D images were performed, starting at approximately 3 seconds after the start of the bolus injection of 0.1 mmol/kg gadodiamide (Omniscan, Hafslund Nycomed, Oslo, Norway).

A new software allowing automated segmentation and quantification of 3D-MRA (University of Leiden) data was used to measure the cross-sections of the common and internal carotid arteries [1]. After loading the series with arterial phase, the MRA data are

CARS 2002 – H.U. Lemke, M.W. Vannier; K. Inamura, A.G. Farman, K. Doi & J.H.C. Reiber (Editors)
ᶜCARS/Springer. All rights reserved.

initially presented as the three orthogonal maximal intensity projection images (MIPs) and a 3D view of the same MIPs. The segmentation algorithm needs a start and end-point to define the vessel of interest. After segmentation and 3D reconstruction of the vessel the software calculates the cross-sections along the vessel pathway as displayed in Figure 1. The results are given in graphical and numeric way. Based on the surface of the cross-sections of the CCA and the ICA at a distance of 1cm from the carotid bifurcation the vessel diameter was calculated.

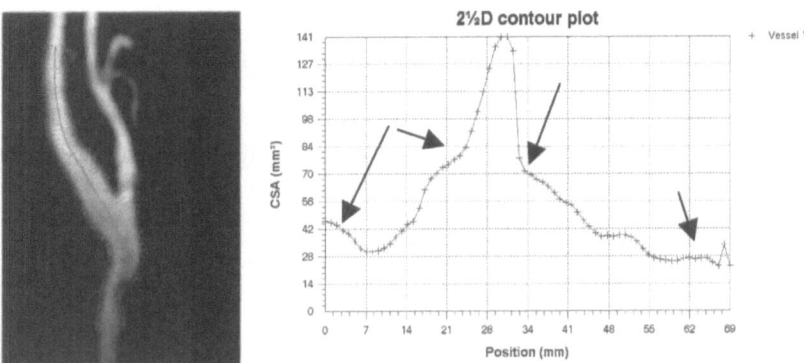

Figure 1: On the left panel a 2D-MIP image of the carotid bifurcation is shown with contours displayed, each representing a cross-sectional measurement along the vessel pathway. On the right panel the corresponding plot is shown with the vessel cross-section [CSA] on the y-axis for each point along the vessel pathway and the relative position [in mm] on the x-axis. CCA, common carotid artery; ICA, internal carotid artery.

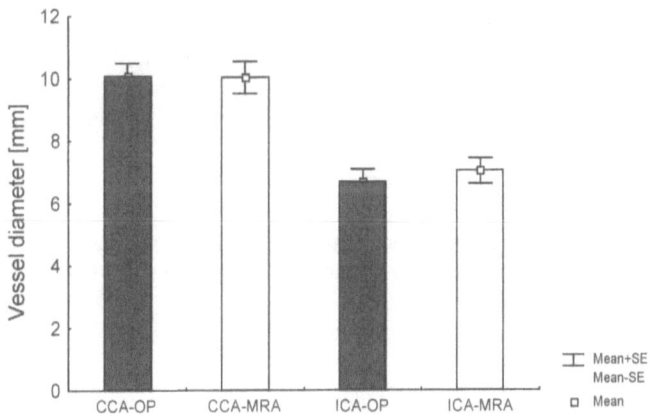

Figure 2: Bar plot showing the mean diameter (±SEM) of the common carotid artery (CCA) and the internal carotid artery (ICA) as measured intraoperatively (-OP) and on 3D-MRA data (-MRA).

CARS 2002 – H.U. Lemke, M.W. Vannier; K. Inamura, A.G. Farman, K. Doi & J.H.C. Reiber (Editors)

920

3. Results

No patient suffered adverse effects from intraoperative vessel measurement or postoperative radiological investigation. The diameter of 15 CCAs and ICAs were available for the statistical evaluation. The mean diameter (±SEM) of the CCA was 10.1±0.4mm as measured intraoperatively and 10.0±0.5mm as calculated on 3D-MRA. For the ICA the mean diameter (±SEM) was 6.7±0.4mm vs. 7.0±0.4mm for intraoperative and 3D-MRA respectively (Figure 2). The mean difference between the intraoperative and 3D-MRA measured diameters for the CCA was 1.43% and for the ICA 10.45%. Statistical analysis showed no significant difference between intraoperative and 3D-MRA diameter determination (Figure 2).

3D-MRA and Intraoperative data were found to be highly correlated with a factor of $r=0.94$ for the common carotid artery (Figure 3) and $r=0.95$ for the internal carotid artery (Figure 4) measurements (95% CI, $p<0.05$).

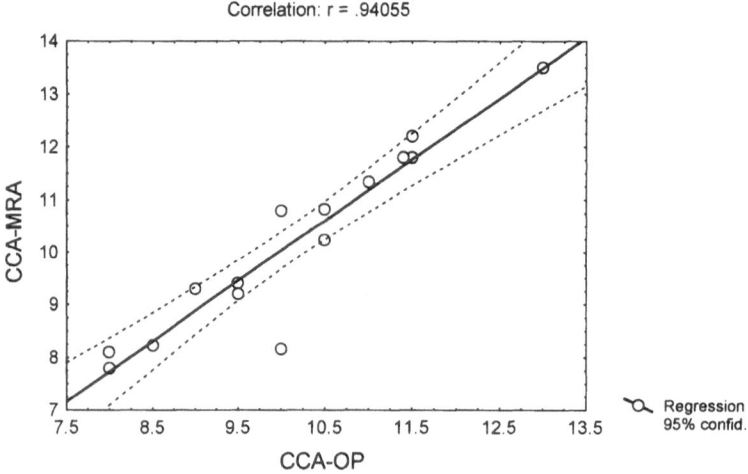

Figure 3: Scatterplot showing the correlation of the diameter as measured on 3D-MRA (-MRA) and intraoperatively (-OP) for the common carotid artery (CCA).

4. Discussion

Surgical quality assessment is an important means to judge for the success of carotid endarterectomy. MRA offers a non-invasive method to investigate the carotid morphology after endarterectomy. Besides the qualitative evaluation of MIPs, we wanted to quantify the vessel lumen expansion after CEA. In view of this question we tested a new software for automated vessel segmentation and quantification based on contrast enhanced 3D-MRA data. In order to prove the accuracy of this segmentation and quantification software we conducted a series of validation studies.

CARS 2002 – H.U. Lemke, M.W. Vannier; K. Inamura, A.G. Farman, K. Doi & J.H.C. Reiber (Editors)

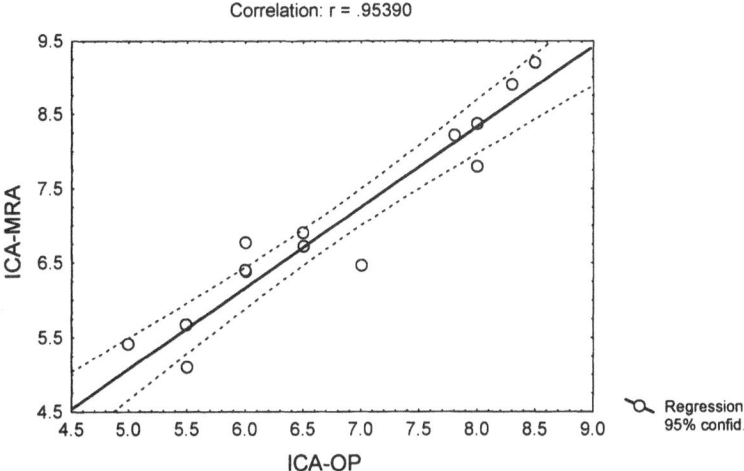

Figure 4 Scatterplot showing the correlation of the diameter as measured on 3D-MRA (-MRA) and intraoperatively (-OP) for the internal carotid artery (ICA).

At the University of Leiden measurements on phantoms were performed, comparing contrast enhanced 3D-MRA with X-ray DSA [1]. It was concluded that the quantification of vessel diameter using the new segmentation software did not differ more than 1% of comparable measurements in X-ray DSA. Thereafter a retrospective clinical validation study on 10 patients was performed, correlating vessel diameter measurements on X-ray DSA, 2D-MIPs and 3D-MRA data using the new software [2]. A statistically significant correlation between X-ray DSA and automated 3D-MRA measurements (r=0.82, p<0.05) was found [2]. Furthermore due to automated evaluation interobserver variability was eliminated. In the present prospective study on 15 patients undergoing CEA for high grade carotid stenosis, we demonstrated that direct intraoperative vessel diameter measurements are highly correlated to vessel diameter obtained with the automated 3D-MRA analysis with a r of 0.95 and a r of 0.94 for the CCA and for the ICA, respectively. Differences between intraoperative measurements which assess the outer vessel diamter and MRA measurements which presumably assess the inner vessel diameter, were found not to alter the outcome. Hence introducing a correction factor for vessel wall thickness did not change the results.

In conclusion we can summarize that quantitative analysis of contrast enhanced 3D-MRA data using this new segmentation software is reproducible and highly accurate in clinical patient data.

CARS 2002 – H.U. Lemke, M.W. Vannier; K. Inamura, A.G. Farman, K. Doi & J.H.C. Reiber (Editors)

922

References

1. J.A. Schaap, P.J.H. de Koning, R.J. van der Geest, J.H.C. Reiber, 3D Quantification and visualization of MRA. In: Computer Assisted Radiology and Surgery 2001. Proceedings of the 15th International Congress and Exhibition. Lemke HU, Vannier MW, Inamura K, Farman AG, Doi K (Eds), International Congress Series (1230); 928-933, Elsevier, Amsterdam, 2001

2. R. Guzman, H. Oswald, A. Barth, P.J.H. de Koning, L. Remonda, KO. Lövblad, G. Schroth, Clinical validation of quantitative carotid MRA. In: Computer Assisted Radiology and Surgery 2001. Proceedings of the 15th International Congress and Exhibition. Lemke HU, Vannier MW, Inamura K, Farman AG, Doi K (Eds), International Congress Series (1230); 934-937, Elsevier, Amsterdam, 2001,

3. A.Barth, L. Remonda, KO. Lövblad, G. Schroth, RW Seiler, Silent cerebral ischemia detected by diffusion-weighted MRI after carotid endarterectomy, Stroke 31 (2000) 1824-1828

4. L. Remonda, O. Heid, G. Schroth, Carotid artery stenosis, occlusion, and pseudo-occlusion: First-pass, gadolinium-enhanced, three-dimensional MR angiography – preliminary study, Radiology 209 (1) (1998) 95-102

CARS 2002 – H.U. Lemke, M.W. Vannier; K. Inamura, A.G. Farman, K. Doi & J.H.C. Reiber (Editors)

Model-based vessel segmentation using an elliptic cylinder

Stewart Young[a], Vladimir Pekar[a], Jürgen Weese[b], Thomas Netsch[a],
Arianne van Muiswinkel[c]

[a] Philips Research Laboratories, Röntgenstrasse 24-26, 22335 Hamburg, Germany
[b] Philips Research Laboratories, Weisshausstrasse 2, 52066 Aachen, Germany
[c] Philips Medical Systems, Veenpluis 4-6, NL-568 DA Best, The Netherlands

Abstract

For viewing vascular structures in 3D MRA with bloodpool contrast agent via maximum intensity projection, it is necessary to suppress other occluding vessels which are also contrasted. These can be located very close to the vessels of interest. In this paper, an automated selection method based on the use of an elliptically cross-sectioned cylinder model is proposed. This model of local shape is used to define the speed function for a front propagation algorithm, which extracts a vessel axis between two selected points. The boundary is then reconstructed using local shape parameters from the fitted cylinder model. A comparison of automated and manual segmentations showed a mean selection accuracy of 94% using elliptical model, and a mean surface deviation of 1.1mm.

Keywords: MRA bloodpool contrast agents, vessel separation, front propagation

1. Introduction

The visualisation and quantification of complex 3D vessel structures in magnetic resonance angiography (MRA) images is important for diagnosis of vascular pathologies such as aneurysms and stenoses. Maximum intensity projection (MIP) is the most common method for viewing this type of data. The use of MRA bloodpool contrast agents, which have an extended intravascular half-life, enables higher spatial resolution since imaging can occur during the steady-state of contrast agent diffusion. However, since both arteries and veins are highlighted, the important diagnostic information can be occluded in the MIP by other large, bright vessels in the same viewing direction.

In order to improve the visualization, the occluding vessels can be segmented and then suppressed during MIP generation. A widespread approach for vessel selection (e.g. [1]) is based on the eigen-values and eigen-vectors of the Hessian matrix, which are used to classify the local image structure. A scale-selection method is needed to detect structures across a range of radii. However, the segmentation of individual vessels is often complicated by the close proximity of other vessels, leading to partial voluming and thus merging of the high contrast image regions corresponding to the separate objects. This effect is amplified at larger scales, leading to problems in distinguishing between separate objects.

We propose an alternative approach for vessel selection that is based on a cylindrical shape model integrated into a front propagation scheme. The method extracts a path along the axis of a vessel of interest, and then measurements of the local shape along this axis are combined to reconstruct the vessel volume. In [2], it was shown that this algorithm

924

(using a circular cylinder model) obtains a significantly more accurate vessel axis estimate, in comparison to a Hessian-based method. Here, the vessel model is extended to include an elliptical cross-section (a so-called elliptical cylinder). While a circular cylinder is a fairly representative local model for a typical vessel section, the cross-sectional profile can also deviate significantly. Although profile shapes which are not well modelled by an ellipse may also occur, the additional flexibility of this model over a circular cross-section leads to a significant improvement in the segmentation, enabling the propagating front to explore vessel sections with highly eccentric cross-section profiles.

2. Methods

A structure of interest is indicated by placing a seed point at each end of the vessel section. The algorithm extracts a path along the vessel between these seed points. The vessel boundary is then reconstructed using measurements determined during path estimation.

2.1 Front propagation
A front propagation approach [3] is used to determine the 'shortest path', with respect to a cost function defined on local image properties, between two seed points within the vessel of interest. The region surrounding each of these points is iteratively expanded according to the local speed response, $F(\mathbf{p})$, and then the time of arrival of the front, $T(\mathbf{p})$, at newly included voxels is determined by the solving following propagation equation

$$|\nabla T|F = 1 \qquad (1)$$

Once the two regions surrounding the seed points meet, the minimal time path is traced to determine the vessel axis estimate. Therefore, to ensure that propagation occurs fastest along the vessel axis, the response measure should be largest on axis and negligible outside the object. We propose the use of a geometrical elliptical cylinder model to define this measure.

2.2 Vesselness response
An elliptical cylinder can be specified via its location, axis orientation, the orientation of the ellipse's major axis, and the major and minor radii (a fixed cylinder length of 4 voxel spacings is used, since the model is valid only locally). In order to define the vesselness response at a given image location, $\mathbf{p}$, locally optimal model parameters are determined via model adaptation. Given an *initial estimate* for the axis orientation, $\mathbf{a}$, a set of feature points, $\tilde{\mathbf{x}}_{i,j}$ (i=1,..,N_i, j=1,..,N_j), on the vessel border are extracted along surface normals, $\mathbf{n}_i$, perpendicular to the axis, at discrete steps, l_j, along the axis:

$$\tilde{\mathbf{x}}_{i,j} = \mathbf{p} + l_j\mathbf{a} + \delta\mathbf{n}_i \underset{k=1...r_{max}}{\arg\min} \{Dk^2\delta^2 \cdot f(\mathbf{p} + l\mathbf{a} + k\delta\mathbf{n}_i)\} \qquad (2)$$

where δ is the sample spacing, D is a weighting parameter and $f(x)$ is an appropriate feature response (e.g. gradient along the normal). An updated axis estimate, $\mathbf{a}'$, is determined using the extracted feature points, according to

CARS 2002 – H.U. Lemke, M.W. Vannier; K. Inamura, A.G. Farman, K. Doi & J.H.C. Reiber (Editors)

$$\mathbf{a'} = \sum_i (\tilde{x}_{i,1} - \tilde{x}_{i,N_j}) \Big/ \Big| \sum_i (\tilde{x}_{i,1} - \tilde{x}_{i,N_j}) \Big| \tag{3}$$

Then the remaining model parameters are computed by projecting the feature points onto a plane perpendicular to this updated direction, and fitting an ellipse. Performing the feature search in a set of planes spaced along the axis provides an important advantage over previously proposed methods (e.g. [4, 5]) where features are extracted in only one plane at a time, since it allows the local orientation to be updated directly.

The adapted model is used to determine the vesselness response, defined using the sum of residual distances between each feature point and the model, combined with the integrated image gradient across the model surface:

$$F(\mathbf{p}) = \exp\left(-\sum_{i,j} (\tilde{\mathbf{x}}_{i,j} - \mathbf{s}_{i,j})^2 \Big/ \mu \mathbf{s}_{i,j}^{\;2}\right)\left\{1 - \exp\left(-\sum_{i,j} f(\tilde{\mathbf{x}}_{i,j}) \big/ \upsilon\right)\right\} \tag{4}$$

where $\mathbf{s}_{i,j}$ are model surface points along the normals, and the parameters μ, υ control the sensitivity to the respective terms. This approach yields the largest response on the vessel axis, as the sum of the residual distances increases as the model centre deviates from the centre of the vessel's cross-section.

Combining this model-based response with a front propagation scheme has some interesting implications. Firstly, the information extracted at one location on the front can be passed to neighbouring locations as the front expands into previously unexplored regions, to provide an initial estimate for the adaptation process described above (at the seed points, the estimates can be derived, for example, by exhaustive search). Another property of the method is that once a path along the vessel has been determined, the local structure parameters at the path points can be used directly to reconstruct the vessel boundary (for example, a mesh representation of the surface). These parameters can also be directly applied to obtain quantitative measurements of the vessel morphology, such as the degree of arterial thinning in a stenotic region.

3. Results

The method was validated via comparison with five manual vessel segmentations, in which the main arteries and veins of a blood-pool MRA data set were delineated. The original images were re-sampled to obtain isotropic data, from original image dimensions of 512x512x60 voxels of size 0.9x0.9x1.8mm. Since it is typically the arteries which are of diagnostic interest, the main venous branches (left and right) were segmented in each image to provide a total of 10 test vessels. An example MIP with both the main venous branches suppressed is shown on the right hand side of figure 1. Seed points were placed in the major veins, the axis path was extracted via front propagation, and then the vessel boundary was reconstructed using the local shape parameters to obtain a triangulated mesh surface representation. The region within this boundary was extracted to define the final vessel segmentation, which was suppressed during MIP generation.

926

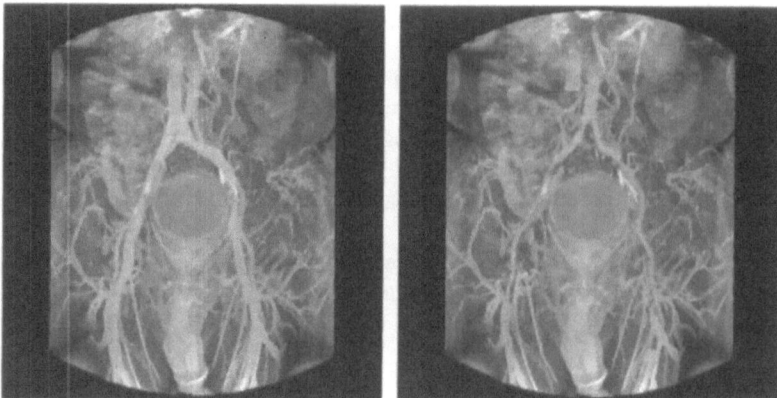

Figure 1: MIPs before (left) and after (right) suppression of the left and right iliac venous branches

A quantitative assessment of the segmentation quality was obtained using the overlap between manually and automatically segmented venous regions. The mean (manually) segmented vein volume was approximately 40,000 voxels. In order to obtain the vessel of interest from the *manual* segmentation, connected branches were first pruned by placing rectangular exclusion regions over the beginning of the branching to obtain a single connected region. Another consideration regards the extent of over-selection of nearby arteries in the automated segmentation. It is important to assess the false positive selection, since suppression of other nearby structures (or parts thereof) can directly affect the visual quality of the resulting MIP (a complete vessel selection could easily be obtained at the expense of selecting large parts of other nearby vessels). To permit comparison of the arterial selection across datasets, the selection fraction was normalised

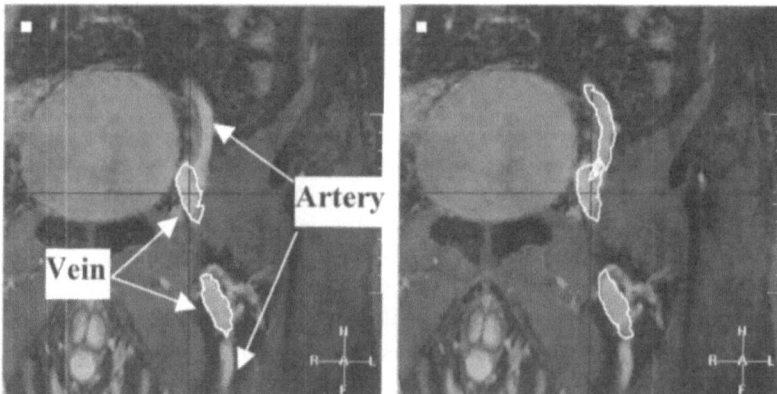

Figure 2: Image slices with the boundaries of the selected regions superimposed in white, obtained using elliptical (left) and circular (right) cylinder models. Note that the path followed by the circular model jumps into the artery, while the elliptical model constrains the path to the vessel of interest.

CARS 2002 – H.U. Lemke, M.W. Vannier; K. Inamura, A.G. Farman, K. Doi & J.H.C. Reiber (Editors)
©CARS/Springer. All rights reserved.

with respect to the total selected *vein* volume. Table 1 compares the selection results obtained using circular and elliptical cylinder models. In two of the ten test cases, while the elliptical model yielded a correct selection, the circular model failed to extract a valid path, instead jumping into the nearby artery for a short section. An example is seen in figure 2. These cases were excluded from the presented results, in order not to bias the comparison statistics. Another consequence of the introduction of the elliptical model is reduced selection of nearby structures. In previously reported results [2], the extracted mesh representation, obtained with the circular cylinder approach, was refined by deformable model adaptation, in order to improve the selection result. However, this adaptation also resulted in increased artery selection. The introduction of the elliptical cylinder improves on the selection achieved using the deformable model refinement, while simultaneously reducing the degree of arterial selection, since mesh adaptation is no longer required.

4. Conclusions

In this paper we present a novel approach for vessel segmentation that allows occluding structures to be suppressed in MIP visualizations. An elliptical cylinder model for local vessel structure is used to achieve discrimination between very closely separated vessel structures. This model is used to define the speed function for a front propagation segmentation scheme. This allows local structure information, such as radius and orientation, to be propagated along the vessel to initialise model adaptation at the next location. The use of an elliptical cross-section improves vessel selection, compared to a circular cross-section, yielding 94% selection. The method also enables the quantification of vessel pathologies, since local shape parameters (radius, eccentricity) are available along the vessel's axis.

Acknowledgements

The authors thank Dr. Toombs and Dr. Flamm from St. Luke's Episcopal Hospital, Houston, USA for providing MRI blood pool contrast images.

References

1. A. Frangi, W. Niessen, K. Vincken, and M. Viergever, "Multiscale vessel enhancement filtering", MICCAI 1998, 130--137, Cambridge, MA, 1998.
2. S. Young, V. Pekar and J. Weese, "Vessel segmentation for visualization of MRA with blood pool contrast agents", MICCAI 2001, 491-498, Utrecht, October 2001.
3. R. Malladi and J. Sethian, "A real-time algorithm for medical shape recovery", Proc. 8th Int. Conf. on Computer Vision, 304-310, Bombay, India, 1998.
4. O. Wink, W. Niessen, and M. Viergever, "Fast delineation and visualization of vessels in 3D angiographic images", IEEE Trans. Medical Imaging, 19(4):337-346, 2000.
5. B. Verdonck, I. Bloch, H. Maitre, D. Vandermeulen, G. Marchal. "A New System for Blood Vessel Segmentation and Visualization in 3D MR and Spiral CT Angiography", CAR'95, 177-182, June 1995.

CARS 2002 – H.U. Lemke, M.W. Vannier; K. Inamura, A.G. Farman, K. Doi & J.H.C. Reiber (Editors)

928

Integration of cath-lab signals and magnetic resonance imaging for postoperative computerized assessment of heart reduction

Andrea Ripoli, Sergio Berti, Nael Olsen[a], Massimo Lombardi, Stefano
Bevilacqua, Mattia Glauber

CNR, Institute of Clinical Physiology, "G. Pasquinucci" Hospital, Massa, Italy

[a] Johns Hopkins University, Department of Radiology, Baltimore, USA

Abstract

To treat end-stage cardiomyopathy, cardiac transplantation is not widely available, mainly because of shortage of donors. A number of non-transplant cardiac operations have been proposed, from partial left ventriculectomy to mitral annuloplasty, from dynamic cardiomyoplasty to endoventricular plasty. The evaluation of the impact of this kind of procedures on left ventricular performance is an important, and as yet elusive, goal. Because left ventricular geometry and volume change significantly after cardiac non-transplant surgery, both regional and global ventricular function result deeply affected by the treatment; moreover, the surgical procedures differently affect systolic and diastolic performance, improving ejection and worsening filling. To assess the effect of a surgical remodeling procedure performed in "G. Pasquinucci" Hospital, the information available from cath-lab study and Magnetic Resonance imaging have been merged in an unique software environment, obtaining a quick and easy to use computerized tool. The regional ventricular function has been investigated exploiting magnetic resonance tagging images; the global function has been studied, according to time-varying elastance theory, processing the pressure-volume loops acquired in cath-lab. The developed software has been exploited to investigate the patients who underwent a ventricular remodeling procedure, furnishing insights about the relation between ventricular shape and function.

Keywords: Magnetic resonance tagging, cath-lab, ventricular function.

1. Introduction

Heart failure represents a world-wide emergency, each year, in the United States alone, more than 500.000 new cases occur, with a 5-years survival of about 50%; these dramatic epidemiological data has pushed clinicians and surgeons towards the investigation of new techniques for the treatment of heart failure [1]. Particularly, in the last years, surgical procedures of left ventricular remodeling have been introduced. In partial left-ventriculectomy [2] a viable muscle section of the open beating heart is excised, and the wound is closed by direct suture; in mitral repair the valve is surgically reconstructed, eliminating the leak towards the atrium by means of an over-corrective mitral ring [3]; in endoventricular patch plasty, the ischemic region is removed and the ventricular shape is

CARS 2002 – H.U. Lemke, M.W. Vannier; K. Inamura, A.G. Farman, K. Doi & J.H.C. Reiber (Editors)

restored inserting a Dacron patch [4]; new devices, to be placed around and inside the heart, have been proposed to contain the dilatation of the failing ventricle [5].

All these procedures aim at a global reduction of dilated ventricular chamber and at a restoration of the normal ventricular geometry. While the reduction of wall stress, the immediate consequence of the volume reduction, appears as the clear improvement furnished by the surgical remodeling, its major effect on the complex relation between shape and function of the heart remains to be evaluated on the single patient. A postoperative adverse shape, resulting in increased regional wall tension, generates mechanical disadvantages, inevitably leading to a new ventricular dilatation; even if all postoperative hemodynamic data show a marked improvement.

In order to establish the net effect of ventricular remodeling, to potentially predict the long-term result of the intervention, a computerized system has been developed for an accurate, quantitative and fast assessment of both global and regional ventricular function, exploiting the pressure-volume loops, acquired during an invasive cath-lab study, and noninvasive tagged Magnetic Resonance Imagining (MRI). By integrating of cath-lab signals and magnetic resonance imaging, the ventricular function can be investigated contemporaneously exploiting the two milestones of cardiac mechanics: the time varying-elastance theory and the stress-strain relationship of ventricular wall.

2. Methods

To assess the global ventricular function on the basis of the time-varying elastance theory, a computerized system for the acquisition and the analysis of the pressure-volume loops has been developed. A fluid-filled catheter was used to measure the aortic pressure. Ventricular pressure has been acquired by means of a catheter-tip piezoelectric transducer (Sentron, Inc.). Ventricular volume has been measured by a 12-electrodes conductance catheter (CardioDynamics, Leycom, Inc.). The conductance catheter was interfaced by a Leycom Sigma-5DF signal conditioner–processor (CardioDynamics, Leycom, Inc.), to continuously estimate left ventricular volume.

To avoid problems regarding safety, the cath-lab acquisition system has been based on a battery powered notebook PC. We used a Pentium ® II 366 MHz, with 256 MB RAM and 3 Gbyte HD. The signals have been acquired by means of a PCMCI 12-bit multifunction DAQCard-700 (National Instruments, Austin, Texas). Both acquisition and on-line processing of the signals have been performed by a program developed in LabView (National Instruments, Austin, Texas) environment.

Due to the critical conditions of the investigated patients, particular attention has been devoted to the fulfillment of a quick and reliable acquisition protocol. A completely automatic calibration procedure for the pressure transducers and for the conductance catheter has been performed; the transient vena cava occlusion, otherwise required for the change of preload, necessary to evaluate the end-systolic and end-diastolic pressure-volume relations, has been avoided, exploiting new developed algorithms. End-systolic elastance has been evaluated by means of a bilinearly approximated time-varying

CARS 2002 – H.U. Lemke, M.W. Vannier; K. Inamura, A.G. Farman, K. Doi & J.H.C. Reiber (Editors)
ᶜCARS/Springer. All rights reserved.

930

elastance waveform [6], while the end-diastolic stiffness has been assessed by the nonlinear fitting of the diastasis part of the pressure-volume loop, using a Levenberg-Marquardt algorithm. The algorithms for beat-to-beat evaluation of left ventricular mechanics parameters have been tested, comparing their results with the ones obtained by well accepted multibeats measurements. The comparison has been performed with the data acquired in two patients, where transient vena cava occlusion has been performed (Figure 1).

The acquired signals (ECG, left ventricular pressure, aortic pressure, total and segmental ventricular volumes) have been on-line displayed and processed, giving important information about the correct placement of the conductance catheter inside the ventricle. On a beat-to-beat basis, all the major parameters of the global ventricular function and energetics have been extracted (end-systolic elastance, end-diastolic stiffness, ventricular dead volume, isovolumic relaxation time, effective aortic elastance, pressure and volume values, mean systolic ejection ratio, time derivatives of the ventricular pressure, stroke work, potential energy, pressure volume area).

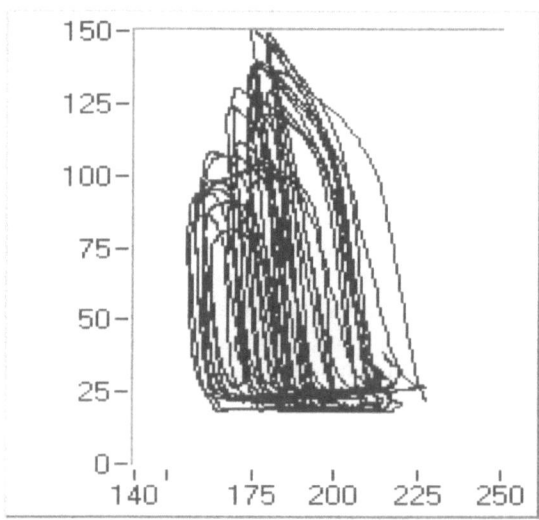

Figure 1. Preoperative pressure-volume loops acquired during transient vena cava occlusion.

To assess the regional function, the Harmonic Phase (HARP) MRI method has been exploited [7]. While tagged MRI of the heart is recognized as a valuable technique for the quantitative noninvasive assessment of regional myocardial performance (Figure 2), its clinical use has been limited by traditional time-consuming and observer-dependent analytical techniques. HARP imaging approach has been demonstrated to overcome these drawbacks, resulting in a fast and automated procedure of analysis. By means of Fourier

CARS 2002 – H.U. Lemke, M.W. Vannier; K. Inamura, A.G. Farman, K. Doi & J.H.C. Reiber (Editors)
ᶜCARS/Springer. All rights reserved.

filtering, specific regions in the spectrum of the tagged images are extracted, producing complex images whose phase values are directly related to the motion; the resulting harmonic phase images can be used to track the motion and measure myocardial strain in both Lagrangian and Eulerian sense.

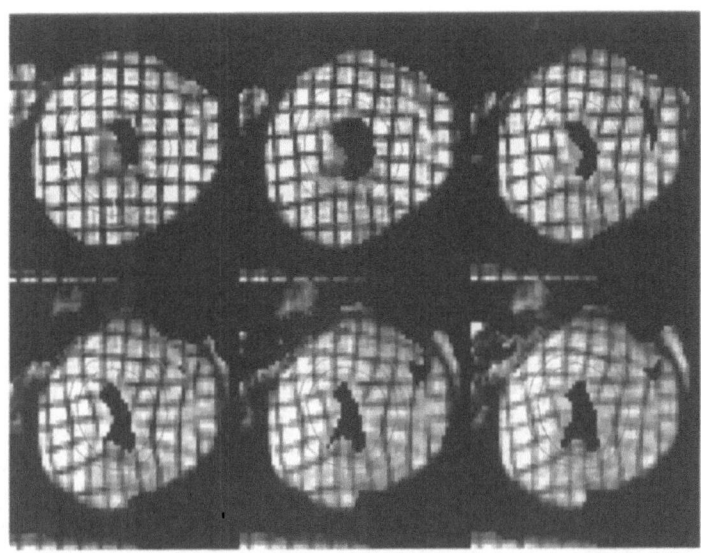

Figure 2. Magnetic resonance tagging: progressive deformation throughout systole.

The acquisition protocol allowed us to imagine 4 slices within 4 breath-holds (from 15 to 20 seconds each). The scanner settings were: field of view 36 cm, tag separation 6 mm, slice thickness 8 mm, TR 6.5 msec, TE 2.3 msec, tip angle 15°, image matrix 256x256, with 7 phase-encoded views per movie frame and cardiac cycle.

The images, acquired on a 1.5-T whole-body magnet (Signa, General Electric Medical Systems), were analyzed by an ad-hoc developed Matlab (The Mathworks, Inc.) program, implementing the HARP method. The software automatically performed the Fourier Transform and the filtering of the tagged images, furnishing, in the selected number of wall segments, Lagrangian and Eulerian, circumferential and radial strain, computed at endocardium, midwall and epicardium. The full assessment of myocardial strains in a single slice took less than 1 minutes, on a Pentium III PC (1GHz).

The same Matlab program performed the off-line processing of the hemodynamic data and a 3D reconstruction (Figure 3) of the ventricle, segmenting by a "snake" algorithm the tagged MR images, in this way realizing an unique integrated assessment environment for the ventricular function. Informed patient consent was obtained for insertion of the catheters and for magnetic resonance analysis.

932

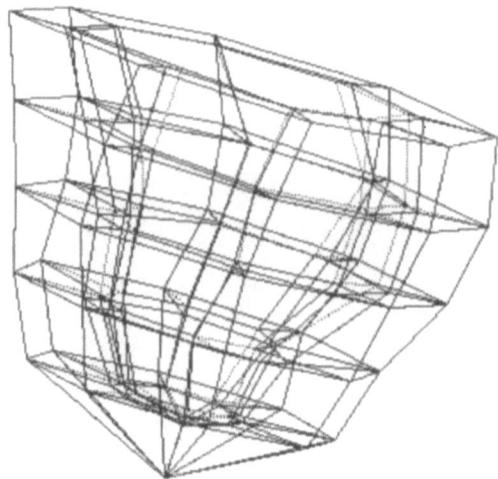

Figure 3. Left ventricular 3D reconstruction from magnetic resonance images.

3. Results

The computerized system has been tested with the preoperative and postoperative studies accomplished on 5 patients who underwent an heart reduction procedure, consisting in an apical reshaping of the ventricular chamber, without the use of Dacron patch. The preoperative studies highlighted, in each patient, a depressed global ventricular function and a marked apical wall motion abnormality. The postoperative studies showed, in each patient, an improvement of systolic function (i.e., an augmented end-systolic elastance) and a further deterioration of the diastolic function (i.e., an augmented diastolic stiffness), with an overall balancing leading to an increase in the global ventricular function, as emphasized by the augmented Frank-Starling relation, computed in two patients by transient vena cava occlusion. The tagging analysis showed that regional function improved both in the apical remodeled zone and in the remote equatorial and basal zone (i.e. a rise of both Lagrangian and Eulerian strain) (Table 1), pointing out a better arrangement of the fibers in the whole ventricle, as a consequence of the apical morphological changes. If the regional improvement happened in each patient, different was its amount in different subjects; in detail, the remote improvement was less significant in patients who had a more marked worsening of global diastolic function. Even if any statistical consideration is obviously premature, the analyzed cases suggest a major attention for the follow-up of patients with a lower increase of remote regional strain and a greater increase of global diastolic stiffness.

	Preoperative	Postoperative
Basis	-0.131 ± 0.0214	-0.163 ± 0.0394
Equator	-0.122 ± 0.0243	-0.178 ± 0.0412
Apex	-0.072 ± 0.0061	-0.152 ± 0.0212

Table 1. HARP computed preoperative and postoperative circumferential shortening.

CARS 2002 – H.U. Lemke, M.W. Vannier; K. Inamura, A.G. Farman, K. Doi & J.H.C. Reiber (Editors)
ᶜCARS/Springer. All rights reserved.

4. Conclusions

The preliminary results of the developed computerized systems are in agreement with the literature reported considerations about the heart reduction procedure, besides furnishing further information, potentially useful to predict the long-term result of the single surgical intervention. The Matlab developed interface and the obtained speed of the computation resulted in an easy to use tool for clinicians and surgeons; the graphical representation of the numerical results, joined to the 3D reconstruction of the ventricular motion, allowed an immediate comprehension of the heart conditions. The general model of ventricular global and regional function (i.e. the time-varying elastance theory and the stress-strain relationship), exploited in the development of the computerized system for the assessment of ventricular state, allows its the use even out of surgically oriented considerations. The accomplished 3D reconstruction of the ventricle volume, by means of the segmented MR images, and the single-beat developed algorithms, for the evaluation of left ventricular function, suggest the possibility of creating a completely noninvasive tool for the assessment of the heart function, evaluating pressure by a noninvasive transducer. A complete noninvasive instrumentation would be of great importance in the study of critically ill patients, before and immediately after the surgical procedure.

References

1. Westaby S, "Non-transplant surgery for heart failure", *Heart*, 83, 603-610, 2000.
2. Batista RJV, Nery P, Bocchino L et al, "Partial left ventriculectomy to treat end-stage heart disease", *Ann Thorac Surg* 64, 634-638, 1997.
3. Bach DS, Bolling SF, "Early improvement in congestive heart failure after correction of secondary mitral regurgitation in end-stage cardiomyopathy", *Am Heart J*, 129, 1165-1170, 1995.
4. Dor V, Sabatier M, Di Donato M, Montiglio F, Toso A, Maioli M, "Efficacy of endoventricular patch plasty in large postinfarction akinetic scar and severe left ventricular dysfunction: comparison with a series of large dyskinetic scars", *J Thorac Cardiovasc Surg*, 116, 50-59, 1998.
5. Burkhoff D. "New heart failure therapy: the shape of thing to come?", *J Thorac Cardiovasc Surg*, 122, 421-423, 2001.
6. Shishido T, Hayashi K, Shigemi K et al, "Single beat estimation of end-systolic elastance using bilinearly approximated time-varying elastance curve", *Circulation*, 102, 1983-1989, 2000.
7. Osman NF, Kerwin WS, McVeigh E and Prince LJ. "Cardiac motion tracking using cine harmonic phase (HARP) magnetic resonance imaging", *Magnetic Resonance in Medicine*, 42, 1048-1060, 2000

CARS 2002 – H.U. Lemke, M.W. Vannier; K. Inamura, A.G. Farman, K. Doi & J.H.C. Reiber (Editors)
©CARS/Springer. All rights reserved.

934

Development of software for four-dimensional cardiac function analysis using multi-slice CT scanner

S. Yamamoto [a, c], S. Hamada [b], H. Naito [c], T. Johkoh [c], M. Miyamoto [d],
J. Masumoto [d], S. Azemoto [d], T. Kanagawa [e], S. Nakanishi [a], H. Nakamura [b]
[a] Department of Radiology, Osaka University Hospital, 2-15, Yamadaoka, Suita
City, Osaka, Japan. E-mail: yamamoto@hp-rad.med.osaka-u.ac.jp
[b] Department of Radiology, Osaka University Graduate School of Medicine.
[c] Department of Medical Physics, Osaka University
[d] Medical Imaging Laboratory, Co. Ltd.
[e] KCO, Ltd.

Abstract

We developed a software for cardiac four-dimensional imaging and semi-automatic ventricular volume estimation by joint research with medical and computer science department. The sequential volume data sets were acquired from retrospective ECG-gating helical scan. Ten and more sequential volume data sets were converted to three-dimensional (3D) image, and these sequential 3D images can be displayed as movie (Four-dimensional cardiac image). It has a potential for the visualization of the aortic valve, left ventricular free-wall motion and coronary artery et al. Moreover, we developed the semi-automatic ejection fraction (EF) and cardiac cycle (%)-volume (ml) curve to estimate the left ventricular motion and volume. As verification of accuracy for area definition in left ventricular lumen, we compared basic statistical method, using the histogram of Hounssfield Unit (HU) values of left ventricular lumen, with manual selection of specific color-coded three-dimensional objects. In the latter technique, we use the opacity function with volume histogram for volume rendering. We introduce our original developed software for cardiac 4D imaging and estimation of ventricular volume.

Keywords: Four-dimensional display, ejection-fraction, multidetector-row CT

1. Introduction

Multidetector-row CT (MDCT) offers good cardiac image quality without motion artifact using ECG synchronized technique [1-5]. Few reports were described about accurate estimation of ventricular volume and motion by using MDCT [6-8]. However, it is difficult to estimate the ventricular motion and volumes on the CT apparatus itself because the large cardiac volume data need high performance images processing. In case of re-constructing the time-series images from the ECG signal, hundreds or thousands of trans-axial images are produced. Interactive reading tool for cardiac CT examination is expected to help efficient diagnosis. In order to estimate the four-dimensional (4D) cardiac imaging and left ventricular volume, we developed a software for 4D imaging and semi-automatic calculation of Ejection Fraction (EF) and Cardiac cycle phase (%)-volume curve by using image and volume histogram analysis. In this work, we show the concept

935

of large volume data acquisition from DICOM network system and introduce the cardiac 4D visualization and estimation of the ventricular motion and volume.

2. Materials and methods

2.1 CT data acquisition system
Four-dimensional (4D) cardiac analysis software was installed on a standard personal computer (PC) with Pentium IV, 1GHz CPU, and 1.5GB RAM. Network interface of the software is a standard viewer for DICOM 3.0 file server (TFS3000, Toshiba, Tokyo, Japan). The software can be connected to any DICOM 3.0 model database (patient, study, series, image), via an Ethernet TCP/IP network. The users can transfer the DICOM images from MDCT (Aquillion VZ: Toshiba, Nasu, Japan and LightSpeed QX/i, GE, Milwaukee, Wisconsin) directly to the 4D workstation with the cardiac analysis software. Also, the users can export images and movies in PC standard format, for local storage, presentation, and print.

2.2 Procedure for cardiac 4D imaging and cardiac function analysis
For each patient, 10 volume data sets were created by using both half-scan and segment reconstruction based on the retrospective ECG gating helical scanning [2]. For the first end-diastolic phase, the image acquisition window was centred on the peak of the R wave.

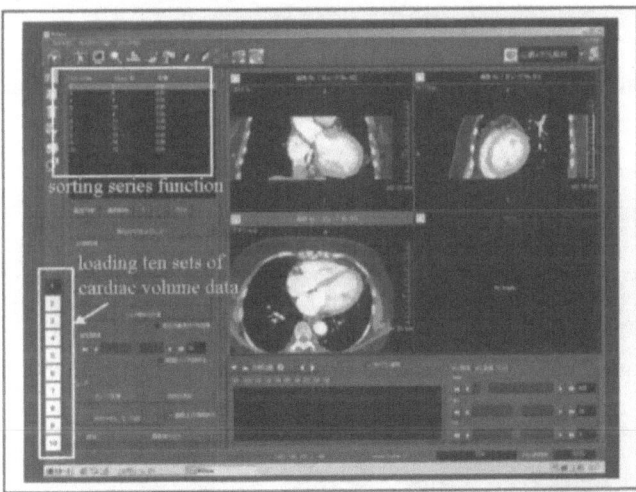

Fig.1: Ten sets of DICOM data acquisition and 2D-CT image display.

For the second data set, the centre was positioned at 10 % of the R-R interval, and for the subsequent data sets, the centre of the image acquisition window was moved toward the end of the cardiac cycle in increments of 10 %. The software can obtain all ten-volume data sets as DICOM series. The numbers of series depend on the memory size of RAM. Sorting series of data set is supported for uncorrected sequential order (Fig.1).

After retrieving ten sets of DICOM series into the PC-Workstation, user can control all of series by manipulating an arbitrary series in case of making 4D cardiac image. (The

936

remaining nine sets of series were processed in sync with a series of interest.) Semi-automated EF calculating procedure is as follows:

(a) Selection of the interactive region of interests (ROIs) around the left ventricular cavity on trans-axial images in end-diastolic phase. (The ROIs were interpolated between all slices where areas have been selected) (Fig.2).

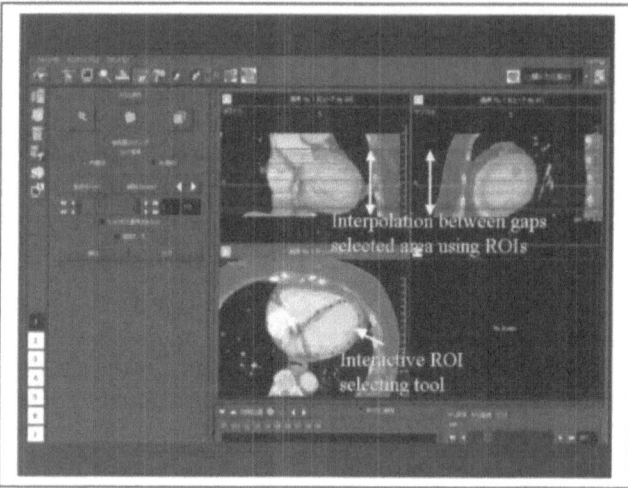

Fig.2 ROI selection around the left ventricular cavity and interpolation among gaps of selected area.

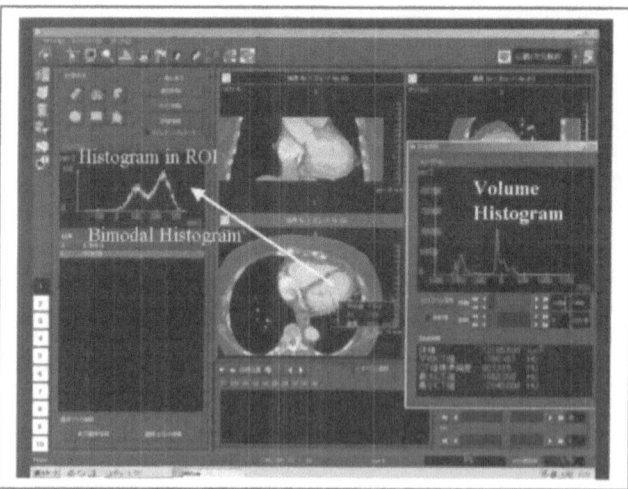

Fig.3 Segmentation of left ventricular cavity using histogram analysis.

(b) Copying ROIs of end-diastolic phase to all the other phases (Left ventricular cavities with all phases were covered by left ventricular cavity at end-diastolic phase).

CARS 2002 – H.U. Lemke, M.W. Vannier; K. Inamura, A.G. Farman, K. Doi & J.H.C. Reiber (Editors)

937

(c) Estimation of threshold Hounsfield Unit (HU) value for segmentation of left ventricular cavity using histogram analysis (Fig.3).

(d) Automatic drawing the cardiac cycle (%) – volume (ml) curve and EF calculation. (Fig.4)

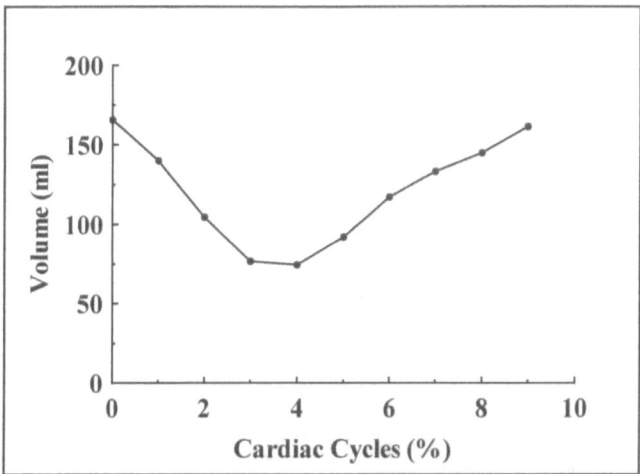

Fig.4 Automatically calculated cardiac cycle-volume curve (EF 55.1%)

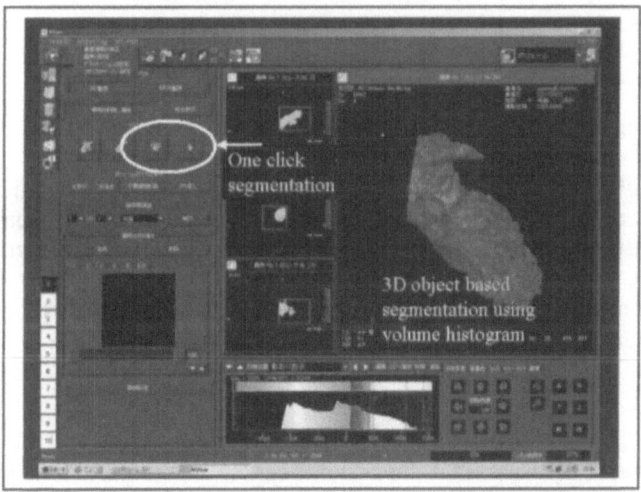

Fig.5 One click segmentation using volume histogram

Two segmentation methods, based on voxel counting, were compared in order to decide the simpler one for left ventricular volumetry of left ventricle. One is the Mode method [9,10] that explains the most basic segmentation using threshold grey level. The left ventricular cavity filled with contrast media were segmented by statistical method (mode value) depending on the HU value histogram. Threshold HU values were decided as a midpoint value between two modes values on bimodal histogram drawing round the ROI of left ventricular cavity. The other is manual selection of specific color-coded left

938

ventricular lumen using volume histogram with volume rendering. Users can measure the volume of 3D object by point and one click segmentation (Fig.5). These two methods were normalized (%) on the basis of pre-calculated volume of the contrast media in the phantom.

3. Results

Four-dimensional cardiac imaging displays were helpful to understand the motion state of coronary artery and left ventricular wall motion (Fig.6).

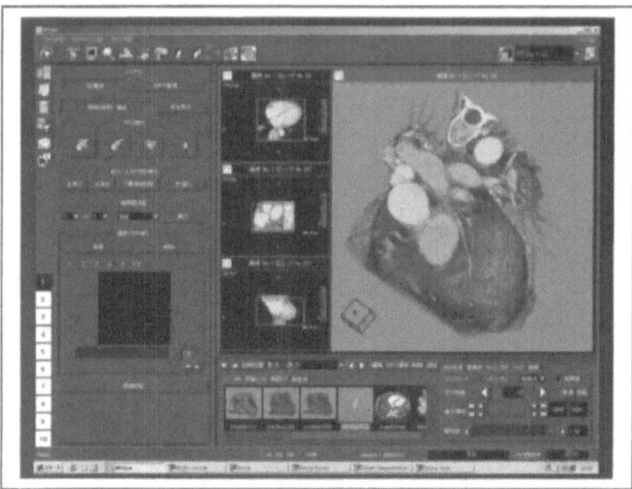

Fig.6 Display of the 4D imaging (end-diastolic phase)

Interactive ROI tool with segmentation of the left ventricular cavity and automatic drawing of cardiac cycle-volume curve improves the volumetry process comparing with slice-by-slice manually selection. In the statistical method using image histogram of one slice CT data, there was approximate 1 % error compared to phantom volume. In the manual selection using volume histogram (point and one click segmentation), there was approximates 4 % error.

4. Conclusion

The DICOM-supported software for 4-dimensional cardiac imaging and function analysis with on-line connection to Multi-slice CT apparatus is useful to comprehend the left ventricular motion and volumes.

Acknowledgements

This work has been supported by Medical Imaging Laboratory, Co, Ltd. and Department of Multi-dimensional Image Analysis, Osaka University Graduate of Medicine

939

References

1. Hayball M, Coulden R. Brown S, Clements L. "ECG Triggered X-ray Computed Tomography using a conventional CT system.", Electromedica, 66: 31-35, 1998.
2. Becker CR, Ohnesorge BM, Schoepf UJ, Reiser MF. "Current development of cardiac imaging with multidetector-row CT.", Europ J Radiol, 36: 97-103, 2000.
3. Klinge beck-Regn K, Schaller S, Flohr T, Ohnesorge B, Kopp AF, Baum U. "Subsecond multi-slice computed tomograpy: basics and applications.", Europ J Radio, 31, 110-124, 1999.
4. Ohnesorge B, Flohr T, Becker C, Kopp AF, Schoepf UJ, Baum U, Knez A, Klingenbeck-Regn K, Reiser MF. "Cardiac imaging by means of electrocardiographically gated multisection spiral CT: initial experience.", Radiology 217,564-71, 2000.
5. Kachelriess M, Ulzheimer S, Kalender WA. "ECG-correlated image reconstruction from subsecond multi-slice spiral CT scans of the heart." Med Phys., 27, 1881-1902, 2000.
6. Mochizuki T, Koyama Y, Tanaka H, Ikezoe J, Shen Y, Azemoto S. "Images in cardiovascular medicine. Left ventricular thrombus detected by two- and three-dimensional computed tomographic ventriculography: a new application of helical CT.", Circulation, 97, 933-934, 1998.
7. Koyama Y, Matsuoka H, Higashino H, et al. "Four-dimensional cardiac image by helical computed tomography.", Circulation, 100, 61-62, 1999.
8. Mochizuki T, Murase K, Higashino H, et.al., "Two- and three-dimensional CT ventriculography: a new application of helical CT." AJR Am J Roentgenol , 174:203-208, 2000.
9. Sahoo, P. K., Soltani, S., Wong, A. K. C. and Chen, Y. C. "A Survey of Thresholding Techniques,Computer Vision, Graphics, and Image Processing", 41, 233-260, 1998.
10. Chow, CK, Kaneko, T. "Automatic Boundary Detection of the Left Ventricle from Cineangiogram.", Computers and Biomedical Research, 5, 388-410, 1972.

8th Computed Maxillofacial Imaging Congress
Chairman: Allan G. Farman, PhD (odont.) (USA)

Image-Guidance in Implantology

CARS 2002 – H.U. Lemke, M.W. Vannier; K. Inamura, A.G. Farman, K. Doi & J.H.C. Reiber (Editors)

943

Clinical evaluation of patient misalignment during CT scans for computer assisted implantology - a new approach for compensation

J. Brief [a], S. Hassfeld [a], W. Stein [a], R. Krempien [b], J. Muehling [a]

[a] Department of Oral and Maxillofacial Surgery, University of Heidelberg
69120 Heidelberg, Germany, Email: jbrief@med.uni-heidelberg.de
[b] Department of Radiology, University of Heidelberg
69120 Heidelberg, Germany

Abstract

Computer assisted implantology relies on good CT data. Therefore a strict protocol for acquiring the CT scan has to be adhered to. Most errors are introduced by misalignment and movement of the patient during scanning. We introduce a new method in terms of software algorithms and of clinical protocol changes, which allows for an optimal patient positioning to reduce movement artefacts and for compensating patient positioning misalignments.

Keywords: Dental implantology, patient misalignment, virtual occlusion plane

1. Methods

After CT scanning a 3D volume data set is reconstructed from DICOM slices. Then the user moves an 3D template of a jaw arc and standard dental planes (occlusion/median/frontal) interactively through the data set to define its optimal position (Fig. 1a-c). This is subsequently used for compensating all alignment errors and for initialising standard views when reconstructing secondary views, e.g. 'cross sectionals'.

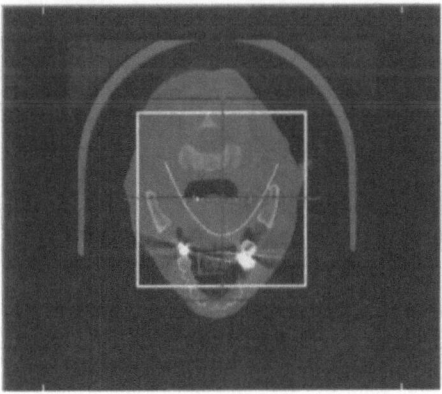

Fig. 1a Patient data set before positioning (cross sectional view).

944

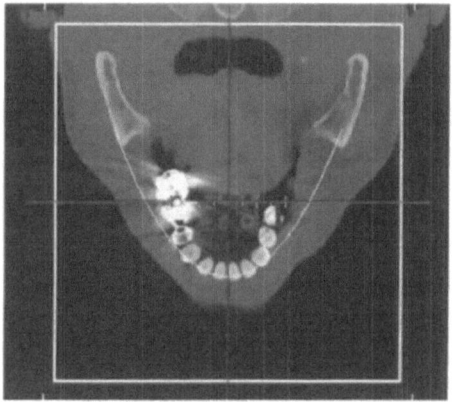

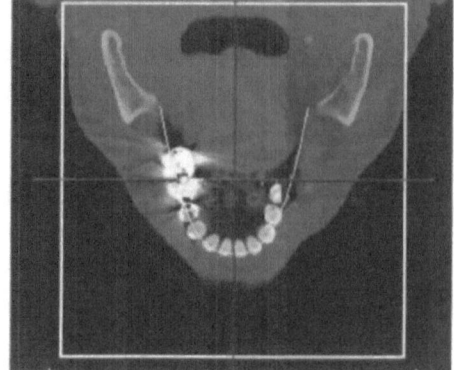

Fig. 1b Patient data set, sub-optimal
(cross sectional view).

Fig. 1c Patient data set, optimal
(cross sectional view).

For evaluating our methods we developed a new '3D Panoramic View', which allows us to simulate all kinds of misalignment and helps for easy comparison with well known dental orthopantomographic x-rays (Fig. 2, 3).

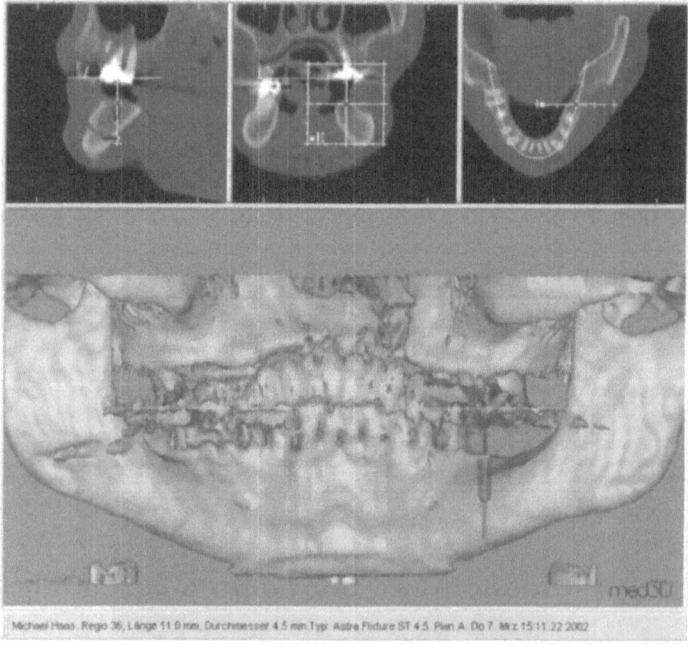

Fig. 2 Implant planning with conventional (cross sectional views in upper pictures) and new developed "3D Panoramic View" (lower picture).

CARS 2002 – H.U. Lemke, M.W. Vannier; K. Inamura, A.G. Farman, K. Doi & J.H.C. Reiber (Editors)

2. Results

We applied our algorithms and clinical protocol to 12 patient data sets and noticed in all of them some positioning misalignment in the CT scan, although our staff put best efforts in placing the patients according to our conventional protocol.

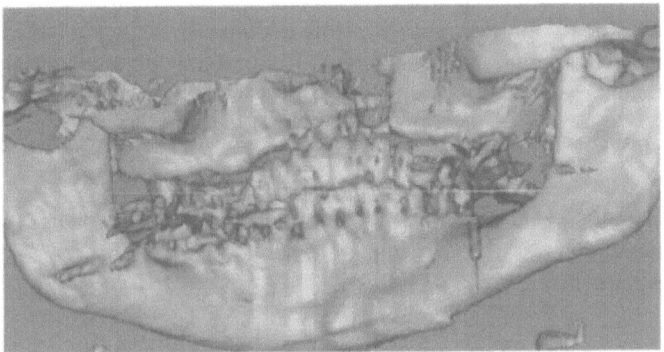

Fig. 3 Positioning misalignment in the CT scan
(3D Panoramic View).

A typically angulation error of $\alpha = 10$ degrees then would result in a deviation of the apex position for an implant with a length of $l = 11$ mm of more than $\Delta x = 1.9$ mm (Fig. 4 a-b).

$$\Delta x = \sin (\alpha) * l$$

This becomes worse for longer implants and stronger misalignments. Our new software algorithms allow for compensating this kind of error.

Erroneous patient movement during scans is very notably reduced, since a patient can be placed in the most comfortable and stable position, because any misalignment to standard protocol's can be corrected, even long after the CT scan has been acquired, thus reducing the need for rescanning the patient.

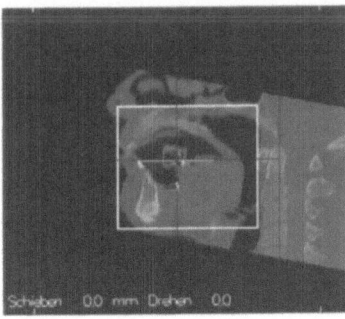

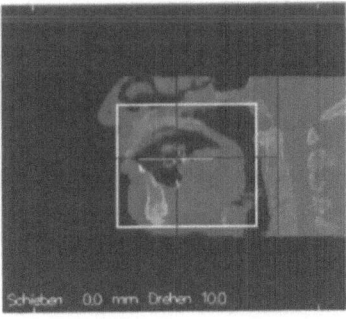

Fig. 4a Patient data set, with an angulation error of 10 degrees. (cross sectional view).

Fig. 4b Same patient data set, after angulation error correction . (cross sectional view).

946

3. Conclusion

The newly developed algorithm '3D Panoramic View' allows for very easy image understanding and evaluation of alignment errors during CT scans. Qualitiy of computer assisted implant planning based on CT data is drastically improved, because alignment errors can be fully compensated and a patient be placed in the best possible and comfortable position during scanning, therefore additionally reducing movement artefacts. Our studies have shown that hardly any patient is 'perfectly aligned' during scans and all these misalignments can be corrected with our newly developed algorithm.

Acknowledgement

The work is being funded partially by the Sonderforschungsbereich 414 "Information Technology in Medicine - Computer and Sensor Supported Surgery" of the Deutsche Forschungsgemeinschaft.

References

1. Brief, J., S. Hassfeld, T. Redlich, C. Ziegler, J. Muenchenberg, S. Daueber, A. Pernozzoli, R. Krempien, P. Slacik, M. Opalek, R. Boesecke, J. Mühling: Robot Assisted Insertion of Dental Implants - A clinical evaluation, CAR 2000, (2000), 932 – 937.
2. Brief J., S. Hassfeld, U. Sonnenfeld, N. Persky, R. Krempien, M. Treiber, J.Mühling: Computer guided insertion of dental implants-a clinical evaluation, CAR 2001, (2001), 696– 701.
3. Hassfeld St., J. Brief, W. Stein, C. Ziegler, T. Redlich, J. Raczkowsky, R. Krempien, J. Mühling: Navigationsverfahren in der Implantologie - Stand der Technik und Perspektiven. Implantologie 4: 373-390 (2000)
4. Hassfeld, St., J. Brief, R. Krempien, J. Raczkowsky, J. Münchenberg, H.Giess, H.P. Meinzer, U. Mende, H. Wörn, J. Mühling Computerunterstützte Mund-, Kiefer- und Gesichtschirurgie. Radiologe 40: 218-226 (2000)
5. Münchenberg J., Brief J., Hassfeld S., Raczkowsky J., Rembold U., Wörn H.: Expert Supported Operation Planning in the Maxillofacial Sur-gery (1998), Proceedings of Computer Assisted Radiology and Surgery (CAR'98), June, 1998, Tokyo, Japan
6. Stein W., Hassfeld S., Brief J., Bertovic I., Krempien R., Mühling J.: CT-Based 3D-Planning For Dental Implantology. Proceedings of Medicine Meets Virtual Reality (MMVR'98). San Diego, 1998, S. 137

CARS 2002 – H.U. Lemke, M.W. Vannier; K. Inamura, A.G. Farman, K. Doi & J.H.C. Reiber (Editors)

The precision of the RoboDent system – an in vitro study

O. Schermeier, T. Lueth, C. Cho, D. Hildebrand, M. Klein, K. Nelson, J. Bier
Clinic for Maxillofacial Surgery and Clinical Navigation and Robotics
Fraunhofer IPK – Charité • Campus Virchow Clinic
Augustenburger Platz 1, 13353 Berlin, Germany, olaf.schermeier@charite.de

Abstract

In this paper, the overall system accuracy of the navigation system RoboDent® is determined for the application in oral implant surgery. The measurements are performed by drilling in five models of the human jaw. The experimental test bed includes all steps of the intervention including image acquisition, registration, planning, instrument calibration and drilling. The results show that the new methods for registration and visualization that are implemented in the system increase the accuracy of navigation systems making the system capable of improving the treatment quality in oral implant surgery.

Keywords: Dental, implant, navigation, accuracy

1. Introduction

In the last few years, the insertion of dental implants has become a standard treatment to replace missing teeth. Therefore, the focus has changed from improving the implants to improving the insertion of the implants, making the procedure surgically safer and optimizing the prosthetic results. The optimal positioning of an implant becomes difficult if all of the following criteria need to be fulfilled. The implant should be in the center of mastication in parallel to the force vector, neighbored implants should be in parallel, the available bone structure is to be used as much as possible, various structures, like the mandible nerve and the sinuses need to be avoided, the patient trauma and the healing time is to be kept as low as possible.

Existing procedures to transfer preplanned implant locations to the patient are complicated and inaccurate. Theses procedures are mostly based on drill guides. These are manufactured by computer driven milling machines, stereo lithography or by dental labs. However, movements of the splint caused through drilling vibrations occur. Therefore, the diameters of drill guides need to be wide enough to inhibit resonance, lowering the accuracy. Other problems occur due to heat, the guidance of only one drill and the missing space for inserting long drills in some regions of the mouth.

An alternative way to transfer preplanned implant positions to the jaw is the usage of robots or navigation systems ([1], [2], [3], [4]). With the aid of these systems, the positioning of the implants becomes ascertainable and predictable. The risk of complications, like nerve injury, opening of the sinuses, and inducing fractures decrease.

The interactive robot system IIH (Intelligent Instrument Holder) was developed in the Clinic for Maxillofacial Surgery and Clinical Navigation and Robotics of the Charité in

CARS 2002 – H.U. Lemke, M.W. Vannier; K. Inamura, A.G. Farman, K. Doi & J.H.C. Reiber (Editors)

948

Berlin [5]. It has been used successfully in the clinical routine to insert extra oral implants in patients with general anesthesia [6]. This sedation method is essential because of the necessary fixation of the patient's head. For the insertion of dental implants, this considerable does not seem to be necessary.

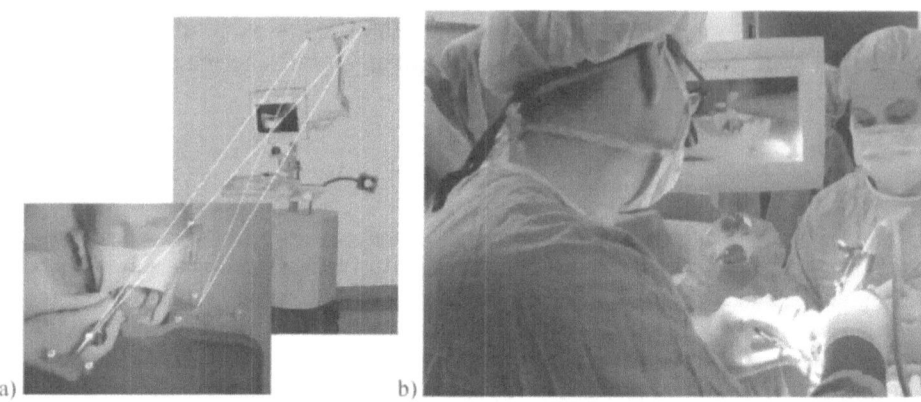

Fig. 1   a) Components of the RoboDent® navigation system, b) navigated insertion of dental implants in the Clinic for Maxillofacial Surgery and Clinical Navigation and Robotics, Charité, Berlin (©2001, RoboDent GmbH).

With the knowledge and experience of an active surgical robot system, the navigation system RoboDent® has been developed for the application in computer assisted oral implantology [1]. It consists of a 3D planning system for inserting dental implants and a treatment system to drill the implant seat guided by sensor data. The system uses an optical passive sensor (Polaris or Ropal, both NDI, Ontario, Canada) to measure the location of the patient and the instrument (Fig. 1a). A highly accurate automatic registration algorithm [7] is used for patient registration without interaction with the user. Since most measurement and calibration procedures are automated, the user interaction is intuitive and simple. The system has the medical approval for the European market and has been proven its practicability in more than 100 successfully navigated implantations (Fig. 1b).

The procedure of implantation begins with the fabrication of a navigation frame that consists of a splint of the individual dental status which is attached to a reference body. The splint of the dental status is supplemented by radio opaque material outlining the future teeth. A radiological CT exam is taken with the navigation splint in place. The images are saved in DICOM format on a CD. Afterwards, the CD is inserted into the RoboDent® system. Here, the surgeon is able to define the implant's size, type, exact position and axis without any intraoperative surprises due to the available information about the bone quality, quantity, structure deviations, and exact location of sensible structures like the mandible nerve, sinuses, and hidden bone cysts. By rendering a 3D model of the jaw with the integrated implant models the implants can be proofread in their location, using the additional approach of planning dental implants according to the layout of the teeth. Instruments for measuring the density and for orienting several implants in parallel enable the user to define the best possible implant location. Prior to surgery the frame is attached to the patient's teeth. The handpiece is calibrated using a pin on the patient tracker, the length of the drill is registered by an indentation on the navigation splint.

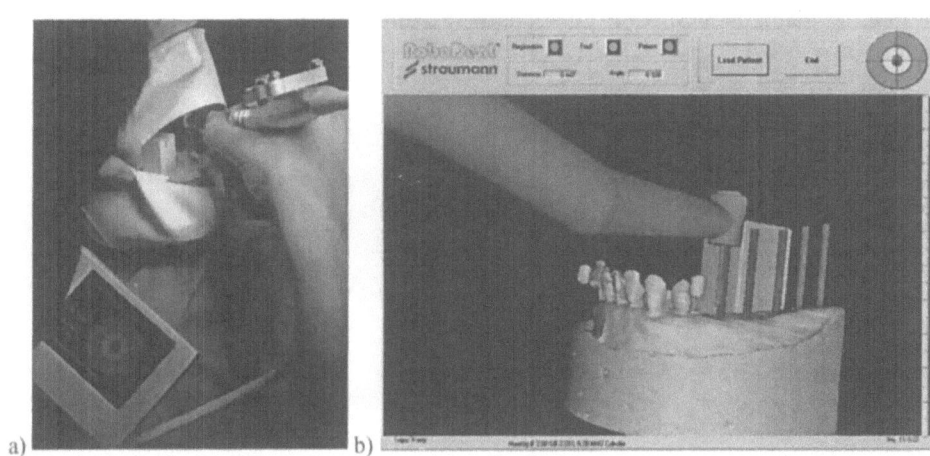

a) b)

Fig. 2 Drilling in a model while observing the target deviation on a) a miniaturized display next to the patients mouth and b) a 3D-Scene of the Instrument, jaw and implant axes model (©2001, RoboDent GmbH).

During the surgery, deviation information between the implant and the drill is displayed on a LCD touch screen (Fig. 2b) as well as on a small screen which is placed next to the patient (Fig. 2a). In this unit information about the position, the angle, and the drilling depth are conveyed. Next to the visual support an acoustic guidance is offered in this system. Warning sounds announce approaching dangerous structures.

2. Purpose

RoboDent® is currently used for the regular patient care by several dentists and surgeons. In patient care, good results are achieved, the accuracy is sufficient adequate for treatment, and all patients have been treated successfully without any system failure. In this study the degree of accuracy of this navigation system is to be displayed by quantifying the total error. The total error consists of the sum of different errors which can be identified as:

$$e_{total} = e_{ima} + e_{cal} + e_{reg} + e_{nav} + e_{hum} + e_{mec} \tag{1}$$

where:

e_{total} - total error
e_{CT} - distortion of the CT and movement of patient during scan,
e_{cal} - error of instrument calibration,
e_{reg} - error of patient registration
e_{nav} - error of sensor of the navigation system
e_{hum} - error of user / surgeon
e_{mec} - mechanical error e.g. clearance of the drill.

To measure the overall accuracy the complete process has to be integrated in the experimental test bed. The planned and finally drilled implant locations have to be

CARS 2002 – H.U. Lemke, M.W. Vannier; K. Inamura, A.G. Farman, K. Doi & J.H.C. Reiber (Editors)

measured in the same reference coordinate system. Since this coordinate system is difficult to define in an in vivo situation, the experiments are performed on a model of a human jaw.

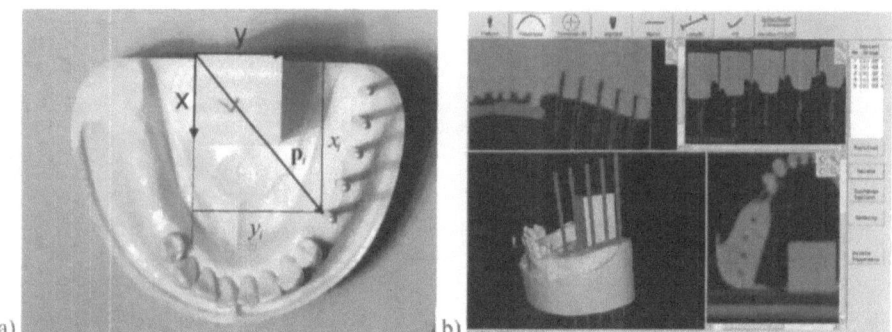

Fig. 3: a) Definition of a cartesian coordinate system in the jaw model and b) planning of the desired drill axes with the RoboDent planning module(©2001, RoboDent GmbH).

3. Methods

A modified KaVo™ phantom jaw made of Biresin-G20 (Sika Stuttgart, Germany) was used for the study (Fig. 3a). A model of a lower bilateral free end situation jaw was created with an integrated 20mmx20mmx50mm rectangular block as a reference. The block builds a rectangular coordinate system. Positions and angles of drill holes in the model can be measured easily and highly accurate with a digital caliper. Six copies of this situation were made. The maximal divergence of the models was 0.1mm.

One of the models was declared as the reference object. Five parallel holes with a diameter of 2mm were drilled in this model using a computer driven milling machine. A dental splint with a reference frame was made. This compound of the reference model and the dental splint was scanned in a CT, Siemens Somatom Plus 4 Volume Zoom (Siemens AG, Munich, Germany), and 140 Slices with a 0.5mm width were generated. These images were saved in DICOM format on a CD and inserted into the RoboDent® system.

The first step includes the planning. The registration markers in the images of the compound are automatically identified. The planning program calculates a surface model. A panoramic line is set through the visible drill holes in the axial slices. Instead of using specific implants, cylindrical pins with a diameter of 2mm were placed into the model, matching the position and orientation of the drilled holes (Fig. 3b).

In the treatment program this planning is used to transfer the situation to the remaining 5 models (Fig. 2). The experienced user's task was to drill the holes which were defined in the planning program, reproducing the axes. The preplanned configuration of the implants was drilled while the visual and acoustic support guided the procedure. The navigation sensor Polaris was used for the drillings.

For the measurements, pins of stainless steel with 2mm diameter are inserted into the drill holes of the original model and in the 5 models that are drilled with the navigation system. The measurements were done with a digital slide gauge with a 0.01mm resolution, and

CARS 2002 – H.U. Lemke, M.W. Vannier; K. Inamura, A.G. Farman, K. Doi & J.H.C. Reiber (Editors)
°CARS/Springer. All rights reserved.

according to the manufacturer, with an accuracy of 0.03mm. The distances of the pins to the block were measured perpendicular in x- and y- direction at two different levels. With these four measurements, the position and the angles of the pins were determinable in the metric coordinate system.

4. Results and conclusion

The deviation between the 24 drillings and the target is shown in Fig. 4. to understand the dimensions, the drill diameter is displayed as a circle in Fig. 4a.

The following values where determined for the mean μ and standard deviation σ of the position deviation (index pi) and angular deviation (index ang):

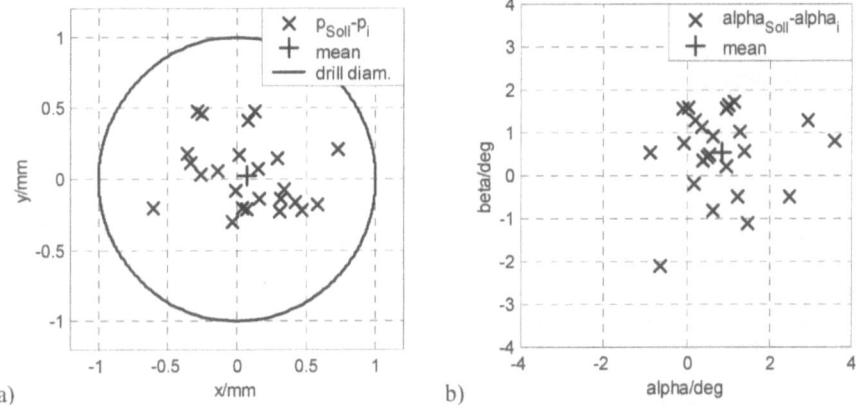

a)   b)

Fig. 4: Deviation between 24 drillings and target axes in a model separated by a) position and b) angle.

$$\mu_{pi} = \sqrt{\mu_x^2 + \mu_y^2} = 0.08 \, \text{mm} \, , \, \sigma_{pi} = \sqrt{\sigma_x^2 + \sigma_y^2} = 0.41 \, \text{mm} \, , \quad (2)$$

$$\mu_{ang} = \sqrt{\mu_\alpha^2 + \mu_\beta^2} = 0.98° \, , \, \sigma_{ang} = \sqrt{\sigma_\alpha^2 + \sigma_\beta^2} = 1.44° . \quad (3)$$

The low mean of the measurements shows, that systematic errors like registration or calibration errors are nearly negligible. The standard deviation shows that the main error of the drillings is caused by non systematic errors like the tremor of the user, inaccuracies in the perception of the human and the noise of the navigation system. However, this experiment shows that excellent accuracy can be reached with the RoboDent® system that can increase the quality in oral implant surgery. It could be shown, that the new methods as described in [7] and [8] increase the usability and the accuracy of the RoboDent system compared to the studies described in [9]. Measurements of the in vivo accuracy of the system are to be published soon.

Acknowledgement

This research work has been performed in the Clinic for Maxillofacial Surgery and Clinical Navigation and Robotics (Prof. Dr. mult. Juergen Bier, Prof. Dr. Tim C. Lueth), Medical Faculty Charité, Humboldt-University Berlin and Fraunhofer IPK. The work has been supported by the Deutsche Forschungsgemeinschaft with the Graduiertenkolleg 331 – Temperaturabhängige Effekte (granted to Prof. Dr. Dr.h.c. R. Felix, PD Dr. N. Hosten) and by the Real-Time Control Group, Prof. Dr.-Ing. Guenter Hommel, of the Technical University Berlin. Parts of the research have been supported financially by the Alfried Krupp von Bohlen und Halbach Stiftung, Deutsche Krebshilfe (granted to Prof. Dr. Dr. J. Bier, PD Dr. P. Wust) and the Berliner Sparkassenstiftung Medizin (granted to Prof. Dr. T. Lueth, Dr. Dr. Ernst Heissler, Prof. Dr. Dr. Berthold Hell). Special thanks to the companies RoboDent, Straumann, NDI, Rohwedder Visotech, Elekta, Metalor and Philips for their support of the project. We would like also to thank Thomas Hölper, Edgar Schüle, Dr.-Ing. Armin Freybott, and W. Scholz. Their personal engagement was the basis for this challenging research.

References

1.   Schermeier, O. (2001): Ein Navigationssystem für die dentale Implantologie. PhD-Thesis, Technical University of Berlin.
2.   Hein, A.; M. Klein, T. C. Lueth, J. Queck, M. Stien, O. Schermeier, J. Bier: (2001): Integration and Clinical Evaluation of an Interactive Controllable Robotic System for Anaplastology. MICCAI 2001, Utrecht, Netherland, 14.-17. Oct.
3.   Birkenfellner W. et. al. (1999): Computer - Aided Implant Dentistry -An early Report-. MICCAI99, Cambridge, pp. 883-891.
4.   Brief, J., S. Hassfeld, U. Sonenfeld, N. Persky, R. Krempien, M. Treiber, J. Mühling (2001): Navigated Insertion of Dental Implants. ISRACAS Fourth Israeli Symposium on Computer-Aided Surgery, Medical Robotics and Medical Imaging, Tel-Aviv, Israel, May 17.
5.   Hein, A. (2000): Eine interaktive Robotersteuerung für chirurgische Applikationen. PhD-Thesis, Technical University of Berlin.
6.   Klein M., T. Lueth, A. Hein, M. Stien, O. Schermeier, S. Weber, H. Menneking, O. Schwerdtner, J. Bier (2001): Robot assisted insertion of craniofacial implants - clinical experiments.. CARS 2001 Computer Assisted Radiology and Surgery Proceedings of the 15th International Congress and Exhibition, Berlin, June 27 - 30, pp. 133-138.
7.   Schermeier, O., T. Lueth, J. Glagau, D. Szymanski, R. Tita, D. Hildebrand, M. Klein, K. Nelson, J. Bier (2002): Automatic patient registration in computer assisted maxillofacial surgery. Medicine Meets Virtual Reality (MMVR), Newport Beach, USA, Jan. 23. - 26.
8.   Schermeier, O., R. Tita, J. Glagau, D. Hildebrand, M. Klein, J. Bier, T. Lüth (2001): Navigierte Insertion von Dentalimplantaten mit dem Behandlungssystem RoboDent. Automed2001, Bochum, Germany, Sep. 17., 18.
9.   Schermeier, O., D. Hildebrand, T.C. Lueth, D. Szymanski, J. Bier (2001): Accuracy of an Image Guided System for Oral Implantology. CARS Computer Assisted Radiology and Surgery, Berlin, Germany, June.

CARS 2002 – H.U. Lemke, M.W. Vannier; K. Inamura, A.G. Farman, K. Doi & J.H.C. Reiber (Editors)

A new method and a clinical case for computer assisted dental implantology

François Goulette[a], Julien Dutreuil[a] and Claude Laurgeau[a]
Jaime Clavero Zoreda[b] and Stefan Lundgren[b]
[a] Centre de Robotique, Ecole des Mines de Paris,
60 boulevard Saint Michel, 75272 Paris Cedex 06, France
{goulette, dutreuil, laurgeau}@caor.ensmp.fr
[b] Department of Oral and Maxillofacial Surgery,
Umeå Universitet, 90187 Umeå, Sweden
jclavero.z@tbc.es, stefan.lundgren@odont.umu.se

Abstract

This paper presents a new method for dental implant surgery. A pre-operative planning software is used to work with CT scanner data. Implant fixtures are placed with the help of a 3D reconstructed model of the patient's jaw. An accurate robot is then used to drill a jaw splint, at the locations determined with the planning software, in order to make a surgical guide. The matching between image and robot referentials is performed with radio-opaque markers attached in a specific way to the jaw splint. A clinical case of this new technique is presented.

Keywords: Dental implants, surgical guide, radio-opaque markers

1. Introduction

Dental implants are used in maxillofacial restoration to replace a tooth or a set of teeth. One implant is composed of three parts: a titanium fixture surgically placed into the patient's jaw, a prosthetic crown replacing the missing tooth, and a mechanical part connected between the fixture and the crown, the abutment.

The success of a dental implantation depends directly on the localisation of the fixture in the patient's jaw bone. Firstly, the good adequacy between the axis of the fixture (surgical axis) and the axis of the prosthetic tooth (prosthetic axis) is critical for the good setting of the implant: the angle between both axes must be as small as possible in order to minimise lateral constraints transmitted from the crown to the abutment and then to the fixture [1]. Secondly, the fixture must be precisely implanted in hard cortical bone to assure a good stability. The surgery also requires great accuracy because of particularly sensitive anatomic structures in the neighbourhood of these implants (the mandibular nerve and the maxillary sinus) [1,2].

954

The new technique we propose improves the accuracy in the fixture placement. It uses a pre-operative planning phase for virtual placement of the fixture, and an accurate robot to drill a jaw splint, exact negative shape of the patient's jaw, in order to create a surgical guide.

Other solutions have already been proposed to improve the accuracy of the fixture placement: using a robot for drilling a splint [1, 3, 4], using stereo-lithography to build the splint from CT scans [5, 6], or using a navigation system during the surgery, coupled with scanner data [7, 8].

2. Method

This method consists in a 4-stage procedure (figure 1):
Stage 1: a denture impression of the patient's jaw is taken. It is used to make a plaster model of the jaw, and a splint on which the missing teeth are replaced by crowns. Radio-opaque balls are placed at precise locations on the splint, to provide scanner markers [9].

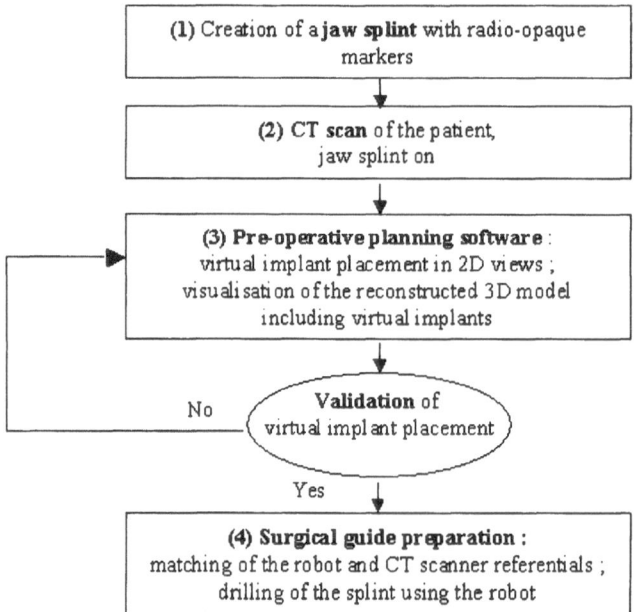

Fig. 1. Sketch of the new method

Stage 2: a CT scan of the patient is taken, with the splint placed in the mouth. The use of CT scans is very classical in dental implantology, because they can provide complete 3D data by tomographic reconstruction, with an excellent sensitivity to bone tissues density [9, 10].　·
Stage 3: a dedicated pre-operative planning software is used, that has been especially developed to be adapted to the needs of dental implant surgeons (Figure 2). The

CARS 2002 – H.U. Lemke, M.W. Vannier; K. Inamura, A.G. Farman, K. Doi & J.H.C. Reiber (Editors)
^cCARS/Springer. All rights reserved.

955

planning stage consists in identifying the best location to place implants inside the patient's jaw, according to the ideal prosthesis, in order to improve the medical result [11]. The software provides tools and cut views interpolated from the data to optimise this location process.

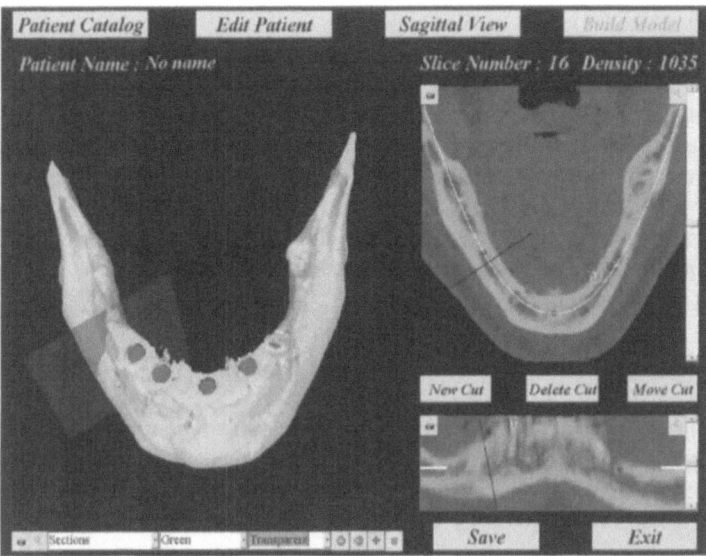

Fig. 2. General view from the pre-operative planning software.

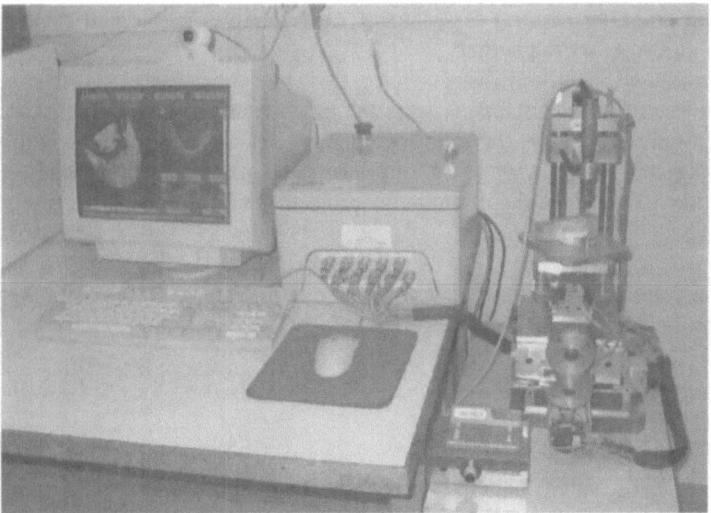

Fig. 3. Complete processing workbench, from pre-operative planning to splint drilling.

Stage 4: the splint is placed on the plaster model which is fixed on the robot work plan. Radio-opaque balls located on the splint are visible directly, on the splint and on the

CARS 2002 – H.U. Lemke, M.W. Vannier; K. Inamura, A.G. Farman, K. Doi & J.H.C. Reiber (Editors)

956

CT scanner data: the matching between the robot referential and the CT data referential may be performed. The result of the matching is combined with the information of the desired implant location, expressed in the scanner referential (stage 3), to compute the implant location in the robot referential. Finally, the splint is drilled by the robot at this precise location to make the surgical guide.

The robot is an accurate numerical command machine, with five degrees of freedom (3 translations and 2 rotations). It has a 0.04 mm translation accuracy, and a 0.15° rotation accuracy (Figure 3). By pointing (mechanical contact) the radio-opaque balls with the robot, the location of these balls in the robot referential is determined with an accuracy close to 0.3 mm ; by pointing them in the CT scanner images, their location in the scanner referential is also determined, with an accuracy close to 0.25 mm (only limited by the scanner definition). We can evaluate that the global accuracy of the complete treatment, from the planning phase to the surgery as presented on figure 3, is lower than 1 mm in location and 1° in orientation.

3. Results

A first case has been treated with this new protocol, at the department of oral and maxillo-facial surgery of Umeå University, in Sweden. The patient was an upper jaw edentulous woman. Because of a strong bone resorption, she had a bone graft before the implant surgery.

It is noteworthy that, even if the patient was treated with our new experimental method, there was no additional risk compared to the classical method, as has been pointed out elsewhere for a similar method [1]: a visual expertise was performed by the surgeon on the surgical guide before the surgery.

A 8-implant treatment was planned, using the pre-operative planning software, visible on figure 4-a ; figure 4-b shows the robot drilling the splint ; on figure 4-c, one can see the patient during the surgery, with the surgical guide placed in the mouth, right before drilling the jaw ; figure 4-d displays the position of the fixture implants placed in the jaw after drilling.

This first operation was a success, validating our method : all implants were precisely placed at the right location.

4. Conclusion

A new method for dental implantology has been presented, which is based on the use of a surgical guide, CT scanner imaging, a pre-operative planning software, a robot to drill the splint and a method based on radio-opaque markers to match the implant virtual positions and the actual drilling directions in the splint.

The first clinical case demonstrated the simplicity and the efficiency of the method. Further work is planned with a clinical validation campaign.

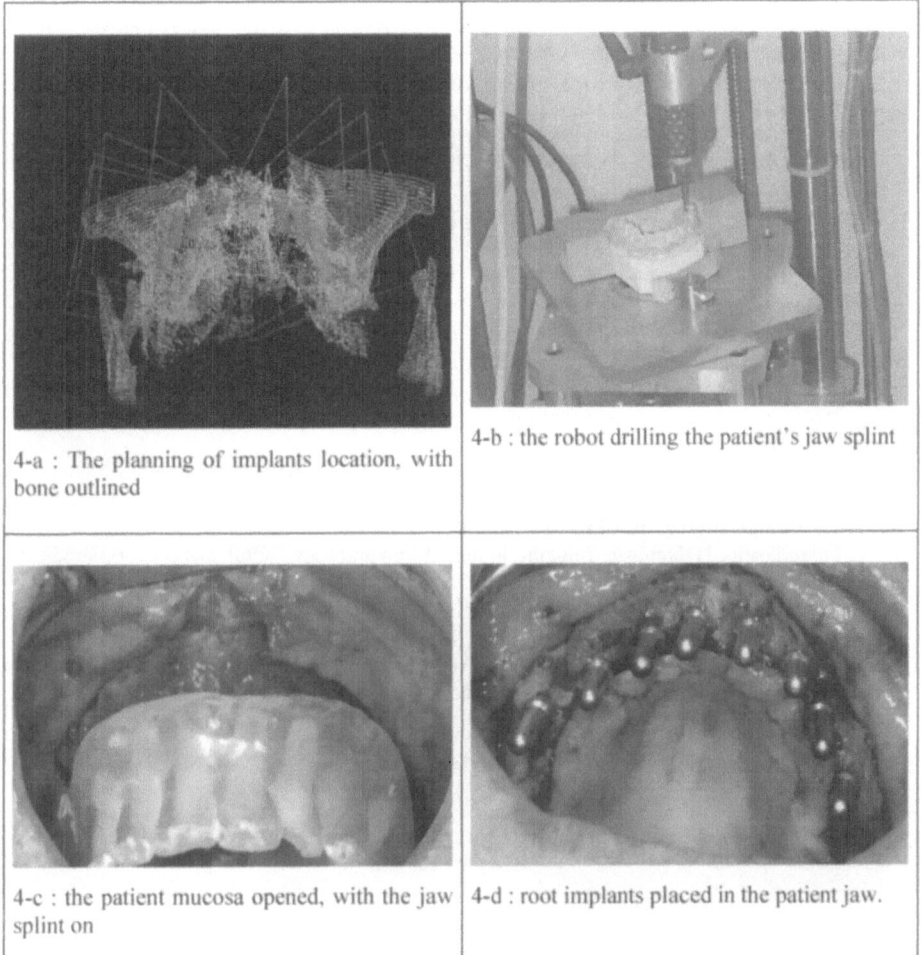

4-a : The planning of implants location, with bone outlined

4-b : the robot drilling the patient's jaw splint

4-c : the patient mucosa opened, with the jaw splint on

4-d : root implants placed in the patient jaw.

Fig. 4. Clinical case.

Acknowledgements

This work has been partly supported by the VISIMPLANT Leonardo da Vinci European program (partners: Ecole des Mines de Paris, Umeå University, Techdent, SFO, Imperial College).

958

References

1. T. Fortin, J.P. Coudert, G. Champleboux et al. : "Computer-assisted dental implant surgery using computed tomography", Journal of image guided surgery, no. 1, p. 53-58, 1995
2. S.L. Bass : "The effects of preoperative resorption and jaw anatomy on implant success: a report of 303 cases". Clin. Oral Impl. Res., no. 2, p. 193-198.
3. G. Champleboux, E. Blanchet, T. Fortin et al. : "A fast, accurate and easy method to position oral implants using computed tomography". In Proc. Computer Assisted Radiology - CAR'98, Elsevier Science, H.U.Lemke Ed., 1998.
4. K. Verstreken, J. van Cleynenbreugel, G. Marchal et al. : "An image guided planning system for oral implant surgery". Proc. of Computer Aided Radiology - CAR '96, p. 888-893, 1996.
5. V. Hietschold, W. Harzer, L. Eckhardt et al. : "Stereolithography of the occlusion plane using MR-tomographic imaging of the set of teeth". In Proc. Computer Assisted Radiology, 1996.
6. J. Lambrecht, C. Besimo, W. Müller et al. : "Precision of presurgical implantological planning with digitised CT and Scanora". In Proc. Computer Assisted Radiology, 1996.
7. P. Solar, S. Rodinger, C. Ulm et al. : "A computer-aided navigation system for oral implants using 3D-CT reconstructions and real time video projection", Int. Conf on Computer Assisted Radiology, 1996.
8. W. Birkfellner, F. Wanschitz, F. Watzinger et al. : "Accuracy of a Navigation System for Computer-Aided Oral Implantology", Proc. MICCAI'00, Lecture Notes in Computer Sciences no. 1935, Springer Verlag, p. 1061-1067, 2000.
9. N. L. Frederiksen : "Diagnostic imaging in dental implantology", Oral surgery, oral medicine, oral pathology, vol. 80, no. 5, p. 540-554, 1995.
10. N. Bellaiche, D. Doyon : "La tomodensimétrie dans le bilan pré-opératoire en implantologie orale", Journal de la Radiologie, tome 73, n°1, 1992.
11. K. Verstreken, J. Van Cleynenbreugel, K. Mertens et al. : "An Image-Guided Planning System for Endosseous Oral Implants", IEEE Transactions on Medical Imaging, 17(5): p. 842-852, 1998

CARS 2002 – H.U. Lemke, M.W. Vannier; K. Inamura, A.G. Farman, K. Doi & J.H.C. Reiber (Editors)

"Image guided implantology" – real-time guidance of dental implant surgery in the operative field using CT-scan image

Lior Shapira

Hebrew University – Hadassah Medical Centers, Jerusalem, Israel

Abstract

The surgical stage of dental implant placement is a complicated one, requires meticulous planning and pinpoint accuracy during surgery. The surgical plan is guided by prosthetic considerations and anatomical structures, which limit the envelope into which implants can be inserted. The transfer of the CT-based planning data to the operative field is still a problem. A new system, IGI, helps to overcome surgical complexities by allowing the practitioner to plan, view and real time navigation of drilling and implant positioning. The CT data is downloaded into the computer, and is used for computer-assisted planning. With the aid of infrared emitters, that are located on the drilling system and the patient, and a camera, the IGI system guides the surgeon "on-line" on the CT-scan image into the appropriate implant position, according to the treatment plan. We used the IGI system to plan and perform implant surgeries on human subjects. Our experience suggests that the use of the IGI system allows minimal flap reflection, resulting in shortening of chair-time and healing period. The computer-assisted control of the surgery, the three-dimensional navigation of the implant into the pre-planned implant location, as well as the ability to alert the user from implant malpositioning, reduces the stress of both the patient and the surgeon.

Keywords: Dental implant, image-guided, CT-scan

1. Introduction

Guidance of surgical procedures by computerized imaging becomes more and more popular procedures. It reduces the invasiveness of the operation and improves localization and targeting during surgery, as well as being a powerful planning tool. The information on the position of the surgical tool is displayed on a computerized image that provides the surgeon with exact information on the anatomical situation. Medical applications of position information for controlling imaging devices include ultrasound [1], fluoroscopy [2] and magnetic resonance [3].

Dental implants are considered today as important part of the rehabilitation of the human dentition [4]. The dental implants are inserted into the bone of the jaws for supporting dental prosthesis. The long-term prognosis of implant-supported dental restorations depends to a large extent on the implant position [5]. Furthermore, the aesthetic, phonetic, and functional aspects of the treated patient in highly depended on the position of the implants in the oral cavity [6]. One of the more accurate and popular approaches for

960

planning of implant placement is computerized tomography (CT) [7-10]. The identification of critical anatomical structures on the CT, such as the inferior alveolar nerve, the maxillary sinus, adjacent teeth and the bone envelope was found to improve the success of surgical performance and to reduce morbidity.

Currently, the transfer of the CT information to the operating field is usually based on the production of a dental template with drill guides [11-13]. However, using the template there is the lack of real-time control during the surgical procedure, and the surgeon can use the guide without any possibility for modifications during the procedure.

Several efforts were done in the last years to transfer the CT information to the surgical field for real-time navigation [14, 15] using magnetic tracking systems. However, the accuracy of this system was far from satisfactory. The use of optical tracking system was found recently to have superior qualities to the magnetic system [16, 17]. The present manuscript describes the use of IGI (image-guided implantology) with an optical tracking system for planning and performing implant surgeries on human subjects.

2. Methods

CT scanning protocol. An impression of the dentition and the edentulous ridges together with the antagonist jaw and bite registration were taken from the patient and the casts were mounted in a dental articulator. An acrylic guide was prepared to be placed on stable teeth adjacent to the implant area. A U-shape registration body was cemented to the guide, parallel to the occlusal plain (Fig. 1). 8-10 ceramic spheres (3 mm diameter) were mounted on the U-shaped body and were used for transferring the location of CT image in relation to the patient mouth, and for the correction of CT distortions. Patients were scanned with the guide using a DICOM format with 1 mm slice thickness.

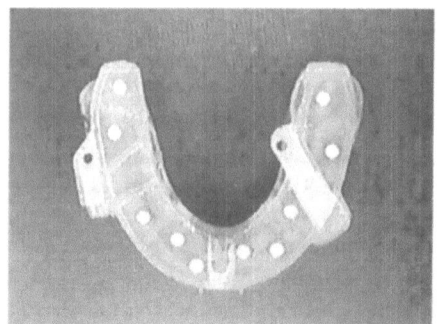
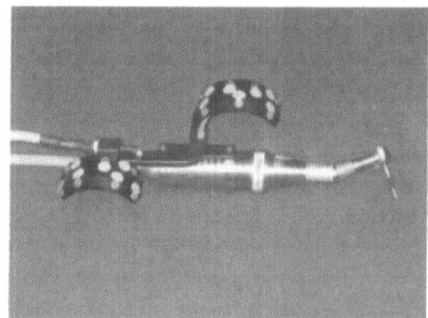

Fig. 1: CT-Guide.   Fig. 2: Surgical Handpiece.

Surgical tools and data acquisition. The position measurement system used is an optical tracker which is an integrated part of the system. The tracker consists of 2 2-D CCDs with an electronic interface to a host computer. The optical tracker determines the position of light emitting diodes (LED), which it computes as the intersection point of 2 lines in the space defined by the photoelectronical sensors of the tracker. The position and orientation

CARS 2002 – H.U. Lemke, M.W. Vannier; K. Inamura, A.G. Farman, K. Doi & J.H.C. Reiber (Editors)

of a tool equipped with at least 3 LEDs can be derived from the measurements provided the tracker sees the LEDs. 14 LEDs are attached to the surgical handpiece (Fig. 2), which determine the position of the handpiece during surgery.

Since the jaw will move during surgery, a sensor assembly with 7 LEDs (referred to as reference body) was developed to update the patient's jaw position continuously (Fig. 3). In the surgical field the reference body is mounted into the guide that is attached to the patient dentition.

Software development and acquisition of position data from the tracking system were done on a PC compatible computer.

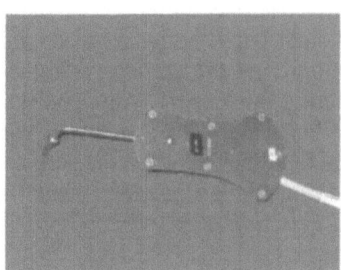

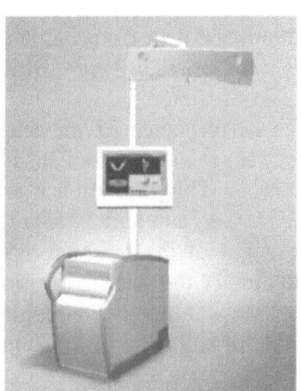

Fig. 3: Reference body.   Fig. 4: Main system.

Surgical protocol. Prior to each surgery, the position of the implants was pre-planned using the IGI software. Pre-operative preparations, including sterile field preparation, pre-surgical medications and local anesthesia were carried out using standard protocol. Registration was performed using the ceramic spheres, and the guide was prepared by cutting out the parts which were in the edentulous areas. The guide was placed together with the reference body on the patient teeth. Each implant was inserted into the jaw bone using standard drilling sequence which was guided by the computerized image on the system screen.

3. Conclusion

Imaging of dental structures using CT is the most accurate imaging modality today for preoperative planning in implant dentistry. Several studies have described the efforts to transfer the planning data to the surgical field [13-16, 18, 19]. Recent data [17] using optical tracking system suggests that both reliable registration and high accuracy can be achieved for computer aided implant surgery.

Our experience of using the IGI navigation system for positioning of dental implants in humans suggests that the system helps to overcome surgical complexities, by allowing the

962

practitioner to better pre-plan the implant position and to trasfer the plan to the operative field. In addition, the system was found to be "user friendly" allowing safe and easy navigation of the insertion route of the bur during the surgery. In case of variance between the plan and the performance, the system alerts the user, thus reducing patient risk. Advantages of the use of image-guided implantology (compared to conventional guide methods) include ability for better planning, the control of implant drill positioning and therefore the possibility for minimal flap reflection, resulting in improved healing.

The technical performance of the IGI optical system provides a good accuracy of approximately 0.1 mm. Using *in vitro* models, the system was found to provide accuracy of 0-1.2 mm (mean 0.5 mm), and 95% of the deviations were found to be below 1 mm [20]. Preliminary data from human studies was found also to be very accurate and the deviations were less than 1 mm, which is acceptable as a standard for implant surgery.

During the performance of the surgeries, we found that one limitation of the optical tracking system is the requirement for a free line-of-sight between the surgical handpiece and the sensors. This limitation was overcome by modifying the seating positions of the surgical team (surgeon and assistant) prior to and during the surgery. Any disturbance in the line-of-sight of the tracking systems was identified by the system, which alert the surgeon to modify the seating position for creating a "free line" between the surgical tools and the sensors. Other technologies such as electromagnetic digitizers, which do not require a line-of sight, are prone to magnetic field distortions [21].

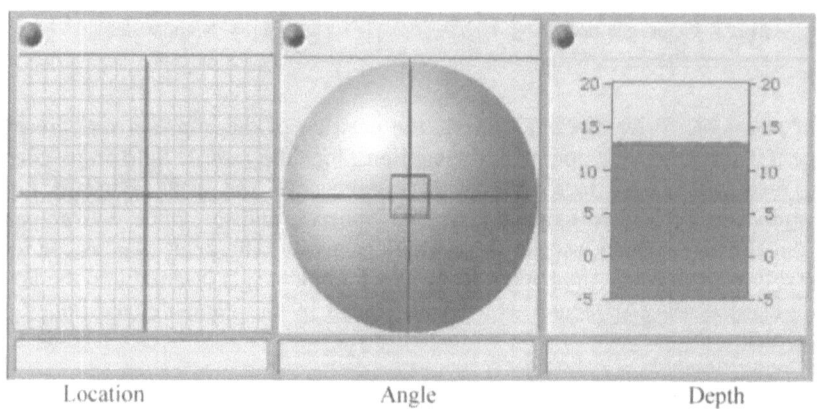

| Location | Angle | Depth |

Figure 5: Navigating screens.

The position of the dental drill can be navigated on the screen using "navigating indicators" (Fig. 5) that guide the surgeon in all 3 dimensions and can also be seen on the CT image (Fig. 6). In our experience the first method is superior during the surgical procedure, assisting the surgeon to position the drill in an accurate site and angle during the drilling procedure. Figure 7 demonstrates 3 dental implants (MIS, Israel) that were positioned using the IGI system.

CARS 2002 – H.U. Lemke, M.W. Vannier; K. Inamura, A.G. Farman, K. Doi & J.H.C. Reiber (Editors)
©CARS/Springer. All rights reserved.

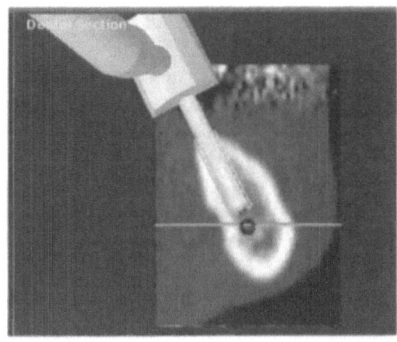 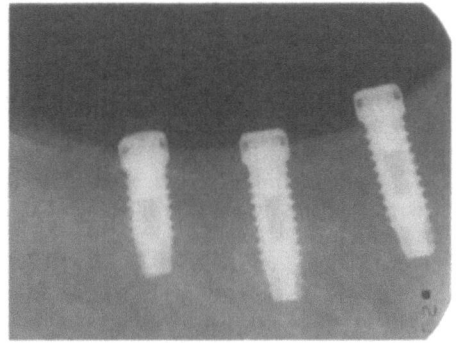

Figure 6: Position of the drill during surgery.　　Figure 7: Dental radiograph of the implants.

In conclusion, the IGI system represents the accuracy and reliability required for the clinical application, improving the safety and efficacy of dental implantology.

References

1. Fenster A & Dwney DB. 3D Ultrasound imaging: A review. IEEE Engineering in Medicine and Biology Magazine 15:41-51, 1996.
2. Joskowicz L, Tockus L, Yaniv Z, Simkin A, Milgrom C. Computer-aided image guided bone fracture surgery: concept and implementation. Computer Aided Surgery 3: 271-288, 1998.
3. Jolesz FA. Interventiaonal and intraoperation MRI: a general overview of the field. J. Magnetic Resonance Image 8:3-7, 1998.
4. Branemark PI, Breien U, Adell R, Hansson BO,Lindstrom H & Ohlsson A. Intraosseous anchorage of dental prostheses. Scand J Plastic Reconst Surg 3:81-100, 1969.
5. Hobkirk JA & Havthoulas TK. The influence of mandibular deformation, implant numbers, and loading position on detected forces in abutments supporting fixed implant superstructures. J Prosthet Dent 80:169-174, 1998.
6. Taylor TD. Prosthodontic problems and limitations associated with osseointegration. J Prosthet Dent 79:74-78, 1998.
7. Rothman SLG, Chaftez N, Rhodes ML & Schwarz MS. CT in the preoperative assessment of the mandible and the maxilla for endosseous implant surgery. Radiology 168:171-175, 1988.
8. Vannier MW, Hildeboldt CF, Conover G, Knapp RH, Yokoyama-Crothers N & Wang G. Three-dimensional dental imaging by spiral CT. Oral Surg Oral Med Oral Pathol, Oral Radiol Endodont 84:561-570, 1997.
9. Jacobs R & van Steenberghe D. Radiographic planning and assessment of endosseous oral implants, Berlin: Springer Verlag, 1998.
10. Quirynen M, Lamoral Y, Dekeyser C, Peene P, Steenberghe DV, Bonte J & Baert AL. The CT scan standard reconstruction technique for reliable jaw bone volume determination. Int J Oral Maxillofacial Implants 5:384-389, 1990.
11. Hussaini S & Canela Pichardo D. Palatal impression template for a fully edentulous arch during stage I implant placement. J Prosthet Dent 77:630-632, 1997.
12. Sicilia A, Noguerol B, Cobo J & Zabalegui I. Profile surgical template: a systematic approach to precise implant placement. A technical note. Int J Oral Maxillofacial Implants 13:109-114, 1998.
13. Fortin T, Coudert JL, Chapleboux G, Sautot P & Lavallee S. Computer-assisted dental implant surgery using computed tomography. J Image Guided Surg 1:53-58, 1995.

CARS 2002 – H.U. Lemke, M.W. Vannier; K. Inamura, A.G. Farman, K. Doi & J.H.C. Reiber (Editors)

964

14. Ploder O, Wagner A, Enislidis G & Ewers R. Computer-assisted intraoperative visualization of dental implants. Augmented reality in medicine. Radiologe 35:569-572, 1995.

15. Solar P, Grampp S & Gsellmann B. A computer-aided navigation system for oral implant surgery using 3D-CT reconstruction and real time video-projection. In: Lemke HU, Vannier MW, Inamura K, Farman AG, eds Computer Assissted Radiology-CAR'96, 884-887, Amsterdam: Elsevier Science, 1996.

16. Watzinger F, Birkfellner W, Wanschitz F, Millesi W, Schopper C, Sinko K, Huber K, Bergmann H & Ewers R. Positioning of dental implants using computer-aided navigation and an optical tracking system: Case report and presentation of a new method. J Cranio-Maxillo-Facial Surg 27:77-81, 1999.

17. Birkfellner W, Solar P, Gahleitner A, Huber K, Kainberger F, Kettenbach L, Homolka P, Diemling M, Watzek G, Bergmann H. In vitro assessment of a registration protocol for image guided implant dentistry. Clin Oral Impl Res 12:69-78, 2001.

18. Verstreken K, Van Cleynenbreugel J, Martens K, Marchal G, van Steenberghe D & Suetens P. An image guided planning system for endosseous oral implants. IEEE Transactions on Medical Imaging 17:842-852, 1998.

19. Verstreken K, Van Cleynenbreugel J, Marchal G, Naert I, Suetens P & van Steenberghe D. Computer-assissted planning of oral implant surgery: A tree dimensional approach. Int J Oral Maxillofacial Implants 11:806-810, 1996.

20. Brief J, Hassfeld S, Sonenfeld U, Persky N, Krempien R, Treiber M, Mühling J. Navigated Insertion of Dental Implants. Proceeding of CARS 2001.

21. Birkfellner W, Watzinger F, Wanschitz F, Enislidis G, Kollmann C, Rafolt D, Nowotny R, Ewers R & Bergmann H. Systematic distortions in magnetic position digitizers. Medical Physics 25:2242-2248, 1998.

CARS 2002 – H.U. Lemke, M.W. Vannier; K. Inamura, A.G. Farman, K. Doi & J.H.C. Reiber (Editors)

Computer based approach for design and treatment of immediately loaded implants

Meyer U.[a], Fillies T.[a], Meier N.[b], Stamm T.[a], Wiesmann HP.[a], Joos U.[a]

[a] Clinic for Cranio- Maxillofacial Surgery, University of Münster, Germany

[b] Institute for Radiology, University of Münster, Germany

Abstract

The survival of implants provide superior stability from a clinical point of view when the implant and bone characteristics match the biological and biomechanical requirements of implants. The design and the placement of implants are important factors governing the long term success. We therefore developed on the basis of finite element calculations a new dental implant system indicated for an immediate loading protocol. To optimise loading and to ease the clinical performance of implant treatment image guided navigation was used to insert implants. Implants were inserted in the mandible of minipigs by the robodent system (Straumann, Germany) according to the boundary conditions used in our FEM analysis. Our results indicate that a good accuracy of implant insertion can be achieved. Immediate placement of prefabricated crowns demonstrated a good occlusal relationship. The maximum deviation between the planned and the realised implant position was 0.6mm. Histological analysis demonstrated a biomechanically stable position of implants. We conclude that the design as well as the insertion and prosthetic treatment of oral implants is improved by computer assisted surgery.

Keywords: Implant, image guided navigation, finite element analysis

1. Introduction

Improved performance of tissue reaction at implant sides which occur at the tissue-implant interface is contributing to a proactive approach of biomaterial design and handling. Computer methods are one tool to improve the production and use of biomaterials which are engineered to elicit specific, desired responses from a patients body. Implant therapy must encompass both anatomical and functional considerations. The long term survival of immediate loaded implants can be obtained when bone loads around implants do not exceed normal bone physiology (1). Whereas previous studies mention that premature loading leads to implant loss, recent studies indicate that it is the excessive bone loading at the implant surface that interferes with bone/implant integration. Bone remodelling is dependent on the effects of bone strains as has been demonstrated in various studies. Frost (2) distinguished a minimum effective strain (500 μstrain) necessary for bone maintenance from supraphysiological strains (>5.000 μstrain) leading to fibrous tissue formation. Strain is the relative elongation of cells, calculated by the ratio between the initial cell length and their elongated length. It is known by finite element calculations that special bone and implant geometries are necessary to achieve a homogenous and physiological strain distribution in bone tissue around loaded implants.

CARS 2002 – H.U. Lemke, M.W. Vannier; K. Inamura, A.G. Farman, K. Doi & J.H.C. Reiber (Editors)

Implant insertion in a proper bone position is an important prerequisite of such an approach. Implants must therefore inserted in an sufficient amount of cortical bone surrounding especially the crestal part of the implant. Computer aided planning and navigation is a new tool to improve the outcome of surgical procedures (3). It is assumed that implant positioning by computer aided surgery is clinically superior in cases of difficult anatomical situations. As immediate loaded implants are dependant on a good bone/implant relation, implant placement can be seen as a difficult clinical approach (4).

The purpose of this study was therefore to test a dental implant in an clinical environment that allows an immediate loading protocol. Two prerequisites should be obtained, the micromotion at the implant surface should not exceed 5.000 µstrain, as assumed by the finite element analysis. Second, the implant should be positioned in mandibular bone in a way that simulates the FE mesh generation.

2. Methodology

An implant was therefore produced on the basis of mathematical calculations and implant placement planning and insertion was performed by a computer aided surgery system (Figure 1a). An experimental animal study was therefore performed to investigate the clinical performance of the implant therapy. Clinical, radiographical and histological investigations of the immediately loaded implants were performed in order to evaluate the success of this approach in an clinical environment.

Mandibular premolars of minipigs were removed and a computed tomography of the skull was performed after healing of extraction sockets. On the basis of CT data the robodent system (Straumann, Freiburg) was used for preoperative planning and intraoperative guidance of implant insertion. The accuracy of the implant position and supraconstruction was evaluated clinically, radiographically and histologically at different time intervals postoperatively. An optical tracking system with specially designed tools allowed implant positioning and immediate prosthetic rehabilitation. Implants were planned by the robodent system to be placed in the second premolar position (occlusal contact) and in the primate gap (non-occlusal contact) (Figure 1b). Planning was performed with special respect given to the bone geometries around the implant and a vertical load protocol. Implants were placed according to the robodent planning system first by the computer assisted navigation in a plaster model of the jaw and single crowns were produced in the dental technician laboratory. For crown production special care was given to allow vertical loads and to avoid tranversal loads on the implants. After production of the crowns implants were then inserted by help of the robodent system in the mandible of anesthesised minipigs according to the preoperative planning (Figure 1c, 1d). Animals were allowed to masticate at the first postoperative day. A CT scan was performed postoperatively to compare the inserted with the planned implant position. After 14 days of mastication animals were sacrified and mandibular bocks explanted to prepare for histological investigations.

3. Data

A new dental implant was designed on the basis of finite element analyses (FEA) in order to gain physiological bone loads at the implant surface. The implants used in this study were screw-shaped implants (max. diameter 4.1mm, length 10 mm). The gross morphology of the implants were designed according to FEA calculations. The FE- mesh was modelled with a specialised computer programme (CAGIG). Models consisting of 10.000 elements were generated. Bone dimensions and bone properties were chosen to simulate mandibular bone. The FE analysis was performed by COSMOS/M and its 8-noded isoparametric volume elements. Loading was performed by application of a vertical load of 150 Newton. Geometrically non-linear and material non-linear calculations were performed. The computed tomography was performed on a Philipps tomoscan and data were stored in a DICOM format. The bone characteristics of the finite element model - compared to the CT data- demonstrated that the alveolar crest in the premolar region matched the bone geometries and properties of minipigs. Implant placement was therefore planned in this region.

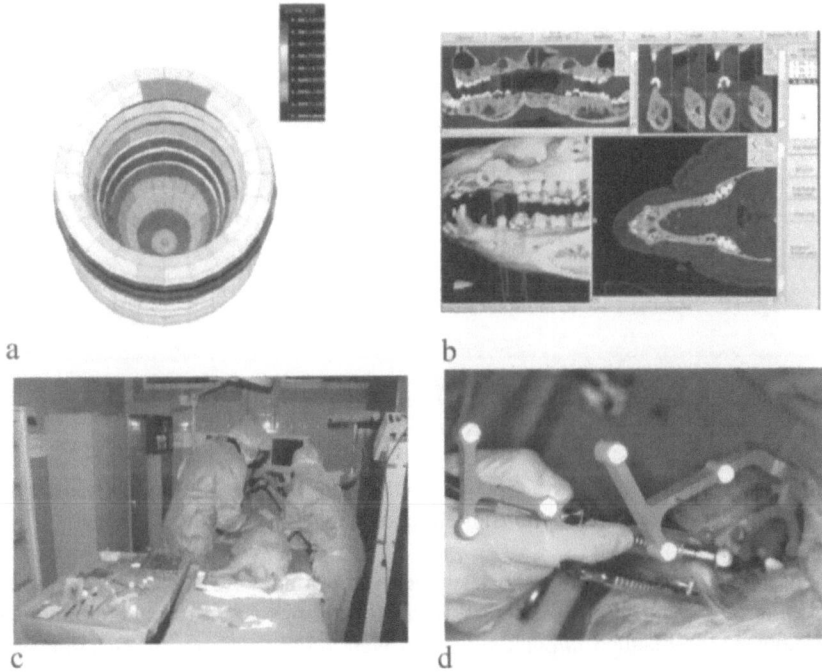

Fig.1: a) Finite element analysis of bone strains adjacent to the implant surface. b) Planned implant positions. c) Image guided surgery. d) Optical tracking of instruments.

4. Results

The mesh generation of bone around the newly designed implant was chosen to lead to a monocortical fixation of the implant. The bone geometries and properties were comparable to bone geometries and densities in the preoperative CT scan of minipigs. The FEA calculations, considering a fixed bond between implant and bone, of vertically loaded implants revealed a homogenous strain distribution at the whole implant surface. Strains were in the range of 1.000 to 3.000 µstrains (Figure 1a). Peak strains did not exceed hyperphysiological values. Strains at the shoulder of the implants did not differ

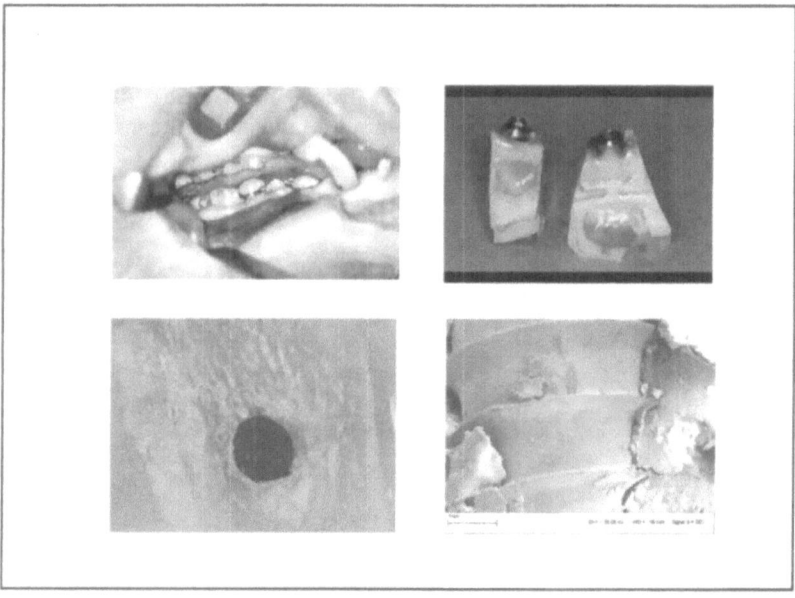

Fig.2: a) Clinical aspect of crown position. b) Explanted specimens. c) Histological cross section d) Implant interface (Scanning electron microscopy).

significantly from those at the tip. Von-Mises stress distribution demonstrated peak stresses at the shoulder and the tip of the implant.

The experimental animal study was designed to investigate the theoretical assumptions in a clinical environment. Preoperative CT scans of minipigs demonstrated an alveolar bone morphology at the planned implant sides that were comparable to the mesh generation of the FE model. Implant insertion under anesthesia was performed in minipigs without clinical problems. The implants could be positioned precisely as preoperatively planned as revealed by postoperative X-rays and CT scans. The accuracy achieved compares well to the resolution of the CT scans used. Maximum deviation of the realised towards the planned implant position was 0.6mm. Implants were inserted in a central alveolar bone position. Immediate prosthetic treatment showed a good occlusal relationship (Figure 2a). Crowns placed on the implants demonstrated a normal contact relation to the neighbour

CARS 2002 – H.U. Lemke, M.W. Vannier; K. Inamura, A.G. Farman, K. Doi & J.H.C. Reiber (Editors)
CARS/Springer. All rights reserved.

teeth as well as a point contact towards the antagonists. Implants were clinically stable after implant insertion by computer aided navigation and remained stable throughout the experimental period. Histological cross sections of explanted mandibular specimens (Figure 2b) revealed a biomechanically stable position of osseointegrated implants. Histology demonstrated a monocortical fixation of implants. Cross sectional views demonstrated a central position of implants in the bone specimens (Figure 2c). There was intimate contact between the implant and the surrounding bone (Figure 2d). The histological picture was similar for the occlusal loaded and non-occlusal loaded implants. Implant positions in the mandibular bone were comparable to the implant position in the finite element mesh.

5. Conclusions

This study was designed to evaluate the possibility to transfer computer based approaches in a clinical environment. Implant design and therapy was performed by the aid of computer technology (4). The results of our study reveal that altering the gross morphology of implants is able to gain homogenous physiological strains at the whole implant surface. Peak loads can be avoided under the assumptions made in our theoretical FE model. Under conditions of good bone quality loading of implants can be performed without excessive micromotion at the implant surface. The experimental results confirm that oral implant insertion and prosthetic treatment is improved by computer assisted surgery (5). Implants can be placed accurately in the planned positions. Due to the high accuracy reached by computer aided navigation it is possible to produce the prosthetic devices prior to surgery. Histological analysis of the early loading phase indicates that occlusal loading can be performed without disturbance of bone physiology. Bone remodeling at the implant surface may be due to a micromovement below the critical strain level. Immediate loading of oral implants may be therefore achieved by a computer based approach.

References

1. Branemark PI, Osseointegration and ist experimental background, J Prosth Dent, 50, 399-410, 1983
2. Frost HM, Mechanical determinants of bone remodeling, Calcif Tissue Int, 36, 56-61, 1984
3. Watzinger F, Birkfellner W., Wanschnitz F, Positioning of dental implants using computer aided navigation and an optical tracking system: case report and presentation of a new method, 27, 77-81, 1999
4. Meyer U, Vollmer D, Bourauel C, Joos U, Sensitivity analysis of bone geometries around oral implants upon loading using finite element method, Comp Meth Biomech Biomed Eng, 4, 143-147, 2001
5. Use of an image guided navigation system in dental implant surgery in anatomically complex operation sites, Sießegger M, Schneider BT, Mischkowski RA, Lazar F, Krug B, Klesper B, Zöller JE, J Cranio Maxillofac Surg, 29, 276-2

CARS 2002 – H.U. Lemke, M.W. Vannier; K. Inamura, A.G. Farman, K. Doi & J.H.C. Reiber (Editors)

970

Surgical simulation of multisegment osteotomies and implant dentistry in cleft palates

Rüdiger Marmulla, Stefan Hassfeld, Joachim Mühling
Dept. of Cranio-Maxillofacial Surgery, University of Heidelberg, Germany

Abstract

So far, multi segment osteotomies have not been realized in the course of threedimensional surgical planning and intraoperative surgical navigation. A new multilayser splint system to achieve this goal is presented.

Keywords: Cleft palate, mid-face hypoplasia, surgical planning, navigation

1. Introduction

Mid-face hypoplasia and maxillary micrognathism in patients with a cleft lip and a cleft palate require complex surgical planning of five single procedures:
- maxillary advancement
- transversal expansion of the maxilla
- osteoplasty of the cleft palate
- dental implantation within the area of the former cleft palate
- prosthetic rehabilitation
A new multilayer splint system for computer assisted surgical navigation of multiple osteotomied maxillary segments is presented.

2. Material and methods

The laboratory unit for surgical simulation (LUCAS) is implemented on a workstation from the surgical navigation network (SNS, Fig. 1). Additional tools for registration and calculation of the target positon of multiple bone segments have been developed with Visual Studio .net from Microsoft and have been implemented as a Surgical Segment Navigator tool (SSN^2) on the surgical navigation network workstation (SNS).

The target position of multiple segments is transferred to a multilayer splint system and to infrared transmitters which are fixed on the multilayers of the splint system.

Surgical planning data define the spatial displacement of the multiple bone segments. These data are transferred via disk or intranet to the SSN^2 system and its infrared localizing system in the operating room. Figures 2 to 6 describe the multilayer splint system that is prepared for computer assisted surgical navigation of multiple bone segments (Fig. 8).

A first surgical simulation of implant dentistry is performed on the simulated post op cast, the final surgical simulation of implant dentistry can be based on a maxillary CT or Cone Beam data set six months after computer assisted repositioning osteotomy of the cleft palate [1, 5].

CARS 2002 – H.U. Lemke, M.W. Vannier; K. Inamura, A.G. Farman, K. Doi & J.H.C. Reiber (Editors)

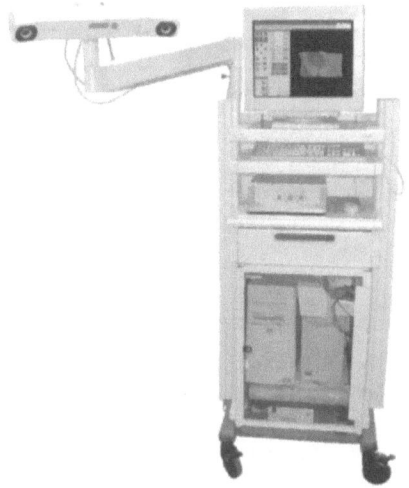

Fig. 1 Additional tools for registration and calculation of the target positon of multiple bone segments have been developed with Visual Studio .net from Microsoft and have been implemented as a Surgical Segment Navigator^2 tool (SSN^2) on the surgical navigation network workstation (SNS). In contrast to the former SSN system, the SSN^2 can be connected as well to a Flashpoint *and* to a Polaris infrared camera system.

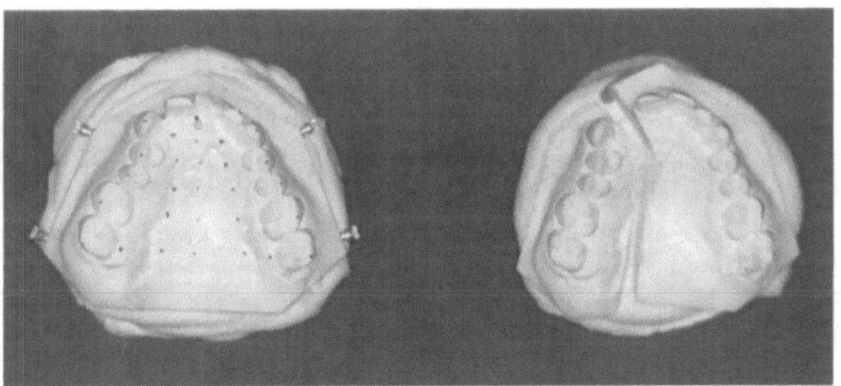

Fig. 2 Surgical repositioning of two maxillary segments is documented in two dental casts. 30 points on the surface of each cast are used for infrared measurement and navigation (Fig. 7). An infrared pointer registers these marked points. Left cast: pre op situation. Right cast: pre op surgical planning with transversal enlargement parallel to the maxillary cleft.

972

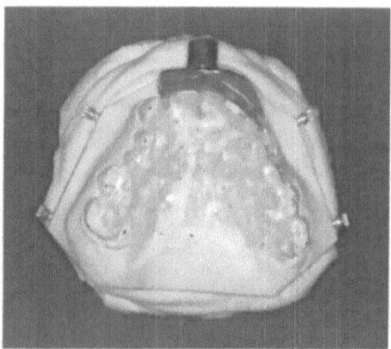 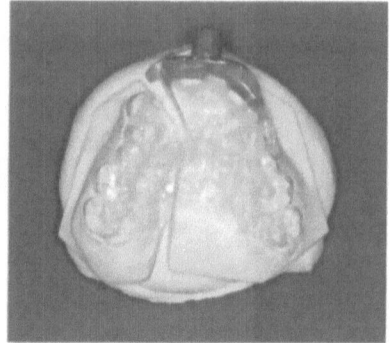

Fig. 3 (left), Fig. 4 (right) A dental splint for repositioning osteotomy is segmented in two parts for the right and for the left segment. Both splint segments fit to the pre op cast (Fig. 3) and the simulated post op cast (Fig. 4). A mechanical interface - to be connected to the infrared transmitters for surgical navigation - is fixed to one of the two splint segments. These two splint segments define a first layer splint system.

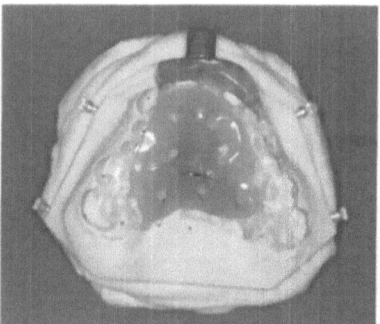 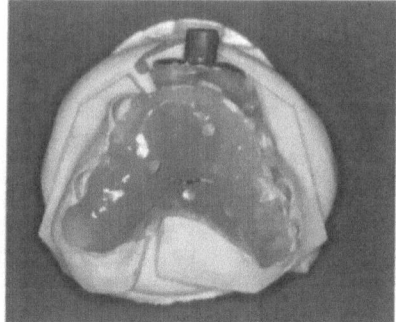

Fig. 5 (left), Fig. 6 (right) Two different sandwich splints define a second layer and can be fixed on the two first layer splint segments via pins. These two second layer sandwich splints define the pre op (Fig. 5) and simulated post op spatial relationship (Fig. 6) between the two first layer splint segments.

CARS 2002 – H.U. Lemke, M.W. Vannier; K. Inamura, A.G. Farman, K. Doi & J.H.C. Reiber (Editors)

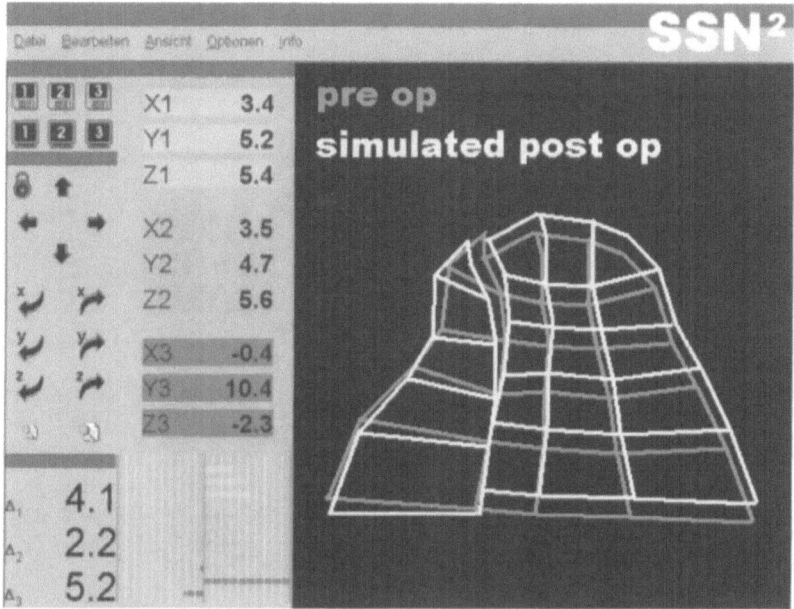

Fig. 7 Threedimensional surgical simulation of a maxillary multisegment osteotomy. The monitor of the SSN² workstation displays the pre op and the post op position of the segments. The data set can directly be used for surgical navigation (Fig. 8).

3. Results

The multilayer splint system with infrared transmitters allows for accurate threedimensional navigation of multiple maxillary segments in relation to the skull base.

Without navigation, it is difficult or impossible to reproduce the surgical plan in three dimensions, especially in the distal area of the upper jaw. The navigation system allows easily to achieve this goal - thus surgical navigation is very helpful to transfer a surgical plan concerning the spatial relationship of segments to the skull base on the one hand.

On the other hand the multilayer splint system allows for the navigation of a block of single osteotomied segments in a mechanical way. The spatial relationship between the single maxillary segments is defined via the second splint layer. This second splint layer is produced with the precision of a dental laboratory that is much higher than the precision achieved by computer assisted surgical navigation - thus surgical navigation is less helpful to transfer a surgical plan concerning the spatial relationship between single maxillary segments.

These two effects are combined in the presented method of computer assisted surgical navigation of multiple maxillary segments fixed by a multilayer splint system.

974

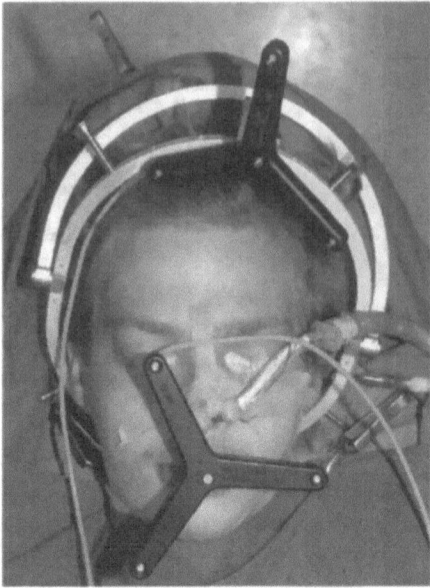

Fig. 8 Surgial navigation of the two maxillary segments is carried out with infrared transmitters which are connected to the presented multilayer splint system. The intra op navigation can be compared to the typical surgical segment navigation that is performed on one bone segment [3]. The multilayer splint system connects the single osteotomied segments.

Computer assisted surgical navigation is useful as long as methods and guiding functionalities are supported that maximize precision, minimize risk and the costs of a surgical approach [2] - this is guaranteed for example for the navigation of segments in relation to the skull base [3, 4] - but this is not guaranteed for the transferration of a surgical plan concerning the spatial relationship between single maxillary segments; here, the information of the spatial relationship between the maxillary segments can easily be put into a second layer splint with the accuracy of a dental laboratory (100 µm and better).

References

1. Hassfeld S, Brief J, Stein W, Ziegler C, Redlich T, Raczkowsky J, Krempien R, M‚hling J:Navigationsverfahren in der Implantologie - Stand der Technik und Perspektiven. Implantologie 8, 373-390, 2000
2. Hassfeld S, M‚hling J, Zˆller J: Intraoperative navigation in oral and m axillofacial surgery Int J Oral Maxillofac Surg 24: 111-119, 1995
3. Marmulla R, Niederdellmann H: Computer-assisted bone segment navigation. J Craniomaxillofac Surg 26, 347-359, 1998
4. Marmulla R: Computergest‚tzte Knochenseg mentnavigation Quintessenz, Chicago, Berlin, 2000
5. Stein W, Hassfeld S, Brief J, Bertovic I, Krempin R, M‚hling J: CT-based 3D-planning for dental implantology. Stud Health Technol Inform 50,137-43, 1998

CARS 2002 – H.U. Lemke, M.W. Vannier; K. Inamura, A.G. Farman, K. Doi & J.H.C. Reiber (Editors)

Computer aided navigation and interactive teleconsultation in dental implantology

K. Schicho [a], A. Wagner [a], R. Ewers [a]

[a] University Hospital of Cranio-Maxillofacial and Oral Surgery, Medical School University of Vienna, Waehringer Guertel 18-20, 1090 Vienna, Austria

Abstract

Utilizing advancements in software technology and clinical practicability computer-aided navigation technology is gaining in significance in the field of dental implantology. This presentation is intended to describe the current state of technical development in the field of implant navigation, particularly focusing on practicability, reliability and work-flow in routine clinical application. Technical requirements, potential and limitations of interactive teleconsultation to support the preoperative planning procedure via internet are depicted. A least-squares error algorithm (as implemented in navigation software) is discussed as a possible approach for improved accuracy control. Computer aided navigation actually proofs to be suitable for practical application and particularly advantageous to comprehensive preoperative planning based on accurate assessment of bone density and structure. The preoperative plan can be realized exactly, avoiding nerve- and teeth- damage. Interactive teleconsultation via internet can provide valuable support especially during the initial phase for surgeons who are not well versed in computer-based planning of implant positions. The accuracy-control algorithm is appropriate to detect systematic registration errors (i.e. mistaken identification of fiducial markers) and cumulative intraoperative errors, but does not separately reflect all components affecting overall quality of system performance.

Keywords: Dental implantology, computer aided navigation, interactive teleconsultation

1. Introduction

Computer-based navigation systems were initially developed for neurosurgical applications [1]. In ENT-Surgery this technology is already established with an ever increasing number of applications [2, 3]. To adapt computer-aided navigation to applications in the field of cranio- and maxillofacial surgery, numerous hard- and software innovations were required. These efforts resulted in successful applications of navigation technology for temporomandibular joint arthroscopy, distraction osteogenesis and in the surgical treatment of post-traumatic deformities of the zygoma [4-6]. Currently navigation in dental implantology is a topic of increasing interest and importance, from scientific as well as from practical aspects. Navigation in dental implantology aims at a comprehensive preoperative planning of implant positions, considering the prosthetic concept, followed by a precise and secure realization of this plan also in case of patients with most difficult implantologic situations (e.g. after ablative tumor surgery). Recently published studies report on promising results in navigated dental implantology [7-10]. The objective of this

976

lecture is to summarize the actual state of development in computer assisted placement of oral implants, to present various 3D visualizations and a workflow for routine application, including an approach to teleconsultation via internet to support the planning procedure.

2. Materials and methods

2.1 Technical setup and workflow

This work is based on investigations by means of the Virtual Patient Implant™ system (Artma Medical Technologies AG, Vienna, Austria) combined with an active optoelectronic tracking system for position- and motion capturing (FlashPoint 3000™, Image Guided Technologies Inc., USA).

In step 1 of the workflow for computer aided implant navigation a plastic imprint splint with markers is prepared for CT scanning (workflow step 2). Preoperative planning of implant positions is performed synchronously using 2D and 3D models calculated from CT images. Prosthetic requirements have to be taken into account. An interactive step-by-step menu structure of the software provides a guideline during the planning phase, which starts with automatically reading of CT data by the system (step 3). After optimizing graphic representation of anatomical structures by setting distinct parameters (e.g. Hounsfield values), a „dental arc" (i.e. a curve following the positions of the teeth, step 4) and (in case of implantation at the lower jaw) the inferior alveolar nerve (step 5) are drawn (Fig.1). As a precaution, definition of the nerve is performed manually, but supported by 2D and 3D views.

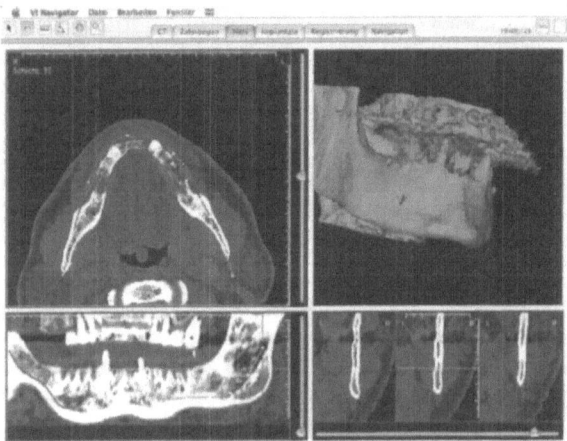

Figure 1. Analysis of bone structure by means of synchronized 2D- and 3D-views in the planning procedure. The inferior alveolar nerve is drawn point-by-point in the axial CT or in the panoramic view. The mental nerve should be marked directly at the mental foramen of the mandible in the 3D view, which can also be switched to a semi-transparent mode to make the nerve clearly perceptible.

In the next preoperative step implants are selected from a list, where they are classified by manufacturer, length and diameter, and moved to the correct position by „drag and drop" (step 6). „Fine-tuning" of implant position and orientation can be carried out in various

CARS 2002 – H.U. Lemke, M.W. Vannier; K. Inamura, A.G. Farman, K. Doi & J.H.C. Reiber (Editors)
ᶜCARS/Springer. All rights reserved.

977

2D and 3D views (Figs. 2a-c), that are synchronized for this purpose. Additional tools for precise measurements during planning are implemented in the software.

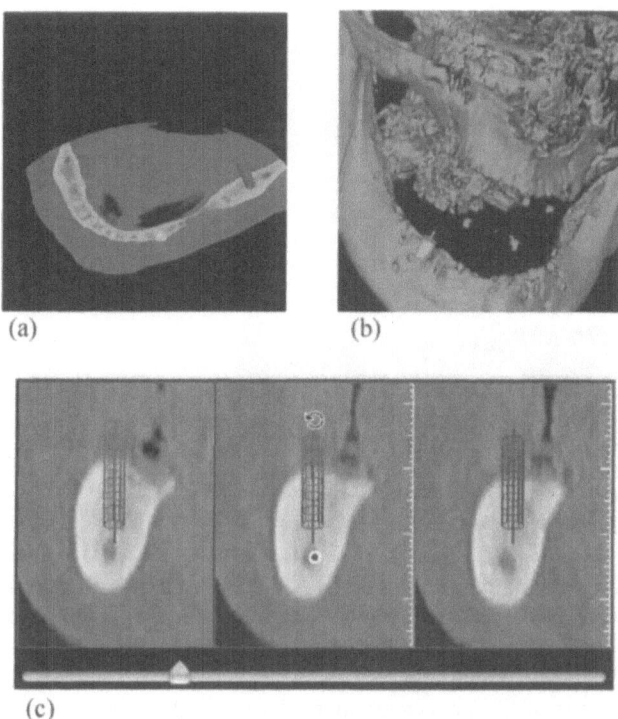

(a) (b)

(c)

Figure 2. Planning and "fine-tuning" of implant positions and orientations in various views.

The planning procedure is comfortable and easy to do from the technical point of view, therefore it and can be performed shortly before the start of the operation. Alternatively, planning can be supported by interactive teleconsultation via internet, e.g. in cases where additional prosthetic advice is desired. For this purpose sufficient capacity of the internet connection is required, e.g. ADSL, ISDN or LAN. At the remote site either a complete planning system or only software for remote control of the navigation system can be used.

During the operation a sensor is rigidly attached to the patient's jaw (step 7). Four distinct fiducial markers of the splint are manually defined on the computer screen and then touched with a digitizing stylus in arbitrary consecutive order (on the splint while it is attached to the patient's jaw – step 8). The plastic imprint splint is removed after initial registration. A least-squares error algorithm calculates a measure for the overall registration-error (section 2.2). Provided that this value remains under a specified limit (usually <2.0mm), navigation can start (step 9). During the operation various 2D and 3D views can be choosen, enabling clearly arranged, precise positioning and orientation of dental implants by means of additional intuitive graphical tools (Fig.3).

CARS 2002 – H.U. Lemke, M.W. Vannier; K. Inamura, A.G. Farman, K. Doi & J.H.C. Reiber (Editors)

978

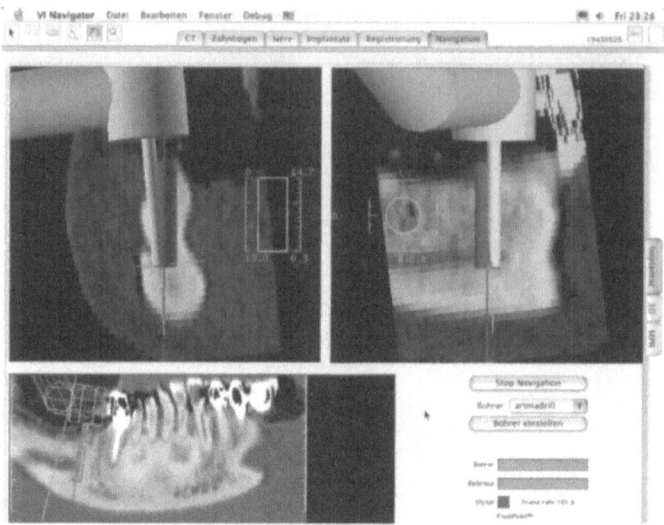

Figure 3. Intraoperative screen showing position and inclination of the drill. Orientation is additionally supported by "spider lines".

2.2 Algorithms for control of overall registration error and overall intraoperative error

An algorithm integrated in the navigation software analyzes deviations between corresponding coordinates of fiducial markers on the splint determined by applying two different methods: 1.: 4 fiducial markers perceptible as points (diameter about 1.5mm) in planar reconstructions of CT-images are manually marked on the screen of the navigation computer. 2.: These 4 fiducial markers are touched with a stylus during the registration process (workflow step 8), leading to coordinate-measurements by means of the digitizing system. Corresponding coordinates are integrated in a least-squares error (LSE) algorithm, i.e.:

$$LSE := \sqrt{\frac{\sum_{i=1}^{4}\left((x_{si} - x_{di})^2 + (y_{si} - y_{di})^2 + (z_{si} - z_{di})^2\right)}{4}} \quad ,$$

with (x_{si}, y_{si}, z_{si}) ... coordinates determined on the screen and (x_{di}, y_{di}, z_{di}) ... corresponding coordinates delivered by the digitizer. Registration is based on 4 fiducial markers, therefore 4 squared deviations are calculated. Applying basic rules of matrix algebra, (x_d, y_d, z_d) are calculated from original digitizer data (ξ, ψ, ζ) with the matrix equation (containing the homogeneous registration matrix):

CARS 2002 – H.U. Lemke, M.W. Vannier; K. Inamura, A.G. Farman, K. Doi & J.H.C. Reiber (Editors)

$$
\begin{pmatrix} x_d \\ y_d \\ z_d \\ 1 \end{pmatrix} = \begin{pmatrix} a_{11} & a_{12} & a_{13} & 0 \\ a_{21} & a_{22} & a_{23} & 0 \\ a_{31} & a_{32} & a_{33} & 0 \\ a_{41} & a_{42} & a_{43} & 1 \end{pmatrix} \cdot \begin{pmatrix} \xi \\ \psi \\ \zeta \\ 1 \end{pmatrix}
$$

Registration errors and additional inaccuracies e.g. resulting from the distances between CT slices and from inaccuracies in the calibration of the drill are cumulatively described by an overall error value that is displayed intraoperatively.

3. Results

Computer-aided implant navigation proves to be feasible for routine clinical application now. The least-squares algorithm for control of registration accuracy and control of intraoperative overall system accuracy theoretically clearly reflects the „dynamic" of cumulative errors, but system-inherent sources of errors respectively inaccuracies affecting overall system performance can not be registered separately.

4. Discussion

Today there are still unabated controversies on advantages of computerized navigation in the field of dental implantology. Some surgeons assure that navigation technology and augmented reality are not required for effective, successful implantation, on the other hand the testing phase of the system used in this study clearly revealed, that navigation is likely to provide valuable support also for experienced surgeons. Computer aided navigation technology enables a detailed assessment of the specific anatomical situation and available bone and can guarantee an exact realization of prosthetic concepts even in complicated cases. The risk of nerve damage is minimized. Nevertheless, correct handling of all components of the system is a fundamental prerequisite.

Implementation of algorithms to control registration- and intraoeprative accuracy can contribute to detection of possible handling-errors timely and improve reliability of implant navigation. However, the least-squares error approach presented in this lecture only allows for a reliable detection of cumulative errors, including systematic registration errors (i.e. mistaken identification of fiducial markers on the splint), digitizer errors and errors in the calibration of the drill, but it can not provide concise information concerning factors affecting system performance separately. This task can hardly be accomplished, because of the large number of factors actually influencing overall system accuracy (e.g. digitizer errors must be expected to be at least > 0.25mm). The fact that fiducial markers have to be identified on the computer screen manually to start calculation of the registration error is not likely to increase the overall system error considerably: Proceeding on the assumption of a display size of 24.5*18.5cm^2 and a resolution of 1024*768 pixel, the center of circular fiducials (diameter on the screen: approximately 1.5mm) can clearly be identified. Howewer, fully automatic detection of fiducials in the registration procedure might be subject of future developments.

5. Conclusion

Computer assisted navigation is a promising technology also in the placement of oral implants. Interactive teleconsultation facilitates and optimizes quality of treatment planning and can therefore be expected to increase acceptance of computer aided navigation systems in dental implantology.

Acknowledgements

We gratefully acknowledge support by Michael Truppe MD, George Varga MS, Ferenc Pongracz DSc and the Austrian Science Foundation FWF P-12489 med.

References

1.   P.J. Kelly. State of the Art and Future Directions of Minimally Invasive Stereotactic Neurosurgery. Cancer Control 1995;2:287-292.
2.   W. Freysinger, A.R. Gunkel, C. Pototschnig, W.F. Thumfart, M. Truppe. New developments in 3D endonasal and frontobasal endoscopic sinus surgery. Kugler Publications, Paris 1995.
3.   W.F. Thumfart, W. Freysinger, A.R. Gunkel, M.J. Truppe. 3D image-guided surgery on the example of the 5,300-year-old Innsbruck Iceman. Acta Otolaryngol 1997;117(2):131-4.
4.   A. Wagner, G. Undt, F. Watzinger, F. Wanschitz, K. Schicho, K. Yerit, C. Kermer, W. Birkfellner, R. Ewers. Principles of computer-assisted arthroscopy of the temporomandibular joint with optoelectronic tracking technology. Oral Surg Oral Med Oral Pathol Oral Radiol Endod 2001;92(1):30-7.
5.   F. Watzinger, F. Wanschitz, M. Rasse, W. Millesi, C. Schopper, J. Kremser, W. Birkfellner, K. Sinko, R. Ewers. Computer-aided surgery in distraction osteogenesis of the maxilla and mandible. Int J Oral Maxillofac Surg. 1999;28:171-175.
6.   F. Watzinger, F. Wanschitz, A. Wagner, G. Enislidis, W. Millesi, A. Baumann, R. Ewers. Computer-aided navigation in secondary reconstruction of post-traumatic deformities of the zygoma. J Craniomaxillofac Surg. 1997;25:198-202.
7.   M. Siessegger, B.T.Schneider, R.A. Mischkowski, F. Lazar, B. Krug, B. Klesper, J.E. Zoller. Use of an image-guided navigation system in dental implant surgery in anatomically complex operation sites. J Craniomaxillofac Surg 2001;29(5):276-81.
8.   Schicho K., Ewers R. Telekonsultation und 3D-Visualisierung in der computerunterstützten Implantologie: Der aktuelle Entwicklungsstand; Implantologie Journal 5/2001:86-88.
9.   F. Watzinger, W. Birkfellner, F. Wanschitz, W. Millesi, C. Schopper, K. Sinko, K. Huber, H. Bergmann, R. Ewers. Positioning of dental implants using computer-aided navigation and an optical tracking system: case report and presentation of a new method. J Craniomaxillofac Surg 1999;27(2):77-81.
10. A. Wagner, F. Wanschitz, W. Birkfellner, K. Zauza, F. Watzinger, K. Schicho F. Kainberger, C. Czerny, H. Bergmann, R. Ewers. Computer-Aided Placement of Endosseous Oral Implants in Patients after Ablative Tumor Surgery: Assessment of Accuracy. Clinical Oral Implants Research, in press

Image-Guided Cranio-Maxillofacial Surgery

CARS 2002 – H.U. Lemke, M.W. Vannier; K. Inamura, A.G. Farman, K. Doi & J.H.C. Reiber (Editors)

3D osteotomy planning in cranio-maxillofacial surgery: experiences and results of surgery planning and volumetric finite-element soft tissue prediction in three clinical cases

Stefan Zachow [a], Evgeny Gladilin [a], Adam Trepczynski [a],
Robert Sader [b], Hans-Florian Zeilhofer [b]

[a] Zuse-Institute Berlin (ZIB), Takustr. 7, 14195 Berlin, Germany
[b] Dept. of Oral & Maxillofacial Surgery, University of Technology Munich

Abstract

In this paper we present the current status of our work on the development of an integrated 3D osteotomy planning system for cranio-maxillofacial surgery. Besides the demonstration of recent finite-element simulations for soft tissue prediction, as a *result* of an osteotomy planning, we introduce a novel technique for an improved planning of the osteotomy itself. In contrast to common approaches that concentrate on bone rearrangements only, neglecting the actual planning of bone cuts, a free-hand osteotomy planning method for arbitrarily shaped cuts is presented. Thus, sagittal split osteotomies of the mandible according to Obwegeser-Dal Pont can be planned correctly under consideration of vulnerable structures, as for instance the mandibular nerve

Keywords: Cranio-maxillofacial surgery, osteotomy planning, soft tissue prediction

1. Introduction

Severe cranio-maxillofacial dysmorphies always require an extensive planning of the surgical treatment. However, in current clinical practice well established techniques on the basis of lateral cephalograms, dental casts, or stereolithographic models are limited to the assessment of functional rehabilitation, i.e. the dental occlusion, or skull symmetry. In computer-assisted 3D osteotomy planning, advanced techniques, based on geometric modeling, image processing and numerical analysis can be combined with conventional planning methods to achieve a better imagination of what a certain treatment will result in. This is especially true for the assessment of different osteodistraction or bone relocation procedures, as well as for the consideration of vulnerable structures like nerves and vessels within the scope of osteotomy planning. Nevertheless, the most appreciated feature of an improved 3D planning is a reliable prediction of the post-operative facial appearance. We present the current status of our work on such an integrated system for 3D osteotomy planning, that will be exemplified on three clinical cases.

2. Material and methods

In our previous work we have shown that osteotomy planning can be improved in several ways [1,2]. Our approach on using patient specific tetrahedral grids of the entire facial tissue, and applying enforced deformations due to relocations of embedded bony structures, has proven to be extremely robust for the prediction of a resulting soft tissue

CARS 2002 – H.U. Lemke, M.W. Vannier; K. Inamura, A.G. Farman, K. Doi & J.H.C. Reiber (Editors)

984

deformation [3]. The generation of adequate patient models is always based on a segmentation stage, followed by a surface reconstruction and an adaptive surface simplification. Finally a tetrahedral grid with controlled aspect ratios is generated from the simplified surface model [4]. A typical head model consists of approx. 200.000 triangles. The soft tissue grid, generated from such a surface model, is made up of 0.5 million tetrahedra and more. The entire model generation usually takes several hours, depending on artifacts, that have to be removed or the number and resolution of anatomic structures, that have to be taken into account for surgery planning. In total we performed our planning on five different clinical cases within the last two years, while developing and optimizing tools and methods for an intuitive and fast operation planning. Currently we are working on enhanced tools for the 3D planning of the osteotomies themselves. Our goal is to provide an intuitive and easy to use interface for surgeons to perform osteotomy planning on individual bone models under consideration of the preservation of vulnerable structures.

2.1 Osteotomy planning

For the planning of osteotomies there exist two different strategies, that have been investigated: i) a definition of a trajectory in 3D for a virtual cutting tool, and ii) a definition of osteotomy lines on top of the 3D bone surface. Both methodologies lead to a surface (i.e. a manifold in R^3), that can be used for cutting the bone model including inner structures. However, the latter method seems to be the most intuitive one, because it reproduces the common practice of drawing osteotomy lines onto a stereolithographic model of a patient's skull *before* cutting it with surgical instruments. A possibility for direct cuts might be of interest for surgical training, but it requires dedicated 3D input and output devices, two handed interaction and force feedback for an immersive look and feel. Even with appropriate devices, VR techniques and the experience or ability to use these things properly, it turned out, that it is pretty difficult to perform correct cuts in a direct manner. In practice it is much easier to draw a contour line onto the bone model's surface.

Drawing osteotomy lines onto the bone model

For the definition of osteotomy lines on a 3D surface model we do not require dedicated input devices or stereo viewing techniques. A contour can simply be drawn onto the polygonal surface model via a standard computer mouse or an electronic pen (figure 1a). The contour line is always automatically attached to the visible surface. One can correct misshaped contour segments, and one can stop and resume drawing a contour for intermediate rotation, translation or zoom of the bone model. Thus, arbitrary cut lines can be defined.

Arbitrary cuts of the bone model

A closed contour in 3D allows us to generate a surface, that can be used for cutting the bone model including all inner structures like nerves and vessels, what of course is not intended to happen during surgery. Within the osteotomy planning stage, however, it is very useful to visualize the interdependencies between cut surfaces and bone models. We implemented two different ways of creating surfaces from contours, having in mind, that a cutting tool must be able to produce such a cut surface. Therefore, one can chose between *minimal surfaces* and so called *ruled surfaces*, to be generated from a given contour [5,6]. Minimal surfaces are suited for flexible cutting tools, while ruled surfaces rather meet the requirements of being a good approximation of surfaces that result from cuts with non-flexible saw blades. Since ruled surfaces are generated by lines that are moved along a

CARS 2002 – H.U. Lemke, M.W. Vannier; K. Inamura, A.G. Farman, K. Doi & J.H.C. Reiber (Editors)

trajectory, a start and an end point must be specified. This is easily done by clicking on the contour or moving appropriate markers along the contour line.

After cut surfaces have been defined by contour lines (or direct sweeps of a cutting tool), these surfaces can still be modified (shifted, deformed or enlarged) to meet all require-ments of a reasonable osteotomy for a specific anatomical situation. The cut surface can be visualized in combination with the bone surface to assess the resulting cut with regard to the protection of vulnerable structures (figure 1b). A surface intersection algorithm finally cuts the bone model with the cut surface, for the individual relocation of separated bone parts, as shown in figure 1c. Cut surfaces can be stored for documentation, further assessment or even as input for a navigated intraoperative use.

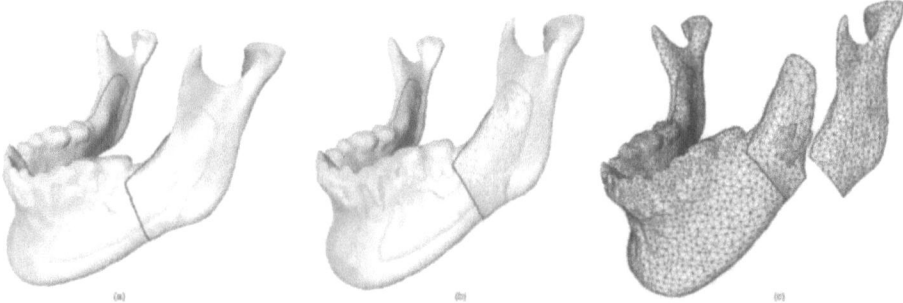

Fig. 1. Sagittal split osteotomy: a) osteotomy line drawn onto the bone surface, b) cut surface in combination with a transparent view of the bone model, c) surface cut

2.2 Relocation of bony structures

The initial bone model for cranio-maxillofacial surgery planning typically consists of the skull and the mandible, with the mandible as the only moveable part, that can be rotated around the mandibular joints as well as shifted a bit forward, backward and sideways. After osteotomies have been performed on the bone model, separated bony structures can also be relocated individually. They can either be rigidly transformed via numeric input (rotation axes, angles and translation vectors) or interactively with any 2D or 3D input device. The transformation of bone parts can be assessed visually with regard to occlusion and symmetry, or quantitatively by a resulting transformation matrix. Such an information is particularly useful for osteodistraction planning, where optimal distraction vectors (magnitude and direction) are to be found.

Osteodistraction

In our studies we performed two plannings for distraction osteogenesis, with unidi-rectional as well as bidirectional distractions. With regard to soft tissue simulation only, an osteotomy planning is not necessarily needed, because the gap between bone fragments will be closed by osseous tissue again. Thus, we do not cut the bone model but mark the osteotomy zone where callus will be generated. The distraction is then modeled by a movement of the bone fragment with mesh relaxation in the vicinity of and within the callus zone (cf. figure 2c). Nevertheless, an osteotomy can be planned as mentioned above for the assessment of the bone structures that are to be cut. For the finite-element simulation of soft tissue deformation, however, the tetrahedral grid will only be stretched, although it would even make sense to generate new tetrahedra within the callus zone to consider bone growth and keep the aspect ratio in an optimal range.

986

Osteosynthesis

For the planning of osteosyntheses (i.e. bone relocation and fixation with mini-plates), a correct osteotomy of the bone model is mandatory for soft tissue simulation, because a bone relocation leads to gaps between bony structures that can be filled with soft tissue. In our studies we performed three plannings for osteosyntheses, with two combined osteotomies, i.e. a (high) Le Fort I osteotomy of the maxilla according to Bell and a sagittal split osteotomy of thew mandible according to Obwegeser-Dal Pont.

For both, osteodistraction and osteosynthesis planning any displacement of bony structures leads to a 3D vector field, that serves as an initial boundary condition, and can be applied to the tetrahedral grid of the patient's soft tissue. The tissue grid, the displacement vectors and a biomechanical model of soft tissue are the basis for our finite-element approximation of the resulting deformation of the entire facial soft tissue [7].

3. Results

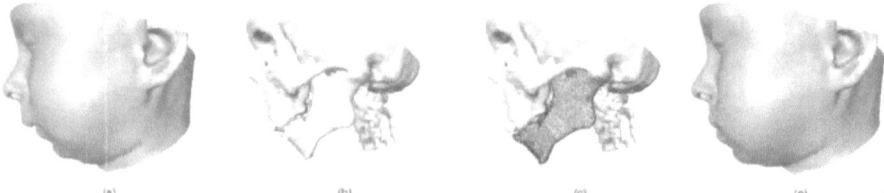

Fig. 2. 3D Planning of a unidirectional distraction of the mandible: left) pre-operative situation and model, right) distraction planning and soft tissue prediction

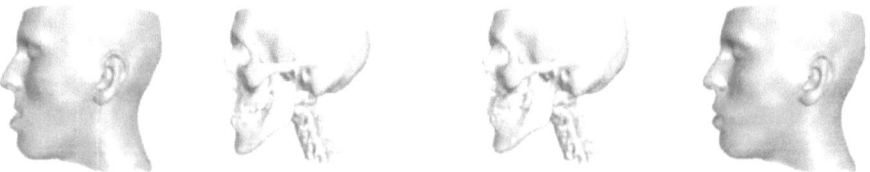

Fig. 3. 3D Planning of a bimaxillary ostetomy: left) pre-operative situation, right) osteotomy planning and soft tissue prediction

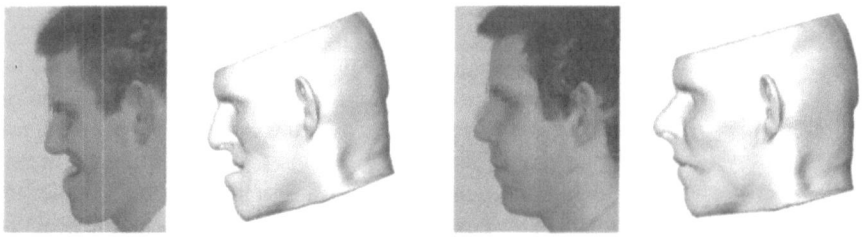

Fig. 4. 3D Planning of a bimaxillary ostetomy: left) pre-operative situation and model, right) post-operative result and simulation

CARS 2002 – H.U. Lemke, M.W. Vannier; K. Inamura, A.G. Farman, K. Doi & J.H.C. Reiber (Editors)

4. Conclusions and future work

Our 3D planning environment including soft tissue prediction has been accepted as a very valuable aid by our cooperating surgeons. Currently we are able to perform a full planning including the generation of an anatomically correct, patient specific model within one or two days, where the planning itself takes only 30 to 60 minutes.

Our free-hand osteotomy planning approach will be further extended in such a way, that the tomographic data can be projected onto the cut surface via texture mapping. Thus, osteotomies can be directly assessed with regard to the preservation of vulnerable structures, without the need of having these structures segmented in advance. Future work is directed to the collaborative use of our planning system, where radiologists or medical assistants evaluate and segment the tomographic data and prepare the 3D patient grid model, and surgeons concentrate on osteotomy planning and bone rearrangement. Due to our volumetric modeling approach the soft tissue prediction comes with no extra costs, as a result of the bone rearrangements. A further extension of our planning system – the simulation of patient specific, anatomy based, and muscle driven mimics – is also in good progress, and will be another valuable criterion for the assessment of a patient's facial appearance after the planning of complex surgical treatments [8].

References

1. Zachow, S ; Gladilin, E ; Hege, HC ; Deuflhard, P: Finite-Element Simulation of Soft Tissue Deformation. In: Lemke, H.U. et al. (eds.): Computer Assisted Radiology and Surgery (CARS), San Francisco, USA, pp. 23–28 (2000)
2. Zachow, S ; Gladilin, E ; Zeilhofer, HF ; Sader, R: Improved 3D Osteotomy Planning in Cranio-Maxillofacial Surgery. Springer Lecture Notes in Computer Science, Proc. Medical Image Computing and Computer-Assisted Intervention (MICCAI), Utrecht, The Netherlands, pp. 473–481 (2001)
3. Gladilin, E ; Zachow, S ; Deuflhard, P ; Hege, HC: Validation of a Linear Elastic Model for Soft Tissue Prediction in Craniofacial Surgery. SPIE Medical Imaging, San Diego, USA, pp. 27–35 (2001)
4. Stalling, D ; Hege, HC ; Zöckler, M et. al.: Amira – An Advanced 3D Visualization and Modeling System, http://www.amiravis.com (2002)
5. Pottmann, H ; Wallner, J: Computational Line Geometry. Springer Series on Mathematics and Visualization (2001)
6. Sethian, JA: Level Set Methods: Evolving Interfaces in Geometry, Fluid Mechanics, Computer Vision, and Material Science. Cambridge Monographs on Applied and Computational Mathematics, no. 3, chapter 13 (1996)
7. Gladilin, E ; Zachow, S ; Deuflhard, P ; Hege, HC: A Biomechanical Model for Soft Tissue Simulation in Craniofacial Surgery. Medical Imaging and Augmented Reality (MIAR), Hong Kong, China, pp. 137–141 (2001)
8. Zachow, S ; Gladilin, E ; Hege, HC ; Deuflhard, P: Towards patient specific, anatomy based simulation of facial mimics for surgical nerve rehabilitation. In: Lemke, H.U. et al. (eds.): Computer Assisted Radiology and Surgery (CARS), Paris, France (2002)

CARS 2002 – H.U. Lemke, M.W. Vannier; K. Inamura, A.G. Farman, K. Doi & J.H.C. Reiber (Editors)

Computer aided planning for orthognatic surgery

Matthieu Chabanas [a], Christophe Marécaux [a,b], Yohan Payan [a], Franck Boutault [b]

[a] TIMC-IMAG Laboratory, Université Joseph Fourier, Grenoble, France
Institut Albert Bonniot, 38706 La Tronche cedex, France
[b] Department of maxillofacial and facial plastic surgery – CCRAO Laboratory,
Hôpital Purpan, 31059 Toulouse cedex, France

Abstract

A computer aided maxillofacial sequence is presented, applied to orthognatic surgery. It consists of 5 main stages: data acquisition and integration, surgical planning, surgical simulation, and per operative assistance. The planning and simulation steps are then addressed in a way that is clinically relevant. First concepts toward a 3D cephalometry are presented for a morphological analysis, surgical planning, and bone and soft tissue simulation. The aesthetic surgical outcomes of bone repositioning are studied with a biomechanical Finite Element soft tissue model.

Keywords: Orthognatic surgery, 3D cephalometry, facial soft tissue model

1. Introduction

Orthognatic surgery, as a part of cranio-maxillofacial surgery, attempts to establish normal functional and aesthetic anatomy for patients suffering from dentofacial disharmony, by repositioning maxillary and mandibular osteotomies.

The current therapeutic protocol is a difficult and laborious process that might be responsible for inaccuracy in comparison with therapeutic planning. It is now well accepted that medical imaging and computer assisted surgical technologies may improve current orthognatic protocol as an aid in diagnostic, surgical planning and surgical intervention. The sequences required for a complete computer assisted protocol in cranio-maxillofacial surgery are well described in the literature since the eighties. Although, in orthognatic clinical practice this protocol still fails on diagnostic and planning in a three-dimensional environment. There is neither three-dimensional skeletal analysis for morphological diagnostic and osteotomy simulation (called 3D cephalometry), nor reliable prediction of post operative facial appearance. This last point is important for surgical simulation as the final soft tissue facial appearance might modify the operative planning. Therefore, the patient also expects a reliable prediction of his post operative aesthetic appearance.

After reminding the sequences of a computer aided cranio-maxillofacial protocol, our own process in computer assisted orthognatic surgery is presented.

CARS 2002 – H.U. Lemke, M.W. Vannier; K. Inamura, A.G. Farman, K. Doi & J.H.C. Reiber (Editors)

2. Method

2.1 Computer assisted cranio-maxillofacial surgery

The different steps and specifications of a computer aided protocol in cranio-maxillofacial surgery are well defined the in literature [1,2,3]. They can be summarized as in figure 1.

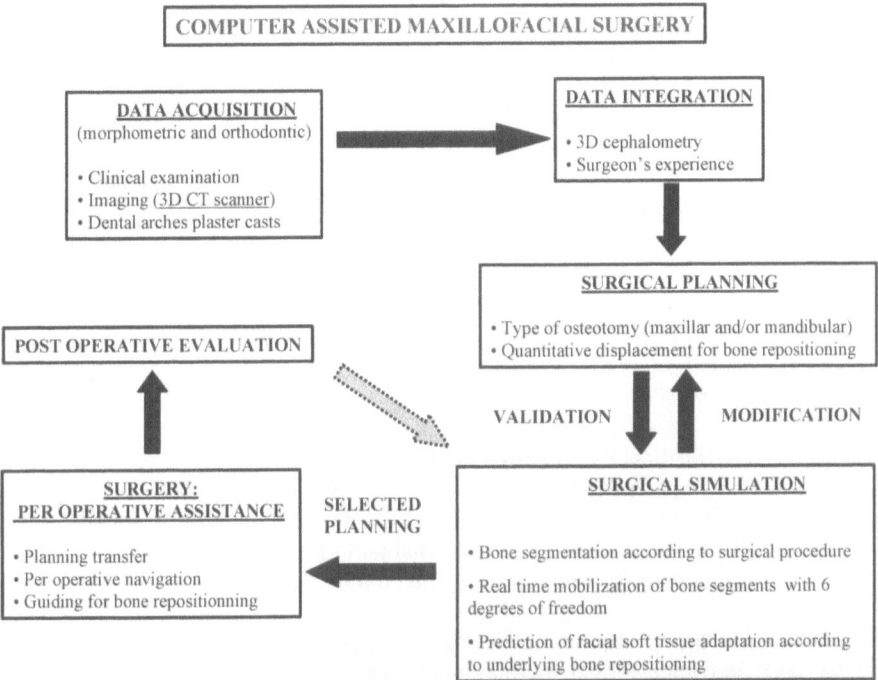

Figure 1. Specifications of a cranio-maxillofacial protocol. The dashed arrow concerns research context only: the post operative evaluation is used for the surgical simulation validation

Different parts of this protocol have been addressed in the literature. Most of them deal with interactive simulation of a surgical procedure on 3D computer generated models and present interesting tools to cut and manipulate bone segments [4,5,6]. However, none of them integrate morphometric and orthodontic data (cephalometric analysis) to establish a surgical planning, and are therefore relevant for clinical practice.

Three-dimensional cephalometric analysis, despite being essential for clinical use of computer aided techniques in maxillofacial surgery, has been studied very little so far. Most of these previous work [1,2], including our group [7], have presented extensions of 2D cephalometry. Cephalometric and orthodontic diagnostic and planning were made in traditional way (on standard 2D teleradiography and plaster dental casts) or with three dimensional constructions from 2D data. One of the most original work has been presented by Treil [8], who introduced a new cephalometry based on CT scanner imaging, anatomic landmarks and mathematic tools (a maxillofacial framework and dental axis of

990

inertia) for skeletal and dental analysis. However, in our point of view, this cephalometric analysis is not relevant for surgical planning and computer guided surgery.

Physical models were also developed to evaluate the aesthetic outcomes resulting from underlying bone repositioning [4,9,10,11]. They commonly use a continuous model based on the Finite Element method, with noticeable differences. According to us, despite their evident scientific interest, most of these works cannot be used in clinical practice since the bone simulation is not clinically relevant and the model generation is highly time consuming.

Our process in computer aided orthognatic simulation emphasises on future applications in a complete clinical protocol, as described in figure 1. In this way, we are developing a facial skeletal model including 3D cephalometry and a Finite Element model of the facial soft tissue for surgical planning and simulation issues.

2.2 Three dimensional cephalometry

A complete computer aided cranio-maxillofacial surgery sequence requires a craniofacial model that enables the morphological diagnostic, supports the surgical bone simulation, integrates the prediction of post operative facial soft tissue deformation, and can be used as interface in computer guided surgical stage.

To be accepted by medical community, this model must be coherent from an anatomical, physiological and organ genetic point of view. A 3D cephalometric tool as an aid in diagnostic is admitted as necessary [1,2,7]. 3D CT scanner imaging is already currently used to apprehend the difficult three dimensional part of this pathology. However, there is no relevant direct three dimensional analysis method of these images (3D cephalometry).

A reliable cephalometry requires to define a referential for facial skeleton orientation, used for intra and inter patient measurements reproducibility and for quantification of bone displacements, and a facial morphologic analysis method for treatment planning decision in comparison to a norm determined as "equilibrated" face. This model should be able to be cut for simulation as in a surgical procedure. The Finite Element facial soft tissue model subsequently described in section 2.3 should also be integrated.

2.2.1 Referential definition

An invariant, reproducible, orthogonal referential composed of 3 planes is proposed (figure 2 left). An horizontal plane is defined, close to the cranio basal planes of previous 2D cephalometries and to the horizontal vestibular plane defined as the craniofacial physiological horizontal plane. Its construction use anatomic reliable landmarks: right and left *capitus mallei* and the middle point between both *foramen supraorbitale*. The medial sagittal and frontal planes are orthogonal to the horizontal one and contain the middle point of both *capitus mallei*. As defined, this referential is independent from the analysed facial skeleton, and is not modified by the surgical procedure.

The x, y and z coordinates of each voxel are transferred from the original CT scanner referential to this new referential. These normalized coordinates allow location or measurement comparison between two patients or in the same one across time.

CARS 2002 – H.U. Lemke, M.W. Vannier; K. Inamura, A.G. Farman, K. Doi & J.H.C. Reiber (Editors)

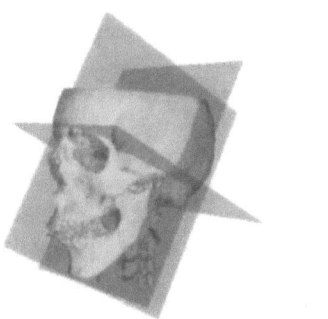 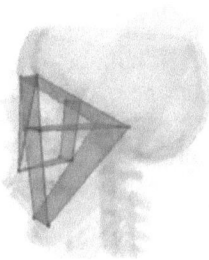

Figure 2. Craniofacial referential (left) and a maxillofacial framework example with anterior and posterior facial surfaces, prefacial surface, upper medium and lower facial surfaces and the palatine surface (right)

2.2.2 Maxillofacial framework for skull analysis
The cephalometric definition requires both a maxillofacial framework for morphologic analysis and a norm defined as an ideal for a pleasant equilibrated face. The operative planning is defined by difference between the current patient state and the norm. This one should be defined as average numeric values in location of special landmarks or as an equilibrated construction.

A maxillofacial framework is presented, composed of 15 anatomic reliable landmarks (*capitus mallei, foramen supraorbitale, foramen infraorbitale, foramen mandibulae, foramen mentale, foramen palatinum majus* and *foramen rotundum* on each side and the *foramen incisivum*) and 8 surfaces (upper and lower anterior facial s., prefacial s., posterior facial s., upper facial (cranio basal) s., medium facial s., lower facial s. and palatine s.). An example of construction is shown in figure 2 (right).

Mathematical tools allow metric, angular and surfacic measurements. Unlike traditional 2D cephalometry, these are direct values and not measurements between projected and constructed points on a sagittal radiography.

2.3 Finite element model of the face soft tissue
Different face models have been developed for simulating the aesthetic outcomes of maxillofacial surgery. Although the first ones were based on discrete mass-spring structures [9], most of them use the Finite Element method [4,10,11] to resolve the mechanical equations describing soft tissue behaviour. These methods are based on a 3D volumetric mesh, generated from patient CT images using automatic meshing methods. Such algorithms are not straightforward to use in this case, as the boundary of the face tissue, i.e. the skin and the skull surfaces, must be semi-automatically segmented, which is highly time-consuming and cannot be used in current clinical activity. Moreover, these meshes are composed of tetrahedral elements, usually less efficient than hexahedral ones in terms of accuracy and convergence.

992

2.3.1 Patient specific mesh generation

Our method [12] is, first, to build one "generic" model of the face composed of 2 layers of hexahedral elements representing dermis and hypodermis. As elements are structured within the mesh, main mimic muscles are modelled. Then, this generic mesh is adapted to each patient morphology, built out of CT scanner data, using a mesh-matching algorithm. This method, based on the octree spline elastic registration algorithm, computes a non-rigid transformation between 3D surfaces, external nodes of the generic model and patient skin surface on one part, and internal nodes of the generic model and patient skull surface on the other part. Elements of the patient mesh are automatically regularised to enable Finite Element computation.

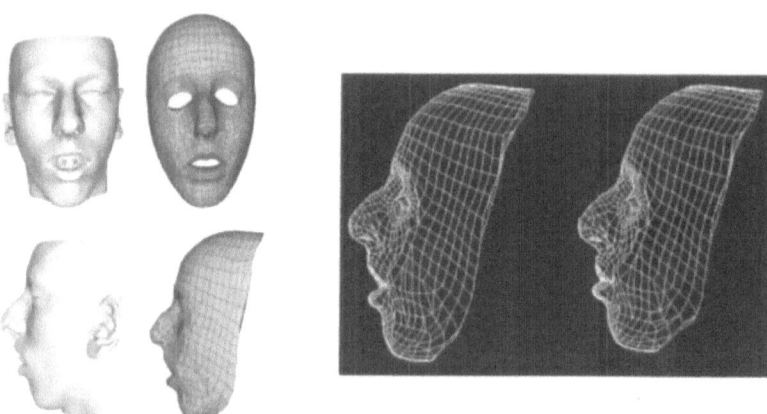

Figure 3. A patient specific finite elements model built from a CT exam (left) and simulation of soft tissue deformation resulting from a bimaxillary osteotomy on this patient

2.3.2 Mechanical properties

In a first approximation, a linear elasticity behaviour is assumed for facial tissues, with a small displacement hypothesis. The facial anisotropy is taken into account by setting linear transverse elasticity in the muscles fibres directions.

3. Results

The 3D cephalometric method allows direct three dimensional morphometrical measurements on CT scanner imaging for patient study. In the same normalized referential, bone displacements from the pathological state to the normalized predicted one are simulated as in the surgical procedure. The displacements of the anatomical landmarks used for the cephalometry are applied to the bone segments where they are located.

The mesh generation method was successfully used to build several patient models with different morphology. The total reconstruction of a patient model is carried out in about 15 minutes. The accuracy given by the matching algorithm is under 1mm. To simulate the aesthetic outcomes of bone repositioning, internal nodes rigidly fixed to the maxilla and mandible are displaced according to the surgical planning. A patient model is presented in figure 3, with a simulation of soft tissue adaptation according to mandible and maxilla repositioning.

CARS 2002 – H.U. Lemke, M.W. Vannier; K. Inamura, A.G. Farman, K. Doi & J.H.C. Reiber (Editors)

4. Discussion

If these models get closer to a clinical application of computer assisted techniques in orthognatic surgery, we are aware of remaining problems. The presented 3D cephalometric model integrates neither basilar mandibular ridge nor gonial angle studies nor dental analysis, which are clinically important. Neither is solved the morphometric norm problem. As no tool for morphometric measurements on 3D imaging exists yet (except Treil's one [8]), no normative data set is available.

The soft tissue model generation is an easy to use, straightforward, almost automatic and fast method. Hence, it is suitable to be used by a surgeon in the current planning elaboration. However, clinical quantitative study must be carried out to validate or modify functional behaviour of the model. It requires the comparison of simulated predictions with real surgical outcomes of the procedure, which has never been done in the literature. These works are currently under development.

References

1. Cutting C., Bookstein F.L., Grayson B., Fellingham L., Mc Carthy J.G., 3D computer-assisted design of craniofacial surgical procedures: optimization and interaction with cephalometric and CT-based models. *Plastic Reconstructive Surgery,* 77, pp. 877-885, 1986.
2. Altobelli D.E., Kikinis R., Mulliken J.B., Cline H., Lorensen W., Jolesz F., Computer-assisted three-dimensional planning in craniofacial surgery, *Plastic Reconstructive Surgery,* 92, pp. 576-885, 1993.
3. Lo L.J., Marsh J.L., Vannier M.W., Patel V.V. Craniofacial computer-assisted surgical planning and simulation, *Clinics in Plastic Surgery,* 21, pp. 501-516, 1994.
4. Zachow S., Gladilin E., Zeilhofer H.F., Sader R., Improved 3D osteotomy planning in cranio-maxillofacial surgery, *MICCAI 2001,* 2208, pp. 473-481, 2001.
5. Barré S., Fernandez C., Paume P., Subrenat G., Simulating facial surgery, *IS&T/SPIE Electronic Imaging,* vol. 3960, pp. 334-345, 2000.
6. Xia J., Ip H.H., Samman N., Wang D., Kot C.S., Yeung R.W., Tideman H., Computer-assisted three-dimensional surgical planning and simulation: 3D virtual osteotomy, *International journal of oral and maxillofacial surgery,* 29, pp. 250-258, 2000.
7. Bettega G., Payan Y., Mollard B., Boyer A., Raphaël B., Lavallée S., A simulator for maxillofacial surgery integrating 3D cephalometry and orthodontia, *Journal of computer aided surgery,* 5, pp. 156-165, 2000.
8. Treil J., Borianne Ph., Casteigt J., Faure J., Horn A.J., The human face as a 3D model : the future in orthodontics, *World Journal of Orthodontics,* 2, pp. 253-257, 2001.
9. Lee Y;, Terzopoulos D. and Waters K. Realistic modelling for facial animation, *SIGGRAPH'95,* pp. 55-62, 1995.
10. Keeve E., Girod S., Kikinis R., Girod B., Deformable modelling of facial tissue for cranio-facial surgery simulation, *Journal of computer aided surgery,* 3, pp. 228-238, 1998.
11. S chutyser P., Van Cleynenbreugel J., Ferrant M., Schoenaers J., Suetens P., Image-based 3D planning of maxillofacial distraction procedures including soft tissue implications, *MICCAI'2000,* 1935, pp. 999-1007, 2000.
12. Chabanas M., Payan Y., Finite element model of the face soft tissue for computer-assisted maxillofacial surgery, proceedings of the Fifth International Symposium on *Computer Methods in Biomechanics and Biomedical Engineering, CMBBE'2001,* Rome, Italy, November 2001.

The exact resection of a tumor and a transplant with the help of 3 D navigation

Schultes G[a]. Kärcher H[a]., Santler G[a]., Gaggl A[a].
University of Graz, Department of Maxillofacial Surgery
Auenbruggerplatz 7 8036 Graz

Abstract

In these case reports we want to show the preoperative and intraoperative procedure to resect a iliac crest transplant in this size we have resected the mandible in tumor surgery. It is possible to resect with a 3 D navigation system an iliac crest transplant after preoperative planning, so you can use it for reconstruct very exactly anatomis structures in head and neck surgery.

Keywords: 3 D navigation, iliac crest transplant

1. Introduction

In the head and neck surgery it is often necessary to resect large structures of the head. Today preoperative it is possible at the CT scan to decide, which structures and the size of these structures have to be removed. With the software of a 3 D navigation system (SNN, Aalen, Germany) we can use the CT scan to plan the resection preoperatively and to transpose this planning exactly intraoperatively. In this paper we want to describe the resections of a tumour (Fig.1) and of a transplant for reconstruction with the 3 D navigation in tumour surgery.

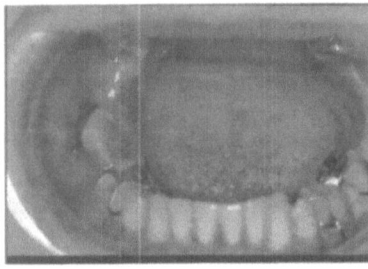

Figure 1 Osteosarcoma of the mandible

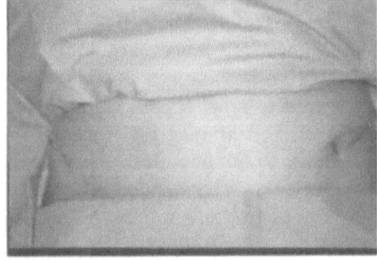

Figure 2 Four Kuerschner wires were inserted in local anaesthesia for reference points

CARS 2002 – H.U. Lemke, M.W. Vannier; K. Inamura, A.G. Farman, K. Doi & J.H.C. Reiber (Editors)
ᶜCARS/Springer. All rights reserved.

2. Material and method

At the CT scan we resect preoperative a part of the mandible and transpose this to the iliac crest. To find these planned structures intraoperatively we have to produce a CT scan of

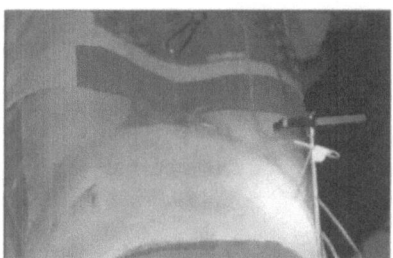

Figure 3 Intraoperatively the insertion at the iliac crest of the "diodes star" for navigation

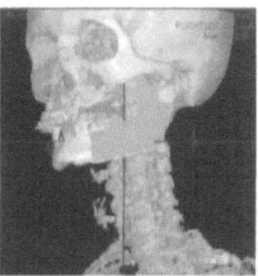

Figure 4 The preoperatively planned resection of the mandible at the 3 D view after CT Scanning

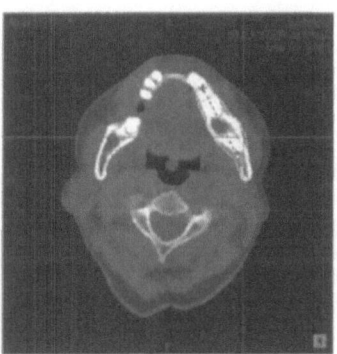

Figure 5 In the axial view of the CT scan the resection of the mandible can be shown

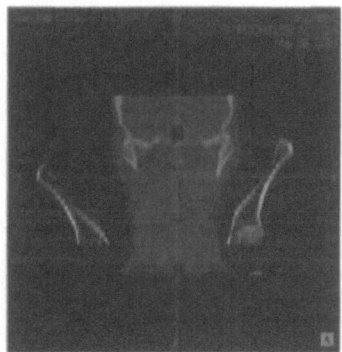

Figure 6 In computer simulation the the transposition of the mandible and the iliac crest is possible

the iliac crest. Before scanning we insert 4 Kürschner wires as reference points in local anaesthesia (Fig 2), two at each side, in the iliac crest. Intraoperatively we insert the „diode star" at the iliac crest (Fig. 3). Before operating we plan the mandible resection at the 3 D scan and transpose this resection to the iliac crest (Fig.4, 5, 6). Intraoperatively we can mark the planned mandible for reconstruction at the iliac crest (Fig. 7). This resected iliac crest transplant can exactly inserted for reconstruction in the mandible defect.

996

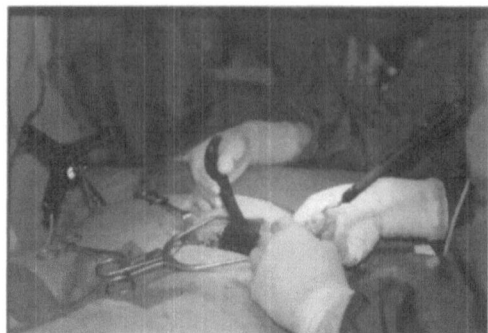

Figure 7 With a pointer the planned resection of the iliac crest can be marked

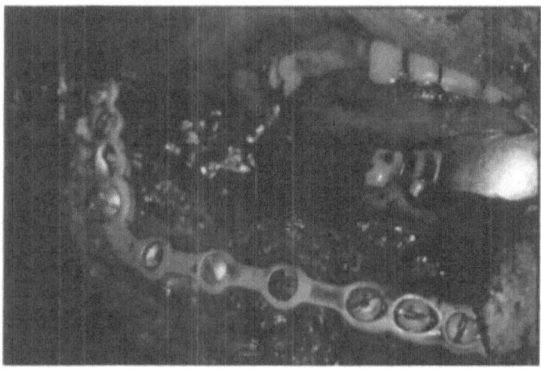

Figure 8 The resected iliac crest transplant inserted for reconstruction of the mandible

3. Result and conclusion

On this way it is possible to resect very exactly a preoperatively planned transplant to reconstruct a mandible defect. So it is a useful help for the surgeon.

CARS 2002 – H.U. Lemke, M.W. Vannier; K. Inamura, A.G. Farman, K. Doi & J.H.C. Reiber (Editors)

997

Assessment of maxillofacial pathological lesions by computed tomography using 3D surface and volume rendering techniques

Marcelo G. P. Cavalcanti[a], Patrícia S. Tossato[b], José Leopoldo F. Antunes[c]

[a,b] Department of Radiology, College of Dentistry, University of São Paulo
[c] Department of Social Dentistry, College of Dentistry, University of São Paulo

Abstract

The objective of this paper was to demonstrate and to compare the application of the 3D-CT surface and the 3D-CT volume rendering techniques for maxillofacial pathological lesions using the computer graphics system. We evaluated CT images from 18 patients with maxillofacial pathological lesions. Axial slices were obtained and were sent to an independent workstation, which used appropriate medical imaging volumetric software to generate 3D images. The surgical observation was considered the gold standard for the diagnosis of pathological conditions. The qualitative and quantitative appraisal indicated the 3D-CT volume technique as allowing more precise and accurate observations than the surface method. In average, measurements obtained by the 3D-CT volume-rendering technique were 6.28% higher than those obtained by the surface method. The sensitivity of the 3D-CT surface technique was lower than the 3D-CT volume technique for all conditions regarding the diagnosis and evaluation of lesions. We concluded that 3D-CT volume rendering technique was more reproducible and sensitive than the 3D-CT surface method in the diagnosis, treatment planning and evaluation of maxillofacial pathological lesions, mainly for those with intra-osseous involvement.

Key words: Tomography, face, pathology

1. Introduction

The surface rendering of 3D images allows the assessment of superficies of anatomic structures [4,5]. Bone structures are associated with light-reflecting surface, and mathematical algorithms estimate the surface of voxels, whose segments reflects a higher or lower intensity of light, dependent on the localization of the observer [4,5]. While studying CT lung angiography Shimizu et al. [6] used as insufficient the information provided by this technique, because of the homogeneous density of superficies visualized, and proposed a technological innovation using multiple colours and transparency, which they called the volume-rendering technique. This tool allows aggregating original data from several concurrent CT axial slices. All voxels are preserved, and 3D images thus reconstructed present a high standard of visual resolution [6]. Furthermore, this technique allows visualizing the interior of bone and tegument structures, such as intra-osseous cavities, articulations, ligaments, muscles and glands [7]. Both the surface- and the volume-rendering techniques were used in several studies assessing different parts of the human body [4,6,7], and also regarding to maxillofacial neoplasms [1-3].

Therefore, the present study aimed at a qualitative and quantitative assessment of 3D-CT surface and volume rendering techniques of maxillofacial lesions, by comparing their results with surgical observations.

2. Methodology

We evaluated 18 patients with different maxillofacial lesions, by using spiral CT. The original data were transferred to an independent workstation, with the software Vitrea®.
The diagnosis of the lesions was confirmed by histopathological examination: 2 cases of dentigerous cyst; 1 ameloblastoma; 4 epidermoid carcinoma; 3 central lesions of giant cells; 3 ossifying fibroma; 1 osteosarcoma; 2 cheratocysts; 1 adenocarcinoma; 1 odontoma. Two examiners trained and calibrated performed independent examinations of surface and volume images in a random order. The surgical observation was considered the gold standard for the diagnosis of pathological conditions.

The precision assessment of a diagnostic tool refers to the inter-examiner agreement. The lower the difference between measures performed by each observer, the higher the technique precision and reproducibility. The validity assessment of a diagnostic tool refers to its ability in distinguishing between who has some characteristic and who does not. Sensitivity refers to the ability of correctly identifying those who have the disorder [8]. Therefore, we especially considered whether the examined techniques correctly identified the lesions diagnosed by the surgical observation. Specificity is the ability of correctly identifying who do not have the disorder. Nevertheless, we also considered whether the examined techniques correctly identified the absence of conditions, which were not confirmed by the surgical observation.

We assessed the sensitivity of the surface and volume techniques by using five different characteristics of lesions: delimitation, localization, expansion and destruction of the cortex, and destruction of hard tissue. We used graphical computation for colour and transparency manipulation of images generated by the 3D-CT volume rendering technique. We used SPSS for gathering the data file and performing statistical analysis.

3. Results

Table 1 synthesises the reproducibility assessment of length measurement by different examiners, both for the surface and volume techniques. In average, the volume technique ranked a lower inter-examiner standard percentage error than the surface method, indicating its higher precision. The comparative analysis between surface and volume measures indicated a standard percentage error higher than values obtained for the inter-examiner comparison of both techniques.

Table 2 systematises the sensitivity assessment of lesions by both techniques, by using surgical observations as the gold standard for the delimitation, localization, expansion and destruction of the cortex, and destruction of hard tissue. The volume technique was more sensitive than the surface method for all categories, with a higher proportion of agreement

CARS 2002 – H.U. Lemke, M.W. Vannier; K. Inamura, A.G. Farman, K. Doi & J.H.C. Reiber (Editors)
©CARS/Springer. All rights reserved.

with surgical observations. Both the surface and the volume techniques presented specificity equivalent to 100%, with no false-positive observation.

Figure 1 presents surface and volume-rendered 3D-CT images of a patient with intra-osseous epidermoid carcinoma of the mandible. The improved delimitation of borders in the volume-rendered image allowed a higher precision of length measurement.

Figure 2 presents surface and volume-rendered 3D-CT images of a patient with multilocular ameloblastoma. The use of transparency and colour devices in images rendered by the volume method enabled an improved delimitation of affected structures, and allowed visualising the greater extent of the lesion.

Table 1. Reproducibility assessment of the 3D-CT surface and volume rendering techniques.

Standard	Inter-examiner comparison		Inter-method comparison
Percentage Error	Volume technique	Surface technique	Surface vs. Volume
Average	1.94%	4.38%	6.28%
Standard Deviation	2.80%	6.12%	8.05%
95% Conf. Interval	0.64 to 3.23%	1.56 to 7.21%	3.65 to 8.91%

Table 2. Sensitivity assessment of the 3D-CT surface and volume rendering techniques.

Characteristics of lesions	Surface	Volume
Localization	66.7%	100.0%
Delimitation of borders	61.1%	88.0%
Expansion of the cortex	61.1%	94.4%
Destruction of the cortex	55.5%	94.4%
Destruction of hard tissue	38.9%	94.4%

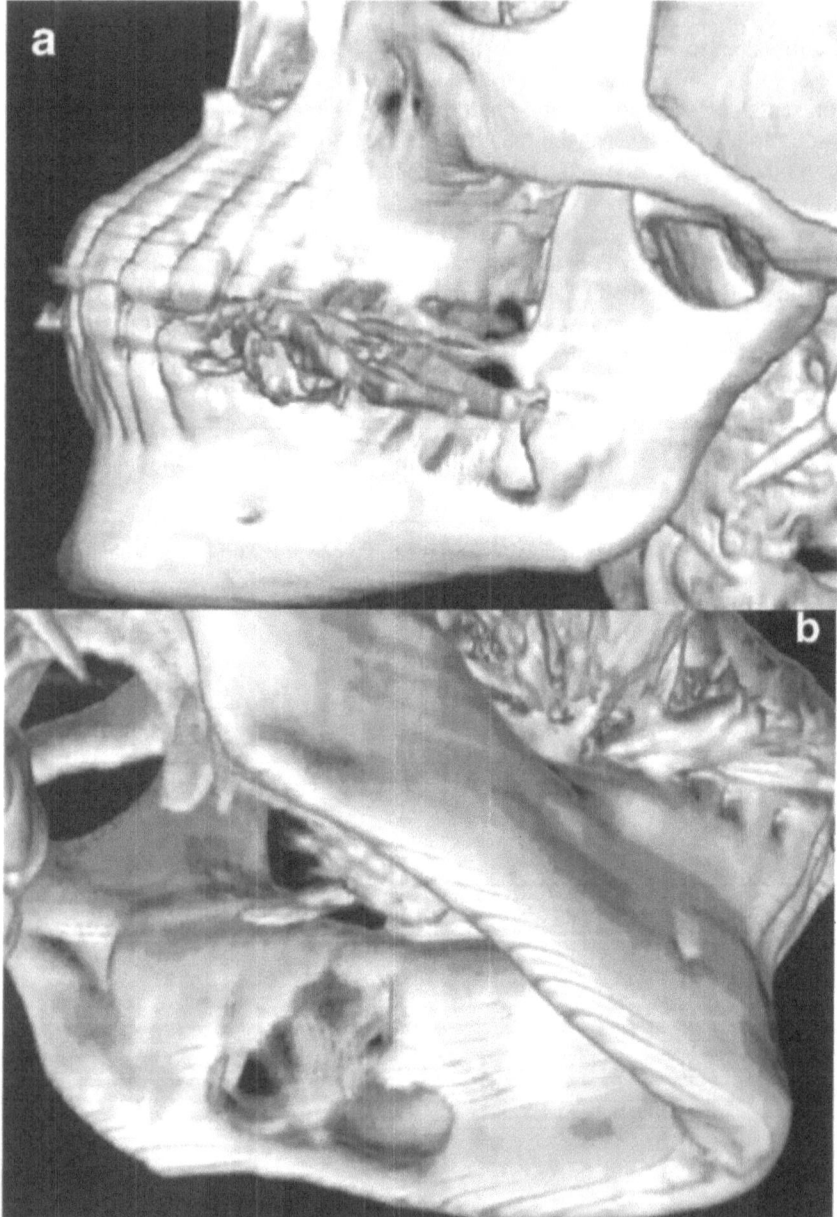

Figure 1 Keratocyst of the mandible. a, b: 3D-CT surface-rendered images showing the destruction of the buccal and lingual cortex of the mandible lateral and inner cortex views respectively.

CARS 2002 – H.U. Lemke, M.W. Vannier; K. Inamura, A.G. Farman, K. Doi & J.H.C. Reiber (Editors)
ᶜCARS/Springer. All rights reserved.

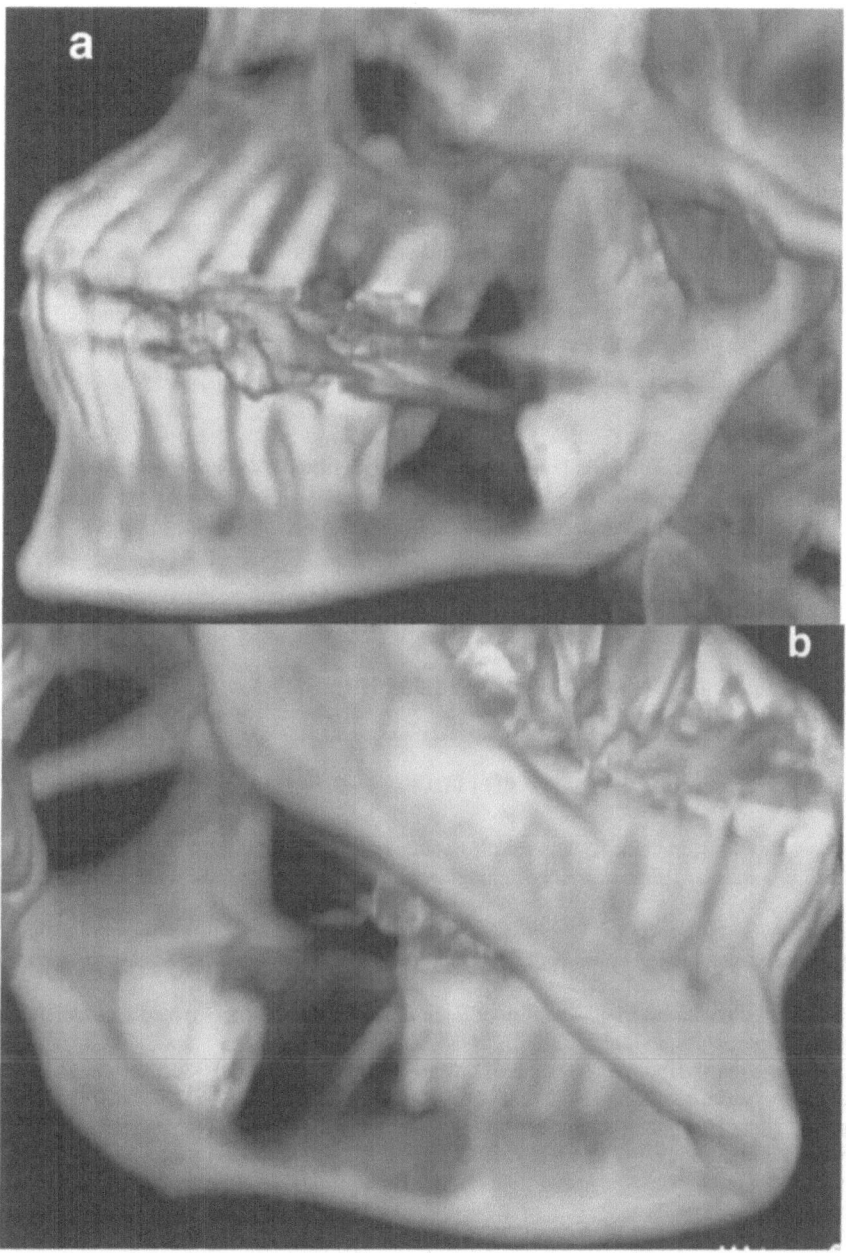

Figure 2 a, b 3D-CT volume images in lateral and inner cortex views respectively depicting a more realistic destruction of the mandible, and the relationship of the third impact molar to the cyst.

4. Conclusions

In the present study, the volume technique qualitatively improved rendered images, refining their visualisation and facilitating the detection of anatomical structures affected by maxillofacial lesions. The reproducibility assessment of 3D-CT images rendered by the volume and surface techniques indicated the former as providing more precise length measurements than the latter, with a lower inter-examiner standard average error.

While the volume technique presented an overall sensitivity of 94.2% for the delimitation of maxillofacial lesions, its localization, expansion and destruction of the cortex, and destruction of bone structures, the average related to the surface method ranked only 46.0%. This observation accounts for the higher validity observed for the volume method, despite both techniques having presented equivalent and satisfactory specificity.

The development of a protocol for the use of these techniques in the diagnosis, surgical planning and therapeutic follow up of maxillofacial lesions may complement previous research evaluating them for other anatomic sites. We have also observed a higher visual resolution of 3D-CT volume-rendered images, which may have contributed for the higher reproducibility and sensitivity of the method.

Acknowledgements

This project is supported by grants from: FAPESP (9910276-4), São Paulo, and CNPq (520425/01-5), Brasília, Brazil.

References

1. Cavalcanti MGP, Ruprecht A, Quests J. Evaluation of maxillofacial fibrosarcoma using computer graphics of spiral computed tomography. Dentomaxillofac Radiol, 28(3): 238-244, 1999.
2. Cavalcanti MGP, Ruprecht A, Quests J. Progression of squamous cell carcinoma evaluated using computer graphics of spiral computed tomography. Dentomaxillofac Radiol, 28(3): 145-151, 1999.
3. Cavalcanti MGP, Vannier MW. The role of three-dimensional spiral computed tomography in oral metastases. Dentomaxillofac Radiol, 27(4): 203-208, 1998.
4. Hooper KD, Tunç Iyriboz A, Neuman JD, Mauger DT, Kasales CJ. Mucosal detail at CT virtual reality: surface versus volume rendering. Radiology, 214(2): 517-522, 2000.
5. Udupa JK, Hung H, Chuang K. Surface and volume rendering in three-dimensional imaging: a comparison. J Digit Imag, 4(3): 159-168, 1991.
6. Shimizu T, Yoshikawa S, Uesugi Y, *et al.* Three-dimensional computed tomographic angiography of pulmonary vessels. Radiat Med, 17(2): 151-154, 1999.
7. Marro B, Valery CA, Sahel M, Zouaoui A, Randoux B, Oppenhein C, Marsault C. Intracranial aneurysm on CTA: demonstration using a transparency volume-rendering technique. J Comput Assist Tomogr, 24(1): 96-98, 2000.
8. 10. Szklo M, Javier-Nieto F. Epidemiology: beyond the basics. Gaithersburg, Md: Aspen, 2000, p. 135.

CARS 2002 – H.U. Lemke, M.W. Vannier; K. Inamura, A.G. Farman, K. Doi & J.H.C. Reiber (Editors)

Application of cone-beam X-ray CT
in dento-maxillofacial region

K. Maki, T.Usui, M.Kubota, H.Nakano, Y. Shibasaki,
K.Araki, T. Okano, K. Ueno[a] and K. Yamamoto[a]
Department. of Orthodontics and Oral Radiology, Showa University,
2-1-1 Kitasenzoku, Ohta-ku, Tokyo, Japan
[a]Hitachi Medico Technology,
Hitachi Hagoromo Bldg, 1-2-10 Uchikanda, Chiyoda-ku, Tokyo, Japan

Abstract

3-dimensional imaging system using a 2-dimensional detector and cone-beam x-ray was developed for dental field. This method reconstructs an isotropic 3-dimensional image from a set of projection images acquired during one rotation scan (9.6 Sec scan time). This system uses high-speed high-precision CCD television camera and Image Intensifier (4.0, 7.0 and 9.0 inches) as a detector and has new techniques to improve image quality and reduce x-ray dose. This system can reconstruct 512x512x512-voxel (130 milion-voxel) image with 0.20-0.35 mm/voxel resolution. Conventional X-ray images such as dental X-ray, panoramic, and cephalogram were reconstructed from volumetric data by image processing software. The application of this new method in dental field was examined with volunteers. From the results, the detailed structures of dento-maxillofacial region (from foramen mentale to TMJ) could be visualized in the 3D images. Bucco-labial extension of periapical lesion, related position of mandibular canal and dental implants, and position of impacted teeth were easy to detect more than conventional x-ray image. Accurate 3-dimensional image of dental arch was also reproduced from serial axial image. This system is widely applicable in dental field and can be used to derive clinically useful information about 3-dimensional maxillofacial structure, tooth position and bone quality.

Keywords: Cone-beam, X-ray CT, dental

1. Introduction

Frequent use of conventional CT is difficult for general dental practitioners because of it had several problems including the high cost, long scan time, necessity of a wide space in which the patient can lay for scanning, and high exposure dose. Moreover, the usefulness of CT is limited in clinical dentistry, which requires minute operations such as prosthetic treatments and endodontic treatment, because of its critical defect, a low vertical resolution. We, therefore, attempted to introduce cone-beam CT using conical X-ray beams and a plane detector to enhance the usefulness of CT in dental diagnosis and treatment.

CT using cone-beam X-ray has been applied in various regions since the late 1990's. Several models have been developed also for the dental region. Conceptually, cone-beam

1004

CT may be compared with conventional CT as follows. By conventional X-ray CT, a cross-sectional image is obtained by rotating a linear detector, and a three-dimensional image is prepared by juxtaposing many cross-sectional images. To achieve a high resolution in the axial direction, in which cross-sectional images are arranged next to one another, a large number of cross-sectional images must be obtained at narrow intervals. Therefore, how to shorten the scan time has been an important problem. The helical scan method, by which the detector is rotated as the patient is moved on the bed in the axial direction, was developed as a measure to shorten the scan time. However, the spatial resolution in the axial direction was still limited by the slit width of the X-ray collimator and the speed of movement of the bed. On the other hand, cone-beam X-ray CT was designed to drastically increase the number of layers of detectors by employing "two-dimensional" detectors and changing the X-ray beam from the fan-shaped beam to the conical beam. Because of this design, cone-beam CT has several advantages compared with conventional CT such as a shorter scan time, better vertical resolution, and low exposure dose.

The objectives of our attempt to develop a new CT system were:
(1) To limit the scanning area to the maxillofacial region
(2) To restrict the area occupied by the system to a square of 2.5 × 2.5 m for general dental offices.
(3) To improve the vertical resolution.
(4) To provide images similar to conventional panoramic images or cephalograms.
(5) To add application software that support orthodontic surgery and implant operations.

2. System and scanning condition

The apparatus developed was an open gantry type CT system exclusively for cone-beam CT, in which the X-ray irradiator and the detector are rotated around the patient (Fig.1). The X-ray tube and the image intensifier (I.I.) are placed in opposite positions in the gantry, and the conical beam rotates 360° around the patient. The X-ray that has penetrated the subject is detected by the I.I., transmitted by a high-resolution CCD camera, and re-constituted with a three-dimensional processor used in the voxel transmission method. The scan time is 9.6 seconds, the I.I. of the detector can be selected from 4.0, 7.0 and 9.0 inches, and 512 projection images of a 512 × 512 matrix are obtained by a single rotation.

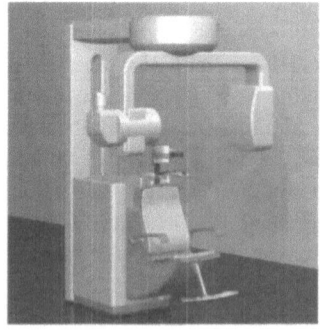

Figure 1. A view of the cone-beam CT. Conical X-ray beam rotates around the patient.

CARS 2002 – H.U. Lemke, M.W. Vannier; K. Inamura, A.G. Farman, K. Doi & J.H.C. Reiber (Editors)
CARS/Springer. All rights reserved.

Also, to increase the usefulness of the system in actual clinical use, the operability of image processing application software was developed.Scanning condition in 5 volunteers is as follows: Tube voltage: 100 kV, Tube current: 15 mA, Voxel size: 340 μm (X=Y=Z), Slice thickness: 340μm, Scan time: 9.6 sec/scan, Field of View (FOV): 174 mm

3. Results of examination

Since the system has a resolution of 512 pixels along all X, Y, and Z axes, clear images are obtained in any cross-section. Very precise images are obtained also in three-dimensional imaging (Fig.2).

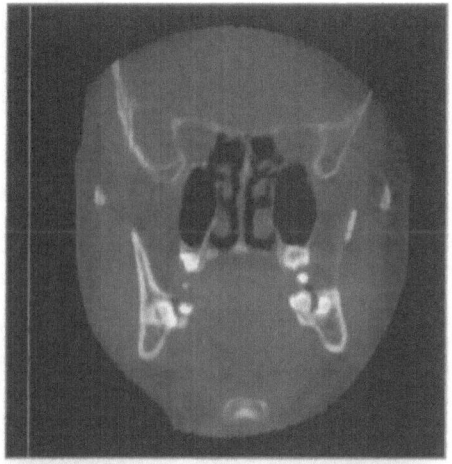

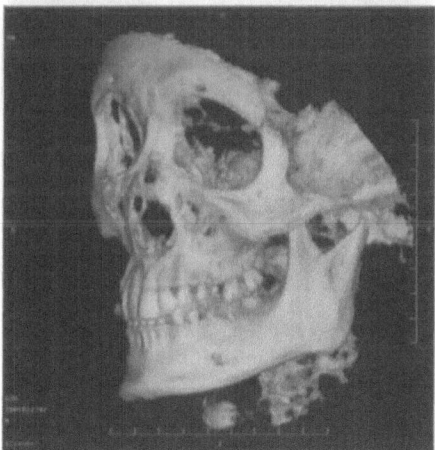

Figure 2. Cross-sectional images and 3D image

The newly developed image-processing software of this system allows adjustment of the window level and width, selection of the display level, accurate marking of soft tissues, and synthetic display of the density distribution [1]. Also, by presenting images along the

CARS 2002 – H.U. Lemke, M.W. Vannier; K. Inamura, A.G. Farman, K. Doi & J.H.C. Reiber (Editors)

1006

dentition using this software, observation practically equivalent to panoramic X-ray imaging becomes possible. The section line can be freely determined (Fig.3). Images similar to cephalograms can also be obtained. The measurement area can be selectively contrasted, and images can be overlain horizontally.

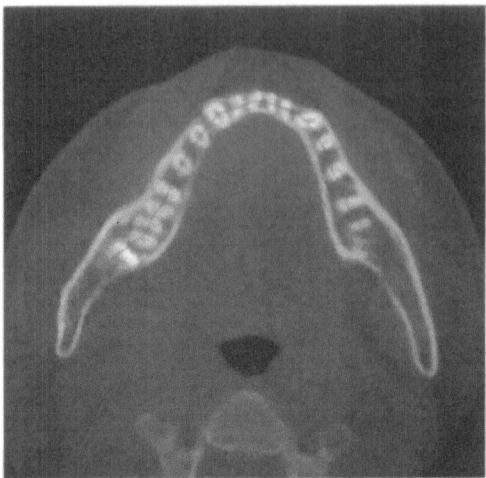

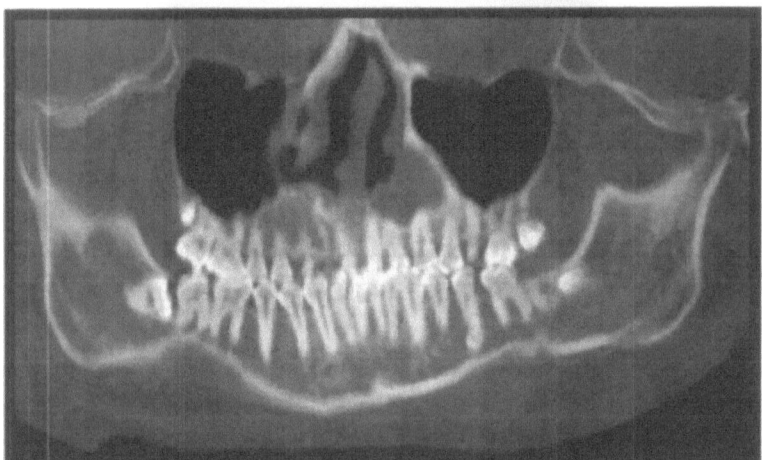

Figure 3. Reconstructed image similar to Panoramic X-ray.
Reference line was settled in axial image as shown in upper.

Furthermore, information of the dental region alone can be selected from the information obtained by a single scan, and the position of the dental roots and the state of the pulp cavities can be examined. These images do not appear to be inferior to the conventional plaster models (Fig.4).

CARS 2002 – H.U. Lemke, M.W. Vannier; K. Inamura, A.G. Farman, K. Doi & J.H.C. Reiber (Editors)

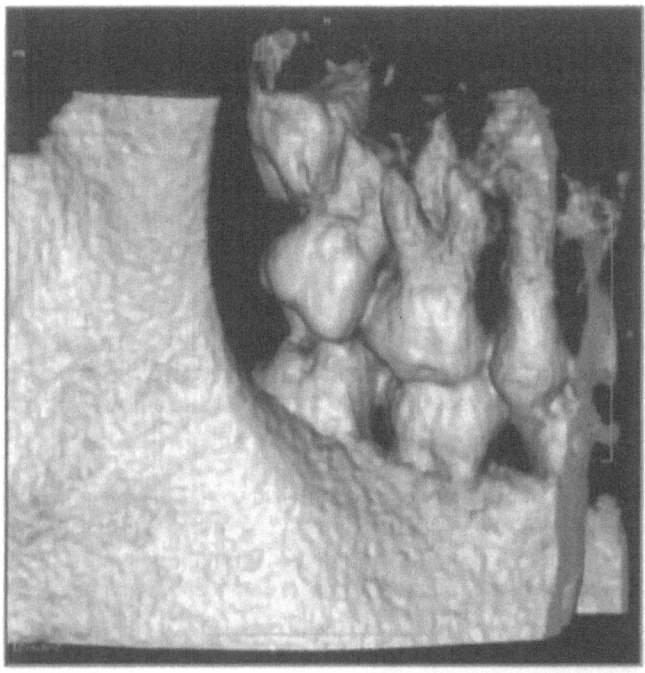

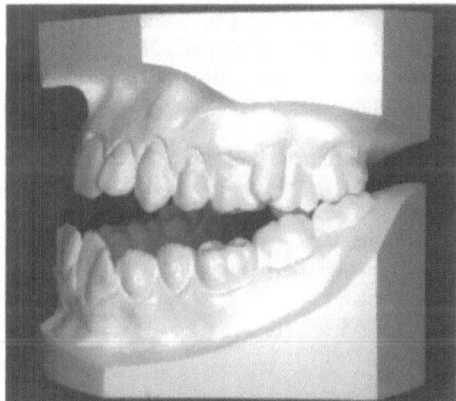 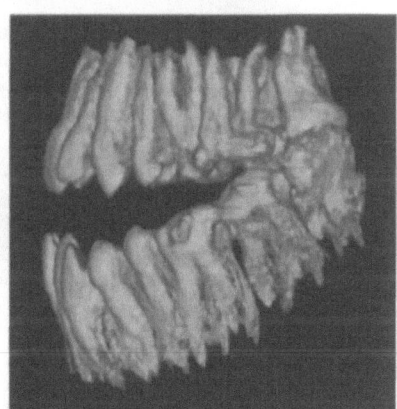

Figure 4. 3D reconstructed images of teeth (Upper) and
dental cast model of an Open bite case and his 3D image (lower).

Three-dimensional models can also be made by using the laser-lithograph technology.
This system, which has made observation at this precision level possible, is considered to
be useful not only as a supportive measure in pulp treatment and implant operations but
also for preparation of prosthetics and robot-assisted treatment in the future. Presently, we
are attempting automatic Finite Element analysis, three-dimensional representation of jaw
movements [2], and preparation of set-up models in orthodontic treatment using
information obtained by this cone-beam CT.

4. Discussion

Three-dimensional images are characterized by depth information along the Z axis in addition to two-dimensional information of the XY plane while information in the depth direction was overlapped in conventional two-dimensional images. Therefore, two-dimensional images extracted from three-dimensional images have a better resolution in the depth direction compared with conventional two-dimensional images. This system is considered to sufficiently fulfill these requirements for a new three-dimensional imaging modality and to provide information with unprecedented precision for various treatments.

Also, by providing images resembling conventional X-ray images, the system is considered to maintain the usefulness of clinical data and knowledge based on experience that have been accumulated to date. If combined with displays of jaw movements and calculation of mastication energy, it is expected to become a powerful tool for evaluation of jaw and oral functions.

At this point, however, the density resolution is low, and the scanning area is restricted, due to the use of the image intensifier. Improvements in the density resolution by the development of imaging techniques and technical improvements in two-dimensional detectors such as the flat panel (plane sensor) are considered to be needed.

References

1. K.Maki, T.Okano, T.Morohashi, S.Yamada, Y.Shibasaki: 3-Dimensional QCT for the Maxillofacial Skeleton and Its Application. J. Dent Maxillofacial Radiol. , 26, 39-44, 1997
2. K.Maki, N.Inou, T.Usui, Y.Toki, Y.Shibasaki: Computer-Aided Biomechanical Simulations for The Diagnosis of Maxillofacial Functions. Computer Assisted Radiology and Surgery, 819-823, 1998, Elsevier (Amsterdam)
3. K.Maki, A.Miller, T.Okano and Y.Shibasaki: Changes in Coretical Bone Mineralization in the Developing Mandible: A Three-Dimensional Quantitative Computed Tomography Study. Journal of Bone and Mineral Research, 15,4, 700-709, 2000
4. K.Maki, A.J.Miller, T.Okano, D.Hatcher, T.Yamaguchi, H.Kobayashi and Y.Shibasaki: Cortical Bone Mineral Density in Asymmetrical Mandibles. Europian Journal of Orthodontics 23, 217-232, 2000

16th International Congress and Exhibition on Computer Assisted Radiology - CAR

CARS 2002 – H.U. Lemke, M.W. Vannier; K. Inamura, A.G. Farman, K. Doi & J.H.C. Reiber (Editors)
©CARS/Springer. All rights reserved.

Survival prediction using artificial neural networks in patients with lung cancer treated by radiotherapy

Masahiro Iinuma, Teruki Teshima, Yuki Iwanaga, Minoru Kawamata,
Makoto Nagayoshi, Kenya Murase
Medical Engineering, Div. of Allied Health Sciences, Osaka University, Suita, Japan

Keywords: Artificial neural networks, lung cancer, radiotherapy

1. Introduction

It is generally known that artificial neural networks (ANNs) may be used for non-linear analysis of complex data. The purpose of this study was to construct the model of prediction using ANNs from radiation oncology database, and to evaluate the usefulness of ANNs for survival prediction in patients with lung cancer treated by radiation therapy.

2. Method

The Patterns of Care Study (PCS) in radiation oncology has over 400 items of factors for radiotherapy of patients with lung cancer. In this study, 822 patients in radiation therapy were selected from 1099 patients in PCS data by a radiation oncologist.

Selected predictive factors are a, histology; b, Given Surgical resection; c, Age;
d, Gender; e, interstitial pneumonitis; f, Karnofsky performance status; g, Stage;
h, Given Total dose; i , Photon energy; j, Maximum radiation field;
k, All fields treated each day; l, Fields reduced during RT; m, Given Chemotheraphy
n, Asthma; o, Pulmonary tuberculosis; p, Pulmonary emphysema; q, Hemosputum

The various combinations were selected by a radiation oncologist for training ANNs. Using the trained ANNs, we predicted the survival in the remaining 411 patients, and compared it with the known 2-year survival. The performance of ANNs was evaluated using receiver operating characteristic (ROC) analysis. The area under the ROC curve (Az) was then used to compare the performance of ANNs.

Combination of prognostic factors:
A: a, b, c, d, e, f, g, h, i, j, k, l, m
B: a, b, c, d, e, f, g, h, i, j, k, l, m, n, o, p, q
C: b, c, d, e, f, g, h, i, j, k, l, m
D: a, c, d, e, f, g, h, i, j, k, l, m
E: a, b, d, e, f, g, h, i, j, k, l, m
F: a, b, c, e, f, g, h, i, j, k, l, m
G: a, b, c, d, f, g, h, i, j, k, l, m

H : a, b, c, d, e, g, h, i, j, k, l, m
I : a, b, c, d, e, f, h, i, j, k, l, m
J : a, b, c, d, e, f, g, i, j, k, l, m
K : a, b, c, d, e, f, g, h, j, k, l, m
L : a, b, c, d, e, f, g, h, i, j, l, m
M: a, b, c, d, e, f, g, h, i, j, k, m
N : a, b, c, d, e, f, g, h, i, j, k, l

3. Results

This summarizes the Az values for various combinations of variables shown above.
A, 0.6708 B, 0.5520 C, 0.5442 D, 0.4825 E, 0.5021 F, 0.5364 G, 0.5438 H, 0.5022 I, 0.5353 J, 0.500 K, 0.4914 L, 0.5029 M, 0.4927 N, 0.5038

4. Conclusion

We have constructed the prediction model using ANNs from radiation oncology database.

CARS 2002 – H.U. Lemke, M.W. Vannier; K. Inamura, A.G. Farman, K. Doi & J.H.C. Reiber (Editors)

1012

Clinical usefulness of multidetector CT angiography : application to the diagnosis of arterial occlusive diseases in lower extermities

N. Hirai, R. Tanaka, Y. Hori, M. Higashi, S. Imakita, H. Naito
National Cardiovascular Center, Osaka Japan

Keywords: Multidetector CT, CT angiography, arterial occlusive disease

1. Introduction
Our goal is to establish the utility of multi-detector row CT angiography (MDCTA) for evaluating arterial stenosis in patients with arterial occlusive disease of lower extremities.

2. Methods
We examined twenty-eight patients (25 men and 3 women, 68+/- 10 years old) with arterial occlusive disease of lower extremities using both MDCTA and DSA. Helical scan was performed with MDCT using "Real Prep helical scanning" from pelvis to ankle with 2.0-mm collimation, 5.5-helical pitch, and scan speed of 0.5-sec/rotation. Contrast material (350 mgI/mL) was injected at the rate of 1.5 mL/sec (total 65-85 mL). The 2.0-mm-thick two-dimensional images were reconstructed every 2.0-mm interval. All images were rendered in maximum intensity projection (MIP), multi-planar reconstruction (MPR), and volume rendering (VR). DSA was performed with "Stepping" or "Bolus chase" method. Data acquisition was performed from pelvis to ankle with continuous single-phase contrast injection. Contrast material (300 mgI/mL) was injected via the catheter at the rate of 7.0-8.0 mL/sec (total 65-75 mL).
Rendered MDCTA images were compared with DSA in anteroposterior view. We segmented the arteries of lower extremity into 8 segments. In each segment, we evaluated the degree of stenosis into four groups on DSA.

3. Results
All 28 patients, 448 arteries were evaluated by both MDCTA and DSA. Two arteries couldn't be evaluated by MDCTA due to strong artifacts from metallic stents. Overall, in 404 out of 446 arteries (90.6%), the degree of stenosis on MDCTA coincided with that on DSA. Twenty-five out of 446 arteries (5.6%) were overestimated by MDCTA and seventeen out of 446 arteries (3.8%) were underestimated by MDCTA.
Twenty-six out of all 42 arteries overestimated or underestimated by MDCTA (61.9%) were below knee arteries and the remaining sixteen arteries (38.1%) had dense calcification or metallic stents.

4. Conclusions
MDCTA with "Real prep helical scanning" is more effective and less invasive method than DSA.

CARS 2002 – H.U. Lemke, M.W. Vannier; K. Inamura, A.G. Farman, K. Doi & J.H.C. Reiber (Editors)

Automatically reducing iodine in contrast head CT scans by image processing

Lijun Yin[a], Ja Kwei Chang[b], Ahmad I. Zainal Abidin [c]

[a, c] Department of Computer Science, SUNY at Binghamton, Binghamton, NY.
[b] Department of Radiology, SUNY Upstate Medical University, Syracuse, NY.

Keywords: Contrast CT scans, image statistics, image detection

1. Introduction

Iodinated contrast agent is commonly used in head CT scans. However, the use of iodinated contrast material may result in an adverse reaction in the patient, and is also relatively expensive. It is therefore of interest to investigate whether it is possible to reduce the amount of iodinated contrast material without any loss of diagnostic information. In this paper, we develop a computer simulation method to study the effect of iodine reduction on clinical image quality. An automatic enhancement and detection of the "difference iodine" images is presented. This research will result in an output of a cost-effective clinical diagnostic system in head CT scans.

2. Methods

We developed an algorithm and software for automatically detecting and monitoring the "difference iodine" image between two scans on the same patient (with and without iodinated contrast). A "guideline curve" for image differences is derived based on image statistics. The "difference iodine" image is reduced in intensity and added back to the non-contrast image to simulate the image that would have been obtained if less iodine had been administered originally. A statistics-based subtraction method is presented to obtain the mean (brightness) and variance (contrast) values [1] of the difference images between the images with and without iodine. The iodine is injected at the rate of 3cc per second, and the total volume of injection is 100cc. 20 CT image frames are scanned. Within each frame, the brain region of interest (ROI) is extracted automatically. Within the ROI, subtraction operation is performed between the current frame and the initial frame. Blending of mean and variance values shows a "peak value" in the mean-variance "guideline curve", which corresponds to a "saturation time" during iodine injections. It shows that the diagnostic information is no longer increased after the saturation time.

3. Results

The result shows that the "saturation time" detected is equivalent to 60% of total iodine injected.

4. Conclusions

The technique based on image subtraction and statistics for the detection of the saturation point reduces the amount of iodine injection by 40%.

References

1. R.C. Conzalez, R. E. Woods, "Digital image processing", 2001. Ptentice-Hall Inc.

CARS 2002 – H.U. Lemke, M.W. Vannier; K. Inamura, A.G. Farman, K. Doi & J.H.C. Reiber (Editors)

1014

Improved visualization of 3D data sets on the example of 3D-rotational angiography

Reiner Koppe[a], Erhard Klotz[a], John Op de Beek[b]

[a] Philips Research Laboratories, Roentgenstr. 24-26, 22335 Hamburg, Germany
[b] Philips Medical Systems PO Box 1000, 5680 DA Best, The Netherlands

1. Introduction

3D-Rotational Angiography (3D-RA) is a new 3D imaging method based on the standard X-ray technique. Since the analysis of the clinically relevant information is often difficult, we have developed tools for improving the 3D visualization.

2. Methods and results

Equalization of grey-values: Contrast medium filled vessels and inserted metallic coils and stents, cannot be viewed simultaneously with a sufficient image quality. In order to improve the visualization, each structure is segmented in different grey-value areas by a level-window transformation and afterwards combined in a new voxel set (fig. 1).

Stereo-mode: Vessel structures like arterio-venous-malformations AVMs often do not allow a sufficient view in depth. The diagnosis can be improved using a stereo presentation (fig. 2). For stereo two data sets are computed from the 3D data set.

Thick slice: The 3D data are usually visualized in the whole-volume mode. Often the views contain information obstructing the ROI. By defining a new VOI by inserting two parallel planes, the disturbing structures in front and behind the VOI are clipped (fig. 3).

Dual cut-volume display: The volume is separated by a cut-plane in 2 sub-volumes. The lower and upper sub-volume (fig. 4) is then displayed together like a "cut apple".

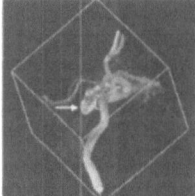 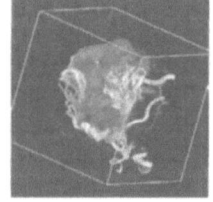

Fig. 1: Coils in an aneurysm   Fig. 2: Complex AVM in stereo-mode

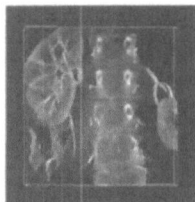 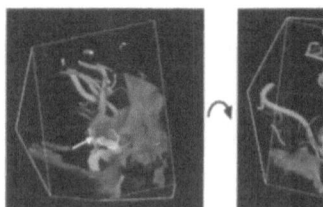

Fig. 3: Renal arteries   Fig. 4: Complex cerebral aneurysm

3. Conclusion

With the visualization tools, the image quality and the analysis of the vessel structures could be improved significantly. The different tools can be combined.

CARS 2002 – H.U. Lemke, M.W. Vannier; K. Inamura, A.G. Farman, K. Doi & J.H.C. Reiber (Editors)
°CARS/Springer. All rights reserved.

EasyTW: computer-aided system for bone age assessment

A.M.M. Da Silva[a], G.L. De Oliveira[b], G.P. Noal[b], C.A.A. Schmitz[b],
L.S.B. Haeffner[b], P.S.P. Antunes[b] , S.D. Olabarriaga[c]

[a] Faculdade de Física, PUCRS, 90016-900, Porto Alegre/RS, Brasil
[b] Hospital Universitário de Santa Maria, UFSM, 97105-900, Santa Maria/RS, Brasil
[c] Instituto de Informática, UFRGS, 90000-900, Porto Alegre/RS, Brasil

Keywords: Bone age assessment, computer-aided system, digital atlas.

1. Introduction

The Tanner-Whitehouse method (TW)[1], considered the most accurate and reliable to assess skeletal maturity, is applied only in a small fraction of cases due to complexity and long examination times. It makes use of bones in the hand-wrist radiograph, which are assigned to a development stage based on some visual features. Each bone is matched with drawings in a specially-prepared atlas and receives a score. The sum of all bone scores corresponds to the TW maturity index, used to determine bone age by comparing with gender-dependent reference tables. We have been constructing a digital hand atlas of healthy Brazilian children to study population differences in skeletal maturity. We developed a computer-aided tool - *EasyTW* - to speed up the skeletal age computation of this large database. This work presents the evaluation study to determine the reliability of *EasyTW* in comparison to conventional TW method, using the printed atlas.

2. Methods

To test *EasyTW* performance, 20 male/female digital radiographs, acquired with computerized radiology (Fuji ACR-3), were evaluated by three physicians (radiologists and pediatricians). Maturity indicators were searched by means of an interactive process to identify shape and texture of 20 bones in hand-wrist. Each image was evaluated by using the software *EasyTW* and the conventional TW method.

3. Results

Using the non-parametric Kruskal-Wallis test, the null-hypothesis was not rejected for the observers in any experiment ($p > 0.7$). There is no statistical significant difference on skeletal maturity results when software *EasyTW* or conventional TW method are applied.

4. Conclusions

EasyTW is a valuable and reliable tool to speed up the analysis of skeletal maturity and growth disorders in large database population studies.

Acknowledgements

This work has the financial support of FAPERGS, CNPq, HUSM.

References

1. J.M. Tanner, M.J.R Healy, H. Goldstein and N. Cameron, *Assessment of Skeletal Maturity and Prediction of Adult Height (TW3 Method)*, 3rd ed., WB Saunders (2001).

CARS 2002 – H.U. Lemke, M.W. Vannier; K. Inamura, A.G. Farman, K. Doi & J.H.C. Reiber (Editors)

1016

3D X-ray imaging of human bones using a mobile C-arm

Jörn Lütjens[ab], Dr. Reiner Koppe[a], Erhard Klotz[a],
Dr. Michael Grass[a], Dr. Volker Rasche[a]
[a] Philips Research Laboratories, Röntgenstr. 24-26, Hamburg, Germany
[b] University of Surrey, Guidford, UK

Keywords: Low-end C-arm systems, cone-beam reconstruction, X-ray imaging

1. Introduction
Motorized high-end C-arm systems can be used for 3D imaging of high contrast objects such as bones [1]. Based on cone-beam data acquisition, careful calibration and cone-beam reconstruction, volume data sets can be obtained that enable an improved insight into 3D structures of bones in order to analyse complex joint fractures or to position prostheses. New developments offer this functionality on hand-moved low-end C-arm systems too.

2. Methods
A mobile surgical C-arm by Philips has been equipped with angle encoders and additional fixation relative to the floor. These changes permit an adjustment to reproducible C-arm positions, a pre-requisite for the indispensable system calibration. Up to 100 images are acquired on a semi-circular trajectory over an angular range of 200°, and passed to a Feldkamp-type cone-beam reconstruction algorithm [2].

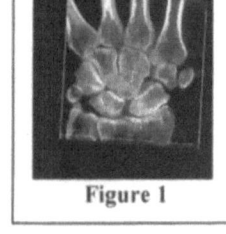

Figure 1

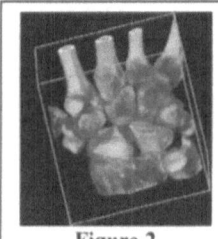

Figure 2

3. Results
First reconstruction results of different parts of a human corpse have been acquired and reconstructed with the methods described above. As an example, the images in Fig. 1 and 2 show grey scale-adjusted volume-rendered views of the reconstructed 3D data of a human wrist. The spatial resolution is in the sub-mm range.

4. Conclusions
The use of a hand-moved, surgical C-arm system for reconstruction of 3D data with previously unachieved spatial resolution comes into the scope of the operation room.

Acknowledgements
This work has been funded by the Philips Research Laboratories Hamburg.

References
1. R. Koppe, E. Klotz, and J. Op de Beck, « 3D vessel reconstruction based on rotational angiography », 1995, Proceedings of the CAR '95
2. L. A. Feldkamp, L. C. Davis, and J. W. Kress. "Practical cone-beam algorithms", *J. Opt. Soc. Am. A*, 6:612—619, June 1984

CARS 2002 – H.U. Lemke, M.W. Vannier; K. Inamura, A.G. Farman, K. Doi & J.H.C. Reiber (Editors)
©CARS/Springer. All rights reserved.

Bone mineral density estimation after soft-tissue effect subtraction in X-ray images

Seunghwan Kim, Sooyeul Lee, Ji-Wook Jeong
Electronics and Telecommunication Research Institute
P.O. Box 106, Yuseong, Daejeon, 305-600 Korea

Keywords: BMD, soft-tissue, x-ray image.

1. Introduction

X-ray imaging is a widespread, routine, and multipurpose screening tool. One of the well-known diseases, which can be screened via x-ray images, is osteoporosis. Osteoporosis is characterized by an abnormal loss of bone mineral density (BMD), which leads to a tendency toward non-traumatic bone fractures or to structural deformations of bone [1]. X-ray image provides rich information about the bone status including BMD. However, BMD estimation from the x-ray image undergoes a severe accuracy error. The most relevant origin of the error is soft tissues that overlap with bones in the x-ray image. In this work, we provide a simple method for soft-tissue effect subtraction in the x-ray image.

2. Methods

Wrist x-ray films of 90 women were obtained under a fixed x-ray condition. Each x-ray film was digitised under 8-bit gray scale. For the comparison, each person was undergone BMD measurement on the wrist using a DEXA. Each image was calibrated using a gray level profile of an aluminium stepwedge. In each image, gray level profiles of soft-tissue region across the wrist were interpolated into the bone region. Then each gray level profile in the bone region was subtracted by the interpolated profile. BMD was simply given by the average gray level over the subtracted gray level in the bone region.

3. Results

The linear correlation coefficient between the above method and the DEXA is 0.96. This result corresponds to 3% accuracy error in determining BMD (g/cm^2). Without the soft-tissue effect subtraction, the correlation coefficient is about 0.73. This is corresponds to 12% accuracy error.

4. Conclusions

In this work, we have provided a simple method for the soft-tissue effect subtraction in the x-ray image and applied the method for the BMD measurement. In case of the wrist, above method provides a highly accurate BMD compared with a DEXA.

Acknowledgements

This work was supported by the Ministry of Information and Communication, Korea.

References

1. S.H. Wasserman and U.S. Barzel, "Osteoporosis: The state of the art in 1987 – a review, *Semin. Nucl. Med.*, vol. 17, pp. 283-292, 1987.

CARS 2002 – H.U. Lemke, M.W. Vannier; K. Inamura, A.G. Farman, K. Doi & J.H.C. Reiber (Editors)

Virtual actors for a patient oriented virtual hospital

J. Wilhelmy[a], S. Märkle[b]

Technical University of Berlin, FG Computer Graphics & Computer Assisted
Medicine, FR 3-3, Franklinstr. 28/29, 10587 Berlin, Germany
[a] j.wilhelmy@nexgo.de, [b] Steffen.Maerkle@TU-Berlin.de

Keywords: Virtual hospital, 3d-interaction, patient oriented information system

1. Introduction

A virtual hospital is realized as an interactive information system based on a 3D- model of
a real hospital. In preparation for a future stay, a patient can visit the location, where later
a therapy may take place, and get a first impression or look at the data in his electronic
patient record, as described in [1]. To be able to experience an almost realistic impression
of the real healthcare process, it is also necessary to offer the patient the possibility to see
and interact with doctors, nurses, administration personnel and also other patients in the
virtual hospital. The authors present a system of virtual actors that can be used to fill the
wards and stations with virtual life. One special purpose for employing virtual actors is
the simulation of diagnostic or therapeutic treatment. For example, to present an
orthopaedic diagnosis, a virtual doctor can take the leg of a virtual patient and make a
reflex test with a rubber hammer.

2. Methods

The virtual actors are based on a simplified hierarchical skeleton model consisting of
bones and joints. The body parts are moved using an inverse kinematics algorithm that is
based on non-linear optimisation. By representing the hierarchical transformations in the
skeleton model as a neural network the algorithm can be reduced to a standard learning
algorithm for feed forward neural networks. The virtual actors can also be animated using
predefined motion data such as captured data from real actors.

3. Results

A prototype of the system has been realized. It is possible to show animated virtual actors,
and interact with them. Several examination scenes have been modelled and can be used
to demonstrate the procedures to a patient.

4. Conclusions

The virtual hospital is intended to be an information system to provide all information
related to healthcare. 3D visualization, animation and interaction techniques can be
employed to give the user a realistic impression of healthcare processes. The presented
virtual actors are an important component to make the visit to the virtual hospital not only
an impressive experience, but also to provide the patient with appropriate information and
demonstrations of diagnostic and therapeutic procedures.

References

1.   S. Märkle, K. Köchy, R. Tschirley, H. U. Lemke. The PREPaRe system - Patient Oriented
     Access to the "Personal Electronic Medical Record". In: Proc. of CARS 2001, pp. 849-854.

CARS 2002 – H.U. Lemke, M.W. Vannier; K. Inamura, A.G. Farman, K. Doi & J.H.C. Reiber (Editors)

User-assisted segmentation of tomographic images

Ardeshir Goshtasby[a] and Martin Satter[b]
[a] Computer Science Dept., Wright State University, Dayton, OH.
[b] Wallace-Kettering Neuroscience Institute, Kettering, OH.

Keywords: Image segmentation, partial volume correction, rational Gaussian (RaG) surface

1. Introduction

Because automated methods that segment tomographic (medical) images often involve errors, editing tools that can rapidly correct the errors are needed. The editing tools presented in this paper may be considered a part of a postprocessing operation that evaluates the accuracy of an automated segmentation and refines the errors.

2. Methods

Given an initial segmentation obtained by an automated method, an environment that enables interactive 3D Region of Interest (ROI) correction of local errors is introduced. The initial segmentation is represented by a parametric surface and the surface is overlaid within the image volume. Orthogonal cross-sections are then displayed and the user is provided with tools to locally displace the surface and refine the segmentation result.

3. Results

The developed editing tools have been tested and optimized for segmentation of CT chest images and MR brain images to rapidly delineate tumors and different organs. Experiments show that once an initial segmentation in the form of a volumetric region is provided, editing of the region to remove the errors takes from a few to several minutes depending on the complexity and size of the region and the severity of the errors.

4. Conclusions

Because automated segmentation methods applied to medical images do not always extract subvolumes correctly, effective tools that can quickly refine segmentation results are needed. Tools for representing and editing 3-D regions are presented. With these tools a user can deform a 3-D region representing an initial segmentation involving some errors to one that represents the final correct segmentation as judged by the user. The tools work with volumetric images rather than with image slices. As a result, the editing process is quick and effective. Typically, editing of a 3-D region requires from a few to several minutes depending on the complexity of the region and the severity of errors.

Acknowledgements

This work was supported in part by the U.S. Air Force Research Laboratory contract no. F33615-98-2-6002.

CARS 2002 – H.U. Lemke, M.W. Vannier; K. Inamura, A.G. Farman, K. Doi & J.H.C. Reiber (Editors)

1020

Quantitative evaluation of medical image fusion algorithms

Uhlemann, F.[a], Sobottka, S.[b], Steinmeier, R.[c]
[a] Institut für Biomedizinische Technik, TU Dresden, Dresden, Germany
[b,c] Klinik für Neurochirurgie, TU Dresden, Dresden, Germany

Keywords: Fusion, matching, accuracy

1. Introduction

A procedure to perform an automated systematic numerical analysis by means of simulated volume data and statistical quality estimates is presented. By employing our technique, objective quantitative comparisons of matching algorithms can be performed.

2. Methods

Our test series were created using a software phantom [1]. This program allows to create medical volume data from a segmented reference image volume by numerically modelling the image retrieval process. Additionally we transformed and used simulated complex MRT and PET brain data [2]. Having full control over all significant imaging parameters, this procedure yields a gold standard volume data set. For the comparison of matching accuracy, various systematic transformations were applied to the PET and MRT data and errors of translation and rotation were determined. Different matching algorithms for rigid affine transformations were examined. One of these was developed by us employing a multiscale approach using normalised mutual information as the quality estimate.

3. Results

Even though all algorithms being investigated rely on sophisticated measures to estimate and optimise the registration accuracy, the achieved results varied significantly. The average error of the newly developed algorithm for translation was 1.8mm and for rotation 1.5 degree (range of applied movements: 0...20mm and 0...45 degree, matching of MRI - PET) compared to an average of 5.3mm and 19.4 degree for the other algorithms.

4. Conclusions

Using the described techniques, a systematic investigation of image fusion algorithms can be performed. This work represents a step towards a standardised highly efficient, repeatable test procedure for an objective, quantitative evaluation of medical image fusion algorithms.

References

1. Uhlemann, F.: Segmentierung, Volumenbestimmung und Visualisierung medizinischer Daten verschiedener Modalitäten. Diplomarbeit, Institut für Biomedizinische Technik, Fakultät Elektrotechnik, Technische Universität Dresden, 2000.
2. Chodkowski, B.: A Simulation of Clinically Realistic PET Data and its Use in the Evaluation of Image Registration Algorithms. Master of Science, School of Engineering and Applied Science of the George Washington University, 1996.

CARS 2002 – H.U. Lemke, M.W. Vannier; K. Inamura, A.G. Farman, K. Doi & J.H.C. Reiber (Editors)

The "Virtual Institute for Computer Assistance in Clinical Radiology" (VICORA): first results of the development of algorithms and applications

S. Krass[a], F. Link[a], T. Boskamp[a], A. Schenk[a], H. Bourquain[a], S. Kohle[a],
R. Rascher-Friesenhausen[a], W. Spindler[a], B. Kümmerlen[a], M. Lang[a], B. Wein[b],
R. Leppek[c], H.-O. Peitgen[a]

[a] MeVis - Center for Medical Diagnostic Systems and Visualization, Bremen
[b] Department of Diagnostic Radiology, RWTH Aachen University Hospital
[c] Department of Diagnostic Radiology, Philipps-University Marburg

Keywords: Algorithms, applications, evaluation

1. Introduction

VICORA was founded in November 2000 as a non-profit institute by six major radiological centers, MeVis, and the two industrial partners Siemens Medical Solutions and MeVis Technology. The mission of VICORA is to develop algorithms and applications for computer assistance in clinical radiology, to evaluate the applications in a clinical environment and to establish them in clinical routine. Initially, VICORA focuses on the development of applications in the areas of vessel analysis, dynamic MRI, and preoperative planning.

2. Methods and Results

To make use of maximum synergy, a number of methodological tasks were identified and solved that are common to most of the clinical projects: Segmentation of tubular structures [1], focal lesions, and parenchymatous organs [2,3], skeletonization of segmented vessels, morphological analysis of tubular structures and focal lesions, contrast agent dynamics, and registration of three dimensional data.

Based on the developed algorithms, three application prototypes were developed for use in the clinical environment: AngioVision, DynaVision and HepaVision2.

3. Conclusion

VICORA incorporates the competence of radiology, computer science, and industry. The first results show the positive effects of synergy in software development and evaluation for medical applications.

Acknowledgements

VICORA is funded by the Federal Ministry of Education and Research (BMBF).

References

1. Morphometric and structural analysis of vasculature in volumetric images. G. Prause, D. Selle, H.-O. Peitgen. Computer Assisted Radiology and Surgery 2001; 947-952.
2. Efficient Semiautomatic Segmentation of 3D Objects in Medical Images. A. Schenk, G. Prause, H.-O. Peitgen. MICCAI 2000; 186-195.
3. Local Cost Computation for Efficient Segmentation of 3D Objects with Live Wire. A. Schenk, G. Prause, H.-O. Peitgen. Proceedings of SPIE 2001; 4322:1357-1364.

CARS 2002 – H.U. Lemke, M.W. Vannier; K. Inamura, A.G. Farman, K. Doi & J.H.C. Reiber (Editors)

1022

Three-dimensional composite images of SPECT/MRI in hydrocephalus

Toshiaki Mito[a], Iekado Shibata[b], Nobuo Sugo[c], Masaaki Takano[d]

[a, b, c, d] 6-11-1, Omori-nishi, Ota-ku, 143-0015, Tokyo, Japan

Keywords: Hydrocephalus, 3D-composite images, SPECT

1. Introduction

Recently programmable valves have been used in many institutions to prevent complications such as subdural hematoma, subdural hygroma and cerebrospinal fluid (CSF) over-or underdrainage in hydrocephalic patients after shunting operation. However, the valves can't be used for MRI, and for patients in whom frequent pressure adjustments are necessary or pressure setting is changeable. We investigated performance of three-dimensional (3D) MRI and SPECT for evaluation of therapeutic effects from morphological and functional aspects using the Orbis-Sigma valve system, a shunt system that automatically controls flow of CSF.

2. Methods

13 patients underwent shunt placement with an Orbis-Sigma valve. SPECT and MRI were performed before surgery and at one month after surgery, and generated 3D SPECT images, voxel graphs and composite SPECT/MR images. SPECT was performed using PRISM 3000 with 123I-IMP. For three-dimensional display and semiquantitative analysis, voxel graphs were generated with the TITAN 2 graphics workstation and the Application Visualization System-Medical Viewer (AVS-MV).

3. Results

One patient who underwent shunt placement with an Orbis-Sigma valve showed underdrainage. On MRI, changes in ventricles by improvement of symptoms were seen in 9 of 13 patients. Changes on 3D SPECT images and voxel graphs were seen in 12 of 13 patients. In composite images, defects in SPECT were reduced with improvement of symptoms. These results show that 3D SPECT images and voxel graphs were better correlated to changes in clinical features than MRI.

4. Conclusions

SPECT was more sensitive to detect clinical changes than MRI. On composite SPECT/MR images, defects imaged by SPECT scans in periventricular regions imaged by MRI were reduced with improvement of symptoms. 3D SPECT images and voxel graphs were better correlated to changes in clinical changes than MRI. Analysis with 3D SPECT images and voxel graphs will provide useful information to elucidate pathology of intractable hydrocephalus. Composite images will contribute elucidation of pathology of PVH because visual assessment of periventricular flow dynamics.

CARS 2002 – H.U. Lemke, M.W. Vannier; K. Inamura, A.G. Farman, K. Doi & J.H.C. Reiber (Editors)

Segmentation of MR brain images using region growing combined with an active contour model

R. Parveen, A. Todd-Pokropek

Dept. of Medical Physics and Bioengineering, University College London, UK

Keywords: MRI segmentation, active contour model, region growing.

1. Introduction
An improved method of segmenting MR brain images has been developed, based on region growing combined with an active contour model. Due to the complexity of getting good segmentation results using region growing, this new algorithm has been tested with various levels of noise. An overlay image with different colours was used in order to locate the segmented information and test the matching with respect to the real data.

2. Tissue segmentation
To extract the brain from the skull, a modified active contour model was used. Instead of using gradient magnitude in the greedy algorithm, an edge-preserving smoothing method implemented by an adaptive smoothing filter was used which provides a balance between edge preserving and noise removal. Using tissue connectivity, initially a 2-D, and latterly a 3-D flood-fill algorithm, was applied on MR brain images to segment out the structures of white matter (wm). The key point in the flood-fill algorithm is 4-connectivity in 2-D and 6-connectivity in 3D. Based on the delineation of wm and intracranial boundary detection, CSF matter was segmented by using the conventional grey level thresholding method. Subtracting CSF and the segmented wm from the brain contour model, was used to extract the grey matter. Examples of segmented tissue slices are shown in Fig. 1.

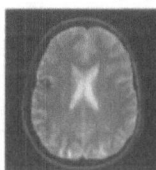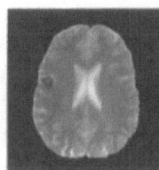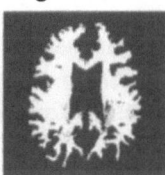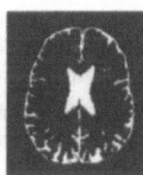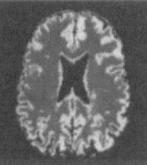

Figure 1. (From left to right) snake fit to the boundary of brain, extracted brain from the skull, white matter, CSF, and grey matter.

3. Results and conclusions
In clinical data, using the region growing method to segment homogeneous regions, the problem of under- or over-selection of brain wm was encountered. To test this, the flood-fill method was applied to segment wm in simulated brain database (SBD) images, adding Gaussian white noise with an S.D, σ of 10.0, 32.0, and 100.0 respectively. For an objective comparison, the segmented wm and the original brain image are merged together to create the overlay image. In the quantitative comparison, we have observed that the flood-fill algorithm can reliably extract the white matter with up to 25% of noise added to the original data values. While visually the results are satisfactory, a more rigorous quantitative validation process is now being undertaken.

Acknowledgements:
Bangladesh Atomic Energy Commission (BAEC) for grants and UCL for financial assistance.

CARS 2002 – H.U. Lemke, M.W. Vannier; K. Inamura, A.G. Farman, K. Doi & J.H.C. Reiber (Editors)

1024

DISCIR: an architecture for high performance distributed and component-oriented image diagnosis applications

C. Alfonso[a], I. Blanquer[a], A. González[a], V. Hernández[a]

[a]Universidad Politécnica de Valencia, Informatics Department (DSIC)

Keywords: Image diagnosis, parallel computing, CORBA.

1. Introduction
The DISCIR (DIStributed Computed Integrated Radiology [1]) is a multi-user, multi-computer, multi-threaded parallel computing software architecture for standard image processing tools, such as 3D segmentation, 3D projection and multiplanar reconstruction. DISCIR runs on a parallel server that provides with high computing power to any standard computer. The DISCIR architecture is completed with a client tool running under MS Windows operating systems that connects to the parallel server via CORBA protocols.

2. Architecture
DISCIR comprises 3 main elements: *The DISCIR Server* constitutes the bridge among the client applications and the parallel computing server. The DISCIR server manages the parallel computing server, controlling the processes and associating them to users. It manages users, fetches studies (through a DICOM gateway), transmits commands to the parallel server and returns results to the appropriate user client through CORBA protocol.

The Parallel Computing Server comprises a variable number of multiprocessor computers and performs the computing-demand operations, such as segmentation or 3D projection. Segmentation is performed either by means of voxel-based methods, such as Region Growing or Thresholding in 3D or by contour extraction methods. Projection is provided in DISCIR by means of different projection engines. DISCIR projection object can be either a 2D projection (a multiplanar projection) or a 3D projection. A 3D projection can be obtained by using one component from each one of the four sets: rendering method (Ray Casting and Splatting); tracing method (Perspective or Orthogonal); interpolation function (Linear and Tri-linear); and projection function (MIP and Surface Shading).

The DISCIR client is the visible part of the system for a user. It is a graphical application that runs on a separate computer and interacts with the server. It provides a user-friendly environment for fetching studies, presenting different images, computing segmentations, 3D projections or multiplanar projections. The DISCIR client does not require large user requirements. Moreover, studies are not downloaded on the local client, but stored on the parallel server. Images are presented only under demand.

3. Conclusions
The architecture DISCIR hides the aspects that depend on the volume distribution, data storage, interpolation, projection mode, etc. to let the programmer concentrate on the particular problem to be solved. Upgrading is easy and it is fully scalable.

References
1.   DISMEDI Project IST-1999-20226, http://www.medicaltech.org

CARS 2002 – H.U. Lemke, M.W. Vannier; K. Inamura, A.G. Farman, K. Doi & J.H.C. Reiber (Editors)

Usefulness of newly developed interactive multiplanar reconstruction viewer for large amount of image sets by multidetector-row CT: evaluation of invasion to surrounding organs of esophageal carcinoma

Takeshi Johkoh [a b], Shuji Yamamoto [a b], Takamichi Murakami [b], Masatoshi Hori [b],
Osamu Honda [b], Takenori Kozuka [b], Mitsuhiro Koyama [b], Mitsuko Tsubamoto [b],
Seiki Hamada [b], Yoshifumi Narum [b], Hironobu Nakamura [b]
[a] Department of Medical Physics, Osaka University Allied Health Sciences
School, Suita, Osaka, Japan
[b] Department of Radiology, Osaka University Graduate School of Medicine

Keywords: Multiplanar reconstruction, interactive viewer, esophageal cancer.

1. Introduction
The objective of this study is to evaluate usefulness of newly developed interactive multiplanar reconstruction (MPR) viewer for the evaluation of invasion to surrounding organs of esophageal carcinoma.

2. Methods
In 49 sites of these 30 patients who were performed surgical operation, invasion to surrounding organs were histologically confirmed (invasion(+); n=18, invasion(-) n= 31). Before operation, postcontrast helical CT was done with 5-mm slice thickness, 2.5-mm X 4 beam collimation, 6:1 pitch, 120kVp, 200mA/rotation, 0.8 second/gantry rotation, and standard algorithm covering whole esophagus using a multi detector-row CT scanner (LightSpeed QXi, GE, Milwaukee, Wi). The volume data for MPR views were reconstructed from above helical CT data with 2.5-mm slice thickness, 1.25-mm reconstruction intervals, and transferred to a newly developed interactive MPR viewer (KaledoScope, KGT, Tokyo, Japan). This MPR viewer can automatically reconstructs coronal and sagittal MPR views immediately after the transfer of volume data. With drawing lines by a pointing device on axial, coronal, and sagittal basic images, observers can promptly make various MPR views which are at right angles to the lines as they like. Using ROC analysis, an observer performance study, in which three observers indicated the confidence level for the determination of invasion or not for each site by axial 5-mm slice thickness postcontrast CT and interactive MPR views, was done.

3. Results
In the determination of invasion or not for each site, observer performance with interactive MPR views (Az=0.921) were superior to that with axial CT (Az=0.851) (P<0.001).

4. Conclusions
This newly developed interactive MPR viewer can improve the detection rate of invasion to surrounding organs of esophageal carcinoma.

CARS 2002 – H.U. Lemke, M.W. Vannier; K. Inamura, A.G. Farman, K. Doi & J.H.C. Reiber (Editors)

1026

Optimization of an anisotropic diffusion method for medical image processing

Kazunori Kawakami, Kenya Murase, Youichi Yamazaki, Masaaki Shinohara,
Minoru Kawamata, Makoto Nagayoshi and Shin-ichiro Iwamoto
School of Allied Health Sciences, Faculty of Medicine, Osaka University, Osaka,
Japan

Keywords: Anisotropic diffusion method, Gaussian and Median filters, statistical noise

1. Introduction

An anisotropic diffusion (AD) method is based on a new concept for image processing, in which smoothing is formulated as a diffusive process and is suppressed or stopped at boundaries by selecting locally adaptive diffusion strengths [1]. It is known that this method is capable of reducing image noise, while preserving the spatial resolution of images. However, the results depend on the parameters used in the diffusion function (DF) adopted in the AD method. Then, this study was undertaken to optimize the parameters used in DF by computer simulations.

2. Method

We generated a simulation map by segmenting the brain MRI of normal volunteers. Gaussian noise was added using normally distributed random numbers with a zero mean and unit variance to give noise levels of 10, 20, 30, 40 and 50%. We calculated the mean and standard deviation of the cerebral blood flow (CBF) values in the gray matter and white matter in the images processed by the AD method with various parameter values in DF. For comparison, we also processed images using Gaussian and Median filters.

3. Result

The images processed by the AD method were more similar to the original image than those processed by the conventional method such as Gaussian and Median filters (Fig.1). The mean CBF values in the images processed by the AD method were close to the assumed CBF values when the parameters in DF were optimized.

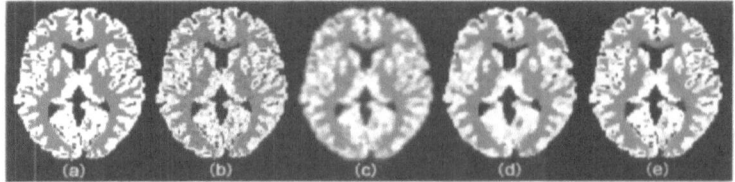

Fig.1 (a) original (b) 20% noise added (c) Gaussian filter (d) Median filter (e) AD method

4. Conclusion

This study will be useful for selecting the parameters in DF when applying the AD method to medical image processing.

References

1.   Perona P and Malik J. *IEEE Trans. Pattern Anal. Mach. Intell.* 1990; 12: 629-639.

CARS 2002 – H.U. Lemke, M.W. Vannier; K. Inamura, A.G. Farman, K. Doi & J.H.C. Reiber (Editors)
CARS/Springer. All rights reserved.

Fast image generation of cerebral perfusion parameters using multi-detector row CT and deconvolution analysis

Kenya Murase[a], Masaaki Shinohara[a], Youichi Yamazaki[a], Kazunori Kawakami[a],
Shin-ichiro Iwamoto[a], Yoshifumi Sugawara[b], Toshihiro Ueda[c], Junpei Ikezoe[b]
[a] Dept. of Medical Engineering, Osaka Univ. Medical School, Suita, Osaka, Japan
[b] Dept. of Radiology, Ehime Univ. Medical School, Onsen-gun, Ehime, Japan
[c] Dept. of Neurosurgery, Ehime Univ. Medical School, Onsen-gun, Ehime, Japan

Keywords: Cerebral perfusion, multi-detector row CT, deconvolution analysis

1. Introduction

Patients with acute cerebral ischemia may be treated by means of thrombolytic therapy within 4-6 hours after symptom onset. As a result, clinical examination and diagnostic imaging must be performed within a short period of time. Then, this study was undertaken to develop a fast method for generation of the maps of cerebral blood flow (CBF), cerebral blood volume (CBV) and mean transit time (MTT) using a multi-detector row CT and deconvolution analysis based on singular value decomposition (DA-SVD).

2. Methods

Dynamic contrast-enhanced CT scans were acquired using a multi-detector row CT (GE Medical Systems, Light Speed QX/i) (1 s/frame x 60 frames) 10 s after injection of contrast medium. The imaging protocol consisted of four contiguous 5-mm sections with a matrix size of 512x512. Acquisition parameters were taken as 80 kVp and 200 mAs. The maps of CBF, CBV and MTT were generated from time-density curves of contrast medium by applying DA-SVD pixel by pixel [1]. The arterial input function was obtained from the anterior cerebral artery automatically using fuzzy c-means clustering [2].

3. Results

Figure 1 shows an example of the maps of CBF (left), CBV (middle) and MTT (right) generated using our method. These images were generated within 5 s using a PC.

Fig. 1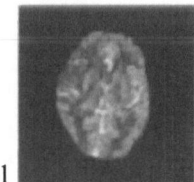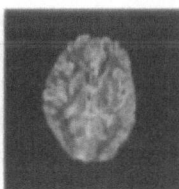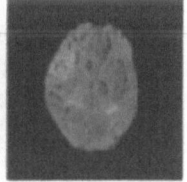

4. Conclusions

Our method allows a fast generation of the quantitative maps of CBF, CBV and MTT, suggesting that it is useful especially for management of patients with acute stroke.

References
1. Murase K, Shinohara M, Yamazaki Y. *Phys. Med. Biol.* 2001; 46: 3147-3160.
2. Murase K, Kikuchi K, Miki H, Shimizu T, Ikezoe J. *J. Magn. Reson. Imaging* 2001; 13: 797-806.

1028

Automated volumetry of lateral entricles in 3-D SPGR MR images using physicians' knowledge represented by fuzzy logic

Syoji Kobashi[a], Yutaka Hata[a], Mieko Matsui[b,c], Hajime Kitagaki[d], Etsuro Mori[b], Tomohiko Kanagawa[e]

[a] Himeji Institute of Technology, Japan
[b] Hyogo Institute for Aging Brain and Cognitive Disorders, Japan
[c] Brain Function Research Institute, Inc., Japan
[d] Shimame Medical University, Japan, [e] KCO Ltd., Japan

Keywords: Automated volumetry, lateral ventricles, Fuzzy logic

1. Introduction

3-D rendering and volumetry of lateral ventricles (LVs) using 3-D SPGR MR images help to diagnose quantitatively and qualitatively many types of cerebral diseases. This work aimed to develop a fully automated method for segmenting lateral ventricles.

2. Materials and methods

20 normal subjects, 20 Alzheimer's disease (AD), and 20 normal pressure hydrocephalus (NPH) were scanned. Coronal 3-D SPGR images were acquired with a FOV of 220mm, 124 by 1.5mm contiguous sections. The method segments the whole brain using software [1], and the CSF by 3-D region growing algorithms. To segment the LVs we introduce a new concept of 'representative line' based on physicians' knowledge. The method segments the whole LVs using the representative line.

3. Results and conclusions

Fig. 1 shows the surface rendered image produced by this study. The mean value of the absolute segmentation error ratio was 1.98%(SD=1.67, CC=0.999). Fig. 2 shows the volumetric relation for patients in the AD, NPH, and the normal group. They were significantly different (P < 0.001). 3-D rendering and volumetric produced by this study can give us a useful tool to assess the brain atrophy.

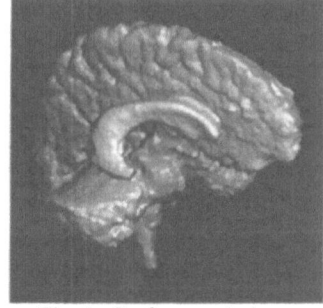

Fig. 1. Surface rendering.

Acknowledgements

This work was supported in part by Ishikawa Hospital Grant, the Ministry of Education, Culture, Sports, Science and Technology, Grant-in-Aid for Encouragement of Young Scientists, and the BISC Program of UC Berkeley.

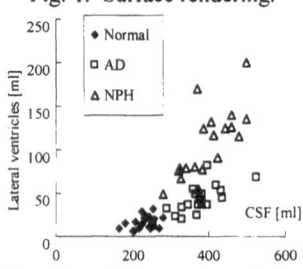

Fig. 2. Volumetric relation between the CSF and the LVs.

References

1. Hata Y, et al. (2000): Automated segmentation of human brain MR images aided by fuzzy information granulation and fuzzy inference, IEEE Trans. SMC-C, 30(3): 381-395, 2000.

CARS 2002 – H.U. Lemke, M.W. Vannier; K. Inamura, A.G. Farman, K. Doi & J.H.C. Reiber (Editors)

Preliminary study for characterizing Legg-Calvé-Perthes disease based on MRI segmentation

P. Pouletaut[a], I. Claude[a], R. Winzenrieth[a], M.-C. Ho Ba Tho[a] and G. Sebag[b],
[a] UMR 6600, Université de Technologie de Compiègne, 60529 Compiègne Cedex
[b] Laboratoire d'imagerie pédiatrique Hôpital R. Debré, 75020 Paris

Keywords: Image segmentation, Legg-Calvé-Perthes disease, hip joint

1. Introduction

Legg-Calvé-Perthes (LCP) disease is defined as avascular necrosis of the femoral epiphysis [1] : it particularly distorts the size and shape of the proximal femur and results in disability and abnormal growth of the hip. We choose magnetic resonance imaging to evaluate the physis deformations. In this paper, we present different segmentation methods for depicting the structures of the hip joint.

2. Methods

Four algorithms have been implemented : (a) dynamic clustering [2], (b) region growing [3], (c) watershed method [4], (d) snakes [5]. Algorithms have been tested on hip images (T2-weighted, coronal plane) to extract the osseous nucleus and to analyse the shape.

3. Results

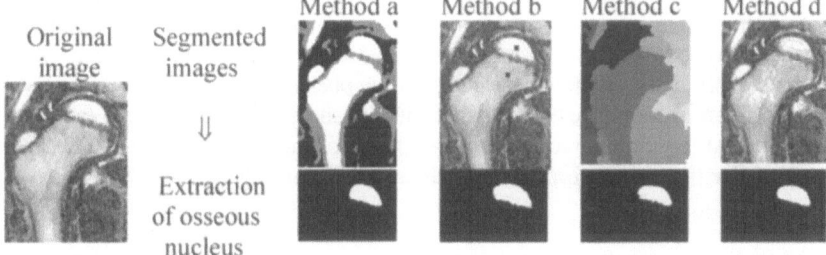

Shape parameters have been calculated to compare the extracted regions.

4. Conclusions

A segmentation tool for MR images of hip has been developed. It provides biometric parameters to evaluate the osseous nucleus abnormalities. Further tests have to be made on pathologic images in order to compare with clinical classifications of the disease.

References

1. Sebag G., Disorders of the hip, MRI clinics of North America, vol.6, n°3, pp. 627-641, 1998.
2. Dubuisson Bernard, Diagnostic et reconnaissance des formes, Hermès, 1990.
3. Adams R. , Bischof L. , Seeded Region Growing, IEEE Trans. PAMI., 16(6), 641-647, 1994.
4. Vincent L., Soille P., Watersheds in digital spaces : an efficient algorithm based on immersion simulations, IEEE Trans. Pattern Anal. Machine Intell., vol. 13, pp.583-598, 1991
5. Xu C., Prince J.L., generalized gradient vector flow external forces for active contours, Signal Processing, 71, pp.131-139, 1998.

CARS 2002 – H.U. Lemke, M.W. Vannier; K. Inamura, A.G. Farman, K. Doi & J.H.C. Reiber (Editors)

Magnetic resonance based biomechanical analysis of the knee joint

M. Siebert[a], K.-H. Englmeier[a], R. v. Eisenhart-Rothe[d], C. Bringmann[b],
F. Eckstein[b], H. Bonél[c], M. Reiser[c], H. Graichen[d]

[a] GSF – Institute for Medical Informatics, Neuherberg, Germany
[b] Musculoskeletal Research Group, Ludwig-Maximilians-Universität München
[c] Institute for Clinical Radiology, Ludwig-Maximilians-Universität München
[d] Research Group for Kinematics and Biomechanics, University of Frankfurt, Germany

Keywords: Open MRT, biomechanics, knee joint

1. Introduction

Insufficiency of the anterior cruciate ligament (ACL) is accused to cause an increase of femoro-tibial translation. This leads to an increase in shear forces which can be relevant for progression of degenerative changes of the meniscus and the cartilage. To quantify the amount of femoro-tibial translation in vivo we developed a new technique using a semi automatic calculated transepicondylar line of the femur for distance measurement [1].

2. Methods

Knee joints of 10 patients with an unilateral, isolated ACL deficiency were examined in an open MR system. After image acquisition, semi automatic segmentation and trilinear interpolation a 3D reconstruction was performed. For determination of femur translation a tibia based local coordinate system was calculated. The posterior parts of the femur condyles are shaped like a part of a cylinder. Two half cylinders surfaces are calculated, that best fit on lateral and medial femur condyles. The center points of the two half cylinders define the transepicondylar line that is transformed in the tibia based coordinate system.

3. Results

During knee flexion (30° to 90°) a posterior translation of the femur and of both menisci relative to the tibia could be measured in all patients, as well during flexing as during extending muscle activity, being significantly higher in ACL deficient knees.

4. Conclusions

In conclusion, we have developed a highly reproducible 3D MR based imaging and postprocessing technique to quantify femoro-tibial translation in vivo. In the future this technique can be used for analysis of the influence of different defects (e.g. additional meniscal tears) on the translation pattern. Further, different treatment options (conservative/operative) can quantitatively assessed in terms of its stabilizing effect in knee joints.

References

1. A. M. Hollister, S. Jatana, A. K. Singh, W. W. Sullivan and A. G. Lupichuk, "The axes of rotation of the knee", Clin. Orthop., 290, pp. 259-268, 1993.

CARS 2002 - H.U. Lemke, M.W. Vannier; K. Inamura, A.G. Farman, K. Doi & J.H.C. Reiber (Editors)

Connected morphological operators for CT-scan images of the abdomen

B. Naegel[a,b], C. Ronse[b], L. Soler[a]

[a] IRCAD 1, place de l'hopital 67091 Strasbourg, France
[b] LSIIT, Pôle API, boulevard Sébastien Brant, 67400 Illkirch Cedex, France

Keywords: Image processing, segmentation, mathematical morphology

1. Introduction

The hepatic cancer is one of the most frequent and the most difficult to operate. Its treatment can be helped by automatic detection of structures of interest in CT-scans. The automatic delimitation of organs close to the liver, of the liver itself, and of its vessels and tumors is a complex task. The aim of this work is to explore the tools of mathematical morphology, and to study how these tools can be used to improve the segmentation.

2. Methods

The classical tool for segmentation in mathematical morphology is the watershed on a gradient image. The first step consists in extracting the minima of the gradient of the image, which are used as markers. However, applying the watershed directly on the gradient image with these markers produces over-segmentation. Image must be filtered in order to remove useless information. To do so, we make a review of powerful morphological operators called "connected operators". These operators are very interesting, because they simplify the image while preserving contours. They interact with the image by means of flat zones. The flat zones of an image are the largest connected components where the grey-level is constant.

3. Results

We use the h-minima operator on gradient image to remove minima that have a low dynamic. The watershed applied on this image produces very good results in term of segmentation, with large flat zones corresponding to organs.

4. Conclusions

Mathematical morphology is a powerful tool for segmentation. In this poster, we have shown how to simplify an image in accordance with visual perception, and how to apply the segmentation paradigm of mathematical morphology on CT-scan images.

References

1. Meyer F. Un algorithme optimal de ligne de partage des eaux. *In 8e RFIA Lyon* (Nov. 1991)
2. Salembier P. and Serra J. Flat zones filtering, connected operators , and filters by reconstruction. *IEEE Trans. on Image Processing 4, 8* (Aug. 1995)
3. Vincent L. *Morphological grayscale reconstruction in image analysis: applications and efficient algorithms. IEEE Trans. on Image Processing 2, 2* (Apr. 1993), 176-201
4. Soille P. *Morphological Image Analysis*, Springer (1999)

CARS 2002 – H.U. Lemke, M.W. Vannier; K. Inamura, A.G. Farman, K. Doi & J.H.C. Reiber (Editors)

Improvement of an automated patient recognition method for chest radiographs using edge-enhanced images

Keisuke Kondo[a], Junji Morishita[a], Shigehiko Katsuragawa[b], Kunio Doi[c]

[a] Kyoto College of Medical Technology, Kyoto, Japan
[b] Dept. General Research Center, Nihon Bunri University, Oita, Japan
[c] Dept. of Radiology, The University of Chicago, Chicago, Illinois, USA

Keywords: Chest radiographs, patient recognition, edge enhancement

1. Introduction

To utilize a large number of digital images in picture archiving and communication system (PACS) environment, it is important that all of images are stored in correct locations such as in the proper patients' folders. We are developing an automated patient recognition method for chest radiographs based on a template-matching technique to prevent such filing errors.

2. Methods

The database used in this study consisted of 2000 posteroanterior chest radiographs that included 1000 current and 1000 previous images for 1000 different patients. We reduced an image matrix size to 64 x 64 in order to reduce the computation time for subsequent image processing. After we obtained edge-enhanced images by using a Sobel filter. Then, we determined the cross-correlation value between a processed current and a processed previous image. If the correlation value was greater than a threshold value, the current image was considered as belonging to the same patient.

3. Results

If a threshold value of 0.383, that is the lowest correlation value for the same patients in our database, is selected for determination of wrong patients, 35.9% of wrong patients in our database can be identified correctly as wrong patients, without any false warning for the correct patient. This performance for identification of wrong patients with the Sobel-filter technique is lower than that obtained from the method without the Sobel-filter technique, 48.8%. However, we found that the distribution of the correlation values with the Sobel filter is different from that without the Sobel filter. Therefore, when we combined the two methods to distinguish the images by a rule-based method, 35.7 % (183/512) of wrong patients which could not be identified as wrong patients by the previous method, were correctly identified with the Sobel-filter technique. Finally, 67.1% of wrong patients in our database can be identified correctly as wrong patients, without any false warning for the correct patient.

4. Conclusions

The combination of our method with and without the Sobel-filter technique indicated that more than 67% of wrong images can be identified correctly. Therefore, we believe that this automated method for patient recognition would be useful in correcting "wrong" images being stored in a PACS environment.

CARS 2002 – H.U. Lemke, M.W. Vannier; K. Inamura, A.G. Farman, K. Doi & J.H.C. Reiber (Editors)

Automatic registration of thoracic FDG-PET and CT for diagnosis and staging of lung cancer

Jane C. Asmuth[a], Richard H. Moore[b], Luca Bogoni[a], Suzanne L. Aquino[bc]

[a]Sarnoff Corporation, Princeton, NJ
[b]Department of Radiology, Massachusetts General Hospital and
[c]Harvard Medical School, Boston, MA

Keywords: Image fusion, image registration, lung cancer

1. Introduction

We developed an application to support physicians in the diagnosis and staging of lung cancer. FDG-PET scans are very sensitive to the existence of cancer. However, due to the relatively low anatomic resolution of PET, clinical scans are usually interpreted accompanied by a separate thoracic CT. Our application registers the PET scan to a pre-existing diagnostic quality helical CT scan of the same patient, making the interpretation of the PET easier and faster.

2. Methods

CT scans were registered with PET transmission scans obtaining a global parametric transformation model using hierarchical coarse to fine techniques. Threshold segmentation was used to identify the chest wall in both the CT and PET transmission scans. Spurious components were eliminated using a 3-D connected component technique. The resulting thresholded volumes were then smoothed to allow registration in a hierarchical coarse-to-fine framework using an intensity-based cost function. We experimented with both affine and quadratic models. The resulting registration parameters were used to warp the PET emission scan onto the CT scan. For visualization, a single fused color volume was created in which intensity represents the CT values and hue represents PET emission values.

3. Results

This technique was applied to 16 clinical cases. Registration speed for each case, including warping, was less than one minute on an Athlon 1.2 GH PC running under LINUX. We obtained consistently satisfactory results in the central thoracic volume. Fused color volumes derived from the CT data and the PET emission data demonstrated more detailed anatomic localization of tumor and physiologic activity when compared to interpretations without image registration. Details of the clinical evaluation are being published separately [1].

4. Conclusions

Our results demonstrated improved diagnostic interpretation with registered datasets when compared to non-registered CT and PET datasets.

References

1.   Aquino SL, Asmuth JC, Moore RH, Weise SB, Fischman AJ, Improved Image Interpretation with Registered Thoracic CT and PET Datasets, In press Am J Roentgenol April 2002.

CARS 2002 – H.U. Lemke, M.W. Vannier; K. Inamura, A.G. Farman, K. Doi & J.H.C. Reiber (Editors)
ᶜCARS/Springer. All rights reserved.

1034

A segmentation method for 3D slice images: searching and bridging

Dongsung Kim[a], Kyobum Ku[a], Jiyoung Park[a]
[a] School of Electronic Engineering, Soongsil University, Seoul, Korea

Keywords: Segmentation, femur segmentation, medical imaging

1. Introduction
Achieving accurate segmentation results is essential for quantitative diagnosis of disease using medical image. This paper proposes a searching-and-bridging method for robust and accurate segmentation of the proximal femur, which is challenging[1] because it has complex shape, ambiguous boundary surfaces, and interference boundary of adjacent acetabulum.

2. Methods
The proposed method segments a volume of interest (VOI) slice by slice with two step modules: searching and bridging. For searching control points, boundary points are sampled from an initial boundary propagated from the adjacent slice. Next, the corresponding control points for the sampled points are searched based on gradient and similarity along a line perpendicular to the boundary curve. Only the confident control points are finally selected and bridged. Bridging control points are performed with a minimum cost path finding method and an active contour method. Adjacent two control points are connected through a minimum cost path, where the cost is computed with gradient and Canny edge magnitude without linking. Zigzag errors occurred in the minimum cost path finding, are overcome by incorporating an active contour method. At the initial slice, user-given control points are bridged with the proposed bridging method.

3. Results
The method successfully segmented the proximal femurs with low contrast areas and interference boundary areas for the three patient CT image data sets; a data set of 110images with 1mm slice thickness, and two data sets of 30 images with 3mm slice thickness. The accuracy of the segmentation results at single slice propagation is more than 97% compared with those of manual segmentation

4. Conclusions
The searching-and-bridging method produced the promising results on segmentation of proximal femurs, and can be extended to segmentations of other organs.

Acknowledgements
This work was supported by KOSEF research project No. R01-2001-00359.

References
1. L.V.Safont, E.M.Marroquin, 3D reconstruction of third proximal femur (31-) with active contours, Proc. of International Conf. on Image Analysis and Processing, pp.458-463, 1999

CARS 2002 – H.U. Lemke, M.W. Vannier, K. Inamura, A.G. Farman, K. Doi & J.H.C. Reiber (Editors)

NEUROCAD: a neurology computer-aided toolkit

L. F. Oliveira[a], L. Cavalcanti[a], M.C. Oliveira[a], G. F. Caetano[a],
P. M. Azevedo-Marques[a]
[a]Image Sciences and Medical Physics Center
Medical School of Ribeirão Preto - University of São Paulo
Av. dos Bandeirantes, 3900 - 14048-900 - Ribeirão Preto - SP - Brazil

Keywords: Image co-register, volumetric analysis, reconstruction

1. Introduction

This work presents NEUROCAD, a neurology computer-aided toolkit. Three modules compose the toolkit, image co-register (MR/CT/SPECT), volumetric analysis and tri-dimensional (3D) reconstruction. All modules aided or in the localization, or in the quantization of brain lesions.

2. Methods

There are three modules in the system. The co-register module uses only two section images of a same plane, which are selected by the specialist. Then, the specialist should place some markers, and its respective pairs in each of the images. The points positioned in the first image serve as a reference, the ones in the second image suffer geometric operations of scale, translation and rotation for the adjustment. In the volumetric analysis module, all the examination images are loaded in sequence. The specialist visualizes the coronal slice, one by one, marking the structures of interest manually, the system stores all the marked objects in the previous image. The Cavalieri's method is applied to do so and it has a principle of the calculation of the area of the selected structure multiplied by the thickness of the image sectioning. The structures marked by the volumetric analysis module may be 3D reconstructed, third module. The images and the coordinates of the structures are interconnected, so we can separate the structures of the images and reconstruct them in three dimensions. With the coordinates we may segment the structures of the images.

3. Results

The co-register has already been used during clinical routine procedures, helping not only the diagnosis but also the planning of invasive surgical procedures. The methods of volumetric analysis and 3D reconstruction are still being tested, but initial results have showed great potential for aided diagnosis in clinical environment.

4. Conclusions

With this system we intend to generate relevant and needed information to the clinical and surgical diagnosis of patients, improving this way the patient's whole treatment in the University Hospital from the Medical School of Ribeirão Preto (HCFMRP) at University of São Paulo (USP), Brazil.

Acknowledgements
FAPESP, CNPq and FAEPA/HCFMRP.

CARS 2002 – H.U. Lemke, M.W. Vannier; K. Inamura, A.G. Farman, K. Doi & J.H.C. Reiber (Editors)
ᶜCARS/Springer. All rights reserved.

Content-based image retrieval using texture features

M. O. Honda, P. M. Azevedo-Marques, J. A. H. Rodrigues
Imaging Science and Medical Physics Center
Medical School of Ribeirão Preto - University of São Paulo
Av. dos Bandeirantes, 3900 – 14048-900 – Ribeirão Preto – SP - Brazil

Keywords: Content-based image retrieval, texture features, BI-RADS™

1. Introduction
This work presents a Content-Based Image Retrieval (CBIR) system, that uses texture features for breast images characterization and computer-aided diagnosis (CAD) based on visual comparison between the investigated image and images previously classified and its clinical information.

2. Methods
A total of 114 consecutive clinical cases was used. Each case containing two mammograms (MLO and CC) of each breast. The image were digitized with "Vidar DiagnosticPro" digitizer. Each case was classified according the Breast Imaging Reporting and Data System (BI-RADS) pattern, by a radiologist of the Medical School of Ribeirão Preto, whom also identified the regions of interest (ROI) into the original films. The ROIs were indexed according to values of texture features (Haralick's features) obtained from spatial gray level dependence (SGLD) matrices. The Principal Components Analysis (PCA) was employed to select the more significant features. The queries are performed with the insertion of a ROI into system, which calculates and normalizes the texture features and searches into database for images with a similar features, inside a degree of approximation defined by the user. The images are presented to the physician who can compare then, verify the diagnosis of retrieved cases and the BI-RADS classification. The evaluation of the system employing the leave-one-out methodology was performed through the quantification of the similarity between the search image and the image retrievals.

3. Results
The initial results obtained from mammograms indexing and retrieval process provided values of Precision of 65% to the evaluation of the ROIs and 60% to the evaluation of the clinical cases with whole images, indicating the potential of the CBIR system to help the diagnostic of the radiologist and correlation with the BI-RADS categories.

4. Conclusions
The results indicate the viability of the utilization of the scheme proposed to help the radiologist, specially on the formulation of queries based on the description of the image content.

Acknowledgements
FAPESP, CNPq and FAEPA/HCFMRP.

CARS 2002 – H.U. Lemke, M.W. Vannier; K. Inamura, A.G. Farman, K. Doi & J.H.C. Reiber (Editors)

Enhancing the diagnostic capabilities of MRCP by high-resolution image acquisition and stereoscopic viewing

Tetsuya Yamagishi, Taku Saito, Kimihiko Abe [a],
Jiro Ishida, Ryuko Nishimura, Tadashi Kudo [b],
Andreas Petersik, Ulf Tiede, Karl Heinz Höhne [c]

[a] Department of Radiology, Tokyo Medical University Hospital, Tokyo, Japan
[b] Department of Radiology, Saiseikai-Kawaguchi Hospital, Saitama, Japan
[c] Institute of Mathematics and Computer Science in Medicine (IMDM),
University Hospital Hamburg-Eppendorf, Hamburg, Germany

Keywords: MRCP, high-resolution (HR) data acquisition, stereoscopic viewing

1. Introduction
Though magnetic resonance cholangiopancreatography (MRCP) is one of the most useful modalities, its capability for precise and realistic description of the biliary system has been inferior to endoscopic retrograde cholangiopancreatography (ERCP). Current MR scanner's spatial resolution of MRCP has become remarkably improved. However, it is time consuming and unpractical to read HR image data as a series of pictures on plain films. This presentation is to show that the combination of HR data and stereoscopic viewing leads to a decisive increase of speed and diagnostic value of MRCP.

2. Methods
The source HR-MRCP data (slice-thickness: 0.8mm, gapless, total 250-270 slices by coronal scanning) of healthy volunteers were obtained by fast spin-echo sequences (TR/ 1639, TE/ 900) with a breath-triggering. A Philips Gyroscan Intera MR scanner (1.5T) was used. Creation of the stereoscopic maximum intensity projection (MIP) on a PC was performed by VOXEL-MAN system developed at Institute of Mathematics and Computer Science in Medicine (IMDM), Hamburg, Germany. The benefit for film-reading and the capabilities for clinical application were then compared with conventional MRCP.

3. Results
The morphological descriptions of detailed contours can be substantially improved on the entire field of the biliary system. The HR data enables a non-cleaved MIP view even in a perpendicular projection compared to the original scanning direction, which is unavailable in the conventional data acquisition of MRCP with thick-slice and slice-interval gaps.

4. Conclusions
Since the presented method reduces the false negative and/ or positive findings of MRCP due to signal overlaps, it may be considered as a reasonable option prior to ERCP in order to cut down the cases of ERCP, which is too invasive as the next modality after screening.

References
1. Karl Heinz Höhne et al, "3D-visualization of tomographic volume data using the generalized voxel-model", Visual Computer, vol. 6, no.1, pp.28-36, 1990

CARS 2002 – H.U. Lemke, M.W. Vannier; K. Inamura, A.G. Farman, K. Doi & J.H.C. Reiber (Editors)

1038

Wavelet de-noising in digital chest radiographs by generalized cross validation

Hideaki Kubota[a], Youichi Yamazaki[a], Masaaki Shinohara[a],
Kazunori Kawakami[a] and Kenya Murase[a]

[a] School of Allied Health Sciences, Faculty of Medicine, Osaka University

Keywords: Wavelet, de-noising, generalized cross validation

1. Introduction
Unlike the "universal threshold" [1], the GCV (generalized cross validation) method [2] has an advantage that the noise-power information is not needed for determining the optimal threshold for wavelet de-noising. The GCV value behaves like MSE (mean square error) with change of threshold. We investigated whether this GCV method would be effective to noise reduction of chest x-ray digital images.

2. Methods
As noise-free images, we used the chest image database created by JSRT in 1998. Zero mean Gaussian noise was added to the noise-free images varying SNR from 10 to 100. We defined the SNR as the ratio of mean pixel value of the noise-free image to SD of the noise value. Then we calculated optimal GCV values and compared them with MSE.

3. Results
The result is shown in Fig.1. As SNR increases, large differences arise in the optimal threshold value determined by GCV and MSE.

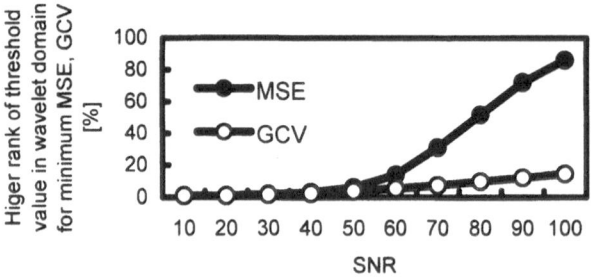

Fig.1 Comparison of MSE and GCV (average of 247 images)

4. Conclusions
The GCV method is valid for large amount of noise (SNR<50) in chest radiographs.

References
1. D. L. Donoho and I. M. Johnstone, "Ideal spatial adaptation via wavelet shrinkage," Biometrika 81, 425-455 (1994)
2. M. Jansen, M. Malfait and A. Bultheel, "Generalized cross validation for wavelet thresholding," Signal Process. 56, 33-44 (1997)

CARS 2002 – H.U. Lemke, M.W. Vannier; K. Inamura, A.G. Farman, K. Doi & J.H.C. Reiber (Editors)
ᶜCARS/Springer. All rights reserved.

A template-based method of ventricle part classification and realistic texturing for virtual ventriculoscopy

I. Goncharenko[a], H. Emoto[b], T. Fujii[b], N. Sugou[c], T. Mito[c], I. Shibata[c],Y. Kanou[a]

[a] 3D Inc., 1-2-12 Bandaicho, Naka-ku, Yokohama 231-0031, Japan
[b] Communication Research Lab., 2-2-2 Hikaridai, Kyoto 619-0289, Japan
[c] School of Medicine, Toho Univ., 6-11-1 Omori Nishi, Tokyo 143-8451, Japan

Keywords: Virtual endoscopy, ventricle, classification.

1. Introduction

A new method for automatic ventricle part subdivision, classification and realistic texturing is proposed to simplify navigation for virtual endoscopy (VE). The method is based on finding distance transformations for input surfaces to fit a template surface. After surface co-registration, each point of the input surface is classified in accordance with the class of the nearest template point and then class-specific textures are applied.

2. Data and methods

Input surfaces are generated by Marching Cube Algorithm applied to pre-segmented 3D MRI volume data of human brains. The template ventricle surface was pre-classified and subdivided into several anatomical parts in accordance with anatomical atlases[1]. Texture samples were captured from video records of real endoscopic operations. After preprocessing of input surfaces, a new template surface is combined from the anatomical model parts based on the best fitness between the input and combined surfaces. At the decomposition step, automatic ventricle part subdivision/classification is carried out. This task is solved as a minimization task in multi-dimensions and it relies on a special fast hierarchical search and the topological similarity of input and template surfaces.

3. Results

Automatic ventricle part sub-division, vertex classification, coloring and texturing were tested for several input data sets. In general, the method classifies successfully the parts of input surfaces if only ventricle-relevant vertices are taken into consideration after preliminary 3D-segmentation. In the case of noisy data, "cleaning" procedures improve the results of classification.

4. Conclusions

The proposed method provides the users of VE systems with the location of concrete anatomical parts closest to the virtual endoscope. The ease of navigation in the VE systems can be achieved by prompting an examiner with the part name and/or switching between textured and coloured modes.

References

1. H.-J. Kretschmann, W. Weinrich. Neurofunctional Systems: 3D Reconstructions with Correlated Neuroimaging. Thieme, Stuttgart, NY. 1998. 150p.

CARS 2002 – H.U. Lemke, M.W. Vannier; K. Inamura, A.G. Farman, K. Doi & J.H.C. Reiber (Editors)

1040

Automatic extraction of cerebral blood vessel and aneurysm from magnetic resonance angiography

Youichi Yamazaki[a], Kenya Murase[a], Masaaki Shinohara[a], Keiichi Kikuchi[b],
Hitoshi Miki[b], Junpei Ikezoe[b]
[a] Department of Medical Engineering, Division of Allied Health Sciences,
Osaka University Medical School, Suita, Osaka, Japan
[b] Department of Radiology, Ehime University School of Medicine, Ehime, Japan

Keywords: Region growing, brain aneurysm, magnetic resonance angiography

1. Introduction
Region growing algorithm has been often used for extracting blood vessels from magnetic resonance angiography (MRA) data. The purpose of this study was to develop an objective method with which cerebral blood vessels and aneurysms are automatically extracted from MRA data.

2. Methods
The extraction method is performed at the following six steps. 1) Binary images were generated from the original MRA data using the threshold value. 2) Statistical noise was eliminated using a labelling process. 3) Vacant regions on the binary image were eliminated prior to the application of a thinning process. 4) Thinning process was applied to the binary image to obtain the skeletons of blood vessels. 5) Blood vessels were extracted using a region growing process with the skeletons being taken as the seeds. 6) The extracted blood vessels were made thin, and they were piled up and displayed in three dimensions. These processes were automatically performed.

3. Results
Figure 1 shows an example of cerebral blood vessels and aneurysms extracted using our method.

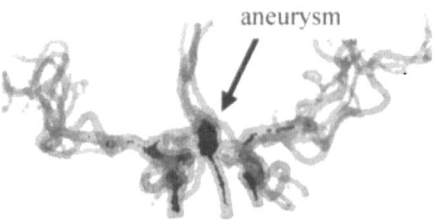

Fig. 1

4. Conclusions
We developed a method for automatic extraction of blood vessels and aneurysms from MRA data. This method appears to be useful for extracting and displaying cerebral blood vessels and aneurysms in a three-dimensional manner.

References
1. Hu X, Alperin N, Levin DN, TanKK, Mengeot M. *J. Magn. Reson. Imaging* 1991; 1: 539-546.

CARS 2002 – H.U. Lemke, M.W. Vannier; K. Inamura, A.G. Farman, K. Doi & J.H.C. Reiber (Editors)

Volume-rendered TOF MR angiography: detection and characterization of intracranial aneurysms

A. Mallouhi, S. Felber, A. Chemelli, A. Dessl, A. Auer, M. Schocke,
W.R. Jaschke, P. Waldenberger
Innsbruck University Hospital, Department of Radiology, Innsbruck, Austria.

Keywords: MR angiography, intracranial aneurysms, volume rendering

1. Introduction

The aim of this study was to compare between volume rendering (VR) and maximum intensity projection (MIP) as post processing techniques of MR angiography in detection and characterization of intracranial aneurysms.

2. Methods

The 3D time-of-flight MR angiography studies acquired in 82 patients were retrospectively evaluated by two blinded independent reviewer teams. Panoramic MIP and VR angiograms were rendered from each data set to investigate the presence of underlying aneurysms. Each detected aneurysm was then interactively evaluated with subvolume MIP and targeted VR to evaluate aneurysm morphology and size.

3. Results

Volume rendering tended to improve the diagnostic confidence (VR, A_z=0.95; MIP, A_z=0.90) and yielded a considerable improvement in sensitivity (VR, 89%; MIP, 71%), particularly in the detection of very small cerebral aneurysms. Regarding aneurysmal morphology, VR performed significantly better than MIP in lobulation detection ($P<$ .001) and slightly better in neck categorization ($P>$.238). Limits-of-agreement analysis showed a trend towards improved assessment of the aneurysm size by VR (-0.31 ± 1.62 mm vs. -1.27 ± 2.84 mm by MIP). Overall image quality and vascular delineation of involved vessels on VR images were rated better than that obtained by MIP ($P\leq$ .012 and $P\leq$ .001, respectively). Evaluation of TOF MRA Data sets was significantly facilitated with VR ($P<$ .001).

4. Conclusions

Volume rendering technique facilitates the evaluation of cerebral TOF MR angiography data sets and allows better detection and more reliable characterization of intracranial aneurysms than MIP.

CARS 2002 – H.U. Lemke, M.W. Vannier; K. Inamura, A.G. Farman, K. Doi & J.H.C. Reiber (Editors)

1042

Accuracy of cerebral blood flow obtained from dynamic susceptibility contrast-enhanced MRI using deconvolution analysis based on singular value decomposition

Masaaki Shinohara[a], Kenya Murase[b], Youichi Yamazaki[a], Masahiro Iinuma[a],
Takuya Enoki[b], Yuki Iwanaga[b], Keiichi Kikuchi[c], Hitoshi Miki[c], Jyunpei Ikezoe[c].

[a] Course of Health Sciences, Osaka University, Suita, Osaka, Japan
[b] Dept. of Medical Engineering, Osaka Univ. Medical School, Suita, Osaka, Japan
[c] Dept. of Radiology, Ehime Univ. Medical School, Onsen-gun, Ehime, Japan

Keywords: Cerebral blood flow, magnetic resonance imaging, deconvolution analysis

1. Introduction

Based on the indicator dilution theory, cerebral blood flow (CBF) can be quantified from dynamic susceptibility contrast-enhanced magnetic resonance imaging (DSC-MRI) by deconvolution between the arterial input function (AIF) and the concentration curve in the brain [1]. There are several methods for performing deconvolution, and an algebraic approach based on singular value decomposition (SVD) has been shown to be one of the most reliable options. The purpose of this study was to investigate the effect of the threshold value for SVD on the accuracy of CBF quantification from DSC-MRI under various conditions.

2. Methods

In this study, the threshold value for SVD was varied from 0.01 to 0.7. A Monte Carlo simulation of 1000 runs was performed for each condition. After 1000 runs, the threshold value giving the mean CBF value closest to the assumed value was chosen as the optimal threshold value. In this simulation, we used three different models for residue function and the effects of dispersion and delay in AIF were also taken into account.

3. Results

Our simulation results indicated that the CBF values obtained by this method largely depend on the threshold value used in SVD. The optimal threshold value changed depending on the model of vascular transport, but did not largely depend on the delay and dispersion in AIF [2].

4. Conclusions

Our results suggest that the threshold value should be carefully considered when quantifying CBF in terms of absolute values from DSC-MRI using deconvolution analysis based on SVD.

References
1. Murase K, Kikuchi K, Miki H, Shimizu T, Ikezoe J. *J. Magn. Reson. Imaging* 2001; 13: 797-806.
2. Murase K, Shinohara M, Yamazaki Y. *Phys. Med. Biol.* 2001; 46: 3147-3160.

CARS 2002 – H.U. Lemke, M.W. Vannier; K. Inamura, A.G. Farman, K. Doi & J.H.C. Reiber (Editors)

A new tool for unsupervised analysis of time series in functional imaging

M. Buerki[a], C. Kiefer[a], A. Nirkko[b], H. Oswald[c], G. Schroth[a]
[a] University Hospital of Berne, Dept. of Neuroradiology, Switzerland
[b] University Hospital of Berne, Dept. of Neurology, Switzerland
[c] T-Systems HCS AG, Switzerland

Keywords: Functional imaging, time series analysis, fuzzy clustering

1. Introduction

The evaluation of time series in medical imaging by means of unsupervised strategies such as the fuzzy clustering algorithm (FCA) is of growing importance. It has been shown that the FCA is a reliable tool for detecting activation patterns in functional MRI[1-2]. Unsupervised analysis allows evaluating complex data without imposing prior assumptions on the results that are searched for and therefore yields a bias-free analysis.

2. Methods

We have developed a software tool for unsupervised analysis of time series in medical imaging that supports the three common file formats Numaris, Analyze and DICOM. It runs as a standalone application under Windows NT and Sun Solaris. This tool implements the fuzzy clustering algorithm with a multiresolution approach to improve the stability and the performance of the computationally very expensive algorithm[3]. The multiresolution FCA has a more straight and stable convergence and does not depend on the initialization of the algorithm. Moreover, preselection methods are implemented to improve the power of the analysis [4]. Preselection aims to discard in a first step those time-courses, where only noise is expected. The preselection options currently available are mean thresholding, spectral peaks and autocorrelation. They can be selected in any combination. Since fuzzy clustering is very sensitive to motion artefacts, an accurate motion correction is needed. We implemented a new FFT-based motion correction that is very stable and accurate and operates nearly in real time[5]. Visualization of the results is implemented by membership maps as well as correlation maps of the time courses with each centroid. Furthermore, the tool supports interactive exploration of the results.

References

1. Fadili M.J., Ruan S., Bloyet D., Mazoyer B., "A Multistep Unsupervised Fuzzy Clustering Analysis of fMRI Time Series", Human Brain Mapping, vol. 10, pp. 160-178, 2000.
2. Buerki M., Oswald H., Lovblad K. O., Schroth G., Gutbrod K., Schnider A., "Evaluation of complex fMRI designs with fuzzy clustering analysis", ISNIP, Bern, Switzerland, 2001.
3. Buerki M., Oswald H., Lovblad K. O., Schroth G., "Additional speed up technique to fuzzy clustering using a multi-resolution approach", In Proc. SPIE, 2001, pp.1141-1150.
4. Somorjai R., Jarmasz M., Baumgartner R., EVIDENT: A Two-Stage Strategy for the Exploratory Analysis of Functional MRI Data by Fuzzy Clustering. National research council, Canada, 2000. http://zeno.ibd.nrc.ca/informatics/pubs/2stagestrategy.pdf
5. Nirkko A., Buerki M., Ozdoba C., Wiesendanger M., Robust and fast (real time) image registration in motion correction of fMRI studies. Swiss Society of Neuroscience, 5th joint annual meeting, Basel, 2000.

CARS 2002 – H.U. Lemke, M.W. Vannier; K. Inamura, A.G. Farman, K. Doi & J.H.C. Reiber (Editors)

1044

Lung MR imaging: robust registration technique of the respiratory phase for quantitative ventilation and perfusion study

Takashi Ueguchi[a,b], Takeshi Johkoh[b], Mitsuhiro Koyama[b], Chikako Tanaka[a],
Masaaki Kawahara[a], and Hironobu Nakamura[a,b]

[a] Osaka University Hospital, Suita, Osaka, Japan
[b] Osaka University Graduate School of Medicine, Suita, Osaka, Japan

Keywords: Lung magnetic resonance (MR) imaging, postprocessing, quantitative analysis

1. Introduction

Recently, an approach by using magnetic resonance (MR) imaging with the inversion-recovery single-shot fast spin echo (IR-SSFSE) sequence has been proposed for assessment of regional pulmonary ventilation and perfusion. In this scheme, more than two images acquired with different conditions are analysed. Therefore, misregistration of respiratory phase between these images is a severe problem, which makes the assessment difficult. In this study, we propose a novel technique for robust respiratory registration.

2. Methods

To describe simply, we introduce our algorithm with an example of ventilation imaging. The electrocardiographically triggered IR-SSFSE acquisition, which sequentially provides 20~50 images, was performed on a 1.5-tesla scanner (Signa Horizon LX, GE Medical Systems) during quiet breathing under air-inhaled and oxygen-inhaled condition, respectively. Then a ventilation map was calculated with using our algorithm. The algorithm is based on a cascade of statistical analysis described below. **Step 1:** Select one image (*image-A*) from air-inhaled images. **Step 2:** Perform correlation analysis to select up to three images (*images-B*; including *image-A*), which have close correlation to *image-A*, from air-inhaled images. **Step 3:** Perform principal component analysis to gather common information (i.e. first principal component) from *images-B* and put it into an image *(image-C)*. **Step 4:** Perform correlation analysis to select up to three images *(images-D)*, which have close correlation to *image-C*, from oxygen-inhaled images. **Step 5:** Perform principal component analysis to create a first principal component image (*image-E*) from *images-D*. **Step 6:** Calculate the ventilation map from *image-C* and *image-E* by a basis of percentage difference of signal intensity.

3. Results and Conclusions

Fig.1 (a) and (b) demonstrates an example of ventilation map with / without the proposed technique, respectively. Excellent image quality without misregistration artifacts was obtained by the proposed technique. Thus, it will be a feasible technique as a first step of the postprocessing of the quantitative lung MR.

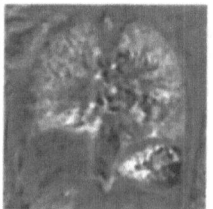 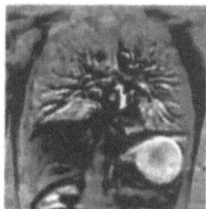

(a) with the technique (b) without the technique

Fig.1 Oxygen-enhanced ventilation map

CARS 2002 – H.U. Lemke, M.W. Vannier; K. Inamura, A.G. Farman, K. Doi & J.H.C. Reiber (Editors)

How to determine the borders of gray matter of young and aged brain on magnetic resonance images

Nobuhiro Tsukamoto[a], Hideo Kumagai[a], Kiichiro Saitoh[a], Masahiko Monma[a],
Yutaka Ando[b], Masayuki Kitamura[b], Osamu Kawaguchi[b]

[a] Dept. of Radiology Sciences Ibaraki Prefectural University of Health Sciences
4669-2 Ami Ami-machi Inashiki-gun Ibaraki Japan

[b] Dept. of Radiology Keio University 35 Shinanomachi Shinjuku Tokyo Japan

Keywords: Human brain, cerebral cortex, volumetric evaluation

1. Introduction

Brain atrophy is related to the severity of the neurological disease. Volumetric evaluation of the barin is useful to make diagnoses and to predict theprognoses. Segmentation of gray and white matter manually is complex and time-consuming. In this study, we propose new strategies for separating gray and white matter from young and aged brain.

2. Methods

Coronal T1-weighted inversion recovery MRI scans were performed on 1.5 tesla Philips Gyroscan MRI system for fifteen males aged 20 to 80 years old with the following parameters: TR=2000msec, TE=15msec, TI=350msec. Each voxel was 0.86x8.6x1.6(mm) = 1.18mm^3 in volume. Relative intensity threshold techniques were applied to select voxels that were expected gray matter. Histograms of signal intensities were made for all voxels in cranial to calculate threshold levels. Median of signal intensities of gray, white matter and CSF were calculated based on the histogram using differential twice. The border of white matter and gray matter, and the border of gray matter and CSF were arranged according to proportions of peak's heights. The gray matter can obtain as voxels have suitable intensities within the two borders, in all sliced images.

3. Results

The distributions of signal intensities showed different pattern depend on ages. For aged brain, the distributions are made clearly three peaks, which meant medians of intensities for gray matter, white matter and CSF. For young, CSF peak was not clear, it made only small hump by the gray matter's mountain-foot. And for child, white matter peak was also unclear, there ware only gray matter's peak with two humps. Differential calculus was effective to determine the borders of signal intensities, which were use as thresholds to select gray matter. It takes to process the images and calculate the volume for in each study about 10 minutes in average, and most processes are performed automatically. It is sufficiently brief to perform in daily MRI studies.

4. Conclusions

We propose a volumetric method for gray matter of brain. It takes about ten minutes without any troublesome hand-drawing processes, so it can be performed in daily MRI studies.

CARS 2002 – H.U. Lemke, M.W. Vannier; K. Inamura, A.G. Farman, K. Doi & J.H.C. Reiber (Editors)

1046

Computerized analysis of magnetic resonance angiography

Allan Z. Wang[a], Shannon Campbell, Qin-yu Chen
[a] Intelligent Optical Systems, Inc., Los Angeles, CA 90505, USA

Keywords: Angiogenesis, computation, MRA

1. Introduction
To develop innovative and user-friendly software for the rapid analysis of magnetic resonance imaging (MRI), focusing on the analysis of angiographies (MRA) that will greatly improve the diagnosis of cancer, vascular diseases, and angiogenesis associated diseases. This new coding technology is required to upgrade the accuracy, speed, image contrast, and user convenience when compared to related existing imaging software.

2. Methods
The first stage analysis of vascular images was automated computation of geometric quantities of the blood vessels, i.e. the length, width, area, and the number of branch points and terminating points. The coding techniques of binarization and thresholding were employed. The next stage analysis was to perform line detection. This was performed by accepting line points that had a second derivative larger than a user specified threshold. Points that had a second derivative smaller than a second user specified threshold were rejected. Then the data were stored in a particular data structure, transferred and calculated. Several other image-processing techniques were also used, including skeletonization algorithm that could readily and quickly compute the number of endpoints and junctions. These quantities were used as inputs to an artificial neural network whose outputs gave a classification in terms of the extent of vascularization.

3. Results
We have successfully applied this coding procedure to binarize, trace, line detect, and quantify the blood vessel on chicken embryo angiography and human brain MRA. The data files for individual vessel segments were automated listed in real-time as the length of each vessel line segment; then the average width followed by standard deviation, and the area along that line segment, as well as the number of branching and ending points.

4. Conclusions
This new computerized technique provides an automatic, reliable, rapid (2-3 seconds per image), sensitive, efficient (the analyses could be performed automatically and continuously without manual operation after initiating a few commands), and accurate analysis of MRA with a high accuracy of over 90% that surpasses existing software for the analysis of vessels or angiognesis, thus effectively assisting the diagnosis of cancer, vascular diseases, and angiogenesis associated diseases.

Acknowledgement
This study was supported by the U.S. grant #DAMD 17-01-C-0020.

CARS 2002 – H.U. Lemke, M.W. Vannier; K. Inamura, A.G. Farman, K. Doi & J.H.C. Reiber (Editors)

Spectral PTF analysis using cine-MRI in normal pressure hydrocephalus

T. Miyati[a], H. Fujita[b], M. Mase[c], T. Banno[c], T. Kasuga[a], K. Yamada[c], K. Koshida[a], S. Sanada[a], H. Imai[a]

[a] Kanazawa Univ. (J), [b] Gifu Univ. (J), [c] Nagoya City Univ. (J)

Keywords: Magnetic resonance imaging (MRI), cine-MRI, flow.

1. Introduction

To clarify intracranial dynamical properties in normal pressure hydrocephalus (NPH), we assessed a spectral phase transfer function (PTF) calculated from the driving vascular pulsation and cerebrospinal fluid (CSF) flow in the aqueduct. Because the PTF is thought to change in accordance with the degree of pressure damping.

2. Methods

On a vertical plane against a mid-point on the long axis of the aqueduct [1], Both CSF flow and blood flow waveforms were measured with cardiac phase contrast cine-MRI. Taking the difference in each cardiac phase between arterial inflow and venous outflow in the brain $[A(t)-V(t)]$ as the input function (driving vascular pulsation)[2], and the CSF flow in the aqueduct as the output function $[C(t)]$, the frequency response function $[G(f)]$ related to the intracranial dynamical properties [2] is obtained from:

$G(f) = C(f) / [A(f) - V(f)]$, $PTF(f) = \tan^{-1}[I(f) / R(f)]$

where $R(f)$ and $I(f)$ are the real and the imaginary parts of $G(f)$.

The PTF was determined in patients (n=9) with NPH after a subarachnoid hemorrhage (SAH-NPH), in an SAH-NPH post-shunt operation group (n=4), and in healthy volunteers (control group) (n=4). The PTF(f)s were also measured 5 min after an intravenous injection of acetazolamide (increase of cerebral blood volume)[1]. The PTF was compared with the pressure volume response (PVR) as an index of the intracranial compliance.

3. Results

The PTF of the 1st harmonic in the SAH-NPH group was significantly larger than in the control group, and the PTF in the SAH-NPH post-shunt operation group tends to be closer to that in the control group than the SAH-NPH group. There was no significant difference in PTF before and after acetazolamide injection at any frequency. A positive correlation was noted between the PTF of the 1st harmonic and PVR.

4. Conclusion

PTF analysis with cine-MRI makes it possible to obtain information noninvasively on intracranial dynamical properties in cases of NPH.

References

1. M. Mase, et al., *Acta Neurochir*, **71**, 350-353 (1998).
2. N. Alperin, et al., *Magn Reson Med*, **35**, 741-754 (1996).

Development of a simple and non-invasive method for measuring cerebral blood flow using Technetium-99m compounds and spectral analysis

Minoru Kawamata[a], Masashi Takasawa[b], Makoto Nagayoshi[a], Takuya Enoki[a], Naohiko Oku[b] and Kenya Murase[a]

[a] School of Allied Health Sciences, Faculty of Medicine, Osaka University, Osaka, Japan

[b] Department of Internal Medicine and Therapeutics, Osaka University Graduate School of Medicine, Osaka, Japan

Keywords: Brain perfusion index, spectral analysis, graphical analysis

1. Introduction

Cerebral blood flow (CBF) can be quantified using the brain perfusion index (BPI), determined from radionuclide angiographic data generated by ^{99m}Tc-HMPAO or ^{99m}Tc-ECD. The BPI is generally calculated using graphical analysis (GA). However, the BPI values obtained by GA (BPI^G) are not in proportion to CBF. In this study, we measured BPI using spectral analysis (SA) (BPI^S), and compared them with BPI^G to investigate the carefulness of BPI^S.

2. Method

Radionuclide angiography was performed on 20 patients with various brain diseases using a bolus injection of ^{99m}Tc-HMPAO or ^{99m}Tc-ECD, followed by sequential imaging (1 s/frame $\times$ 100 frames). Regions of interest were drawn over the left and right brain hemispheres and the aortic arch. The BPI^G and BPI^S values were calculated from time-activity curves in these regions using GA and SA, respectively [1]. The interobserver variabilities of BPI^G and BPI^S between two observers were also investigated.

3. Result

There was a significant correlation between BPI^S (x) and BPI^G (y) (r=0.752, y=0.530x+0.032 for ^{99m}Tc-HMAPO; r=0.886, y=0.568x+0.013 for ^{99m}Tc-ECD). There was a good correlation between the BPI^G values obtained by observer 1 (x) and those obtained by observer 2 (y) (r=0.976, y=1.043x-0.012 for ^{99m}Tc-HMPAO; r=0.987, y=1.010x+0.004 for ^{99m}Tc-ECD). There was also a good correlation between the BPI^S values obtained by observer 1 (x) and those obtained by observer 2 (y) (r=0.992, y=0.965x+0.029 for ^{99m}Tc-HMPAO; r=0.978, y=1.034x-0.025 for ^{99m}Tc-ECD).

4. Conclusion

Our method using SA will provide a more reliable BPI for quantifying CBF using ^{99m}Tc-HMPAO or ^{99m}Tc-ECD than the conventional procedure using GA, with a satisfactory interobserber variability.

Reference

1. Murase K et al. Eur. J. Nucl. Med. 1999; 26: 1331-1339

CARS 2002 – H.U. Lemke, M.W. Vannier; K. Inamura, A.G. Farman, K. Doi & J.H.C. Reiber (Editors)

A multi-resolution retinal vessel tracker based on directional smoothing

K.-H. Englmeier[a,] S. Bichler[a], K. Schmid[a], M. Maurino[b], M. Porta[b], T. Bek[c],
B. Ege[d], O.V. Larsen[d], O.K. Hejlesen[d]

[a] GSF- Institute of Medical Informatics, Ingolstaedter Landstr. 1,
85764 Neuherberg, Germany

[b] Department of Internal Medicine, University of Turin, Torino, Italy

[c] Aarhus University Hospital, Department of Ophthalmology, Aarhus, Denmark

[d] Department of Medical Informatics and Image Analysis, Aalborg University,
Fredrik Bajersvej 7D, 9220 Aalborg, Denmark

Keywords: Vessel course tracking, vessel contour, color fundus photographs

1. Introduction

To support ophthalmologists in their routine and enable the quantitative assessment of vascular changes in fundus photographs vessel extraction techniques have been developed. A multi-resolution approach was developed which segments the vessel tree efficiently and precisely. Our method has been applied to fundus photographs showing different levels of diabetic retinopathy in different resolutions.

2. Material and method

We developed a method to detect blood vessels in digital images of the retina. The algorithms starts at seed points, found in a preprocessing step and then follows the vessel, iteratively adjusting the direction of the search, and finding the center line of the vessels. As an addition, vessel branches and crossings are detected and stored in detailed lists. Every iteration of the Directional Smoothing Based (DSB) tracking process starts at a given point in the middle of a vessel. First rectangularly windows for several directions in a neighbourhood of this point are smoothed in the assumed direction of the vessel. The window, that results in the best contrast is then said to have the true direction of the vessel. The center point is moved into that direction 1/8th of the vessel width, and the algorithm continues with the next iteration. The vessel branch and crossing detection uses a list with unique vessel segment IDs and branchpoint IDs. During the tracking, when another vessel is crossed, the tracking is stopped. The newly traced vessel segment is stored in the vessel segment list, and the vessel, that had been traced before is broken up at the crossing- or branchpoint, and is stored as two different vessel segments.

3. Results and conclusion

This approach has several advantages: With directional smoothing, noise is eliminated, while the edges of the vessels are kept.. DSB works on high (3000 x 2000 pixel) and low-resolution images (900 x 600 pixel), because a large area of the vessel is used to find the vessel direction. For the detection of venous beading the vessel width is measured for every step of the traced vessel. With the lists of branch- and crossing points, we get a network of connected vessel segments, that can be used for further processing the retinal vessel tree.

CARS 2002 – H.U. Lemke, M.W. Vannier; K. Inamura, A.G. Farman, K. Doi & J.H.C. Reiber (Editors)

Two-year experience in using a telediagnostic regional network

O. Barbero, C. Rúbies, J. Fernández-Bayó, J. Valls, I. Périz, J. Puig, L. Donoso
Digital Medical Imaging Center, UDIAT Diagnostic Centre
Corporació Sanitaria Parc Taulí, Parc Taulí s/n, 08208 Sabadell, Spain
e-mail: obarbero@cspt.es

1. Introduction
The goal of the project is to show a variety of uses and scenarios of teleradiology, as well as the lessons learnt for over two years of an experience in a continuous process of evolution.

2. Methods and results
The system is used in the area of Catalunya (north-east of Spain) for exchanging digital CT examinations using a variety of technologies. These are the different scenarios:

Radiologist on duty for remote hospitals
The system is used to send exams from three remote hospitals (located at 10 Km, 50 Km and 140 Km), where there is no radiologist either on duty or on call, to a reference hospital (UDIAT Diagnostic Center, Corporació Parc Taulí, Sabadell) where a resident radiologist is on duty. Images are sent using the standard DICOM protocol, saved at the DICOM archive of the reference hospital, reviewed and reported by the radiologist. Loss-less image compression techniques are used to preserve image and diagnostic quality and to gain transmission speed. Two ISDN lines are used to send the images. This provides a speed of 256 Kbps, enough for this type of exams.

The system is redundant for robustness: a second and parallel system is used in case of failure. For images, two totally alternative ways are set: sending computers, ISDN routers and lines, DICOM archives, network lines, etc. For reports, everything made is sent by encoded e-mail to the referring hospital using the Internet.

Radiologists and neurosurgeons on call
The system is used to send exams from UDIAT Diagnostic Center, where a resident radiologist is on duty, to senior radiologists and neurosurgeons on call. The system is used to support the resident radiologist on duty in UDIAT. In case of doubt, images can be sent for consultation to the senior radiologist or neurosurgeon on call. The neurosurgeon will decide to go to the hospital and operate the patient on. Mobile phone technologies like GPRS and UMTS, when available, are also intended to be tested in the future for use with laptop computers.

A collaboration agreement between two hospitals for a neurosurgery service
The system is used to send exams from UDIAT, without neurosurgery service, to another hospital, Mutua de Terrassa (20 Km away), where the neurosurgeons will review the exams and decide whether to go to the UDIAT to operate the patient on.

3. Conclusion
In our experience the key factors for a successful operation of teleradiology systems are: Simplicity, redundancy, user training and continuous user feedback and improvement.

CARS 2002 – H.U. Lemke, M.W. Vannier; K. Inamura, A.G. Farman, K. Doi & J.H.C. Reiber (Editors)

Interactive (stereoscopic) DICOM image access on mobile devices

Melzer, K.[a]; Lipinski, H.G.[a,b]; Grönemeyer, D.H.W.[c]
[a] University of applied sciences, Dortmund, Germany (kaymelzer@gmx.de)
[b] Institute for Technical Systems, Dept.of Computational Biotechnology
[c] Grönemeyer Institute for Microtherapy, Bochum, Germany

Keywords: Stereoscopy, DICOM, mobile devices

1. Introduction

Accessing medical images everywhere and everytime on mobile hardware is very important for both routine diagnostic and research. Therefore, we developed an application for mobile devices, which are increasingly present like pencils.

2. Methods

Java Mobile-Information-Device-Profile (MIDP) was selected for development [1]. For data-transfer the standard-http protocol is used. The image data (e.g. CT) is available in the dicom file standard. There is no need of special data-preparation before file access. Stereoscopic images were generated with our previously developed medical interactive stereo-3D visualisation tool [2] (supports many stereo standards: filter, glasses, hmd, d4d).

3. Results

Java was used because of the growing range of java-enabled hardware like mobile phones (e.g. Siemens, Motorola, Nokia), personal-digital-assistants (e.g. palm m505, compaq ipaq) and tablet-pc´s. The new MID-Profile is especially for limited devices. Our reference application is running a 16bit-color Palm. Imagefiles (or sets) can be accessed through wireless (wifi, bluetooth, ir, umts, gprs, gsm) or wired (serial, usb, lan, memory cards) connections. The well known http protocol is good enough for serving the image and interaction requests (security with known standards). Once the data is retrieved from a server, the data can be viewed, edited, and saved. Stereo-3D viewing is possible with the chromatek mode [3]. 3D-Interactivity can be supported through servlets.

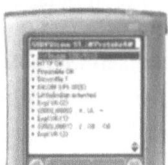 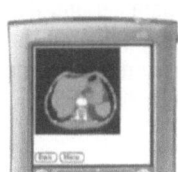 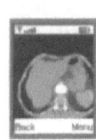 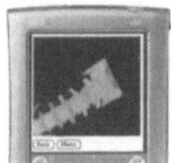

Fig. 1-4. Dicomtags, CT-Image on Palm, CT-Image on Phone, 3D-Chromatek-Image

References

1. http://java.sun.com/products/midp
2. http://www.kaymelzer.de.tf
3. http://www.chromatek.com

CARS 2002 – H.U. Lemke, M.W. Vannier; K. Inamura, A.G. Farman, K. Doi & J.H.C. Reiber (Editors)

1052

Fast volume rendering endoscopy based on semi-automatic path generation

S. M. Kwon^a, J. Yi^a, S. H. Kim^b, J. K. Kim^a, and J. B. Ra^a
^{a}Department of EECS, KAIST, Yuseong, Daejeon, Korea
^{b}Technical Research Institute, KBS, Seoul, Korea

Keywords: Virtual endoscopy, automatic path, bronchoscopy

1. Introduction

In virtual endoscopy, it is very important to observe a target organ with a rapid and easy way. In this paper, we propose a virtual endoscopy system that adopts a fast volume rendering scheme based on perspective ray casting [1] and a semi-automatic path generation scheme to navigate a hollow organ along a centerline.

2. Methods

The basic procedure consists of three steps: (1) the selection of starting viewpoint and view direction by a user, (2) centerline-tracking from the selected starting viewpoint to the next branching point, and (3) automatic navigation through the tracked center line. And this procedure is repeated again until the viewpoint reaches the end of hollow organ.

Normally automatic navigation stops whenever the viewpoint arrives at the next branching point, to prompt a user input. Then, the user only needs to select which branch is the one that he or she wants to navigate through. Between two successive branching points (or the starting and branching point), no user input is needed, since all viewpoints and corresponding view directions are automatically decided. During the navigation, a user can pause anywhere to correct the view direction or viewpoint in detail.

3. Results and conclusions

We evaluate the proposed method by using 3D bronchus and colon data sets taken from a 3DX-ray CT. The data sets include 283 slices of 256x256 pixels and 127 slices of 512x512 pixels, respectively. Both sets have a slice interval of 1mm. Evaluation is performed on a standard desktop PC. The proposed virtual endoscopy system provides prospective results. The fast rendering algorithm can reduce the rendering time, without a loss of image quality, by 74% for the bronchus data set and 81% for the colon data set on average compared with the brute-force ray-casting scheme. It means that it is faster than the other conventional fast algorithms up to 2.5 times. And the proposed semi-automatic path-generation method generates reliable centerlines and helps users to navigate complex organs with many branches.

Acknowledgements

This research was supported by Korea Science and Engineering Foundation (KOSEF) and Virtual Reality Research Center (VRRC).

References

1. S. H. Kim, J. K. Kim, and J. B. Ra, "Fast volume rendering in a virtual endoscopy system," *To be appeared in Proc. SPIE Medical Image 2002*, San Diego, CA, Feb. 23-28, 2002.

CARS 2002 – H.U. Lemke, M.W. Vannier; K. Inamura, A.G. Farman, K. Doi & J.H.C. Reiber (Editors)

Evaluation of PC-based 3D virtual colonoscopy

Junghoon Kim[a], Sanghoon Lee[b], Sangjoon Kim[c]

[a] R&D Team of TechHeim Corporation, Seoul Korea
[b] Dept. of Biomedical Eng., School of Medicine, Dankook University
[c] Dept. of Radiology, School of Medicine, Dankook University

Keywords : 3D, virtual colonoscopy, polyp

1. Introduction

We developed PC-based 3D model creation and navigation program which has diverse functions. It can be easily installed to PC and connected to network system. Through the internet or LAN, the users can examine virtual colon or discuss by navigating inside the 3D object simultaneously. The performance of virtual colonoscopy is evaluated by calculating sensitivity of simulated polyp which is made artificially inside the pig's colon and checked its clinical feasibility.

2. Methods

1) System configuration and data acquisition
2) Development Image Viewer
3) 3D model creation
4) Measurement of sensitivity of virtual colonoscopy

3. Results

The performance characteristics of virtual colonoscopy for simulated polyp detection was evaluated and its total sensitivity is 76%. Grouping according to polyp's diameter, the sensitivity for detection of polyps 10 mm or larger was 100%(40 of 40); 5.0-9.9 mm, 90.0(90 of 100); and smaller then 5 mm, 36.7%(22of 60). Table 1. shows the results and sensitivity for the polyp detection and in the polyps larger than 6 mm, its sensitivity is 98%.

Polyp Diameter(mm)	Sensitivity
Overall	76%(152/200)
Smaller than 5	36.7%(22/60)
5.0 – 9.9	90%(90/100)
1.0 or larger	100%(40/40)

Table 1. Sensitivity of polyp detection

CARS 2002 – H.U. Lemke, M.W. Vannier; K. Inamura, A.G. Farman, K. Doi & J.H.C. Reiber (Editors)
©CARS/Springer. All rights reserved.

1054

Normalized cuts for spinal MRI segmentation

Julio Carballido-Gamio[a], Serge J. Belongie[b] and Sharmila Majumdar[a]

[a]University of California, San Francisco, San Francisco, CA, 94143, USA
[b]University of California, San Diego, La Jolla, CA, 92093, USA

Keywords: Normalized cuts, MRI, segmentation

1. Introduction

Segmentation of bony structures plays an important role in image-guided surgery of the spine. In this paper we give a first approach to the segmentation of vertebral bodies from 2D sagittal MR images of the spine using the normalized cuts (Ncut) segmentation technique [1], and the Nyström approximation method [2].

2. Methods

Due to the fact that Ncut readily admits combinations of different features, we decided to apply this segmentation technique in two different ways to T1 weighted MR images of the spine. 1) The features of interest were windowed histograms of intensity. 2) The features of interest were position, intensity, and windowed histograms of textons [3].

3. Results

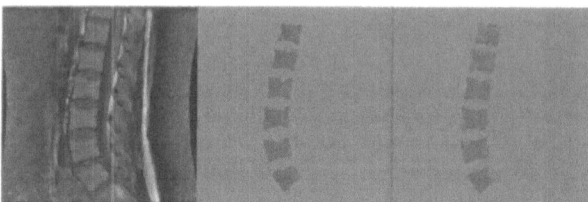

Fig 1. Original slice (left); vertebral bodies segmented with windowed histograms of intensity (center); and with intensity, position, and windowed histograms of textons (right).

4. Conclusions

In this paper we have shown that Ncut combined with the Nyström approximation method provides promising segmentation results on MR images of the spine, although we do believe that a final "accurate" segmentation will require the use of high-level features such as shape in the segmentation algorithm.

Acknowledgements

David Newitt. This work was support in part by a UC-Conacyt and Fulbright scholarships (to JCG). This was also supported by NIA-RO1-AG17762.

References

1. J. Shi and J. Malik. Ncut and image segmentation. IEEE Trans. PAMI, 22(8):888–905, August 2000.
2. C. Fowlkes, S. Belongie and J. Malik. Efficient Spatiotemporal Grouping Using the Nyström Method. CVPR 2001, Kauai, HI, pp.231-238 vol. 1.
3. J. Malik, S. Belongie, T. Leung and J. Shi. Contour and Texture Analysis for Image Segmentation. International Journal of Computer Vision, January 2000.

6th Annual Conference of the International Society for Computer Aided Surgery - ISCAS

CARS 2002 – H.U. Lemke, M.W. Vannier; K. Inamura, A.G. Farman, K. Doi & J.H.C. Reiber (Editors)

1057

Three dimensional colour coded visualization of differences between CT patient data and resulting stereolithographical models

E. Schwaderer[a], F. Dammann[a], M. Heuschmid[a], J. Hoffmann[b], C.D. Claussen[a]
[a] Department of Diagnostic Radiology, [b] Dept. of Oral and Maxillofacial Surgery
University Hospital Tübingen, email: erwin.schwaderer@med.uni-tuebingen.de

1. Introduction
Since stereolithographical models serve for surgical planning procedures the knowledge of overall and detail accurracy of the model is crucial. However the standard quality control procedure of point to point comparison of anatomical landmarks is time consuming and delivers rather unintuitive results.

2. Methods
To obtain detailed surface datasets we compared the generic CT data of patient scans with a CT scan of the corresponding stereolithographical models using a Siemens Volume-Zoom multislice CT scanner. The resulting CT scan data were segmented and then the extracted surfaces were transformed into the stl (stereolithography) output data format. Both stl datasets were imported into the imageware RP (Rapid Prototyping) software (sdrc) (Fig.1,2) and registered within one to three minutes (Fig.3).

3. Results
By using a comparison function we colour coded the deviations between the corresponding datasets onto the surface of the re-scanned stereolithographical model. The colour code shows the qualitative and quantitative results by stepwise changing colours depending on preselected deviation-thresholds (Fig.4).

4. Conclusions
After our first experiences we assume that deviations above 0.5mm can be detected when calibration is done and only bony structures are to be assessed.

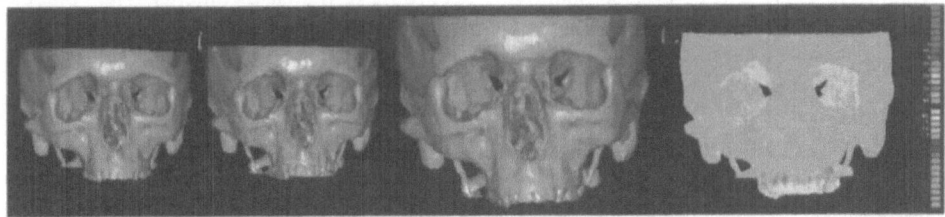

Fig.1: Anatomical   Fig.2: Patient   Fig.3: Registered overlay   Fig.4: Colour coded
    model   of both datasets   result

Acknowledgements
This project is funded by the grant AKF 60-0-0 of the University Hospital Tübingen.

CARS 2002 – H.U. Lemke, M.W. Vannier; K. Inamura, A.G. Farman, K. Doi & J.H.C. Reiber (Editors)

1058

Information integration and management for computer assisted orthopaedic surgery over Internet

T. Wu[a], C. Huberson[b], A. Zimolong[a], G. Müller[c], K. Radermacher[a], G. Rau[a]

[a] Helmholtz-Institute for Biomedical Engineering, RWTH Aachen, Germany
[b] Institut Albert Bonniot, Université Joseph Fourier Grenoble, France
[c] GEMETEC, Aachen, Germany

Keywords: CAOS (Computer Assisted Orthopaedic Surgery), Internet, database

1. Introduction

Because the CAOS is still a relative new technique, it is very important to make the knowledge of experienced surgeons available to the communities of other surgeons. A medical database called "Virtual Observatory" (VO) is developed to integrate, manage and disseminate the information about successful applications of CAOS technique.

2. Methods

The XML (Extensible Markup Language) and DTD (Document Type Definition) were used to enable the multi-centric case information submission. The VO database provides also an interface to output the case information in HTML files so that the remote users can access the VO database through Internet with the common browsers (Fig 1.).

A VOEU-DTD was defined to standardize the contents to be stored in the database. The XML file is generated according to the DTD and serves as a repository to describe the CAOS cases in a structured way. After the XML file being validated by DTD, the case information will be added into the database with the help of an XML reader which establishes a mapping between the XML file and the data model of the database.

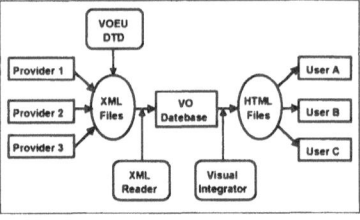

Fig 1 The Structure of the VO Database

The hierarchical structure of the DTD is used by the "Visual Integrator" which has the function of searching and visualizing the case information. A navigationbar based on the structure of DTD will be created adaptively according to the case contents. The concrete information of the case will be extracted from database and then interpreted as plain texts, images, videos or URLs according to the declaration of DTD element in the XML file.

3. Results

A core DTD dealing with the common aspects of CAOS and several specific DTDs for different CAOS techniques have been elaborated. A stored procedures has been implemented to read the content of the XML file into the SQL Server database. The realization of the "Visual Integrator" has been done by a set of Active Server Pages (ASP) which provide users dynamically generated HTML files.

4. Conclusions

The VO database will help to produce a reviewed and consensual CAOS expertise. It is also very useful for surgical education and training.

CARS 2002 – H.U. Lemke, M.W. Vannier, K. Inamura, A.G. Farman, K. Doi & J.H.C. Reiber (Editors)

1059

A novel system of 4-dimensional motion analysis after total hip arthroplasty

Keisuke Hagio[a]; Nobuhiko Sugano[b]; Takashi Nishii[b]; Hidenobu Miki[b]; Yoshito Otake[c]; Asaki Hattori[c]; Naoki Suzuki[c]; Toshihiko Sasama[d]; Yoshinobu Sato[d]; Shinichi Tamura[d]; Kazuo Yonenobu[e]; Hideki Yoshikawa[b]; Takahiro Ochi[a]
Departments of [a]Computer Integrated Orthopaedics and [b]Orthopaedic Surgery, Osaka Univ. Graduate School of Medicine
[c]Institute for High Dimensional Medical Imaging, Jikei Univ. School of Medicine
[d]Div. of Interdisciplinary Image Analysis Osaka Univ. Graduate School of Medicine
[e]Department of Orthopaedic Surgery, Osaka Minami National Hospital

1. Introduction
We have developed a novel system of 4-dimensional motion analysis after total hip arthroplasty that can assess safe ranges of motion for each patient for daily activity to prevent dislocation of the hip.

2. Materials and methods
This system uses 3D-skeletal structure and motion capture data for each patient. Five reflective markers for infrared-light were attached to characteristic points of the skin on each patient and CT images were obtained from the pelvis to the femur. Each 3-D skeletal model was reconstructed from CT data and reflective markers were used for fiducial markers to track and capture position of the pelvis and femur using infrared 3D position sensors. Combining these data, we analyzed motions of getting up and down from a chair in 12 patients (17 hips) who underwent THA. The angle between captured position and impingement points was calculated on the computer monitor. To assess the accuracy of measurements in this system, position of skin markers against bones in various postures was evaluated for five volunteers using open MRI.

3. Results and conclusions
Mean angle at the point of maximum hip flexion was $69 \pm 7°$ for flexion, $-12\pm11°$ for adduction, and $-7\pm12°$ for internal rotation during the activity. Mean angle from the point of maximum hip flexion to the point of impingement between bones and/or implants was $46\pm17°$ for flexion, $53\pm12°$ for adduction, and $54\pm11°$ for internal rotation. No impingement between bones and/or implants was found during the activity in any cases. However, both angles were different for each patient. For each static posture, error in hip angle using the current system was within $\pm10°$ for flexion, adduction, and internal rotation according to the open MRI study. The functional position of the pelvis during daily activities must be taken into account when assessing the real risk of dislocation. The current system enables dynamic analysis in terms of not only alignment of components and bones of each patient, but also individual differences in characteristics of daily motions by analyzing motion capture data for each patient. Further investigation of daily activities using this system will reveal safe ranges of motion for preventing hip dislocation, leading to precise guidance for each patient regarding postoperative activities.

CARS 2002 – H.U. Lemke, M.W. Vannier; K. Inamura, A.G. Farman, K. Doi & J.H.C. Reiber (Editors)

A cadaveric study of robotically assisted spinal needle placement versus manual placement

Kevin Cleary[a], Kevin Ruitort[b], Vance Watson[c]

[a] Imaging Science and Information Systems Center, Department of Radiology, Georgetown University Medical Center, Washington, DC
[b] Georgetown University School of Medicine, Washington, DC
[c] Neurointerventional Radiology, Department of Radiology, Georgetown University Hospital/MedStar Health, Washington, DC

Keywords: Medical robotics, spine, needle placement

1. Purpose

To compare the ability of an experienced physician in performing perispinal nerve and facet blocks on a cadaver using a joystick-controlled robotic needle driver versus manual placement of the needle.

2. Methods

Using C-arm fluoroscopy and manual placement, a 22-gauge needle was placed a total of eight times into the lumbar perispinal region of an elderly male embalmed cadaver. This procedure was repeated using a robotic needle driver for a total of sixteen needle placements. Small metal B nipple markers 1 mm in diameter were percutaneously inserted to serve as targets near the lumbar nerve roots and facet joints. The physician then attempted to place a needle to hit the target points, both manually and using the robot. Radiographs were obtained after each placement to assess the accuracy of placement while the time and number of re-adjustments required to place the needle were measured. The time was measured starting from the initial needle placement until the physician was satisfied with the final placement. A re-adjustment was defined as a withdrawal and re-orientation of the needle.

3. Results

Using *manual placement*, the average time for needle placement was 99.5 ± 29.9 seconds with an average of 3.50 ± 1.41 re-adjustments (n=8). Using *robotically assisted placement*, the average time for needle placement was 58.0 ± 22.4 seconds with an average of 0.38 ± 0.52 re-adjustments (n=8).

4. Conclusions

Using *robotically assisted placement*, an experienced physician can reduce the time to place a needle in the spine compared to the conventional, manual method. The reduction in time is a result of the decrease in the number of times the needle trajectory needs to be re-adjusted. Clinical studies are required to further investigate the advantages and disadvantages of this system for interventional needle procedures.

Acknowledgements
This work was funded by U.S. Army grant DAMD17-99-1-9022. The content of this manuscript does not necessarily reflect the position or policy of the U.S. Government. The robotic needle driver was designed and built by the URobotics Laboratory at Johns Hopkins Medical Institutions under the direction of Dan Stoianovici, PhD.

CARS 2002 – H.U. Lemke, M.W. Vannier; K. Inamura, A.G. Farman, K. Doi & J.H.C. Reiber (Editors)

Accuracy of the 3D angular position of vertebrae reconstructed by low dose digital stereoradiography

A. Le Bras[a], R. Dumas[a], M. Savidan[a], D. Mitton[a], J.A. de Guise[a,b], W. Skalli[a]

[a] Laboratoire de Biomécanique, ENSAM-CNRS Paris, France
[b] Laboratoire de recherche en Imagerie et Orthopédie, ETS-CHUM, Montréal, Canada

Keywords: 3D reconstruction, vertebral orientation, low dose stereoradiography

1. Introduction

The scoliotic spine can be reconstructed in 3D by stereoradiography [1,2,3]. The geometrical reconstruction error of vertebral shape has already been reported as 1.1 mm in average [2]. Few studies [3] reported the accuracy of the 3D angular position of the reconstructed vertebrae and they considered only 6 landmarks. The purpose of this study was to evaluate the accuracy of the 3D orientations when considering a 178 point vertebral model obtained by NSCP technique [1].

2. Methods

Three dry lumbar vertebrae were fixed on separate holders. Each vertebral holder contains 4 markers which define a reference axis system $R^f_{(Li)}$. The holders could be placed in different constructs yielding several orientations (combined rotations) which were quantified a posteriori. Five different constructs were considered. One corresponded to the reference with the vertebrae positioned parallel to a global reference frame. Each construct was X-rayed (2 orthogonal views) in a low dose digital X-ray imaging device from *Biospace Instruments*, France. The 3D models were obtained using a previously defined algorithm based on NSCP method [1].

3. Results

The results of angular errors between the reconstructed markers and the reconstructed vertebrae are presented for the 12 orientations cases in Table 1:

Table 1:	Angular Error for 6 points/vertebrae model		Angular Error for 178 points/vertebrae model	
	Mean	SD	Mean	SD
Lateral Rotation (range: 37.6 °)	1°	0.7°	0.5°	0.7°
Flexion-extension (range: 36°)	1.3°	2.4°	0.5°	0.6°
Axial Rotation (range: 25.4°)	3.6°	2.1°	0.7°	2.3°

4. Conclusions

Stereoradiographic method provides both accurate geometry and correct orientation thus it can be used in clinics to assess the spine curvature in an upright position. The 178 points vertebral model provides more accurate orientations than that based only on 6 landmarks.

Acknowledgements

The authors thank *Biospace Instruments* for their financial assistance.

References

1. Mitton D., de Guise J.A. et al. (2000) Med. Biol. Eng. Comp. 38, 133-139.
2. Mitulescu A., Skalli W. et al. (2001) Med. Biol. Eng. Comp. 39, 152-158.
3. Pearcy (1985) Acta. Orthop. Scan. 212(56), 1-45.

CARS 2002 – H.U. Lemke, M.W. Vannier; K. Inamura, A.G. Farman, K. Doi & J.H.C. Reiber (Editors)

Ultrasound guidance for spinal radiosurgery

Timothy C. Ryken[a], S.L. Meeks[b], J.W. Haller[c], J.M. Buatti[b]

[a] Department of Neurosurgery, University of Iowa
[b] Department Radiation Oncology, University of Iowa
[c] Department of Radiology, University of Iowa

Keywords: Radiation oncology, image-guided therapy

1. Introduction

Difficulty in accurately tracking extracranial targets has limited the development of stereotactic radiosurgery in extracranial applications. The ability to track extracranial structures in real time with ultrasound images allows a system to upgrade and interface pre-treatment volumetric images for extracranial applications. We describe this technique for the treatment of localized metastatic spinal disease.

2. Methods

This extracranial stereotactic system consists of an optically tracked ultrasound unit registered to a linear accelerator coordinate system. Stereotactic ultrasound images are acquired following patient positioning based on a pretreatment CT simulation. The soft-tissue shifts between the virtual CT based treatment plan and the actual treatment was determined and used to correct the treatment plan.

3. Results

The ultrasound based stereotactic navigation system is accurate to within approximately 1.5 mm on average based on testing with an absolute coordinate phantom. A radiosurgical patient treatment was delivered using the system for localization of a metastatic spinal lesion. Compared with the virtual CT simulation, the actual treatment plan isocenter was shifted 12.2 mm based on the stereotactic ultrasound image. The patient was treated using noncoplanar beams to a dose of 15.0 Gy to the 80% isodose shell in a single fraction.

Depth (mm)	Anteroposterior Distance (mm)	Lateral Distance (mm)	Axial Distance (mm)
30	1.8 ± 0.3	0.8 ± 0.4	0.3 ± 0.2
60	1.1 ± 0.3	0.4 ± 0.3	0.2 ± 0.2
110	1.3 ± 0.6	0.6 ± 0.4	0.6 ± 0.3
All depths	1.4 ± 0.5	0.6 ± 0.4	0.4 ± 0.3

Table 1: Accuracy of image guided 3D-ultrasound as a function of the depth of the target. Results are given in term of the distance in the AP, lateral, and axial directions.

4. Conclusions

A system for high-precision radiosurgical treatment of metastatic spinal tumors has been developed, tested, and applied clinically. Optical tracking of the ultrasound probe provides real-time tracking of the patient anatomy and allows computation of the target displacement prior to treatment delivery. The patient reported here supports the feasibility and safety of the technique.

CARS 2002 – H.U. Lemke, M.W. Vannier; K. Inamura, A.G. Farman, K. Doi & J.H.C. Reiber (Editors)

1063

Endoscopic treatment of intraventricular lesions in virtual reality

Novák Z., Krupa P., Chrastina J., Říha I.
Faculty Hospital St.Ann´s Brno, Czech Republic

Keywords: Neuroendoscopy, virtual reality, third ventricle

1. Purpose
The embryonic development of the ventricular system is extremely complex and as a result congenital anomalies are observed extremely frequently. Therefore endoscopy appears suitable in the treatment of hydrocephalus or lesions of the ventricles.

2. Methods
Since 1997, neuroendoscopic system Wolf is employed at the Dpt. of Neurosurgery, combined with the frame-based navigation system utilising software Stereoplan Plus or Praezis (Leibinger). CT navigation was used for the first cases (titanium frame Zamorano Dujowny), nowadays MRI – derived data (Siemens Symphony) are preferred (ceramic frame Leibinger). Data integration in the computer workstation Marconi creates presurgical virtual reconstruction. Intraoperative endoscopy updates the surgical picture.

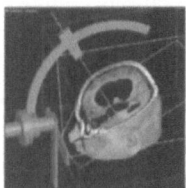 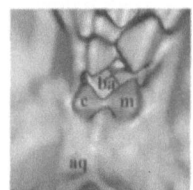 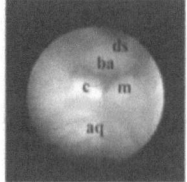

Fig. 1a surgical trajectory   Fig. 1b 3D reconstruction   Fig 1c endoscopic view

3. Results
The surgical series consists of 173 patients, treated endoscopically using virtual reality environment. Ventriculocisternoanastomosis supplements the intraventricular surgeries to assure liquor pathways patency not only in hydrocephalic patients, but in tumors and intraventricular bleeding, too. Navigated septotomy enables the surgeon to work in both lateral ventricles. Histological samples are taken throughout the surgery.

4. Conclusions
Endoscopic procedures, as well as intraoperative ultrasound or MRI actualises the preoperative virtual reality. Bloodless field is an absolute prerequisite as well as postoperative CT or MRI control. Creating a virtual reality image of the ventricular system is a difficult task due to the pulsatory movements of the ventricular walls, causing inaccuracy even in the preoperative decision making. The relationship between the surrounding anatomical structures and neurovascular ventricular structures builts up virtual reality, which is transferred with endoscopic image to the surgical reality. The differentiating ability of the neuroendoscopic system Wolf enables the surgical team to perform step–by–step safe surgery within the closed intracranial space.

CARS 2002 – H.U. Lemke, M.W. Vannier; K. Inamura, A.G. Farman, K. Doi & J.H.C. Reiber (Editors)

1064

PC-based deep brain recording system for functional neurosurgery

J. Tejeiro, R.J. Macías, G. López, J.M. Morales, L.M. Alvarez, E. Guerra, C. Maragoto, E. Alvarez, I. García, W. Bouza
International Neurological Restorative Center, Havana

Keywords: Signal processing, deep brain recording, functional neurosurgery

1. Introduction
The "Neurosurgical Deep Recording System" (NDRS) is a software for physiological targeting during stereotactic and functional neurosurgery using deep brain recording [1]. It substitutes with a personal computer (PC) complex equipment for signal recording.

2. Methods
The NDRS software has been made using a combination of two programming languages: Pascal and Assembler (for the on-line working modules). The NDRS allows to record, show, process and store up to two simultaneous signals. The signal display is carry out on-line with its acquisition, emulating a digital oscilloscope [1]. The recorded signals can also be reviewed and processed off-line. The behavior of several physiological variables can be shown on a 2D- and 3D-representation of the electrode track into the brain, with the corresponding planes of an anatomic atlas [1]. The system also allows the virtual representation of each therapeutic lesion, in order to select the best option before it be made inside the brain of the patient.

3. Results
Several versions of this software have been developed at the International Neurological Restorative Center in Cuba since 1993. Each one of them has been validated, registered and certified by the Medical Equipment Regulatory Agency of the Cuban Health Ministry. This system has already been used successfully in more than 300 neurosurgeries in Cuba, Chile and Spain [1]. The behavior of the brain activity, displayed on the electrode track with the brain atlas, makes easier and safer the identification of different brain structures and the location of specific neuronal groups in each patient, that will be surgical targets.

4. Conclusions
The NDRS has already been used successfully in different countries for deep brain recording as an effective guide for the stereotactic and functional neurosurgery to control different symptoms of Parkinson's disease and other involuntary movement disorders. It allows to substitute with a PC complex electronic equipment, including automatic and graphic facilities, that increases the accuracy and safety of the surgical targeting.

References
1. Macías R, Teijeiro J, Torres A, Alvarez L. Electrophysiological targeting in stereotaxic surgery for Pakinson's disease. In: Obeso JA, DeLong MR, eds. *The basal ganglia and new surgical approaches for Parkinson's disease. Advances in Neurology*, Philadelphia: Lippincott-Raven, 1997: vol.74, pp. 175-182.

CARS 2002 – H.U. Lemke, M.W. Vannier; K. Inamura, A.G. Farman, K. Doi & J.H.C. Reiber (Editors)

Evaluation of a stereotactic neurosurgical robot (NeuroMate™)

C. Edlinger, J-Ph. Perrin, S. Baffert, E. Charpentier, E. Fery-Lemonnier
CEDIT, AP-HP, 3 Avenue Victoria, 75100 RP Paris

Keywords: Computer-assisted surgery, surgical robotics, health technology assessment

1. Introduction
The CEDIT (Committee for the Evaluation and Diffusion of Innovative Technologies) is in charge of technology assessment of medical innovations at the 50 hospitals of Paris area's regional university hospital group (AP-HP). In 2000, the CEDIT has been asked to assess the neurosurgical robot NeuroMate™.

2. Methods
We reviewed the technical, medical, economic and financial aspects of this technology. A systematic review of the literature was carried out. Also five neurosurgeons were committed as experts.

3. Results
Technical aspects
The NeuroMate™ (Integrated Surgical Systems Inc.) is a computer controlled image-guided Neurosurgery multijointed arm for the spatial positioning of an instrument holder or tool guide, usually guiding standard neurosurgical instruments. The system software provides image-based surgical planning and visualization of anatomical structures, brain targets and trajectories proceeding from 3-D image data (CT, MR).
Medical aspects
The literature in the field is mainly descriptive (feasibility studies). The range of applicability of NeuroMate™ concerns small volume cerebral lesions located in deep or highly functional areas. This robot is dedicated to stereotactic biopsy, functional Neurosurgery (pain surgery, Parkinson disease, pharmacoresistant epilepsy) and neuroendoscopic surgery.
Economical aspects
The investment cost of a NeuroMate™ system is 281 K€ (VAT included) for the stereotactic machine frame version. The maintenance contract is 48 K€ per year. One single-use operative cover is necessary per act. The additional cost in supplies is 174 € per act. The large investment cost of this device requires a fairly important level of activity in stereotactic Neurosurgery.

4. Conclusion
The CEDIT recommends the diffusion of NeuroMate™ in Neurosurgery centres which are addressing a large number of patients in stereotactic surgery and are involving Neurology, Neuroradiology, Neurosurgery, and Neurophysiology.

CARS 2002 – H.U. Lemke, M.W. Vannier; K. Inamura, A.G. Farman, K. Doi & J.H.C. Reiber (Editors)
ᶜCARS/Springer. All rights reserved.

An improved fMRI analysis for detecting motor cortex activity near brain tumors

J.W. Haller [a,d], T.A. Gallagher [b], T.C. Ryken [c], K.J. Ahn [a], M.W. Vannier [a,d]

[a] University of Iowa, Department of Radiology
[b] Loyola University Stritch School of Medicine
[c] University of Iowa, Department of Neurosurgery
[d] National Institutes of Health

Keywords: Image guided surgery, surgical planning, functional imaging

1. Introduction

Functional magnetic resonance images (fMRI) typically represent a correlation of the hemodynamic response in a region of the brain that is associated with a stimulus or task; and is used to elucidate areas of neural activity. An inadequate model of the hemodynamic response function (HRF) may prevent the detection of regional brain activity, particularly in brain regions distorted by tumor or other pathology. Thus, *idealized* HRFs may not provide good models of hemodynamic response in brain regions near a tumor, and subject-specific and/or region-specific HRFs are needed.

2. Methods

Functional MR images from one brain tumor patient and three normal subjects were obtained with a GE 1.5 Tesla scanner. Right and left hands were exercised independently during 30 sec squeeze/rest blocks for 5min, during which 5 mm thick, echo planar images (5 slices) were obtained through the motor cortex. Generation of fMRI data using the Analysis of Functional NeuroImages (AFNI) (1) is outlined below.

1. A gamma type HRF + robust correlation from normal ROI → voxels of activation
2. voxels of activation → patient/regionally specific HRF
3. patient/regionally specific HRF derived from tumor-free ROI used with fMRI data from contralateral tumor-infiltrated ROI →functional intensity correlated (fico) voxels (rΣ 0.7)

3. Results

Regions of brain activity using the algorithm above were correlated 0.7 or higher in regions where idealized models of HRF typically provided poor correlations in subjects' normal brain and brain tumor regions.

4. Conclusions

Identification of HRFs in regions of normal brain tissue and their implementation in the analysis of contralateral regions infiltrated by tumor provided a more sensitive method for correlating signal changes associated with hand movement.

Reference

(1) RW Cox. AFNI: Software for analysis and visualization of functional magnetic resonance neuroimages. Computers and Biomedical Research, 29:162-173, 1996.

CARS 2002 – H.U. Lemke, M.W. Vannier; K. Inamura, A.G. Farman, K. Doi & J.H.C. Reiber (Editors)

Combined image-guided surgical navigation and ultrasound images for cranial surgeries

T.C. Ryken[a], M. Barua[a], J.W. Haller[b]

[a] Department of Neurosurgery, University of Iowa
[b] Department of Radiology, University of Iowa

Keywords: Neurosurgery, craniotomy, central nervous system

1. Introduction
Real-time intraoperative ultrasound images were fused with the preoperative anatomic images (either CT or MRI) to assess intraoperative shifts of brain tissue. Preoperative localization with high resolution MRI or CT provides the detail needed for determining surgical trajectories. The shift of intracranial structures following dural opening is visualized with intraoperative ultrasound that is co-registered with preoperative images.

2. Methods
Fifty consecutive cranial procedures (18 metastatic and 32 primary lesions) were analyzed in which preoperative anatomic images and intraoperative ultrasound images were combined. In each case, a series of merged ultrasound and preoperative anatomic images were obtained prior to dural opening and following the completion of the procedure to measure the shift of adjacent intracranial structures.

3. Results
Measure of shift ranged from 0.3 to 3.0 cm in many cases, depending on the extent of the procedure. There were no major complications with this technique. The figure shown highlights the correlated MRI and US images.

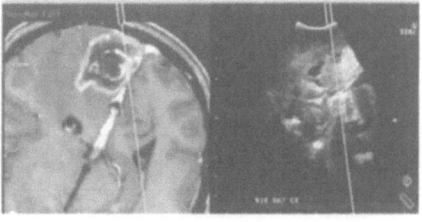

4. Conclusions
While reliance on point localization, as used with standard image guidance, would have resulted in significant misinterpretation of localization, the ability to enhance the real time ultrasound images allowed reliable identification of location despite major structural shift. Ultrasound-assisted image-guided cranial surgery is a valuable tool for assessing intraoperative brain distortion in relation to preoperative images.

Acknowledgements
The authors gratefully acknowledge the support and assistance of Medtronic/Surgical Navigation Technologies (Louisville, CO) and Aloka Co. Ltd., (Tokyo, Japan).

A hybrid navigation system for reliable navigation surgery - microscopic optical tracking and electromagnetic suction tube tracking

Junji Yamada, Amami Kato, Haruhiko Kishima, Masayuki Hirata, Toshiki Yoshimine
Department of Neurosurgery, Osaka University, Japan
Hanwa Memorial Hospital, Osaka, Japan

Keywords: Hybrid navigator, trouble

1. Introduction
To avoid navigation system troubles, we combined the 2 different navigational systems, namely, hybrid navigation system. This system consists electromagnetic tracking of suction tip (CANS), and optical tracking of microscope(EVANS). On this poster, we present the error rate of this navigation system.

2. Methods
From 1998 to 2001, 78 navigational surgery was performed in our institute. We investigate the causes of the failure of the navigation system, they contain the following, missing of fiducial marker, computer troubles(software or hardware),unacceptable calibration error due to dislocation of fiducial skin markers,missing disinfectant.

3. Results

Errors	n	ratio
Missing fiducial skin marker	2	2.16%
Computer trouble	12	11.11%
CANS	4	
EVANS	8	
Caribration error	1	0.93%
CANS	1	
EVANS	0	
Mispreparation of instruments (CANS)	2	2.16%

The causes of navigator system malfunction were computer/software trouble (CANS; 4, EVANS 8), and mispreparation of instruments (CANS; 1). Among these malfunctions, navigator-guided surgery was not able only in 2 cases due to unrecoverable malfunction of both trackings. We also experienced erased fiducial skin markers in 2 cases, when we reregistered those markers with another active navigator.

4. Conclusions
By combining 2 different trackings, the trackings navigation guided surgery became more reliable. The reliability of the system must be further improved.In the pratical use of the navigator, the manpower for preparing the system was also to be improved, and we need much more efforts for avoiding troubles of navigation systems.

References
1. Kato A, Yoshimine T, Hayakawa T, et al: A frameless, armless navigational system for computer assisted neurosurgery. J Neurosurg 74:845-849, 1991.

CARS 2002 – H.U. Lemke, M.W. Vannier; K. Inamura, A.G. Farman, K. Doi & J.H.C. Reiber (Editors)

Open MRI compatible HivisCAS video microscope system for neurosurgery

K. Nambu[a,b], H. Iseki[a], Y. Muragaki[a], T. Maruyama[a], T. Taira[a], R. Mochizuki[c], M. Sugiura[a,d], K. Naemura[a], T. Hori[a], K. Takakura[a]

[a] Tokyo Women's Medical University, 8-1 Kawatacho, Tokyo, [b] Toshiba Corp. Medical Systems Company, [c] NHK Engineering Service, [d] Hitachi Corp.

Keywords: Intraoperative-MRI, video-microscope, navigation

1. Introduction

We are developing a video microscope system "HivisCAS (High Definition Visual Computer Aided Surgery system)", which guides the surgeon by enhancing the live microscope image with superimposed computer graphics of the surgical plan map in 0.5 mm accuracy[1]. On the other hand, we have introduced an intraoperative MRI (AIRIS II 0.3T; Hitachi, Tokyo). To update the surgical plan map by intraoperative images, we modified the video microscope to be compatible with the open MRI, and evaluated its problems and performance.

2. Methods

We replaced major steel parts of the microscope by stainless steel, lead, and plastics. To prevent careless errors, we attached thick and soft plastic films to cover the MRI aperture. Then we examined magnetic attraction by MRI when the video microscope went close to it. After tests in the operating room, we applied the system for a case of frontal glioma. For the patient, we explained the mechanism, merit, and demerit of the system carefully, and informed consent was obtained. Based on presurgical X-ray CT and MRI, we constructed a plan map including the extent of the tumor, and locations of major vessels. To avoid noise during MRI imaging procedure, we disconnected all cables between the computer and the video microscope.

3. Results

The MRI attractted small steel parts of the video microscope weakly, but the microscope stand can remain them stationary. However, if the microscope went close to the aperture of MRI when all the stand joint clutches were out, the MRI may quickly attract it. So we set the stand at a place where the microscope cannot reach to the MRI, even if the stand joints were fully extended. The system worked without any problems in the clinical application. It provided accurate position sensing and fine video view of surgical field with the navigating map. HivisCAS computer system received the intraoperative MRI images in 10 minutes, and we could modify the map based on the updated images.

4. Conclusions

Our video microscope worked in open MRI operating theatre safely by minor modifications. Since the system was not fully compatible with MRI, we had to turn it off during the imaging, and careful setting was necessary. Therefore, we are designing a video microscope that is fully compatible with MRI, as the next step.

References

1. Iseki H, Takakura K, et.al., Three-dimensional video-microscope system in neurosurgery, Proceeding of 11th International Congress of Neurological Surgery, pp.701-705,1997

CARS 2002 – H.U. Lemke, M.W. Vannier; K. Inamura, A.G. Farman, K. Doi & J.H.C. Reiber (Editors)
ᶜCARS/Springer. All rights reserved.

1070

The results of image guided surgery with magnetic and optical hybrid navigation system

A. Kato[a], J. Yamada[a], M. Hirata[a], N. Hirabuki[b], T. Yoshimine[a]
[a]Dept. of Neurosurgery and [b]Radiology, Osaka University, Osaka, Japan

Keywords: Neurosurgery, navigation surgery, clinical results

1. Introduction
In recent years, the image guided surgery including surgical navigators is regarded as a standard technique in the neurosurgery. Only a few papers, however, studied its clinical usefulness in detail. In this paper, we describe the results of our image guided surgery with magnetic and optical hybrid navigation system in comparison with the conventional operations.

2. Methods
Among consecutive 152 neurosurgical operations with computer assisted image guidance, 36 operations were gliomas in and around the functionally eloquent areas (NAV group). The surgical technique applied includes; functional mapping with MEG (synthetic aperture magnetometry), 3D reconstruction of anatomical images for preoperative planning, continuous monitoring of suction tip with electromagnetic tracking, optimal setting of the navigational microscope with optical tracking, intraoperative stimulation mapping and awake surgery, as well as the conventional preoperative examinations. Following parameters were assessed; the removal rate of the tumor, neurological deficits (assessed with Karnofsky scale), operation time, amount of bleeding, surgical achievement (actual removal rate of the tumor divided by planned removal rate) and patient's survival. These results were compared with a group of 31 surgeries operated without navigator (WONAV group). The histopathology, tumor location, age and sex of both groups were approximately matched in both groups.

3. Results
In NAV group, the removal rate of the tumor, surgical achievement, and postoperative Karnofsky scale were significantly better than those in WONAV group, while the operation time was prolonged. There was no significant difference in the amount of bleeding and patient's survival in both groups.

4. Conclusions
Image guided neurosurgery was effective in operation of gliomas in and around the functionally eloquent areas with higher removal rate and reduced risk of neurological deficits. The efficacy to the patient's survival remains to be studied.

References
1. Kato A, Yoshimine T, Hayakawa T, et al.: A frameless, armless navigational system for computer assisted neurosurgery. J Neurosurg 74:845-849, 1991.

CARS 2002 – H.U. Lemke, M.W. Vannier; K. Inamura, A.G. Farman, K. Doi & J.H.C. Reiber (Editors)
ᶜCARS/Springer. All rights reserved.

A new method for 3D modeling of neurosurgical procedures

I. Köster[a], A. Samii[b], T. Brinker[b], H.K. Matthies[a]
[a]Department of Medical Informatics, Hannover Medical School, Hannover
[b]Department of Neurosurgery, Nordstadt Medical Center, Hannover, Germany

Keywords: Neurosurgery, computer aided design, three-dimensional modeling

1. Introduction
This new method shows how to generate quantitative three dimensional models of neurosurgical procedures.

2. Methods
A computer assisted surgery device (MKM© of Zeiss, Germany) is used to scan optically discrete points of the outlines of surgically relevant structures in order to obtain 3D co-ordinates of the surgical scene. This data are applied to a computer aided design (CAD) software which allows quantitative 3D modeling. For demonstration of the method a fixed cadaver head was used to simulate the surgical procedure for the removal of an acoustic neuroma via a suboccipital retrosigmoid craniotomy. A high resolution bony CT scan with 1 mm slice thickness was performed at a gantry = 0. After registration the retrosigmoid approach was performed. During that "navigated dissection" the CAS device was used for measurement of 3D co-ordinates of selected anatomical structures ("scanning of anatomy"). The above mentioned data were then applied to the 3D polyline function of Auto-CAD. The resulting 3D CAD-model was then analyzed in different views, including the perspective through a virtual camera, which was positioned according to the measured data on the optical axis of the microscope. Furthermore quantitative measurements within the model were performed.

3. Results
Using these data we obtained a CAD model of the surgical scene, which represents not only the intraoperative anatomy, but in addition information from the preoperative imaging. For the first time, it was also possible to measure the position of the microscope and of surgical instruments and to use these data for modeling of surgical procedures.

4. Conclusion
This new method of modeling neurosurgical procedures enables a documentation of surgery with quantitative properties and is therefore unique compared to conventional film and photo documentation. The resulting model can be used to simulate different perspective views and to perform measurements within the model like exact localization and size of a craniotomy, spatula position and optical axis of the microscope at different stages of a surgery. Thus, this new method of modeling neurosurgical procedures allows accurate 3D documentation of intraoperative anatomy and surgical manipulation. It therefore provides basis data necessary for 3D modeling and simulation of neurosurgical procedures.

CARS 2002 – H.U. Lemke, M.W. Vannier; K. Inamura, A.G. Farman, K. Doi & J.H.C. Reiber (Editors)

1072

Monte Carlo simulation for anisotropic error prediction in frameless stereotaxy

P.W.A. Willems,[a] H.J. Noordmans,[b] J.W. Berkelbach van der Sprenkel,[a]
M.A. Viergever[c] and C.A.F. Tulleken[a]
[a] Department of Neurosurgery, [b] Department of Medical Technology
[c] the Image Sciences Institute
University Medical Center Utrecht, the Netherlands

Keywords: Frameless stereotactic accuracy, Monte Carlo simulation, error anisotropy

1. Introduction

Typically, frameless stereotactic systems present a crosshair indicating the localisation of an instrument relative to preoperative images. We aim to develop a model that enables three-dimensional graphical presentation of confidence intervals at the instrument's position, during a surgical procedure. This requires the prediction of frameless stereotactic accuracy confidence intervals at any position within the surgical volume.

2. Methods

A Monte Carlo simulation model was designed to incorporate errors involved in fiducial localisation in image space (FL-I), fiducial localisation in surgical space (FL-S) and target digitisation in surgical space (TD-S). These accumulate and result in the final application accuracy. The true magnitude of these errors can only be determined in a phantom set-up. We assumed the magnitude of the FL-S- and TD-S-errors to be equal. In this initial study, the known phantom-target-positions were used rather than their image-positions, resulting in a negligible FL-I-error. 133 accuracy measurements were performed using the STN system (Carl Zeiss, Germany) and a phantom containing 19 fiducial/target positions. These results represented the magnitude of the FL-S- and TD-S-errors and were used in the Monte Carlo simulation. The simulation consisted of 10000 iterations, each simulating the accumulation of error in a single frameless stereotactic procedure. To evaluate the correctness of the resultant 'point cloud', each accuracy measurement was analysed in relation to its 'own' simulation. Since ideally n% of the measurements should lie within the nth percentile of the simulated point clouds, a plot should approximate x=y.

3. Results

Figure 1 demonstrates only a slight overestimation of frameless stereotactic accuracy. Figure 2 demonstrates a typical point cloud generated by the simulation.

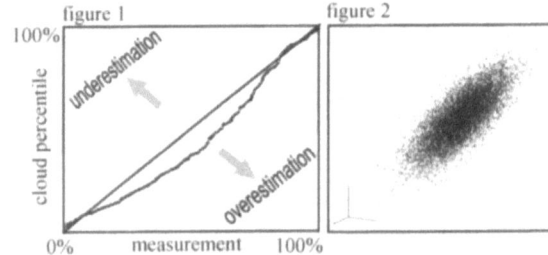

4. Conclusions

We have shown that one can simulate frameless stereotactic accuracy using a Monte Carlo technique, preserving its anisotropy. The results can be evaluated in comparison to actual accuracy measurements. Intraoperative three-dimensional visualisation of the simulation results is a relatively easy next step.

CARS 2002 – H.U. Lemke, M.W. Vannier; K. Inamura, A.G. Farman, K. Doi & J.H.C. Reiber (Editors)
^cCARS/Springer. All rights reserved.

Education tools for surgery: a simulator for pelvic surgery

Raphaël Martin[a], Mario Valderrama[a], Lucile Vadcard[a,b], Jérôme Tonetti[d],
Stéphane Viera[a,c], Jocelyne Troccaz[a,d]
[a] TIMC Laboratory, Faculté de Médecine, Domaine de la Merci,
38706 La Tronche cedex, France - [b] LEIBNIZ Laboratory, Grenoble
[c] INRIA Grenoble, [d] Grenoble University Hospital

Keywords: Computer-Aided Surgery, simulation, orthopaedics.

1. Introduction

This poster presents a simulator dedicated to learning a computer-aided pelvic surgery procedure. Such a technique allows to position screws in the iliac bone minimally invasively (see [1]). The objective of the simulator is to make the clinical diffusion of such new techniques integrating intra-operative data acquisition for registration easier.

2. Methods

The computer-aided procedure operates in three stages. Pre-operative planning is based on a CT acquisition. Intra-operatively, an ultrasonic probe is equipped with localizing features allowing to get 3D images of the pelvic bone. After registration of the US and CT data, the planned trajectory can be transferred to the intra-operative conditions. Finally, a navigation interface allows the surgeon to analyse the position and orientation of the surgical tool relatively to the anatomical structures and to the planned trajectory. The simulator focuses on the two first stages: planning and US acquisition. The US acquisition for registration which is a critical stage is learnt from recorded cases. A virtual US probe is positioned on a haptic device (a Phantom^{TM} from Sensable devices, Inc.). From the position of the probe, a US image is re-sliced in a pre-recorded US volume of data. In parallel, a tactile feedback allows the surgeon to feel the virtual contact of the probe against the model of the patient's body from which the US volume has been reconstructed. The simulator helps the surgeon to make the US acquisition in a way that data will result in an accurate registration from which depends the quality of guidance during navigation.

3. Results and conclusion

The simulator has been integrated and tested and the implemented method allows to have an easy planning and a real time production of US images and tactile feedback. Based on this integration, we are in the process of evaluating the simulator with clinicians.

Acknowledgements

This work is supported by the IST European VOEU project.

References

1. J. Tonetti, O. Clopet, M. Clerc, L. Pittet, J. Troccaz, P. Merloz, J.-P. Chirossel, Optimal placement of the iliosacral screws: 3D computer tomography simulation, Rev Chir Orthop, 86, pp194-198, 2000

CARS 2002 – H.U. Lemke, M.W. Vannier; K. Inamura, A.G. Farman, K. Doi & J.H.C. Reiber (Editors)

1074

Toward modelling and simulation of tearing and cutting in laparoscopic training environment

Shahram Payandeh[a], Hilary Zhang[a], Naoufel Azouz[b]

[a] School of Engineering Science, Simon Fraser University, BC, CANADA
[b] Centre d'Etudes de Mecanique d'Ile-de-France, 91020 Evry, FRANCE

Keywords: Tearing, cutting, mass-spring systems

1. Introduction

This poster presents some of the initial research and results of modeling the cutting and tearing of compliant objects. The modeling of these basic tasks is essential for surgical training environments. Our Learning Training Environment (SFU-LTE) is currently being developed at Simon Fraser University.

2. Methods

Currently, two main approaches exist for modeling compliant objects. These are mass-spring model and finite element methods [1]. To enhance the main approaches, various alternatives were proposed such as using subdivision methodologies to simplify the computation involved [2]. This poster demonstrates these alternatives for tearing and cutting tasks.

3. Results

Figure 1 shows some of our results. The image to the left shows a model of tearing, where an object is being teared away from another object. The modeling is based on a set of non-linear mass spring models. The center image shows an example of cutting a tensional surface using mass-spring model and a novel subdivision scheme, where the original mesh is subdivided as a function of cutting directions. The image to the left demonstrates the simulation of cutting based on the finite-element method.

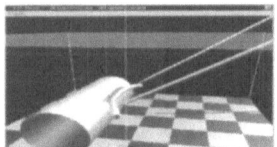 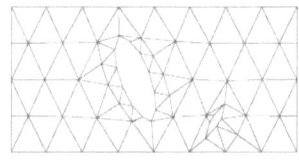 

Figure 1 - Some examples of the tearing and cutting tasks.

4. Conclusions

Development of realistic training environment for tearing and cutting of tissue and organs are challenging problems. This poster presents some intermediate modeling approaches.

References

1. Payandeh, S., Azouz, N., "Finite elements, mass-spring-damper systems and haptic rendering", Proceedings of 2001 IEEE CIRA conference, pp. 224-230.
2. Azouz, N., Payandeh, S., "An efficient finite-element modelling tool for surgical simulation: The ε-mesh radius", Proceedings of 2001 ASME Design Engineering Conference, pp. 71-79.

CARS 2002 – H.U. Lemke, M.W. Vannier; K. Inamura, A.G. Farman, K. Doi & J.H.C. Reiber (Editors)
ᶜCARS/Springer. All rights reserved.

CT fluoroscopy using navigation and automated registration

Waldemar Zylka, Leonid Tafler, and Henning Vohwinkel
University of Applied Sciences Gelsenkirchen
http://pt.fh-gelsenkirchen.de/zylka_voffice

1. Introduction

Image Guided Surgery establishes a new level of treatment.. However, registration of images to the patient is an additional long lasting inaccurate and complex clinical step. We have combined a CT scanner and a tracking device into a system for navigation with automated registration. As a result fluoroscopic interventions can be performed with reduced radiation exposure.

2. Materials and methods

A Windows based PC, a TomoScan M/EG CT scanner (Philips Medical Systems), and a optical position measurement device are combined to a TomoGuide system. CT gantry is equipped with a tracker to measure its position. A suitable calibration procedure is performed to determine the image plane.

On the CT table, markers are attached to the patient. A scan is made based on radiological requirements. Both, gantry and patient are tracked during acquisition. Flexible camera placement allows sufficient volume of interest and almost no disturbances of the clinical procedure. The CT scanner automatically triggers the position measurement. All data are transferred to a workstation using DICOM protocol. As opposed to the marker based registration, our approach allows for an automated registration of the patient and the image without markers.

A planning mode is based on acquired 3D image acquired. As a first application fluoroscopic biopsy will be investigated. After defining the target and the entry point a biopsy needle equipped with markers for the optical position system can be positioned on the entry point and accurately guided along the straight line to the target. At any time in the procedure additional CT scans can be acquired and can replace a previous scan.

3. Results

We have created a laboratory setup, using a CT scanner and a tracking device and implemented a Windows-based user interface. The system is suitable for biopsy, pain therapy or orthopedic applications. Advantages are accurate planning and guidance to the entry point, less exposure to radiation, higher security as well as more time efficiency due to a automatic registration.

4. Conclusion

A new surgical navigation system for fluoroscopic applications based on a in-room combination of a CT scanner and a position measurement system has been designed. The flexible design allows the use of CT scanner or another tomographic modality, such as MR. Current development directs towards the detection of image distortions and the implementation of the spiral mode.

CARS 2002 – H.U. Lemke, M.W. Vannier; K. Inamura, A.G. Farman, K. Doi & J.H.C. Reiber (Editors)

1076

The meaning of precision in computer assisted surgery

M. Wehmöller[a], S. Weihe[b], H. Eufinger[b]

[a] Inst. of Production Systems

[b] Dept. of Oral & Maxillofacial Surgery, Ruhr-University Bochum, Germany

Keywords: CAS, resection, robotics

1. Introduction

From the very start of the development of the TICC-processing chain the technique of prefabricating individual craniofacial implants based on geometric data. The subsequent use of this technique in navigation and robotics requires experiments on the precision of the involved techniques [1].

2. Methods

Experimental studies showed the precision of the necessary steps and gave an idea of the meaning of precision in computer assisted surgery [2].

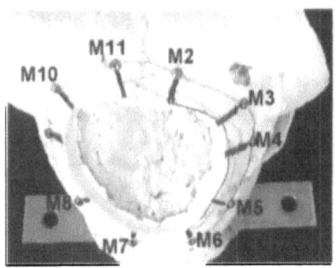 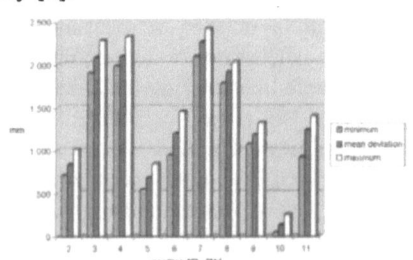

Figure 1. Robot resection in an ovine cadaver skull performed at the Inst. for Process Control & Robotics at the University of Karlsruhe, *left*: positions M2 – M11, right: evaluation of precision at positions M2 – M11

3. Results and Conclusions

Each single step of computer assisted surgery has its own range of deviations, but for the whole processing chain the result is not simply the sum of all theoretical deviations. In contrast, deviations of up to 4 mm have been found in clinical practice for these systems, whereas our own experimental evaluation could demonstrate intraindividual and interindividual deviations of up to 2.42 mm with an average of 1.36 mm.

Acknowledgements

Supported by a grant of the German Research Foundation (DFG - Eu 49/1-2).

References

1. H. Eufinger, M. Wehmöller: Anwendung und Technik der computerunterstützten Implantatversorgung, Planung und Umsetzung geführter Resektionen. In W. Maßberg, G. Reinhart, M. Wehmöller (eds.): Neue Technologien für die Medizin, ISBN 3-8265-7399-4

2. S. Weihe, M. Wehmöller, et al.: Synthesis of CAD/CAM, robotics, and biomaterial implant fabrication: single-step reconstruction in computer aided frontotemporal bone resection. Int. J. Oral Maxillofac. Surg. 29, 2000, p 384

CARS 2002 – H.U. Lemke, M.W. Vannier; K. Inamura, A.G. Farman, K. Doi & J.H.C. Reiber (Editors)

Practical clinical experience with microscopic 3D–navigation at the skull base

W. Freysinger, F. Kral, A. R. Gunkel, W. F. Thumfart

ENT Clinic, University of Innsbruck, Anichstr. 35, 6020 Innsbruck, Austria

Keywords: Skull base, head-up display, microscopic navigation

1. Introduction

Skull base is a challenging task for ENT surgeons, especially when large pathologies are present. 3D-computer assisted navigation techniques provide a very valuable source of intraoperative information. Therefore we have, especially when approaching the internal ear canal or the clival region, optimized our registration and the clinical protocols. Currently, we can routinely navigate in a these areas with an application accuracy to support microscopic surgery, viz. a clinically determined accuracy of ~ 1 mm.

2. Methods

The SNS SNN 3.0 system (SNS, Canada) and a Zeiss OPMI 2000 (Carl Zeiss, Germany) on an NC4 floor stand provide intraoperative orientational support. We use axial 1 mm CT/MR scans and 0.5 mm high-resolution CT images for the petrous bone. Contrast agent is applied according to the surgeon's needs. External and intrinsic landmarks are used for referencing the patient, attached to the VBH-mouthpiece [1] which carries the dynamic reference frame of the navigation system.

3. Results

The system has been used for acoustic neuromas, facial nerve re-routing, facial nerve decompression, removal of a retroclival chordoma, revision cholesteatoma surgery and an orbital meningioma. In all cases the application accuracy stayed constant throughout surgery and critical information was supplied to the surgeon by the structures shown in the head-up display of the microscope. Fused CT-MR data-sets provided optimal surgical support with respect to tumor localization and extent, and superior tissue characterization means. The complementary 3D-video display was helpful for the nurse and teaching puposes, even though the reading of the graphical superpositions demanded long learning curves to be beneficial for the audience.

4. Conclusions

High-fidelity radiologic imaging, navigation with a microscope and touchless referencing and navigation have demonstrated an enormous clincal value. Currently, this system is meeting the surgeon's demands, however much work will have to be spent on the display of graphical information in order to be easily perceptible and intuitive.

References

1. Gunkel AR, Vogele M, Martin A, Bale RJ, Thumfart WF, Freysinger W. Computer-Aided Surgery in the Petrous Bone. Laryngoscope 1999; 109(11):1793-1799.

CARS 2002 – H.U. Lemke, M.W. Vannier; K. Inamura, A.G. Farman, K. Doi & J.H.C. Reiber (Editors)

1078

A fast and accurate method of ultrasound probe calibration for image-guided surgery

J. N. Welch, M. Bax, K. Mori, T. Krummel, R. Shahidi, C.R. Maurer, Jr.
Image Guidance Laboratories, Stanford University
300 Pasteur Drive, Room S-008, Stanford, CA 94305-5327

Keywords: 3D ultrasound, image-guided surgery, calibration

1. Introduction

In 3D ultrasound systems that form a 3D image by tracking the ultrasound probe, calibration is the process of computing the transformation between the coordinate system of the 2D image and the tracking device attached to the probe. Several different approaches to calibration have been used successfully for 3D systems. The cross-wire phantom method produces accurate calibrations but is extremely time intensive. We present a new calibration method that produces calibrations that are as accurate as those produced by the cross-wire phantom method and are much faster and easier to perform.

2. Methods

Our phantom consists of multiple wires with random positions and orientations stretched taut between two parallel plates. When the ultrasound transducer generates an image of the wires, the position of the tracking device mounted rigidly to the transducer is recorded. The locations of the intersection of each wire with the image plane are used to register the image plane with the phantom, and subsequently with the tracking device. We use the Besl & McKay iterative closest point algorithm to solve the rigid-body point-to-line registration problem. To assess the accuracy of the system, for each set of calibration parameters, we reconstruct a phantom of 8 small steel balls arranged in a 2x4 grid from 5 different views. For 20 sets of calibration parameters, the 10 inter-ball distances are estimated 25 times, resulting in 5000 observations.

3. Results

The multi-wire phantom generates reconstructions with the standard deviation of 0.9543mm for 5000 measurements of inter-point distances. Worse case error is 3.5mm. CPU time for performing Besl & McKay iterative closest point algorithm is less than 1s.

Table 1. Reconstruction Accuracy

	Cross-wire gold standard	Multi-wire
Number of Observations	5000	5000
Standard Deviation (mm)	1.3578	0.9543
RMS (mm)	1.3945	1.0146
Mean (mm)	0.3184	0.3449
Max (mm)	5.1226	3.4669

4. Conclusions

Our calibration method is accurate, easy, and fast and thus is potentially useful for image-guided surgery using 3D ultrasound.

CARS 2002 – H.U. Lemke, M.W. Vannier; K. Inamura, A.G. Farman, K. Doi & J.H.C. Reiber (Editors)
©CARS/Springer. All rights reserved.

A clinical prototype system for projector-based augmented reality: calibration and projection methods

H. Hoppe[a], C. Kübler[a], J. Raczkowsky[a], H. Wörn[a], S. Haßfeld[b]
[a] Institute for Process Control and Robotics, Universität Karlsruhe (TH),
Kaiserstraße 12, 76128 Karlsruhe, Germany
[b] University of Heidelberg, Department of Oral and Maxillofacial Surgery,
Im Neuenheimer Feld 400, 69120 Heidelberg, Germany

Keywords: Augmented reality, calibration, computer assisted surgery

1. Introduction

In the last two years, the Institute for Process Control and Robotics has developed a prototype system for projector-based augmented reality in cranio-maxillo-facial surgery. The system essentially consists of two CCD cameras and a common video projector. These are used to track the patient, registrate his position (coded light) and to directly project the preoperatively defined planning data onto his surface.

2. Methods

System Calibration: While Tsai's method [1] seems to be gold standard, we have developed a new and easy to implement calibration model for cameras and video projectors. The model parameter set consists of the optical center, two vectors that align with the pixel edges, two scalars to describe the location of pixel (0,0) and two scalars to consider radial lense distorsion. The model parameters can easily be found by iteratively solving an overdetermined linear equation system. The necessary point correspondences for the projector are generated by using the coded light phase shift approach both horizontically and vertically.

Projection methods: Before the planning data are projected onto the patient's bended surface, an appropriate surface representation has to be calculated. This step is performed each time, the surface significantly changed. Thereby, we defined six projections modes dealing with different visualization requirements (e.g. an access path, viewpoint etc.).

3. Results and Conclusions

Comparing Tsai's to our model, we found out, that our model fits the calibration data better than Tsai's model and is much easier to implement. The chosen projection methods and projection modes showed to be most suitable for all tests during development. They will now have to prove themselves in the forthcoming clinical testings. Our results will be of special interest for all scientists dealing with recurrent problems like camera or video projector calibration.

References

1.   R. Y. Tsai: A Versatile Camera Calibration Technique for High-Accuracy 3D Machine Vision Metrology Using Off-the-Shelf TV Cameras and Lenses, IEEE Journal of Robotics and Automation, vol. RA-3, no. 4, 1987.

CARS 2002 – H.U. Lemke, M.W. Vannier; K. Inamura, A.G. Farman, K. Doi & J.H.C. Reiber (Editors)

Evaluation of a computer aided planning and surgical robot system for craniofacial surgery

Dirk Engel[a], Arno Pernozzoli[b], Oliver Schorr[a], Jakob Brief[b], Thorsten Heurich[b],
Joerg Raczkowsky[a], Stefan Hassfeld[b], Heinz Woern[a], Joachim Muehling[b]

[a] Institute for Process Control and Robotics, Universität Karlsruhe (TH)
Engler-Bunte-Ring 8, 76131 Karlsruhe, Germany
[b] Department of Oral and Maxillofacial Surgery, University of Heidelberg
Im Neuenheimer Feld 400, 69120 Heidelberg, Germany

Keywords: Computer-aided operation planning, robot-assisted surgery, evaluation

1. Introduction

Craniofacial surgery requires skillful and experienced surgeons. Due to the vicinity to vital parts and the great impact of bone repositionings at the complex anatomic structures of the skull, the interventions have to be conducted with high precision. Therefore, we have developed two systems: KasOp, an operation planning system on the basis of 3D-patient-models and RobaCKa, a surgical robot system. After several tests using dummies and animal experiments, which prove the overall system to be safe and accurate, a first test has been conducted on a human test subject.

2. Methods

Firstly, the self-adhesive MRI landmarks were fixed to the test subject's head as well as to a dental adapter. Afterwards, a MRI was taken and a 3D-model generated. On the basis of this 3D-model the planning was conducted with the KasOp system. Using the planning system, several different drill holes and a complex trajectory placed at the forehead of the test subject were planned. Intraoperatively, the test subject was fixed to the operating table using a vacuum cushion and a dental adapter. After the registration procedure, the robot moved along the planned trajectory supervised by the surgeon and also was guided to the preoperatively planned drill holes. Subsequently, the robot was relocated and the registration procedure as well as the intervention were repeated. Finally, the test subject was moved and the registration as well as the intervention were repeated once more. In future experiments, the repetition of the registration procedure should be lapsed because of a new controlling method considering the patient position in relation to the robot position.

3. Results and Conclusions

Since the registration was done using self-adhesive MRI landmarks instead of implanted titanium screws, the evaluation was initially intended to value the overall system integration, the workflow and the usability. Nevertheless, the execution was as accurate that the drawn points and lines coincided exactly after relocating the robot position and moving the test subject (either followed by a new registration procedure).

Acknowledgements

Deutsche Forschungsgemeinschaft (DFG), collaborative research center SFB 414.

CARS 2002 – H.U. Lemke, M.W. Vannier; K. Inamura, A.G. Farman, K. Doi & J.H.C. Reiber (Editors)

Robotic manipulator system for microsurgery (first report)

Hiroyuki Gotani M.D., Yoshiki Yamano M.D.
Dept. of Orthopaedic Surgery Osaka city Univ. Osaka, Japan

Keywords: Microsurgery, manipulator, operation

1. Introduction

Only trained surgeons can suture small vessel of which the diameter is less than 1mm. If many trained other surgeons can perform micro surgical technique with robotic system, it will contribute to many patients those require microsurgical operation. We will present robotic microsurgery system based on master-slave arm method and it will contribute to the field which require microsurgical technique such as hand, plastic and reconstructive surgery.

2. Methods

The manipulator has a seven axis and moves according to the command from master arm. The master arm also consists of 7 axis and it has a self balance mechanism. We selected AC servo motor as an actuator and harmonic drive as a reducer. High resolution optical encoder is selected for informing the movement of master arm of the host computer. Manipulation of an operator is transmitted to encoders of master arm and transferred to the servo driver through counter IC. We used the vessels of 10 rat tails and silastic vessel as materials and evaluated following points. 1) Working area(10x10x10cm), 2) Hold and change the direction of micro vessel and nerve 3) Dilate the vessel 4) Release the vessel from soft tissue 5) Cut the vessel 6) Make a small hole on the vessel 7) Insert the 9-0 and 10-0 nylon into the vessel 8) Assist surgeon during making suture on the vessel and nerve.

3. Results

1) For the purpose of replantation of amputated digits, the limitation of working area is not a problem. In this study, the tip of the instruments could reach whole length of the rat tail.
2) It was easy to hold vessel and nerve at any points. But there were some specific points when we failed to change the direction of vessels upwards. This was mainly due to the size of holder of instruments. 3)4)In order to control precisely, it was necessary to change the proportion of movement electrically between the master and slave arm. 5)6) With the view of microscope, there was no danger to injury other tissues. But it was difficult to give the information of the force of the micro scissors to the operator.7)8) In this experimental circumstance, control of slave arm was easy and precise. Normally operator should keep the unfavorable position of himself during microsurgery. Manipulator system enable operator to do microsurgery in more relaxed position.

4. Conclusions

Based on advanced motor technology , precise movement of manipulator tip was possible. In the experiments, it was comfortable to manipulate the system. In the next step we will try to make the system smaller to match the real operating field for clinical use. We believe that this study will lead to more advanced computer assisted manipulator system for microsurgery.

CARS 2002 – H.U. Lemke, M.W. Vannier; K. Inamura, A.G. Farman, K. Doi & J.H.C. Reiber (Editors)

1082

A distributed system for 3D anatomical structures visualization and surgical planning

C. Koehl[a], L. Soler[a], J. Marescaux[a]

[a] Ircad/Eits, 1 Place de l'hôpital 67091 Strasbourg France

Keywords: Real-time 3D visualization, surgical simulation and training, pre- and intra-operative imaging/visualization

1. Introduction

The progress made in medical imaging has led to enhanced diagnostic capabilities. Nevertheless, the analysis of the complex information contained in a set of 2D CT-Scan or MRI slices is a hard task : physicians have to mentally rebuild the images to obtain a 3D view of a patient's organ. The proposed system is a secure PACS (Picture Archiving and Communication System) including a 3D visualization interface consists of a set of tools which helps the physician in his pre- and intra-operative strategy.

2. Methods

The present system is a distributed architecture allowing secure storage and 3D visualization of anatomical structures reconstructed from CT-Scan and MRI images. Patient information and data are stored in distant databases accessible through the hospital network by using a user-friendly visualization interface. This surgical planning tool consists of : a virtual resecting tool allowing for simulation of surgical procedures, permitting insertion and manipulation of virtual laparoscopic tools, display of security margins, calculating 3D distance, and computation of organ volume.

Finally, one major advantage of the visualization interface is that it works on a simple laptop, which can be temporally disconnected from the hospital network, allowing for consultation of reconstructed exams in the operating room.

3. Results

In the scope of hepatic surgery, the 3D real-time navigation function allows for understanding of liver anatomy, and exact location, size and volume computation of liver tumors of a given patient. The margin tool is used to appreciate the relation of tumors to hepatic and portal veins, and to facilitate therapeutic decision making. The resection tool allows the surgeon to precisely plan, preoperatively, his operative strategy. In the anesthesia field, the system is able to simulate, from an CT airway exam, a difficult endotracheal intubation. While these tools are presently being used for interventions like radiology imaging-guided puncture or radio-frequency ablation, cholangiography analysis or virtual colonoscopy navigation, they have the potential to be used for any other organ.

4. Conclusions

This system, which is a very helpful surgical planning tool, can also form the foundation of augmented reality environments, and can already be used in the scope of computer assisted teaching. Moreover, coupled to force feedback devices, it can be used in realistic surgical simulation systems or in robot-assisted surgery.

CARS 2002 – H.U. Lemke, M.W. Vannier; K. Inamura, A.G. Farman, K. Doi & J.H.C. Reiber (Editors)

1083

A unified process for computer assisted surgery

O. Schorr, A. Pernozzoli, J. Raczkowsky, H. Wörn

Institute for Process Control and Robotics, Universität Karlsruhe (TH)

Keywords: Distribution, unification, model

1. Introduction

Classification and definition of standards for medical data is only one step necessary to interconnect applications and to allow readability. In regard to the increasing demand for distribution, it is necessary to take processes and the structure of applications into account as well. Therefore, we present in this paper a completely new approach of structuring computer assisted surgery by classification of processes. Important aims of our definition are simple interoperability, exchangeability, extensibility and maintenance.

2. Methods

We started to analyse how an architecture of a surgical application or device should look like in order to use communication methods and found that modules in applications for computer assisted surgery can be divided into six semantic groups. The most abstract group of modules is called phase level and contains modules referring to the actual phase (pre-, intra and postoperative phase) of the operation. Groups followed with decreasing degree of abstraction are workflow level, application level, processing level, abstraction level and transportation level. The lowest, transportation level, is responsible for the transportation of any kind of data necessary for surgical interventions. In the corresponding process model each of this levels build a shell (circle) where the outermost shell is the transportation shell and the core of the model is the phase shell.

3. Results

For the organization of the shells and its modules the most important elements are the so called ShellEngines. ShellEngines are organizing units, which keep information about the presence of single modules. They are responsible for information transfer between different shells and act similar to service access points known from layer models. Data, requests and acknowledge-

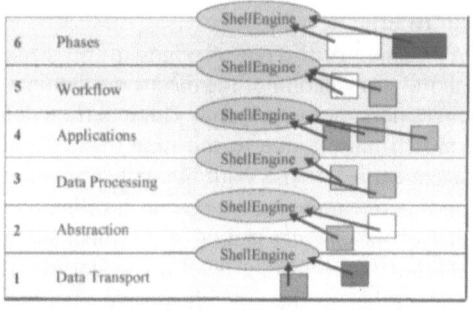

ments are exchanged through the ShellEngines, which are the only access point for information transfer between neighbored shells and modules. Therefore, modules can be located on arbitrary computers. Modules need to register their presence at the ShellEngine during initialization. Once done, information about the presence of modules is shared among all other present ShellEngines of the same level. Information to be exchanged between modules of the same level need to be put through the LayerEngine as the location of other modules is hidden and could be on a different computer thus.

Acknowledgements

This work is funded by the Deutsche Forschungsgemeinschaft (DFG) grant SFB 414.

CARS 2002 – H.U. Lemke, M.W. Vannier; K. Inamura, A.G. Farman, K. Doi & J.H.C. Reiber (Editors)

A novel computer-based approach to diagnostic imaging in the gut

R. Miftakhov

Dept. of Radiology, University of Iowa Hospitals and Clinics, Iowa, 52241, USA

Keywords: Computer model, gut, imaging

1. Introduction
The goal of improved visualization in medical imaging, especially intraoperatively, presently guides computer technology. Accurate diagnosis rests not only on images but also on a conception of pathophysiological processes. Our goal is to build a computer-based diagnostic tool that can aid in the interpretation of MRI and CT images of the gut.

2. Methods
We have developed a model that incorporates major physiological and biomechanical processes involved in gut motor function. A segment of the gut is modeled as a soft biological shell with properties of general orthotropy. Deformations of the shell are finite. Constitutive relationships are nonlinear. The enteric plexus of nerves is formed of multifunctional neurons arranged in ganglia and spatially distributed to form a planar neural network. Synapses provide chemoelectrical and electrochemical neuro-neural and neuromuscular links. The ubiquitous self-oscillatory feature of the syncytium, manifest as electrical slow waves and high frequency spikes results from the activity of ion channels. The gut is activated by the discharge of the interstitial cells of Cajal.

3. Results
A segment of the gut responds to the discharge of a pacemaker with the generation and aboral propagation of the electromechanical wave of deformation. As a response, the shell first undergoes expansion. There is time delay in the generation of the active force by the smooth muscle due to the time needed for the activation of an intracellular cascade of chemical reactions. With the development of contractions, the radius of the gut decreases and a concomitant increase in intraluminal pressure is observed. The latter deformation causes the depolarization of the mechanoreceptors of the primary sensory neurons, if it reaches the threshold level of excitation. The signal is transferred to the motor neurons and further to the smooth muscle elements. The above changes lead to self-sustaining electromechanical activity in the segment.

4. Conclusions
High-resolution digital CT/MRI images of the gut combined with electrophysiological and biochemical studies will provide the input data required in running simulations of gut motor function. Computational results will offer unique insights into physiological processes and will provide otherwise-inaccessible information on mechanical changes observed radiographically. Such an approach should increase diagnostic accuracy, may help understanding of the causes of certain diseases (primary motor dysfunction), and may allow one better to plan therapeutic intervention.

CARS 2002 – H.U. Lemke, M.W. Vannier; K. Inamura, A.G. Farman, K. Doi & J.H.C. Reiber (Editors)
°CARS/Springer. All rights reserved.

Using distance transformations to determine safe needle/probe paths during interventional procedures

Lars Aurdal[a], Ole Jakob Elle[a], Eigil Samset[a], Hugues Fontenelle[b], Tormod Omholt-Jensen[c], Tom Mala[a], Bjørn Edwin[a]

[a] The Interventional Center, Rikshospitalet, 0027 Oslo, Norway
[b] SimSurgery AS, Sognsveien 75B, 0865 Oslo, Norway
[c] Norwegian University of Science and Technology, 7491 Trondheim, Norway

Keywords: Distance, probe, placement

1. Introduction
This article reports on a method for planning probe placement in the liver during interventional procedures so as to avoid large hepatic vessels.

2. Methods
Based on a segmented CT image volume V of the liver and its vessels, a distance map D giving the shortest distance from any voxel in the liver to the hepatic vessels can be calculated. Given D, traverse V and for every voxel in V do:
1) Assume that the voxel is the insertion point for a probe following a linear path P from the insertion point to some target in the liver.
2) Interpolate along P in D to find the shortest distance along P to any voxel in the vessels.
3) Store all such shortest distances in a new volume R.

Calculate a triangulation of the liver surface, and colour each face using a colour derived from R, the result is a rendering of the liver surface coloured so as to show the minimal distance a probe would pass from intrahepatic vessels if inserted at a given point on the liver surface and made to follow a linear path to some intrahepatic target (see figure 1).

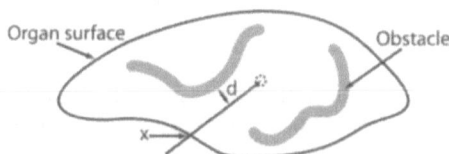

Figure 1: The probe is inserted at **x** and made to follow a linear path to the target. At **x**, the organ surface is coloured according to **d**, the minimal distance from probe to obstacle.

3. Conclusions
We propose a method for determining safe probe insertion areas on the liver surface. The method provides results in good correspondence with radiological findings. The method has potential for use in the planning of highly different interventional procedures.

Acknowledgements
The work of authors one, three and six was financed by the Research Council of Norway.

CARS 2002 – H.U. Lemke, M.W. Vannier; K. Inamura, A.G. Farman, K. Doi & J.H.C. Reiber (Editors)
ᶜCARS/Springer. All rights reserved.

1086

Multi-slider linkage mechanism for endoscopic manipulator

Hiromasa Yamashita[a], Kim Daeyoung[a], Nobuhiko Hata[a], Takeyoshi Dohi[a]
[a] Graduate School of Information Science and Technology,
The University of Tokyo, Tokyo, Japan

Keywords: Multi-slider linkage, endoscopic, manipulator

1. Introduction

Our new proposal in this paper is a slider linkage mechanism to achieve high mechanical performance and applicability to endoscopic surgical tools. Unlike previously reported wire-driven mechanism [1], the newly method requires less maintenance while realizing better mechanical performance including low backlash and higher stiffness.

2. Methods

We have designed and fabricated a prototype of 2-DOFmanipulator with five frames and four joints in-between. The first two joints from the tip can rotate +/- 45 deg respectively to achieve +/- 90 deg of vertical rotation, and the second two enables horizontal rotation. Rotation of joint is available by pulling/pushing the adjacent element by sliding linkage in a fixed order. 1-DOFmotion is realized by the actuation of a slider-linkage driven by an air cylinder at the bottom of this tool. Based on the signal from a user interface, a personal computer-based control unit determines the opening/closing pattern of the electromagnetic valves in the air system to control air cylinders. Correlation between the displacement of piston rods and bending angle is in pre-mapped to simplify control.

3. Results

We examined the relationship between driving time of air cylinder and bending angle in each DOF. S.D. of 10 measurements at bending 0 to 90 deg was 1.3 deg in horizontal bending and 0.9 deg in vertical bending. We also measured generated force from bending motion and the result was a maximum of 0.1675 kgf.

4. Conclusions

In conclusion, we developed a multi-slider linkage mechanism for rotating 2-DOF joints of the endoscopic manipulator. From the result we are sure of high reproducibility of S.D. about 1 deg of this bending mechanism, however, generated force was less design value.

Acknowledgements

A part of this work is supported by Research for the Future Program "Development of Surgical Robot", administered by Japan Society for the Promotion of Science.

References

1. Ryoichi N. et al: Multi-DOF Forceps Manipulator System for Laparoscopic Surgery-Mechanism miniaturized & Evaluation of New Interface-, *Proc of Fourth International Conference on Medical Image Computing and Computer assisted Interventions*, October, 14-17, 606-613, 2001

CARS 2002 – H.U. Lemke, M.W. Vannier; K. Inamura, A.G. Farman, K. Doi & J.H.C. Reiber (Editors)
°CARS/Springer. All rights reserved.

Clinical application of 3D-CT angiography for laparoscopic colorectal surgery

Junji Okuda, M.D., Kanji Nishiguchi, M.D., Keitaro Tanaka, M.D., Sang-Woong Lee, M.D., Masao Toyoda, M.D., Nobuhiko Tanigawa, M.D.
Department of General & Gastroenterological Surgery, Osaka Medical College

Keywords: 3D-CT, laparoscopic surgery, colorectal cancer

1. Introduction

The purpose of the study was to examine the role of three dimensional helical CT angiography (3D-CTA) as an adjunct to laparoscopic surgery for colonic carcinomas. For the resection of sigmoid and upper rectal carcinomas under laparoscopy, we routinely perform lymph node dissection around root of IMA with preserving the left colic artery. In addition, for right sided colon carcinomas, we perform lymph node dissection exposing so called the surgical trunk (superior mesenteric vein). For either of these procedures performing safely, it is important to know the precise individual vascular anatomy bearing their variations.

2. Methods

The 3D-CTA of 25 patients were examined (13: left, 7: right, 5: transverse). These images were compared with intraoperative findings.

3. Results

For left sided cancers, we were able to accurately visualize the left colic artery as well as ascertain its relationship to sigmoidal branches using the 3D-CTA for all patients. For all patients with right sided carcinomas, we were able to assess branches of the superior mesenteric artery as well as determine the presence of right colic artery. These findings were not only confirmed intraoperatively, but knowledge of this anatomy actually facilitated the dissection of these difficult regions.

4. Conclusion

Our experience with the 3D-CTA is that it can accurately determine the surgical vascular anatomy important in the treatment of all portions of carcinomas. With further improvements in imaging quality of the 3D-CTA, it is likely that this will replace standard contrast angiography in the preoperative setting, and may play an important part in the preoperative planning of cancer operations.

CARS 2002 – H.U. Lemke, M.W. Vannier; K. Inamura, A.G. Farman, K. Doi & J.H.C. Reiber (Editors)

1088

The basis of magnetic navigation system for surgery

Junichi Shimada [a], Makoto Kawakami [b], Seiji Endoh[b],
Fumiaki Ikeda[c] , Masaaki Nagahara[d] , Yutaka Yamamoto[d]

[a] Division of Surgery, Kyoto Prefectural Yosanoumi Hospital
[b] Electronic Components Development Dept. Sumitomo Special Metals Co., Ltd
[c] PHOTON Co., Ltd
[d] Department of Applied Analysis and Complex Dynamical Systems, Graduate School of Informatics, Kyoto University

Keywords: Magnetic navigation system, micro fluxgate sensor, video assisted surgery

1. Introduction
It has even been reported that in up to 70% of the cases of lung cancer discovered by x-ray diagnosis, the discovery was too late for surgery. For this reason, there has been a strong demand for a technology, or a surgical system, for the discovery of a micro-tumor in the respiratory system such as lung cancer in units of millimeters such that it can be surgically removed.

2. Methods
The emitted signal is in the form of magnetic fields. We have selected the intensity of magnetic field generated from the transmitter as a signal for indicating the position of the transmitter itself. A surgical micro-tumor tracking system includes a signal transmitter inserted near or at a tumor inside a patient's body, forceps each having a receiver attached at its tip for receiving signals transmitted from the transmitter, a position calculating device for determining the position of the transmitter from signals received by these receivers, and a display device for displaying the position of the transmitter determined by the position calculating device.

3. Results
This system can be the first basic system about real-time magnetic navigation system for surgery to point out the tumor location.
1) Our fluxgate magnetic sensor can measure the feasible intensity of magnetic field, less than 1 mG. This sensor is the highest capability for detecting the magnetic field in the world.
2) The component of 3 dimensional magnetic sensors gives real-time data of magnetic field where it exists.

4. Conclusions
This basis of the "Magnetic Navigation System" will enable us to point out where the tumor exists and give the chance for us to find a way to minimum invasive surgery.

Acknowledgements
This research is supported by Grants in Aid for Scientific Research B, Encouragement of Young scientists (A), and Fujita Memorial Research Funds from Japan Society for the Promotion of Science.

CARS 2002 – H.U. Lemke, M.W. Vannier; K. Inamura, A.G. Farman, K. Doi & J.H.C. Reiber (Editors)
°CARS/Springer. All rights reserved.

Study on bending forceps manipulator with electric-cautery function for laparoscopic surgery

Y. Kim[a], T. Oura[a], D. Kim[b], E. Kobayashi[a], T. Tsuji[a], H. Inada[c],
T. Dohi[b], I. Sakuma[a]

[a] Graduate School of Frontier Sciences
[b] Graduate School of Information Science and Technology
[c] Graduate School of Engineering, the University of Tokyo

Keywords: Forceps manipulator, wire driven, electric cautery

1. Introduction

We have developed a wire driven Multi-DOF forceps manipulator, which has two DOF of bending on the tip of forceps. The purpose of this study is to realize position feedback control of the forceps realizing the smooth motion of the forceps. We also investigated cautery system installed on forceps manipulators that can occlude large vessels such as bile duct securely. The basic data for design of electrodes were corrected.

2. Methods

In the previous system, large friction between rigid bodies at rolling parts led to poor dynamic characteristics [1]. To overcome this, we used a new bending mechanism where force's point of action was positioned closer to the center of bending motion. In addition, a pre-tension mechanism with springs was introduced. We also studied a bending angle measurement system consisting of a light emitting diode (LED) and a phototransistor (PT) placed on both ends of bending parts of forceps. By measuring change in the electric current in PT, we could estimate the bending of forceps. We evaluated the characteristic of the bending mechanism and the measurement system. As for electric cautery system, we investigated condition for secure occlusion of bile duct by electric cautery by changing parameters as follows: method of holding bile duct, patterns of electrode plates, applied voltage and cauterizing time. Porcine bile ducts were used as specimens. To measure strength of occlusion, pressure was applied by injecting air into the occluded bile duct and measured the maximum pressure tolerated before its burst.

3. Results and Conclusion

The displacement of wires was efficiently converted to bending without change in tension of wires in the new mechanism. More stable bending control was realized by reduction of stick-slip. However hysteresis was still large. With the measuring system using LED and PT, bending angle could be measured in the range between $45°$ and $60°$. About condition for secure occlusion by electric cautery, the parallel holding mechanism and plural thin electrode plates positioned in parallel showed superior performance for occlusion of porcine bile ducts. Measurement of electric impedance of tissue appeared to be effective for determining the optimal endpoint of electric energy application. This study is supported by the Research for the Future Program JSPS-RFTF 99I00904.

References

1. R. Nakamura, E. Kobayashi, K. Masamune, I. Sakuma, T. Dohi, T. Tsuji, D. Hashimoto: Development of Forceps Manipulator System for Laparoscopic Surgery, CARS2000: pp.105-110

CARS 2002 – H.U. Lemke, M.W. Vannier; K. Inamura, A.G. Farman, K. Doi & J.H.C. Reiber (Editors)
ᶜCARS/Springer. All rights reserved.

1090

A laparoscope positioning system based on the real-time visual tracking of surgeon's face and surgical instruments

A. Nishikawa[a], S. Asano[a], F. Miyazaki[a], M. Sekimoto[b], M. Yasui[b], M. Monden[b]
[a] Department of Systems and Human Science, Graduate School of Engineering Science, Osaka University, 1-3 Machikaneyama-cho, Toyonaka 560-8531, Japan
[b] Department of Surgery and Clinical Oncology, Osaka University Graduate School of Medicine, 2-2 Yamadaoka, Suita 565-0871, Japan

Keywords: Laparoscopic surgery, human interface, instrument tracking

1. Introduction
We have devised a laparoscope positioner with the surgeon's face image-based human-machine interface towards the realization of "solo surgery"[1]. Currently we aim at improving the performance and expanding the potentialities of our system by integrating the surgeon's explicit commands inputted through the human-machine interface with the surgeon's implicit messages extracted from the scope images.

2. Methods
We improved our laparoscope positioning system [1]. The new system is based on the real-time visual tracking of not only the surgeon's face but also the colour-marked surgical instruments (see Fig. 1). In the current version, the instrument tracking function becomes valid if and only if the surgeon directs the robot to insert/retract the laparoscope for providing the required target magnification. In this case, the surgeon's face motion is transformed into the scope zooming-in/out commands while the pan/tilt camera motions are automatically generated based on the instrument tracking results such that the surgical point of interest (POI) verges toward the centre of the scope image.

3. Results and Discussion
An in-vitro task (running the rope, dropping nuts into lidded boxes) was performed with either the old system [1] or the new one, by four subjects. As a result, the total camera work time was shorter for the new system compared to the old one, for all subjects (see Fig. 2). This demonstrates the effectiveness of appropriate integration of the surgeon's explicit commands through human-machine interface (face motion) with the surgeon's implicit messages (POI on the scope image). An in-vivo test is one of the future works.

References
1. A. Nishikawa et al., CARS 2001, pp.165-170.

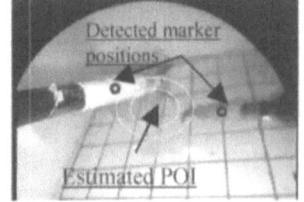

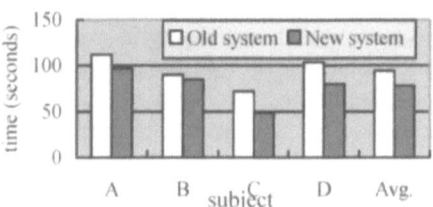

Fig. 1 Visual tracking of colour-marked instruments   Fig. 2 Laparoscopic camera operation time

CARS 2002 – H.U. Lemke, M.W. Vannier; K. Inamura, A.G. Farman, K. Doi & J.H.C. Reiber (Editors)

Feasibility of image-guided abdominal interventions using a novel magnetic position sensing device in an interventional radiology suite

Filip Banovac[a], Michael Jay[a], David Lindisch[a], Neil Glossop[b], Kevin Cleary[a]
[a] Imaging Science and Information Systems Center, Department of Radiology,
Georgetown University Medical Center, Washington, DC
[b] Traxtal Technologies LLC, Bellaire, TX

Keywords: Magnetic tracking, respiratory motion, abdominal interventions

1. Purpose
This was an initial study to evaluate the accuracy of a new magnetic localizing system (AURORA™) in the interventional radiology environment. This work is part of our research effort to incorporate magnetic tracking in an image-guided system for minimally invasive abdominal interventions.

2. Methods
A novel robot was used in an interventional radiology suite to accurately position a magnetically tracked needle at seven locations over a 100 by 40 by 40 mm volume. The robot was considered to be much more accurate than the magnetic localization system. Distances between repositioning attempts were determined by root mean square calculations between successive points.

3. Results

Table 1: Magnetically measured displacement of the robot positioning device.

axis	Robot Displacement (n=7)	Magnetically determined displacement (mm)	Standard Deviation
x	0 mm to 100 mm	100.45	0.40
	100 mm to 0 mm	100.46	0.58
y	0 mm to 20 mm	19.88	0.10
	20 mm to -20 mm	39.28	0.02
	-20 mm to 0 mm	19.43	0.04
z	0 mm to 20 mm	19.99	0.02
	20 mm to -20 mm	40.06	0.05

4. Conclusions
Based on this initial study, the AURORA magnetic tracking system appears accurate enough for use in the interventional radiology suite. Further studies with a larger number of data points and other studies such as cadaver tests are warranted to further investigate this technology.

Acknowledgements
This work was funded by U.S. Army grant DAMD17-99-1-9022. The content of this manuscript does not necessarily reflect the position or policy of the U.S. Government. Thanks are due to Northern Digital Inc. for the loan of the AURORA.

CARS 2002 – H.U. Lemke, M.W. Vannier; K. Inamura, A.G. Farman, K. Doi & J.H.C. Reiber (Editors)
°CARS/Springer. All rights reserved.

Reconstruction of intrahepatic vessel trees from three-dimensional freehand ultrasound-scans

P. Hassenpflug[a], M. Vetter[a], G. da Silva Jr.[b], I. Wolf[a], M. Thorn[a], G. M. Richter[b],
W. Lamadé[c], M. W. Büchler[c], H.-P. Meinzer[a]

[a] Div. Med. and Biol. Informatics, DKFZ Heidelberg, Germany
[b] Surgical and [c] Radiological Clinic, University of Heidelberg, Germany

Keywords: Three-dimensional ultrasound, hepatic vessel reconstruction

1. Introduction

This contribution describes a component of ARION™, an augmented-reality system for intraoperative navigation in oncological liver surgery. In this component, intrahepatic vessels are reconstructed from three-dimensional (3D) intraoperative ultrasound (IOUS).

2. Method

A linear ultrasound probe is used to scan a set of Doppler images of the surgical volume of interest by means of a 3D freehand ultrasound acquisition software [1]. The pixels of each ultrasound image are available in world coordinates of the applied electro-magnetic tracking system (Minibird 500, Ascension Technology Corp., Burlington, VT, USA). Large patches of Doppler artifacts are filtered from the ultrasound images via form factors. If the automatic classification result is uncertain, the radiologist decides interactively about classifying a selection as artifact or blood flow signal. The thus preprocessed Doppler data are used to determine seed points for a local raytracing method to segment the vessel contours slice by slice. The three-dimensional reconstruction of the vessels from their two-dimensionally segmented contours is done by the means of an evaluation function. It decides for each pair of vessel contours from adjacent slices about their topological connectivity. If a pair of vessel contours of two adjacent slices is classified as connected, two corresponding nodes with the respective vessel features are added to the vessel graph. By this means, an intraoperative vessel graph is created, which can be registered with the preoperatively acquired vessel graph.

3. Results

The method introduced in this paper enables the symbolic reconstruction of intrahepatic vessel trees from 3D Doppler IOUS. The current procedure requires an average of less then three seconds for processing a single slice. Therefore, the herein described component for symbolic reconstruction of intraoperatively acquired blood flow signals is an essential prerequisite for an efficient registration with the preoperative vessel graph.

Acknowledgements

This work is funded by BMBF grant 01EZ0008.

References

1. R. W. Prager, A. Gee, and L. Bermann: Stradx: real-time acquisition and visualization of freehand three-dimensional ultrasound. Med Image Anal 3(2):129-40, 1998.

CARS 2002 – H.U. Lemke, M.W. Vannier; K. Inamura, A.G. Farman, K. Doi & J.H.C. Reiber (Editors)
©CARS/Springer. All rights reserved.

Development of AR navigation system for laparoscopic surgery using magneto-optic hybrid sensor: experiences with 3 cases

Kozo Konishi[1], Makoto Hashizume[1], Masahiko Nakamoto[2], Masaki Miyamoto[2],
Mitsuo Shimada[3], Yoshinobu Sato[2], Shinichi Tamura[2], Keizo Sugimachi[3]

[1]Department of Disaster and Emergency Medicine, [3]Department of Surgery and Science Graduate School of Medical Sciences, Kyushu University.
[2]Division of Interdisciplinary Image Analysis, Osaka University Graduate School of Medicine

Key Words: AR image, magneto-optic hybrid sensor, 3D-US

1. Introduction

The purpose of this study is to develop and assess the feasibility of 3D US system using an accurate magneto-optic hybrid sensory system utilized for laparoscopic surgery.

2. Method

The complete system consists of a laparoscope, two different 3D digitizers (Northern Digital Inc, Canada), US device SSD5500 (ALOKA, Japan), and a workstation. A 5D miniature magnetic sensor is combined with an 6D optical sensor outside the body to perform 6D tracking of the .flexible US probe tip in the abdominal cavity. The system was used in 3 cases. (2 hepatectomies and 1 splenectomy)

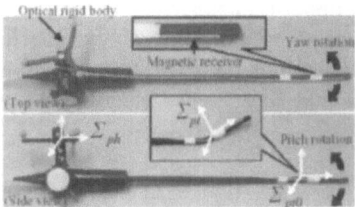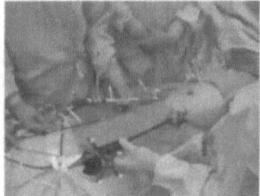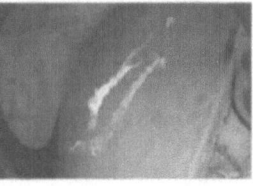

Figures US probe for laparoscope and AR image

3. Results

All procedures were performed safely and postoperative courses were uneventful. AR visualization, which superimposed the visualized 3D-US images onto captured laparoscopic live images was successfully achieved. Display latency were so short that any operative procedures were disturbed.

4. Conclusion

We developed and used the AR navigation system for laparoscopic surgery. However, a further study is necessary.

References

1.   Nakamoto M et al., Magneto-optic hybrid 3-D sensor for surgical navigation, LNCS, 1935 (Proc. MICCAI 2000), 839-848(2000)

CARS 2002 – H.U. Lemke, M.W. Vannier; K. Inamura, A.G. Farman, K. Doi & J.H.C. Reiber (Editors)
ᶜCARS/Springer. All rights reserved.

1094

Evaluation of an augmented reality system for intraoperative data presentation – preliminary results

Tobias Salb[a], Jakob Brief[b], Thomas Welzel[c], Oliver Burgert[a], Tilo Gockel[a],
Robert Krempien[c], Stefan Hassfeld[b] and Rüdiger Dillmann[a]
[a] Universität Karlsruhe (TH), Institute for Computer Design and Fault Tolerance
Haid-und-Neu-Str. 7, 76131 Karlsruhe, Germany
Email: salb@ira.uka.de, WWW: http://wwwiaim.ira.uka.de/
[b] University of Heidelberg. Department of Oral and Maxillofacial
[c] University of Heidelberg. Department of Radiology
Im Neuenheimer Feld 400, 69120 Heidelberg, Germany

Keywords: Augmented reality, head-mounted display, evaluation

1. Introduction

For intraoperative support of surgeons and reduction of clinical risks we developed an augmented reality system called INPRES – "INtraoperative PRESentation of surgical planning and simulation results".

2. Methods

A see-through head-mounted display is used for data visualization and superposition over the surgical field of view. Key tasks are optical tracking of surgeon and patient, registration of virtual data with the patient and detection of occlusions [1]. For the evaluation of INPRES several tests are performed in order to check accuracy, speed, usability and overall quality of our approach. Clinical indications modeled on a phantom skull are a cyst on lower jaw, a tumor in the cerebral area and access planning for a Frontal Orbital Advancement surgery.

3. Results

Results are determined with accuracy and speed measurements and with a questionnaire.

4. Conclusions

Details about the test setup and test results will be presented on our poster.

Acknowledgements

This work is funded by the Special Research Area 414 "Information Technology in Medicine - Computer and Sensor supported Surgery" of the Deutsche Forschungsgemeinschaft.

References

1. Salb, T., Burgert, O., Gockel, T., Brief, J., Hassfeld, S., Mühling, J. and Dillmann, R., "Risk Reduction in Craniofacial Surgery using Computer-based Modeling and Intraoperative Immersion." *Medicine Meets Virtual Reality (MMVR), Newport Beach, CA,* J. Westwood et. al., Studies in Health Technology and Informatics, vol. 85, pp. 441-447, IOS Press & Ohmsha, Amsterdam, 2002.

4th International Workshop on Computer-Aided Diagnosis - CAD

CARS 2002 – H.U. Lemke, M.W. Vannier; K. Inamura, A.G. Farman, K. Doi & J.H.C. Reiber (Editors)

A detection method of ground glass opacities from chest X-ray CT images

Hotaka Takizawa[a], Shinji Yamamoto[a], Tohru Matsumoto[b],
Yukio Tateno[b], Takeshi Iinuma[b], Mitsuomi Matsumoto[c]
[a] Toyohashi Univ. of Tech.
[b] National Institute of Radiological Science
[c] Tokyo Metropolitan Univ. of Health Sciences

Keywords: Computer aided diagnosis, detection of ground glass opacities, chest X-ray CT images

1. Introduction

Detection of Ground Glass Opacities (GGO), which are early stages of lung cancers, becomes to be more important. In order to detect them exactly, we make our Quoit filter [1] more sensitive. By this change, all the GGO's can be detected, but the number of the false positives is increased from about 30 [shadow/patient] to about 200 [shadow/patient]. Thus we develop a new recognition method of lung cancers, specially GGO's, using discriminant functions derived from statistical decision theories.

2. Methods

The recognition process consists of two phases. One is a training phase, the other is a testing phase. In the training phase, first, sample shadows are classified into 8 sub-groups according to their sizes and positions in the lung areas. Next, we (our medical doctor staffs) divide each shadow group into some clusters such as cancers, blood vessels and partial volume effects (PVE). Average feature vectors and co-variance matrices of these clusters are calculated from the feature vectors of the clustered shadows. In the testing phase, we determine the abnormality of the shadow candidate using a mahalanobis distance derived from the average feature vector and co-variance matrix.

3. Results

We apply our Quoit filter to 38 sample images, and all cancer shadows are extracted correctly with about 200 false positives per patient. Next we apply the new method described in this paper. The number of the false positives is decreased to be only about 15 [shadow/patient].

4. Conclusions

In this paper, we described a new recognition method of GGO shadows using discriminant functions derived from statistical decision theories. By applying our new method to actual CT images (38 patient images), good results has been acquired.

References

1. S.Yamamoto et al. "Quoit Filter: A New Filter Based on Mathematical Morphology to Extract the Isolated Shadow, and Its Application to Automatic Detection of Lung Cancer in X-Ray CT", Proc. 13th Int. Conf. Pattern Recognition II, 3--7,1996.

CARS 2002 – H.U. Lemke, M.W. Vannier; K. Inamura, A.G. Farman, K. Doi & J.H.C. Reiber (Editors)

1098

Automated polyp detection from colon MRI images

Julien Lamy[a,b], Christian Ronse[b], Luc Soler[a]

[a] IRCAD, 1, place de l'hôpital, 67091 Strasbourg, France
[b] LSIIT, Pôle API, boulevard Sébastien Brant, 67400 Illkirch Cedex, France

Keywords: Image processing, segmentation, mathematical morphology

1. Introduction

Prevention of colon cancer is achieved today through colonic polyp detection. However, most of the methods are sub-optimal. MRI imaging circumvents most of the drawbacks, being more sensitive than occult blood detection, less invasive than coloscopy or CT-scan imaging, and non-irradiating.

2. Methods

On the input MRI image, the colon lumen is bright, and the surrounding areas as well as the polyps are not contrasted. Hence, the polyps appear as depressions in the colon lumen. We can extract the lumen by automatic thresholding: on the histogram, it corresponds to the rightmost peak. We then use the lumen mask for polyp detection : first, we extract all dark and narrow areas using a closing top-hat [1]. Then, we seek the 2D holes on X, Y and Z slices of the MRI image, and perform a binary reconstruction of the top-hat image in each of the hole image. Finally, we merge the three binary reconstructions using a logical or. The result is refined further using shape criteria [2].

3. Results

This method has been tested on a dozen cases, and is currently undergoing medical validation. The lumen segmentation was hampered by a partially-filled colon in most of the cases, leaving air zones not included in the lumen mask. To overcome this limitation, two images are acquired : one where the patient lies in dorsal decubitus, then in ventral decubitus. We can then use both partial reconstructions to reduce the number of undetected polyps.

4. Conclusions

We have developed a novel method for automatic lumen and polyps detection in colon MRI images, based on morphological and geometrical criteria. The result still has to be examined by an expert, as other structures can look like polyps, e.g. small air bubbles or remaining fecal matters. Other methods to detect polyps, based on topology and registration, are currently under investigation.

References

1. P. Soille, *Morphological image analysis*, Springer Verlag, 1998.
2. L. Soler, H. Delingette, G. Malandain, J. Montagnat, N. Ayache, C. Koehl, O. Dourthe, B. Malassagne, M. Smith, D. Mutter, J. Marescaux, *Fully automatic anatomical, pathological, and functional segmentation from CT scans for hepatic surgery*, Computer Aided Surgery, vol. 6, num. 3, pp. 131-142, August 2001.

CARS 2002 – H.U. Lemke, M.W. Vannier; K. Inamura, A.G. Farman, K. Doi & J.H.C. Reiber (Editors)

Three-dimensional analysis of pulmonary nodules using thin slice helical CT data: automated nodule classification and estimation of malignancy

K. Murao[a], K. Awai[b], A. Ozawa[a], T. Yamanaka[c], M. Komi[b], S. Hori[b]

[a] Fujitsu Ltd, 1-9-3, Nakase, Mihama-ku, Chiba 261-8588, Japan
[b] Izumisano Hospital, 2-23, Rinku-Ourai-Kita, Izumisano, Osaka 598-8577, Japan
[c] Fujitsu Ltd, 1-17-25, Shin-Kamata, Oota-ku, Tokyo 144-8588, Japan

Keywords: Pulmonary nodule, lung cancer, malignancy

1. Introduction
Pulmonary nodules are commonly encountered radiological findings. Although 60-70% of pulmonary nodules have benign causes, many represent early stage cancer, which show relative good prognosis. Thus, accurate differential diagnosis of pulmonary nodules is the important issue. With the wide spread of the helical CT, it became easy to obtain three-dimensional data using consecutive 1.00-1.25mm thickness CT images of pulmonary nodules, and analyze it quantitatively. The purpose of this study was to develop a CAD system to quantify three-dimensional morphological features of pulmonary nodules and estimate their malignancy using artificial neural networks.

2. Methods
We selected 26 malignant nodules and 42 benign nodules which were pathologically or clinically diagnosed. Helical scans of the pulmonary nodules were obtained with a multidetector row helical scanner at 1.25-mm thickness.
After indicating the regions of interest manually, we analyze them as follows.
1) segmentation of the nodules (elimination of vessels, thoracic walls, mediastinum, etc)
2) extraction of 3D image features
3) establishment of neural network using the image features and the corresponding pathological data
When we examine the causal relationship between each feature and the malignancy, we perform the lateral inhibitory learning and observe the network chart in order to enhance the binding between each layer.

3. Results
The network converged in relatively small number of learning iteration within 10% admissible error. This means that malignancy rate was more than 0.9 for all the malignant nodules and below 0.1 for benign ones. From the analysis with the neural network, important parameters for determining malignancy were irregularity index and deviation of CT number inside the nodule.

4. Conclusions
CT lung cancer analysis with thin slice CT is performed using 3D image processing and the neural networks. Preliminary results showed that this method is promising technique for finding the relation between the image features and the malignancy.

CARS 2002 – H.U. Lemke, M.W. Vannier; K. Inamura, A.G. Farman, K. Doi & J.H.C. Reiber (Editors)

Sonographic diagnosis of fatty liver using computer-aided quantification

Seunghwan Kim, Ji-Wook Jeong, Sooyeul Lee
Electronics and Telecommunications Research Institute
P.O. Box 106, Yuseong, Daejeon, 305-600 Korea

Keywords: Ultrasound, fatty liver, normalized gray level

1. Introduction

We investigated the B-mode ultrasound (US) images of abdomen obtaining the normalized gray levels (NGL's) of the liver with the representative gray levels of the liver, adrenal cortex, subcutaneous fat, blood vessel of the hepatic portal vein (HPV) in the ultrasound images to quantify fatty interfiltration of liver (FIL). We also compared the NGL's of the liver with the clinical diagnosis of FIL showing good correlation between them.

2. Methods

The representative gray levels of liver, adrenal cortex, subcutaneous fat, blood vessel of HPV, and blood were obtained by the various image processing methods leading to the two NGL's in the region of interest of the liver: one (NGL1) is the relative gray level of the liver between the representative gray levels of the adrenal cortex and subcutaneous fat. The other (NGL2) is the relative glay level of the liver between the representative gray levels of the blood vessel of HPV and the blood. With the US images of 95 patients ranging from normal to severe grade of FIL, the NGL1 and NGL2 of liver were compared with the clinical diagnosis of FIL.

3. Results

From the statistical distributions of the NGL's in the US images, we found that the NGL's increase monotonically as the clinical estimations of the severity of the FIL is severer. The calculated standard deviation of the NGL1 for the images is about 0.13. The calculated linear correlation coefficient between the NGL1 and the clinical estimation of the severity of the FIL is 0.79. The calculated linear correlation coefficient is 0.69 between the NGL2 and the clinical estimation of the severity of the FIL.

When we use two NGL's of the liver simultaneously, the ambiguity in the diagnosis for the FIL could be fairly reduced compared to the case without the NGL's.

4. Conclusions

From the results, we conclude that the two NGL's of liver could play a role of indices of FIL to enhance the diagnostic accuracy of FIL in clinic. We need to elaborate the NGL's of liver to increase the correlation coefficient between the NGL's of liver and clinical diagnosis of FIL.

Acknowledgements

This work was supported by the Ministry of the Information and Communications, Korea.

CARS 2002 – H.U. Lemke, M.W. Vannier; K. Inamura, A.G. Farman, K. Doi & J.H.C. Reiber (Editors)
©CARS/Springer. All rights reserved.

Detection of abnormal tissue in HRCT scans of the chest

I.C. Sluimer, B. van Ginneken

Image Sciences Institute, University Medical Center Utrecht, the Netherlands

Keywords: Computer-aided-diagnosis, high-resolution computed tomography, texture

1. Introduction
We develop tools to aid the physician in the diagnostic process of high-resolution CT (HRCT) scans of the chest. This abstract presents a method for classifying patches of lung tissue from such scans as normal or abnormal. The classification is performed by comparison to a set of reference cases.

2. Methods
Each patch is represented by a vector of features. In order to obtain these features, the patch is convolved with a set of filters based on the Gaussian and its derivatives. These filters can be considered spot, edge, and line detectors, and they are all calculated on multiple scales. Classification in feature space is performed by a k-nearest-neighbours (kNN) classifier: the classification of a patch is determined by the class to which the majority of its k neighbours belong. The kNN classifier also allows for the system to be used for retrieval of similar images [1].

3. Results
From a set of 42 scans collected from daily clinical practice, 60 patches were segmented by hand. They had the size of about 1/3 of a lung field in a single slice. The categories normal/abnormal contained 30 instances each. For each patch a set of 96 features was calculated, out of which a subset of maximally 40 was selected automatically to increase performance. A leave-one-out experiment yielded a classification result of 82 % (sensitivity : 73 %, specificity : 90 %). We believe that the obtained classification accuracy is limited by the size of our dataset: for certain pathological categories the dataset contains only a single instance and therefore in a leave-one-out experiment the feature selection on the remaining set of datapoints will not be able to account for the patterns displayed in the excluded image.

4. Conclusions
A method was described to detect abnormal pieces of lung tissue in HRCT images of the lung. We perform the classification by means of a feature-based nearest-neighbour pattern classifier. Features are extracted using filters based on the Gaussian and its derivatives. Experiments performed on a set of 60 patches of lung tissue yielded a classification result of 82 %. This result is suspected to be limited by the small size of the current dataset.

References
1.   Shyu, Brodley, Kak, Kosaka, 1999. ASSERT : A Physician-in-the-loop Contents-Based Retrieval System for HRCT Image Databases. Computer Vision and Image Understanding, 75(1,2) : 111-132

CARS 2002 – H.U. Lemke, M.W. Vannier; K. Inamura, A.G. Farman, K. Doi & J.H.C. Reiber (Editors)
°CARS/Springer. All rights reserved.

1102

Development of automated detection methods
for architectural distortions on mammograms

T. Matsubara[a], D. Yamazaki[b], T. Hara[b], H. Fujita[b], S. Kasai[c], T. Endo[d], T. Iwase[e]

[a] Nagoya Bunri University, 365 Maeda, Inazawa-cho, Inazawa-shi 492-8520, Japan
[b] Gifu University, 1-1 Yanagido, Gifu-shi 501-1193, Japan
[c] Konica Corporation, 1 Sakura-machi, Hino-shi 191-8511, Japan
[d] National Hospital of Nagoya, 4-1-1 Sannomaru, Naka-ku, Nagoya-shi 460-0001,Japan
[e] Aichi Cancer Center Hospital, 1-1 Kanokoden Chikusa-ku, Nagoya-shi 464-8681, Japan

Keywords: Architectural distortion, mammogram, computer-aided diagnosis

1. Introduction

The architectural distortion is a very important finding in interpreting breast cancers as well as microcalcification and mass on mammograms. In addition, it sometimes appears at the previous stage of obvious mass shadow. In despite of the importance for detecting architectural distortions, few algorithms for detecting them have been reported. The purpose of this study is to develop a new detection method for the area of architectural distortion existing around skinline in order to detect breast cancer at an early stage.

2. Methods

The contours of normal glandular tissue around skinline are tend to be smooth lines, on the other hand, those of distorted one are depressed.
Firstly, the dynamic-range compression technique is carried out within the breast regions in order to remove the background density from the breast thickness. Secondly, the thick mammary gland regions are extracted by using binarization technique and local discriminant analysis. The threshold at this process is determined by referring to the density of pectoral muscle region in order to be less susceptible to the condition of mammography. Thirdly, the top-hat processing based on morphological operators is applied to determine the suspect depressed regions. In our experiments, we have chosen linear structures in seven directions to fit to the shape of outlines. Finally, the false-positive candidates are eliminated by the features of their locations and sizes. The residual candidates are indicated by circles as "true" architectural distortions.

3. Results

Our image database with architectural distortions consists of 51 cases. The sketches and comments in details of all cases were made by an experienced radiologist. As a result, the sensitivity was 92% with 3.8 false-positive detections per image.

4. Conclusions

We have developed an automated detection method of architectural distortions on mammograms based on the top-hat processing. It is concluded that our approach is effective because the performance shows high sensitivity. For the future work, it is necessary to decrease the false positives and to collect the images in order to perform the validation test for this detection approach.

CARS 2002 – H.U. Lemke, M.W. Vannier, K. Inamura, A.G. Farman, K. Doi & J.H.C. Reiber (Editors)

Some results on the preprocessing of mammograms for microcalcification detection

Enrique Nava[a], Raúl Mata[b], Francisco Sendra[a], Esther Ristori[a]

[a] Universidad de Málaga, Spain, en@uma.es

[b] Universidad de Jaén, Spain

Keywords: Computer-aided-diagnosis, wavelet, microcalcification

1. Introduction

In this work, it is presented a new algorithm to pre-process mammograms that contains microcalcifications using wavelets and some statistical analysis, that can be useful in an early stage of a detection algorithm, or as a method to remove 'not-interesting' regions. The main purpose of this work is, of course, to obtain an automatic method to extract all microcalcifications of a mammogram, but this project is not finished now. In spite of this, we have an strong feeling that some ideas or results can be useful to other researchers.

2. Methods

The method used to pre-process the mammogram involves three phases: an initial phase is an usual pre-processing technique: the mammogram is divided in 400x400 pixels size, contrast enhanced, filtered and background removed. A second phase is a wavelet decomposition (similar to [1]) to detect size range objects and to remove fibrograndular tissue background. In the third and final phase, small regions in each level image are tested looking for a 'typical luminosity' characteristics of a microcalcification, modelled using classical statistical parameters of microcalcification.

3. Results

Over a selected set of ROIs with a size of 400x400 pixels obtained from the USCF mammogram database, between 80 and 90% of pixels were removed, with none mistakes, leaving pixels grouped (90%) in a single or few compact regions (clusters) or in sparse regions (10%) showing isolated microcalcifications. The final stage of the automatic detection algorithm is not finished now and it's expected to be working in one year.

4. Conclusions

The proposed method is useful to pre-process a mammogram that contain microcalcifications. A considerable percentage of pixels can be removed with none further processing, improving both single and clustered microcalcification detection algorithms.

Acknowledgements

This work was supported in part by TIC-128, Junta de Andalucia, PAI research funds.

References

1. M. J. Lado, P. G. Tahoces, A. J. Méndez, M. Souto, J. Vidal, "A wavelet-based algorithm for detecting clustered microcalcifications in digital mammograms", Med. Phys. 26 (7), pp 1294-1305, July 1999.

2002 International Symposium on Cardiovascular Imaging - CVI

CARS 2002 – H.U. Lemke, M.W. Vannier; K. Inamura, A.G. Farman, K. Doi & J.H.C. Reiber (Editors)

A multiscale medial axis detection of coronary arteries in X-rays angiographies

Benoit Tremblais[a], Bertrand Augereau[a], Michel Leard[a]
[a] Laboratoire IRCOM-SIC UMR 6615 CNRS, BP 30179,
86962 Futuroscope Chasseneuil Cedex, France

Keywords: X-rays angiography, scale-space, medial axis

1. Introduction

In the present work we are concerned with the assistance to the diagnostic of coronaries stenosis from X-rays angiography modality. We are treating here the problem of the 2D multiscale medial axis segmentation.

2. Methods

Using differential geometry we can characterize locally the medial axis of arteries as the image surface bottom lines of valleys. As Lindeberg [1], we use a normalized scale-space based approach to regularize the calculation of derivatives. Then, we can easily compute a local measure of valley for each scale of the process. The detection of the medial axis position is made searching the local maxima of the measure of valley in the direction of the first principal curvature. Then the medial axis and valley measure scale-spaces are used to obtain the 2D mutliscale medial axis of the coronary arteries. Then, the medical practitioner can choose the arteries of most interest for the future 3D reconstruction.

3. Results

We have tested our process on several angiographies. The medial axis is well extracted even in the case of strong stenosis. Furthermore, using the whole scale-space we limit the discontinuities of the medial axis detection. And, the computation cost is quite low.

4. Conclusions

In this communication we have proposed a multiscale medial axis detection. We have shown that with a low interaction of the medical practitioner and a low computational cost we obtain an attractive tool for segmentation of the coronarian tree. We feel that this tool is a first step toward a promising 3D reconstruction .

Acknowledgements

We thank the F.I.S.C consortium (Fluids Images Signal and Cardiology), and the region Poitou-Charentes (France) for the financing of this work.

References

1. Tony Lindeberg, Edge detection and ridge detection with the automatic scale selection, Computer Vison and Pattern Recognition, pp. 465-470, 1996.

CARS 2002 – H.U. Lemke, M.W. Vannier; K. Inamura, A.G. Farman, K. Doi & J.H.C. Reiber (Editors)
^cCARS/Springer. All rights reserved.

1108

Model-based segmentation and visualization of IVUS images for radiation treatment planning in cardiovascular brachytherapy

F. Weichert [a], C. Wilke [b,c], P. Spilles [a], A. Kraushaar [a],
H. Müller [a], U. Quast [c] and D. Wegener [b]
University of Dortmund, [a] Computer Science VII and [b] Institute of Physics,
[c] Essen University Hospital, Clinical Radiation Physics

Keywords: Segmentation, ultrasound, brachytherapy

1. Introduction
Within the last few years intravascular ultrasound (IVUS) has become a standard for the diagnosis of cardiovascular diseases [1]. Besides giving imaging informations of the coronary artery anatomy, IVUS data can also be used for cardiovascular brachytherapy. This task requires precise segmentation of the different layers of the coronary artery.

2. Methods
After having acquired a 3D-stack of 2D-IVUS-images, segmentation starts with the application of a gradient-based edge detector [2] to determine relevant contours. The goal of edge detection is the extraction of feature points, which can be assigned to a definite coronar structure with high probability. These sets of weighted feature points are now transferred into closed vessel contours, representing the corresponding arterial layers.
For this purpose, a parameterized elliptical template is used which resembles a vessel shape not excessively deformed by arteriosclerosis. The idea for fitting ellipses to scattered data was first proposed by Rosin [3]. The desired spatial model of vessel sections is represented by a voxel model, the results of segmentation by contours. Both results can be visualized by methods of combined volume and polygon rendering.

3. Results and Conclusion
Physicists and physicians should be supported by a semi-automatic method, which is capable of differentiating vessel structures in straight vessel sections with stent efficiently and quickly, and by visualizing the result by 3D graphics.
Based on current results, we expect that both demands could be fulfilled. In order to improve on the quality of the distinction of vessel structures, the contours found should serve deformable models as a base of a more correct approximation.

Acknowledgements
This work has been supported by grant Qu 39/16-1, Deutsche Forschungsgemeinschaft.

References
1. R. Erbel, J. Roelandt, J. Ge, G. Görge: Intravascular Ultrasound, Martin Dunitz Limited, (1998)
2. J.R. Parker: Algorithms for image processing and computer vision, Wiley, New York, (1997)
3. P.L. Rosin: A note on the least squares fitting of ellipses, Pattern Recognition Letters, Vol. 14, p.799-808, (1993)

CARS 2002 – H.U. Lemke, M.W. Vannier; K. Inamura, A.G. Farman, K. Doi & J.H.C. Reiber (Editors)
°CARS/Springer. All rights reserved.

Hydatid cyst of heart contribution of two-dimensional echocardiography

S. Ernez-Hajri, G. Jeridi, H. Bouraoui, T. Filali, A. Mahdhaoui, H. Ammar

Department of Cardiology, Hospital Farhat Hached of Sousse, Tunisia

Keywords: Heart, hydatid cyst, echocardiography

1. Introduction

Cardiac location of Hydatid cysts is rare representing 0.5 to 2 % of all hydatid cysts in humans. Diagnosis is difficult because the presenting symptoms are variables and non-specifics. The aim of our study is to clarify the role of echocardiography in the disease (Hydatid cysts in the heart)

2. Methods

Into eleven years period (1991-2001) we reviewed seven patients who had cardiac Hydatid cysts. The mean age was 29 ± 19 years with a range of 4 to 56 years. One patient of our series was asymptomatic, and six patients complained of symptoms (dyspnea atypical chest pain, palpitations, urticaria). In two cases the cyst was revealed by a pulmonary embolism. Clinical investigation included in all cases chest X-ray, ECG, echocardiography and computed tomography (CT) scan.

3. Results

The diagnosis and the location of the cyst were obtained by echocardiography.

Patients	1	2	3	4	5	6	7
Location of the cyst in the heart	Left ventricle	Right ventricle	Inter ventricular septum	Pericardium	Left atrium	Right atrium	Left ventricle
Other visceral localisation of the cyst	Hepatic Pulmonary renal	Pulmonary		Pulmonary		Pulmonary hepatic	pulmonary

The diagnosis of hydatid cyst was confirmed by positive hemagglutination test. Two dimensional echocardiography provided a rapid anatomical an topographic diagnosis, completed by CT scan. There was two hospital death do to pulmonary embolism, but in the other five patients, surgical resection was performed and the outcome was good.

4. Conclusion

These seven cases illustrate the diagnostic value of two dimensional echocardiography in Hydatid cyst of the heart as a diagnostic tool. The combination echocardiography and computed tomography allowed a precise topographical inventory, reducing the need for magnetic resonance imaging to the complicated cases and to the rare cases of inconclusive results by echo-CT scan.

CARS 2002 – H.U. Lemke, M.W. Vannier; K. Inamura, A.G. Farman, K. Doi & J.H.C. Reiber (Editors)

1110

Demonstration of three-dimensional visualization techniques for coronary artery evaluation using EBCT – a case study

P.M.A. van Ooijen[a], P.J. de Feyter[b], M.Oudkerk[a]

[a]Dept. of Radiology, University Hospital Groningen, Groningen, The Netherlands
[b]Thoraxcentre, University Hospital Rotterdam, Rotterdam, The Netherlands

Keywords: Electron beam computed tomography, 3D visualization, coronary arteries

1. Introduction
A variety of visualization techniques, both established and recently developed, can be used for evaluation of the coronary arteries and identification of stenotic lesions. Using a single contrast enhanced electron beam computed tomography (EBCT) scan the results and drawbacks of these techniques will be shown.

2. Methods
Forty two-dimensional slices were acquired with prospective triggering (80% of the RR-interval) on an Evolution XP-150 (Imatron, San Francisco, CA) EBCT scanner. The acquisition started just cranial to the left main coronary artery. To enhance the contrast of the coronary lumen, 120-180 ml of contrast medium was injected into the antecubital vein at 3-4 ml/second. Three commonly used visualization techniques are used for the evaluation of the coronary artery tree, Multi Planar Reformation (MPR), Maximum Intensity Projection (MIP) and Volume Rendering (VR). The basics of these techniques are well established and frequently described in literature [1,2].

3. Results
The techniques mentioned before are all performed on the same dataset clearly showing the advantages and drawbacks of each technique. Beside the standard algorithms alternative applications are shown demonstrating the use of elaborate segmentation and virtual intra-vascular visualization [3].

4. Conclusions
Despite the drawbacks we feel that clinical and diagnostic value of volume rendering combined with – automated – extensive segmentation and intravascular visualization will increase with the increase of spatial and temporal resolution. However, clinical application will mainly depend on availability within the radiology or cardiology department of workstations to perform the visualizations described above.

References
1. Bendib K, Poirier C, Croisille P, Roux JP, Revel D, Amiel M. *Characterization of arterial stenosis using 3D imaging. Comparison of 3 imaging techniques (MRI, Spiral CT and 3D DSA) and 4 display methods (MIP, SR, MPVR, VA) by using physical phantoms.* J. Radiol. 80(11)1561-1567.
2. Calhoun PS, Kuszyk DB, Heath DG, Carley JC, Fishman EK. *Three-dimensional volume rendering of spiral CT data: theory and method.* Radiographics 19(3)745-764.
3. Ooijen van PMA, Oudkerk M, van Geuns RJ, Rensing BJ, de Feyter PJ. *Coronary artery fly-through using electron beam computed tomography.* Circulation 102(1)e6-e10.

CARS 2002 – H.U. Lemke, M.W. Vannier; K. Inamura, A.G. Farman, K. Doi & J.H.C. Reiber (Editors)

Left ventricular perfusion/function differences between ischemic and dilated cardiomyopathy assessed by SPECT myocardial imaging: visual and quantitative computer analysis

J. Maksimovic[a], M. Vavlukis[b], I. Peovska[c], D. Pop Gorceva[d], V. Majstorov[e]

a, b, c Clinical Center, Institute for Heart Disease, Skopje, Republic of Macedonia

Key words: Myocardial perfusion imaging, dilated cardiomyopathy, ishemic heart disease

1. Introduction

The aim of the study was to evaluate the myocardial perfusion imaging (MPI) scans in patients (pts) with ischemic (ICM) and dilated cardiomyopathy (DCM) and to assess the role of SPECT MPI in the diagnosis and differentiation of the above mentioned cardiomyopathies.

2. Methods

10 pts (Gr.I) with DCM and 21 pts (Gr.II) with ICM, age (56+/- 12 years), with LVEF <40%, underwent Tc-99m MIBI one-day dipyridamole rest/stress MPI. The angiography was performed in all pts in order to exclude or diagnose coronary artery disease (CAD) (luminal stenosis >50%). All pts with DCM had normal angiographic findings. We have evaluated 620 segments, using 20 segment model analyses with 5 point scoring system (0=normal; 4= no uptake) for estimation of defect severity. Semiquantitative analysis was done using summed stress score (SSS), summed rest scores (SRS) and summed differential or reversibility score (SDS). Wall motion (WM) was evaluated using 6 point scoring system (0-normal motion, 5-dyskinetic). LVEF was estimated echocardiographicly at rest. We have performed visual and quantitative analysis.

3. Results

In pts with DCM we have found: global hypokinesia, symmetric WM abnormalities with inhomogeneous, lower regional uptake of the tracer, more often mixed defects, average WM an LVEF were lower compared to ICM, more often enlarged right and left ventricle. In pts with ICM findings were as follows: segmental hypokinesia, akinesia and diskinesia were more prevalent, clearly cut defects, larger regional asymmetric WM and uptake abnormalities, higher SSS and SDS, enlarged LV.
DCM (n=10): Normokinetic 0/200; Hypokinetic 184/200 (92%); Akinetic 12/200 (6%); Diskinetic 4/200 (2%) LVEF 25+/-8; SSS 7+/-3; SRS 3+/-1; SDS 4+/-2. **ICMP (n=21):** Normokinetic 29/420 (7%); Hypokinetic 273/420 (65%); Akinetic 84/420 (20%); Diskinetic 37/420 (8%); LVEF 33+/-5; SSS 20+/-11; SRS 12+/-5; SDS 7+/-6

4. Conclusions

Assessment of regional perfusion/function by Gated SPECT is useful for diagnosis and differentiation of ICM and DCM. Reversible defects in DCM are probably due to microvacular abnormalities. After performing the SPECT imaging in pts with DCMP the angiography could be avoided.

CARS 2002 – H.U. Lemke, M.W. Vannier; K. Inamura, A.G. Farman, K. Doi & J.H.C. Reiber (Editors)

Heart phantom
a simple elastomechanical model of ventricle

Wahju Sediono, Olaf Dössel

Institute of Biomedical Engineering, Universität Karlsruhe (TH), Kaiserstr. 12,
76131 Karlsruhe, Germany

Keywords: Elastomechanics, numerical simulation, hyperelasticity

1. Introduction

In this paper a simple heart phantom made of silicon rubber is presented. This phantom can be placed into a machine that is able to mimic the pump movement of the heart. If the elastomechanical properties of the rubber material and the external forces are well known the complete stress and strain distribution inside the moving heart phantom can be determined. Using this phantom various imaging techniques can be tested.

2. Methods

At first the elastomechanical parameters of the rubber material that is subject to the law of hyperelasticity must be determined. The determination can be accelerated with the aid of computer simulations. The simulation and the following numerical analysis are performed with an existing FE software package. For further validation through imaging techniques a precise knowledge of the stress and strain tensors inside the phantom is very important. This is only available if external forces can be applied in a wellknown and reproduceable manner. The movement machine consists basically of a rotating piston. The moments are created pneumatically. In parallel an investigation was carried out, to what extent the elastomechanical properties of a real heart can be modelled with the Mooney-Rivlin material. A systematic analysis of stress-strain curves reported in the literature is carried out and the best compromise to model the heart is found. [1][2]

3. Results

The hyperelastic properties of the heart phantom are determined. The machine that moves the phantom is fabricated and tested. Stress and strain distribution inside the phantom are calculated using a FE software package. The simulation of torsion test shows that the nodal reaction forces are distributed concentrically.

4. Conclusions

A simple heart phantom made of silicon rubber is fabricated. Its elastomechanical properties are determined and described using the Mooney-Rivlin model. Stress and strain distribution are applied and calculated. They can serve as a golden standard for imaging techniques like e.g. tagged MR Imaging. In addition a reasonably good description of the elastomechanical properties of the heart using the Mooney-Rivlin approach was achieved.

References

1. Huisman, R. M., Sipkema, P., Westerhof, N., Elzinga, G.: "Comparison of models used to calculate left ventricular wall force", *Med. Biol. Eng. Comp.* 18:133-144, 1980.
2. Hunter, P. J., McCulloch, A. D., ter Keurs, H. E. D. J.: "Modelling the mechanical properties of cardiac muscle", *Prog. in Biophys. Mol. Biol.* 69:289-331, 1998.

8th Computed Maxillofacial Imaging Congress - CMI

CARS 2002 – H.U. Lemke, M.W. Vannier; K. Inamura, A.G. Farman, K. Doi & J.H.C. Reiber (Editors)

Image post-processing for optimization of photostimulable phosphor cephalograms

West KD, *Farman TT, Scheetz JP, Silveira A, Johnson BE, Farman AG
School of Dentistry, The University of Louisville, Louisville, KY, USA

1. Purpose and methods

To evaluate 16-bit PSP cephalogram images for orthodontist-perceived quality of cephalometric landmark clarity at baseline and with three different image enhancements (emboss, inverse, and inverse/emboss). This presentation concerns results limited for detection of Porion and Pronasale. These two landmarks were evaluated in view of being extremes in contrast requirements. A Sectagraph (Denar Corporation, CA) was used with the DenOptix storage phosphor system (Dentsply/Gendex, IL). Images from 48 patients (plus 12 repeats) were presented randomly and simultaneously to 10 observers engaged in orthodontics. Each observer independently rated Porion and Pronasale detection (1 = poor; 2 = satisfactory; 3 = excellent). Equal numbers of images having single and double peak histograms were included. Enhancements used in the study were: (1) emboss; (2) inverse; and (3) inverse/emboss.

2. Results and conclusions

For double peak images inverse/emboss was favored for Pronasale (mean 2.60), and inverse images were rated lowest (mean 2.23). For double peak images, inverse/emboss enhancement was preferred for Porion (mean 1.58), with baseline images least favored (mean 1.35). For single peak images emboss was the preferred enhancement for Porion (mean 1.55), and inverse was rated lowest (mean 1.13). For single peak images, baseline and the inverse were equal and preferred for Pronasale (mean 1.23), with emboss the least favored enhancement (mean 1.05). Significant differences in rating were found between single and twin peak images for the following enhancements - Porion: inverse ($p = .002$), inverse/emboss ($p = .027$); Pronasale: baseline ($p = .000$), emboss ($p = .000$), inverse ($p =.000$), inverse/emboss ($p = .000$). Hence, twin-peak histogram images were favored over single-peak histogram images for detection of Pronasale and were further rated as being improved by inverse/emboss enhancement. Use of the inverse/emboss enhancement was also preferred for twin-peak images in detection of Porion.

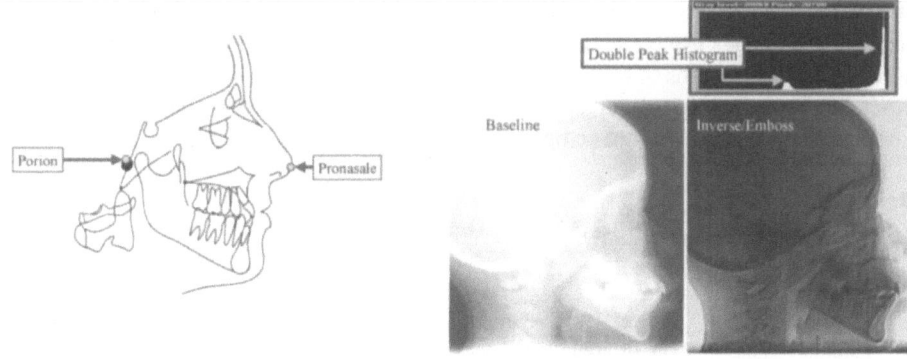

CARS 2002 – H.U. Lemke, M.W. Vannier; K. Inamura, A.G. Farman, K. Doi & J.H.C. Reiber (Editors)

1116

Evaluation of sensitivity of 3D-CT for diagnosis of craniofacial fractures

Marcelo G. P. Cavalcanti [a], Adriana Paula A. Costa e Silva [b]

[a,b] Department of Radiology, College of Dentistry, University of São Paulo, São Paulo, Brazil

Keywords: Tomography, face, fractures

1. Introduction

Three-dimensional imaging (3D) is a imaging technology, which has been developed in a stage of high quality, and represents an important advance in the treatment of craniofacial fractures [1]. The purpose of this study was to demonstrate the importance 3D-CT for diagnoses of craniofacial fractures using an independent workstation.

2. Methods

We analysed 20 patients with craniofacial fractures who were submitted to a multislice CT. The original data were transferred to an independent workstation using the Vitrea® software to generate 3D images. Then the images were interpreted using the 3D software tools, by 2 radiologists who required the 3D technique in cases that axial 2D-CT was not clarified. The surgical findings were considered the gold standard corroborating the diagnosis of the craniofacial fractures and its anatomical localization. In this study, the validity assessment of a diagnostic tool methodology named sensitivity was studied.

3. Results

The 2D-CT findings were equal to the surgical examination in 40% of cases. The results demonstrated that 60% of the 2D-CT needed the 3D-CT images. Also in the same case we found the 3D-CT technique to be equivalent with the surgical examination. The sensibility of the 3D-CT was higher than in 2D-CT for the orbital fractures in 75%, and in 37,5% for the sphenoid fractures. The 3D-CT images also added valuable information in cases of zigomatic and the relationship between the condyle and the glenoide fossa. For the other anatomical structures the 2D-CT demonstrated same results than 3D-CT.

4. Conclusions

The 3D-CT images using an independent workstation with multislice CT added important information in relationship to 2D-CT images for the final diagnosis of craniofacial fractures, especially for orbital and for sphenoid fractures. We also concluded that 2D-CT should not be substituted, but complemented with the 3D-CT technique.

Acknowledgements

FAPESP, São Paulo, CAPES and CNPq, Brasília, Brazil.

References:

1. Cavalcanti MGP, Haller JW, Vannier MW. Three-dimensional computed tomography landmark measurement in craniofacial surgical planning: experimental validation in vitro. J Oral Maxillofac Surg, 57(6):690-694, 1999.

CARS 2002 – H.U. Lemke, M.W. Vannier; K. Inamura, A.G. Farman, K. Doi & J.H.C. Reiber (Editors)
©CARS/Springer. All rights reserved.

Tuned-Aperture Computed Tomography (TACT®) to assess impacted teeth using 2D slices and 3D pseudo-holograms

Kazuhiro Yamamoto[a], Yoshihiko Hayakawa[a], Norio Kobayashi[a], Yuji Kousuge[a],
Mamoru Wakoh[a], Hiroshi Sekiguchi[b], Masashi Yakushiji[b], Allan G. Farman[c]
[a]Dept. of Oral and Maxillofacial Radiology, [b]Dept. of Pediatric Dentistry,
Tokyo Dental College, Chiba 261-8502, Japan
[c]Health Sciences Center, The University of Louisville, Louisville, Ky, 40292, USA

Keywords: TACT, dento-alveolar imaging, impacted teeth

1. Introduction

The purpose of this clinical study was to compare the diagnostic information yield of interactive TACT 3D pseudo-holograms, 2D TACT slices and conventional dento-alveolar images for the imaging and localization of impacted maxillary incisor teeth.

2. Methods

With IRB approval, 20 patients were examined. TACT image sets (both 3D pseudo-holograms and 2D slices) were compared for diagnostic utility against available conventional radiographs including periapical, occlusal, rotational panoramic and/or lateral cephalograms. Sixteen dentists independently evaluated the image clarity of the impacted tooth and selected surrounding anatomic details. Estimation of confidence in clinical assessment was made together with determination of TACT's potential for effecting treatment plan modifications. Both TACT 2D slices and 3D pseudo-hologram were studied. The number of component projections per TACT reconstruction was either five or six and a conical beam-projection array was employed in every case. The fiduciary marker was an X-Spot lead pellet (Beekley, USA). The detector was an RVG-ui (Trophy Radiology, France/Yoshida Dental Corporation, Japan).

3. Results

TACT significantly improved depiction of the buccal/palatal position of the impacted tooth and its relationship with adjacent teeth ($p<0.0001$) irrespective of the availability of lateral cephalograms. Subjective assessments for clinical decision-making approximated a 10 % increase in confidence ratings with TACT. The added diagnostic yield with TACT varied from case to case. Morphology and position of vertically impacted teeth were clearly demonstrated by TACT; however, horizontal impactions occasioned less perceived information gain. The 3D pseudo-hologram method was superior to the TACT 2D slices in cases where the impacted tooth was horizontally oriented bucco-lingually.

4. Conclusions

Interactive 2D TACT slices were perceived to be diagnostically more informative for assessing impacted maxillary incisor teeth and their relation to surrounded tissues than conventional methods in some but not all cases. TACT occasionally altered treatment option selection. 3D pseudo-hologram were preferred to 2D slices in horizontal impaction.

Acknowledgement
Supported by grant #12671839 from Japanese Society for the Promotion of Science.

CARS 2002 – H.U. Lemke, M.W. Vannier; K. Inamura, A.G. Farman, K. Doi & J.H.C. Reiber (Editors)

1118

Development of new tomography equipment with magnification

A. Satoh[a], R. Yamato[a], M. Tada[a], H. Nakahama[a], N. Takahashi[a], Y. Okumura[a]

[a] Department of Radiology, Meikai University of Dentistry, Saitama, Japan

Keywords: Magnification, image reconstruction, linear movement

1. Introduction

At present, a curved layer tomography generated by panoramic equipment and plane tomography derived from multi-orbital tomographic techniques are employed in the production of radiographic tomograms in the medical field. However, tomographic images obtained from this type of equipment require that the x-ray tube and film revolve about a fixed point functioning as a central axis. Therefore, radiography must be repeated in order to photograph different tomograms.

Tomography with magnification, which we developed, is comprised of fairly simple equipment. That is, an x-ray tube is closely aligned with image detecter system (intensifying screen and CCD camera); additionally, the photograph is produced with linear movement. Consequently, this technique is able to incorporate image information of a subject plane tomogram. We report the development of this equipment, which features the abstraction of an arbitrary tomogram with a single photograph with digitization.

2. Methods

Image reconstruction fixes the tomogram magnification. As a result, scaling treatment was performed on each frame image in order to adjust the standard and gray scale transformation processing. Consequently, each frame image was superimposed, and a standardized image of the tomogram was abstracted. These components are coupled with fixed photo acceptance equipment, which consists of an intensifying screen and CCD camera in opposition to an x-ray tube occurring at a distance of 1030 mm. Therefore, a linear path is created against the subject. Five model plates are employed as the subject; moreover, the surface of each plate is arranged in the direction of the incident x-ray. Furthermore, the models are positioned at 45 degree angles at intervals of two cm against the direction of the incident x-ray.

3. Results

This method could incorporate the image information of plane tomography with only one radiograph with linear movement; consequently, it could shorten radiographic time. Furthermore, due to the arbitrary standardization of image restructuring associated with tomography, signal intensities on x-ray of the tomograph were accurate and could be abstracted. Other tomographs displayed blurred images when heterolytic signal intensities occurred on x-ray. The thickness of the tomograph was approximately 2cm.

4. Conclusions

In the present experiment, we were able to develop new tomography equipment with magnification. It appears that x-ray equipment based on this principle will be applicable not only in the field of dentistry, but also in the medical field in the future.

CARS 2002 – H.U. Lemke, M.W. Vannier; K. Inamura, A.G. Farman, K. Doi & J.H.C. Reiber (Editors)

Computer simulation of an intraoral radiography using perspective projection of CT data

Kazutoshi Okamura[a], Kazunori Yoshiura[b], Kenji Tokumori[b], Takemasa Tanaka[a], Shigenobu Kanda[b]

[a] Dept. of Oral & Maxillofac. Radiology, Kyushu Univ. Dental Hospital
[b] Dept. of Oral & Maxillofac. Radiology, Faculty of Dental Science, Kyushu University, Japan

Keywords: Computer simulation, intraoral radiography, computed tomography

1. Introduction

Though the intraoral radiography is most frequently and widely used in clinical dentistry, this method is very special comparing with other extraoral radiography for jaw bones. The radiographer must consider a lot of factors, such as, the anatomical form of maxilla or mandible unique to each patient, direction and size of the tooth, the position of the film, and the position and angle of the cone-head. It is not easy to master this technique because of these factors associated with this technique. Computer-assisted training system may be useful to learn the effects of these factors on the radiograph. The purpose of this study was to develop a computer simulation system for intraoral radiography by a projection from point focus using the three dimensional data of the head with CT scanner.

2. Methods

A dried skull was scanned with multidetector CT (Aquilion TSX-101A,Toshiba Medical System Inc.). This data and some clinical data of the patients such as impacted tooth or cyst were transferred to the workstation OCTANE (Silicon Graphics Inc.). We applied the program AVS Express Developer (Advanced Visual Systems Inc.) to create intraoral radiographic images. We have simulated intraoral radiographic images using perspective volume rendering projection with average value algorithm.

3. Results

Using the present method, simulated images of intraoral radiography with perspective projection instead of parallel one were constructed. In contrast to the simulated images of a dried skull, simulated intraoral radiographic images of the patients were not clear enough. However, these images were useful to understand the radiographic appearances of the lesions on the ordinary intraoral radiographs.

4. Conclusions

Computer simulation system of intraoral radiography with present method may be useful for the training and education of an intraoral radiographic technique for students. It was suggested that intraoral radiographic images of some lesions could be simulated by our method to understand the typical radiographic appearances of the lesions.

CARS 2002 – H.U. Lemke, M.W. Vannier; K. Inamura, A.G. Farman, K. Doi & J.H.C. Reiber (Editors)
°CARS/Springer. All rights reserved.

1120

44 years of temporomandibular ankylosis

Marcos Anchieta[a], Frederico Salles[b]

[a, b]ARTIS - Prototipagem Biomédica, Brasília, Brazil

Keywords: Ankylosis, stereolithography, 3D

1. Introduction

A rare case of traumatic temporomandibular ankylosis started when the patient fractured his right condyle at age of 14. Briefed about the risks of an osteotomy next to the skull fossa, he postponed surgery until age of 58, undergoing it only after the authors built the stereolithographic model of his skull and explained the safety such technology provides.

2. Surgical technique

All steps were made previously in the model [1]; consisting of: 1) the mandibular fossa and the condyle contours were drawn on the model; 2) burs lengths and angulations were set by visualizing their directions through the transparence of the model and were intended to avoid compromising the anterior wall of the inner ear conduit and of the skull fossa; 3) burs in position, a surgical guide was built in metal; 4) the depth of each bur was set by a stopper; the precision of the osteotomy enabled to engrave the osseous mass into condyle, eliminating the need for a graft; 5) a vertical osteotomy of the ramus was made keeping the medial pterygoid muscle inserted, in order to provide the access and the engraving. 6) a temporalis muscle and fascia flap was made and placed between the new mandibular fossa and the new condyle [2]. Surgical model, miniplates and screws were autoclaved in order to be used in the surgical field.

3. Discussion

The surgical time lasted 6 hours, saving about 2 hours. Postoperative intensive care required only 8 hours. A day after surgery the patient could open his mouth spontaneously and begin a light diet, progressively to solid, having immediately started physiotherapy. Models can provide safety for the surgical team; increase of patient's trust in the team and, consequently, reduction of preoperative stress; reduction of hospital costs; and reduction of postoperative trauma and care [3].

4. Conclusions

3D models are an evolution of preoperative exams, representing the state of the art in the surgical planning. This technology, also called rapid prototyping, can convert a very difficult and potentially dangerous procedure into a simple surgery.

References

1. W. J. James, M. A. Slabbekoorn, W. A. Edgin, and C. K. Hardin: Correction of Congenital Malar Hypoplasia Using Stereolithography for Presurgical Planning. J Oral Maxillofac Surg 56:512-517,1998.
2. S. Omura and K. Fujita: Modification of the Temporalis Muscle and Fascia Flap for the Management of Ankylosis of the TMJ. J Oral Maxillofac Surg 54:794-795, 1996.
3. D. M. Erickson, D. Chance, S. Schmitt and J. Mathis: An Opinion Survey of Reported Benefits From the Use of Stereolithographic Models. J Oral Maxillofac Surg 57:1040-1043,1999.

CARS 2002 – H.U. Lemke, M.W. Vannier; K. Inamura, A.G. Farman, K. Doi & J.H.C. Reiber (Editors)

1121

Context sensitive visualized information in cranio-maxillofacial navigation systems

Rüdiger Marmulla, Stefan Hassfeld, Thorsten Heurich, Joachim Mühling
Dept. of Cranio-Maxillofacial Surgery, University of Heidelberg, Germany

Keywords: Displayed information, monitor view, computer assisted surgery

1. Introduction

During surgical navigation, the view on a monitor or inside of a headmounted display provides the surgeon with different types of visualized information, such as two- or threedimensional aspects of the data set, graphical bars, polygons, cylinders or numerical boxes to display the distance from a target. The different types of visualized information are compared, stressing the most helpful view for each different intraoperative procedure.

2. Methods

The surgical navigation network workstation (SNN), the surgical segment navigator (SSN), the Aesculap-Orthopilot and the Robodent system are compared. Different demands on the navigation systems, such as the localization of instruments, the navigation of implants and bone segments, are regarded. The different types of visualized information are displayed alternating. The display mode which is utilized by the surgeon is recorded .

3. Results

Threedimensional visualization of data sets are most helpful for the first adjustment of localized instruments. For the fine adjustment of instruments, selected twodimensional slices in two or three orthogonal ascpects are preferred. The first adjustment in the early stage of a navigation of bone segments is mostly performed with polygons which are to be matched. For the fine adjustment, graphical bars which have to be minimized are preferred. The surgeon usually controls the last phase of a segment navigation via numerical boxes which display the distance from the target position in millimeters. In implant dentistry a first adjustment phase with threedimensional visualization of the surgical site is commonly not required. The surgeon usually finds the approximated position of the implant bed spontaneously. Graphical bars and cylinders are commonly viewed and matched for the fine adjustment of the drilling guide and the last phase of an implantation. Improved ergonomics are found in the Robodent system that provides the surgeon with an additional monitor view near to the surgical site.

4. Conclusions

Different displayed information is usually preferred for different phases of a navigation. A context sensitive and specific automatic alteration of the monitor view, emphasing different types of displayed information, depending on first and fine adjustment requirements in each stage of the procedure, is recommended. This context sensitive automatic alteration can be adapted to special and individual demands of each surgeon and each surgical procedure.

CARS 2002 – H.U. Lemke, M.W. Vannier; K. Inamura, A.G. Farman, K. Doi & J.H.C. Reiber (Editors)

1122

3D-imaging for the assessment of volume changes of the human face

Emeka Nkenke[a], Xavier Laboureux[b], Michaela Benz[b], Tobias Maier[b], Gerd Häusler[b], Peter Kessler[a], Jörg Wiltfang[a], Friedrich Wilhelm Neukam[a]

[a]Department of Oral and Maxillofacial Surgery, University of Erlangen-Nuremberg, Glueckstr. 11, 91054 Erlangen, Germany, [b]Chair for Optics, University of Erlangen-Nuremberg, Staudtstr. 7, 91058 Erlangen, Germany

Keywords: Phase measuring triangulation, volume determination, orthognathic surgery

1. Introduction

It was the aim of the study to determine the accuracy of the assessment of volume changes of a non-contact, non-invasive, optical 3D-imaging method in vitro and in vivo for patients, who underwent mid-facial distraction.

2. Methods

For the measurements an optical sensor was used. For validation, the volume of a phantom with dimensions was determined. The visible volume changes were assessed in 10 volunteers who received subcutaneous injections of 2 ml of saline solution in the malar area and 5 patients who underwent mid-facial distraction.

3. Results

While the theoretical measurement uncertainty for the volume determination of the phantoms was 0.3 %, it turned out to be 0.4 % in reality. A volume of injection of 2 ml showed a visible volume increase of 2.06±0.5 ml. 6 months after mid-facial distraction the patients showed a visible soft-tissue volume increase of 4.5 up to 17.6 ml on each half of the face. The volume increase showed no correlation to the distance of distraction. After 2 years the distance of distraction remained constant. In 2 grown-up patients the soft-tissue volume was stable, while in 3 growing patients there was a reduction of the visible volume change. In one case, the volume was even less than in the pretreatment situation.

4. Conclusions

Optical 3D-measurements can be used with an adequate precision for the assessment of volume changes in vivo that has not been reached with non-contact methods before. The results of the follow-up of visible volume changes after mid-facial distraction reveal that in such situations a prediction of soft-tissue changes is difficult to achieve.

Acknowledgements

This study was granted by the "Deutsche Forschungsgemeinschaft" (Sonderforschungsbereich 603 – Teilprojekt C4).

References

1. Nkenke E., X. Laboureux, G. Häusler, J. Wiltfang, P. Kessler, F.W. Neukam: Assessment of visible volume changes in soft tissue after distraction osteogenesis of the mid-face. J Cranio Maxillofac Surg 28 (Suppl 1): 55-56 (2000)

CARS 2002 – H.U. Lemke, M.W. Vannier; K. Inamura, A.G. Farman, K. Doi & J.H.C. Reiber (Editors)

Evaluation of the exophthalmia reduction with a finite element model

Vincent Luboz[a], Annaig Pedrono[b], Frank Boutault[c], Pascal Swider[b], Yohan Payan[a]

[a] Laboratoire TIMC, Faculté de Médecine, 38706 La Tronche, France, vluboz@imag.fr
[b] Laboratoire biomécanique, [c] Hôpital Purpan, BP 3103, 31026 Toulouse, France

Keywords: Exophthalmia surgery, computer-aided planning, FE model

1. Introduction

The exophthalmia is a pathology defined by an excessive forward protrusion of the ocular globe [1]. For disthyroidy exophthalmia, a surgery is usually needed, once the endocrinal situation has been stabilized. A classical surgical technique consists in decompressing the orbit [2] by opening the walls, and pushing the ocular globe in order to evacuate some of the fat tissues inside the sinuses. This work aims at proposing a biomechanical model of the complete orbit in order to help the clinician in the definition of his surgical planning.

2. Methods

In order to provide a precise and patient-specific modelling, our method is based on:

a) A generic biomechanical model manually elaborated: CT data are used for the extraction of the orbital cavity, fat tissues, ocular muscles and nerve. From this segmentation, a volumetric mesh is manually built and a Finite Element (FE) poro-elastic material is introduced to model the orbital soft tissues. The simulation of the wall orbit osteotomy and of the pressure applied to the globe, is modelled with specific boundary conditions: nodes located in the osteotomy hole region are fixed, while pressure forces are applied to the nodes that are in contact with the ocular globe.

b) Patient data acquisition, through segmentation of CT images.

c) Local elastic deformations of the generic FE mesh to fit each patient morphology. The Mesh Matching algorithm [3] is used to automatically generate patient FE models.

3. Results

This study aims to assist the surgical planning by estimating (1) the influence of the hole size and location onto the backward globe displacement, and (2) the mechanical behavior of orbital soft tissues, especially in the hole region. Four FE models corresponding to four patients geometries were generated. For each patient, four different holes were simulated, assuming two locations and two sizes for the degree of osteotomy. Our simulations provided heterogeneous results: (1) for the same hole size, different levels of globe backward displacement are observed depending on the location of the hole, and (2) for a given hole size and location, different globe backward displacements and different soft tissues volumes evacuated through the hole are observed according to patient geometries.

References

1. Saraux H., Biais B., Rossazza C., 1987. *Ophtalmologie*. Masson Eds. Chap. 22 : Pathologie de l'orbite, pp.341-353
2. Wilson W.B., Manke W.F., 1991. Orbital decompression in Graves' disease. The predictability of reduction of proptosis. *Arch. Ophthalmology.*, vol. 109, pp. 343-345.
3. Couteau B., Payan Y., Lavallée S., 2000. The mesh-matching algorithm: an automatic 3D mesh generator for finite element structures. *Journal of Biomechanics*, vol. 33, pp. 1005-1009.

CARS 2002 – H.U. Lemke, M.W. Vannier; K. Inamura, A.G. Farman, K. Doi & J.H.C. Reiber (Editors)

1124

Digital x-ray mini-panel dental-planning outcomes for MRDD inpatients

[1]Allan G. Farman, [2]Henry Hood, [1]Brian Horsley, [1]Edward Warr
[1]School of Dentistry, The University of Louisville, Louisville, KY, USA
[2]Hazelwood Center Dental Services Clinic, 1800 Bluegrass Ave.,
Louisville, KY 40214, USA

1. Purpose and methods

Severely and profoundly mentally retarded and developmentally disabled (MRDD) patients are unable to communicate disease symptoms. This study evaluated the dental treatment planning impact of radiographic mini-panels for MRDD patients. With IRB approval, and the informed consent of the legal guardian, digital series of six periapical radiographs were achieved on 72 MRDD inpatients residing at Hazelwood out of 74 on whom this survey was attempted. The panel consists of images of the posterior teeth on both sides of the maxilla and mandible (four images) made using a parallel detector to tooth relationship. For the anterior teeth in both arches (two images) the detector was placed along the occlusal surface and a topographic projection was performed. Patients' charts and video images were studied both with and without the radiographic series in to assess the series impact on treatment planning.

2. Results and conclusions

Conditions noted radiologically are indicated on the histogram (below). Radiographic panels made on MRDD patients were found to affect treatment planning in more than 60%. In more than 30%, the detected condition potentially caused pain and suffering. This discomfort could not be described by the patient and had probably been ascribed to behavioural disorders. Dental inspections of MDDR patients are incomplete if radiographs are not made. Such inspections can be aided by use of a digital imaging system that permits minimization of dose followed by image post-processing to improve image density and contrast. [Supported by NIH DE 07171-13 and the WHAS Crusade for Children.]

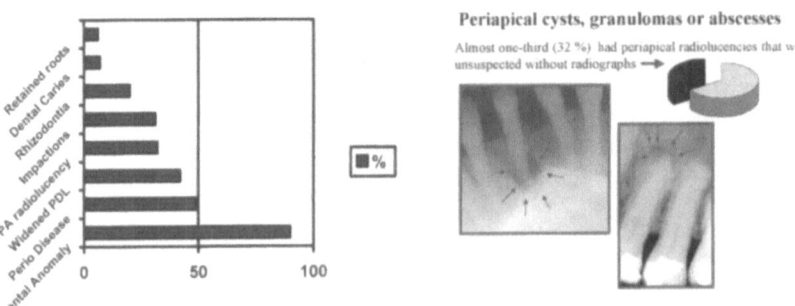

Periapical cysts, granulomas or abscesses

Almost one-third (32 %) had periapical radiolucencies that were unsuspected without radiographs ➔

CARS 2002 – H.U. Lemke, M.W. Vannier; K. Inamura, A.G. Farman, K. Doi & J.H.C. Reiber (Editors)

The need for model generation and validation in craniofacial prosthodontics: a feasibility study

Zafrulla Khan, Aly A. Farag, Taeko T. Farman, Allan G. Farman
The University of Louisville Schools of Dentistry and Engineering and the James
Graham Brown Cancer Center, Louisville, Kentucky 40292, USA

1. Purpose

This paper reports case studies that demonstrate the problems facing the maxillofacial prosthodontist. Such cases can benefit from 3-D modeling and the use of rapid prototyping.

3D Model Building: Based on CT/MRI and other images made for diagnosis and treatment it is possible to generate a 3D model of the face. This model can be enhanced with data generated by video images. Shape extraction algorithms including Shape From Shading (SFS) and Space Carving to extract 3D depth information from 2D images can be used to enhance the model. Image segmentation methods are used to isolate the required organ(s) from the 3D data, and CAD tools are able to fit a closed surface model for these organs.

Software Validation: Once a 3D model has been generated, it is imperative for a Maxillofacial Prosthodontist to work with a software technician to select the desired shape for the prosthesis. Tools for shape deformation (such as active surfaces and deformable models) can be used to generate the desired shape. The shape then must be calibrated using the specifications of the sensors used in the model generation. Immersive visualization tools such as stereoscopic imaging or the Immersa Desk at the CVIP Lab in the Electrical Engineering Department of the University of Louisville can be used to generate a virtual 3D model for the organ with all metric information displayed. This enables the Prosthodontist to initiate the fabrication process.

Rapid Prototyping: Once a calibrated model is generated in the computer, the 3D file can be converted into a suitable format for the rapid prototyping machines that are readily available. The School of Engineering at the University of Louisville has three rapid prototyping units that can generate model from various materials.

2. Results

Retrospective study of patients treated in the Dental Oncology Unit of the James Graham Brown Cancer Center, determined that there are more than 50 new cases of oral cancer treated each year and that many require prosthetic repair following surgical removal of the tumor. As the success rate for the treatment oral cancer means that most of the patients are living greater five years, there is also the periodic need for replacement prostheses. We have succeeded in the development of a system to overlap sequences of images using an intra-oral camera, and fitting a surface mesh to specific registration points to create 3-D models. We are in process of integrating this method with CT and MRI databases in a manner that can be applied to cancer patients requiring maxillofacial prosthodontic repair. We are in process of determining the ideal properties for materials to be used in the rapid prototyping of maxillofacial prostheses. Such materials need to be biologically compatible, structurally strong and also provide the opportunity of developing excellent esthetic results.

3. Conclusions

Need for the development of 3-D modeling processes for maxillofacial prosthodontics has been demonstrated by retrospective evaluation of patient's data. Development of appropriate video modeling methods and 3-D reconstruction from CT and MR data sets has been achieved. Future directions involve the use of these models as the basis for rapid prototyping.

Index auf Authors

Index of Authors